Delmar's Radiographic Positioning & Procedures

Volume I: Basic Positioning and Procedures

Joanne S. Greathouse, EdS, RT(R)(ARRT), FASRT

Associate Professor and Chair
Department of Radiation Sciences
Virginia Commonwealth University
Richmond, Virginia

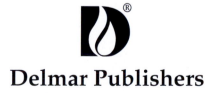

Delmar Publishers

an International Thomson Publishing company

Albany • Bonn • Boston • Cincinnati • Detroit • London • Madrid
Melbourne • Mexico City • New York • Pacific Grove • Paris • San Francisco
Singapore • Tokyo • Toronto • Washington

Notice to the Reader

Cover Design: Bill Finnerty

Delmar Staff

Publisher: Susan Simpfenderfer
Acquisitions Editor: Marlene McHugh Pratt
Developmental Editor: Melissa Riveglia
Project Editor: William Trudell
Art and Design Coordinator: Rich Killar
Production Coordinator: Cathleen Berry
Marketing Manager: Darryl L. Caron
Editorial Assistant: Maria Perretta

COPYRIGHT © 1998
By Delmar Publishers
a division of International Thomson Publishing Inc.

The ITP logo is a trademark under license.

Printed in the United States of America

For more information, contact:

Delmar Publishers
3 Columbia Circle, Box 15015
Albany, New York 12212-5015

International Thomson Publishing Europe
Berkshire House 168-173
High Holborn
London WC1V 7AA
England

Thomas Nelson Australia
102 Dodds Street
South Melbourne, 3205
Victoria, Australia

Nelson Canada
1120 Birchmount Road
Scarborough, Ontario
Canada, M1K 5G4

International Thompson EditoresCampos
Eliseos 385, Piso 7
Col Polanco
11560 Mexico D F Mexico

International Thomson Publishing GmbH
Konigswinterer Strasse 418
53227 Bonn
Germany

International Thomson Publishing Asia
221 Henderson Road
#05-10 Henderson Building
Singapore 0315

International Thomson Publishing—Japan
Hirakawacho Kyowa Building, 3F
2-2-1 Hirakawacho
Chiyoda-ku, Tokyo 102
Japan

Library of Congress Cataloging-in-Publication Data

Delmar's radiographic positioning and procedures.
     p. cm.
   Contents: v. 1. Basic positioning and procedures / [edited] by Joanne S. Greathouse—v. 2. Advanced imaging procedures / [edited] by Cynthia Cowling.
     ISBN 0-8273-6782-1 (v. 1. : alk. paper).—ISBN 0-8273-6317-6 (v. 2. : alk. paper)
  1. Radiography, Medical—Positioning. I. Greathouse, Joanne S. II. Cowling, Cynthia. III. Title: Radiographic positioning and procedures.
[DNLM: 1. Technology, Radiologic. 2. Posture. WN 160 D359 1997]
RC78.4.D44 1997
616.07'572—DC21
DNLM/DLC
for Library of Congress

97-43449
CIP

Contents in Brief

Contents in Detail

CONTENTS

Chapter 6   **Ribs and Sternum**   **315**

Dennis F. Spragg, MSEd, RT(R)(ARRT)
Joanne S. Greathouse, EdS, RT(R)(ARRT), FASRT

CONTENTS

CONTENTS

Foreword

If you have been searching for a user friendly, visually stimulating textbook to use in your basic radiographic procedures course, this book is for you! It provides clear, concise material on the most frequently used radiographic positions and procedures without the overload of content found in similar texts which may be more appropriate later in the curriculum after the student has developed, implemented, and refined the basic positioning skills.

The author, Joanne Greathouse, and the distinguished group of contributing authors, have demonstrated their professional and clinical experience in the depth of the content and the simplicity of the format of the text. The learner's attention is focused on the essential elements of each procedure. Visual learners will be particularly stimulated by the excellent line drawings included in the text which are most often accompanied by photographs and/or radiographs for comparison. Among the most unique features of this text are the icons used with each position that visually demonstrate the needed radiation protection measures, film size, and proper film placement. The special considerations sections at the end of each unit incorporates conditions or events which may require some deviation from the routine as well as some discussion and comparison of other imaging modalities.

The entire text is easy to read, sequenced in a logical order with defined objectives for each section, and review questions that reflect the intent of the objectives. Beginning students will benefit from the pronunciations of medical terms included in the text.

This is an exciting new positioning book for all levels or types of educational programs in the Radiologic Sciences. It is a "back to basics" kind of text that students will appreciate in the introductory positioning course. Experienced technologists who are re-entering the field or the radiology department after an extended absence will find this a valuable reference book. It is my considered opinion that this text will provide beginning students with an easy to use format for learning the basics of radiographic positioning and procedures that will challenge and encourage their interest in the art of radiography.

Nadia Bugg, PhD, RT(R)(ARRT), FAERS
Professor and Graduate Coordinator, Radiologic Sciences
Midwestern State University
Wichita Falls, Texas

Preface

T he study of radiographic positioning and procedures is at the core of any radiography curriculum. Technology that can replace accurate positioning of the patient by the radiographer has not yet been envisioned. Students usually approach this foundation course with a great deal of anticipation and enthusiasm because it is often one of the first courses in the professional curriculum. The excitement can fade fast when the student is faced with a text that is dull or unchallenging or that offers an encyclopedic approach to the topic.

This text is designed to bring excitement and challenge to the study of radiographic procedures. To aid the student faced with an enormous amount of information, the text is categorically organized and concisely written to facilitate management of the huge quantity of information.

Each chapter begins with an outline, objectives and, after the first chapter, continues with a review of relevant anatomy. A list of routine and alternative positions covered in the chapter precedes each positioning section to present the contents in capsule form. Each position is clearly outlined, providing sufficient coverage of important details without redundant or superfluous information that can distract the beginning student from more important concepts. Variations are included in the tips section at the end of the presentation of a position, allowing the instructor to use as much of it as is required at the time or delaying all of it until a later time when the student has mastered the essentials contained in the basic presentation. Chapters conclude with review questions, which provide students with an opportunity to check their learning progress. Important terms to know are bold on their first appearance in the text. The definitions for these terms can be found in the glossary.

Learning positioning is a highly visual process. This is reflected in the text, which provides over 1500 illustrations, including photographs of positions, radiographic images, and line drawings to help in identifying relevant anatomy on the images. To facilitate visual learning, icons are used to illustrate various aspects of positions including film size, indicated radiation protection measures, and phototiming.

Another key feature of the text is the special considerations section. This section underscores the need to make appropriate adjustments necessitated by age considerations or pathologic conditions. A brief discussion of selected pathology adds interest and provides the students with a view of the larger context of positioning. A presentation and brief discussion of correlated images again provides a view of the larger imaging context, including comparison of the different imaging modalities.

In addition to the text, an ancillary slide series has been developed to meet educators' needs for quality visual aids. A student workbook, which correlates closely with the text, assists students in organizing their study of the topic and provides additional opportunities for self-checks of learning progress.

Radiographic positioning and procedures is a critical and challenging subject for students in the radiologic sciences. The author and contributing authors hope that this text conveys the excitement and challenge of the subject and that it will facilitate the students' mastery of this important content.

Joanne S. Greathouse, EdS, RT(R)(ARRT), FASRT

This book is dedicated to the memory of my parents, Mike and Mary Ludwig,
who taught me the value of hard work and doing things right.

Acknowledgments

No book is produced without the contributions of many people whose names do not appear on the title page. This book is no exception. I would like to express my sincere gratitude to the following individuals who contributed significantly to this project.

First and foremost, to my husband, George, for his support and forebearance.

To the original focus group for agreeing on the need for a book of this type and for their initial guidance in focusing the project: Mike Adams, PhD, RT(R)(ARRT); Cynthia Cowling, BSc, MEd, MRT(R), ACR; Rick Carlton, MS, RT(R)(CV)(ARRT), FAERS; Ronald Griffith, RT(R)(ARRT); Nancy Lavin, MEd, RT(R)(ARRT); Mike Madden, PhD, RT(R)(ARRT); and Anita Slechta, MS, BSRT(R)(M)(ARRT). A special thanks to Mike Madden who was a major contributor in the beginning of the project and deserves a great deal of credit for the final product.

To all of the staff at Delmar Publishers, especially to Melissa Riveglia, Developmental Editor and Rich Killar, Art and Design Coordinator for their support and contributions in bringing it all together.

To the radiography students (Class of 1999) at the Medical College of Virginia/Virginia Commonwealth for their willingness to serve as photographic models and their patience during the process: Amy Adams, Kim Clark, Candice Crouch, Kenneth Lawson, Salah Lefta, Amber Mason, Jeff Mullins, John Peters, and Tracey Sattelmaier.

To the faculty and staff in the Department of Radiation Sciences at the Medical College of Virginia/Virginia Commonwealth University for their support and encouragement throughout the years it took to bring this project to completion.

To all of those who helped acquire the many radiographic images vital to a text such as this, particularly to Mary Hagler, MHA, BA, RT(R)(N)(M)(ARRT) and Ann O'Connor, BS, RT(R)(M)(ARRT) at rtAdvancements, Linda Croucher, MS, RT(R)(ARRT) and Ferell Justice, BSRT(R)(ARRT). Also, appreciation is extended to the facilities that supplied images for the text: Navidad Medical Center, Salinas, CA; Salinas Valley Radiologists, Salinas, CA; Valley Radiology, San Jose, CA; Medical College of Virginia, Virginia Commonwealth University, Richmond, VA; St. Francis Hospital and Medical Center, Topeka, KS; Colmery-O'Neil VA Medical Center, Topeka, KS; Methodist Hospital, Merrillville, IN; St. Mary's Hospital, Richmond, VA; and Children's Hospital, Richmond, VA.

To the photographer, Jerry Margolycz, and the medical illustrator, Joe Chovan, for their excellent photography and art work.

To the following reviewers for their comments and suggestions which added immeasurably to the quality of the book.

Nadia Bugg, PhD, RT(R)(ARRT)
Professor/Graduate Coordinator
Radiologic Technology
Midwestern State University
Wichita Falls, Texas

Mark Hagy, MS, RT(R)(ARRT)
Assistant Professor
East Tennessee State University
Elizabethton, Tennessee

Sandra Ostresh, MEd, RT(R)(ARRT)
Program Director/Coordinator
Radiologic Technology Program
Quinsagamond Community College
Worcester, Massachusetts

Anita Phillips, BS, RT(R)(ARRT)
Program Director
Radiologic Technology
Wake Technical Community College
Raleigh, North Carolina

Gary Watkins, PhD, RT(R)(ARRT)
Associate Professor
Department of
  Radiographic Science
Idaho State University
Pocatello, Idaho

Ray Winters, MS, RT(R)(ARRT)
Director, Radiologic
  Sciences Programs
Arkansas State University
State University, Arkansas

And, finally, to all the radiographers, radiologists, and students out there with whom I have worked, because I have undoubtedly learned something from each of them.

Contributors

Michael Patrick Adams, PhD, RT(R)(ARRT)
Associate Dean of Health, Mathematics, and Science
Pasco-Hernando Community College
New Port Richey, Florida

Linda Croucher, MS, RT(R)(ARRT)
Associate Professor
Washburn University
Topeka, Kansas

Sarajane Doty, MSEd, RT(R)(ARRT)
Associate Professor
Lexington Community College
Lexington, Kentucky

Terri Laskey Fauber, EdD, RT(R)(M)(ARRT)
Assistant Professor/Assistant Director
Virginia Commonwealth University
Department of Radiation Sciences
Richmond, Virginia

Joanne S. Greathouse, EdS, RT(R)(ARRT), FASRT
Associate Professor and Chair
Department of Radiation Sciences
Virginia Commonwealth University
Richmond, Virginia

Mary J. Hagler, MHA, BA, RT(R)(N)(M)(ARRT)
Clinical Coordinator
Radiologic Technology Program
Cabrillo College
Aptos, California

Robin Jones, MS, RT(R)(ARRT)
Lecturer, Radiologic Sciences Program
Indiana University Northwest
Gary, Indiana

M. Ferell Justice, BSRT(R)(ARRT)
Senior Radiologic Technologist
Department of Radiology
Virginia Commonwealth University
Richmond, Virginia

Jeffrey Legg, MH, RT(R)(ARRT)
Senior Radiologic Technologist
Virginia Commonwealth University
Richmond, Virginia

Michael Madden, PhD, RT(R)(ARRT)
Director, Radiologic Sciences
Fort Hays State University
Fort Hays, Kansas

Anita Marie Slechta, MS, BSRT(R)(M)(ARRT)
Professor, Health Science
Program Director, Radiologic Technology
California State University Northridge
Northridge, California

Dennis F. Spragg, MSEd, RT(R)(ARRT)
Associate Professor/Clinical Coordinator
   of Radiography
Lima Technical College
Lima, Ohio

HOW TO USE THIS TEXT

Radiographic positioning and procedures is an exciting and challenging subject. Delmar's Radiographic Positioning and Procedures, Volume I: Basic Positioning and Procedures presents a thorough overview of the procedures most common in the day to day operation of a typical radiology department. The text is designed with efficient learning in mind rather than as comprehensive coverage of every topic. The text has many unique features which will make it easier for you to learn and integrate theory and practice, including:

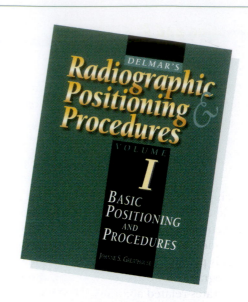

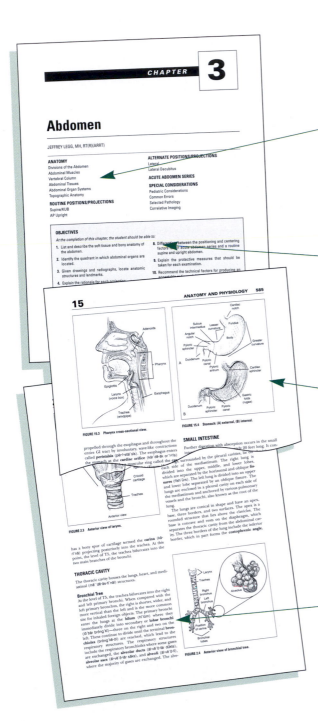

Chapter Outline

1 At the beginning of each chapter is an outline listing the main headings covered within the chapter. Review these headings of topic areas before you study the chapter. They'll be a roadmap to the material in the chapter.

Objectives

2 Learning objectives identify the key information to be gained from the chapter. Use these objectives, together with the review questions, to test your understanding of the chapter's content.

Anatomy and Physiology Section

3 Each body system chapter includes an overview of the structure and function of that particular system. Numerous line drawings with labels help differentiate human structures and organs and explain physiological processes. The full-color anatomy and physiology figures, which can be found near the front of the text for easy reference, further assist you in visualizing and understanding anatomy and physiology concepts.

Key Terms

4 Important terms to know are presented in bold throughout the text. These terms are defined in the glossary at the end of the text. Phonetic spellings follow terms that may be difficult to pronounce the first time they appear in the text.

Routine and Alternative Positions/Projections

5 A comprehensive list of routine and alternative positions/projections for each body region is included.

Positions/Projections

6 Each position/projection is presented in a bulleted format with icons to show film size/placement and indicated radiation protection measures. A photo of the patient position is presented first, followed by the corresponding radiograph. Line art (drawn from the radiograph) illustrates related anatomy. The tips section includes variations of basic positioning.

Special Considerations

7 This section emphasizes the need to make appropriate adjustments necessitated by age considerations or pathologic conditions. The presentation of correlated images provides a comparison of different imaging modalities.

Review Questions

8 Various types of review questions are presented to test your knowledge of the chapter content.

References and Recommended Reading

9 This listing includes both the references used in each chapter and additional sources for further study.

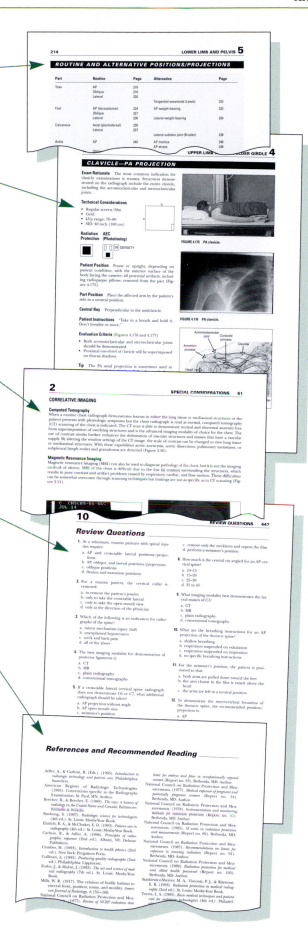

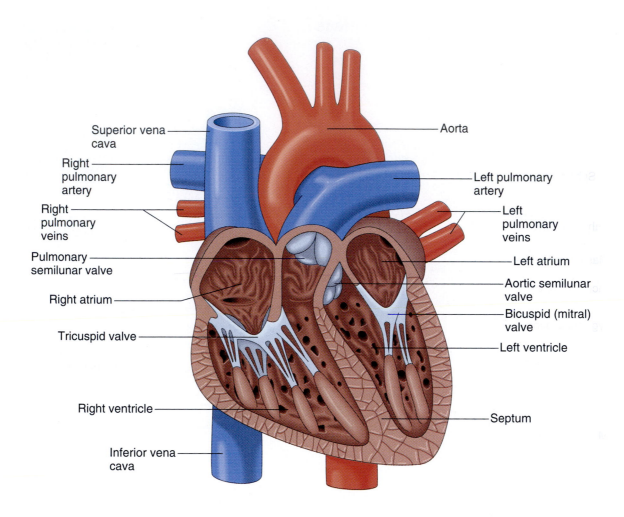

Superior vena cava

Right pulmonary artery

Right pulmonary veins

Pulmonary semilunar valve

Right atrium

Tricuspid valve

Right ventricle

Inferior vena cava

Aorta

Left pulmonary artery

Left pulmonary veins

Left atrium

Aortic semilunar valve

Bicuspid (mitral) valve

Left ventricle

Septum

ILLUSTRATION 1   Anterior Internal View of Heart

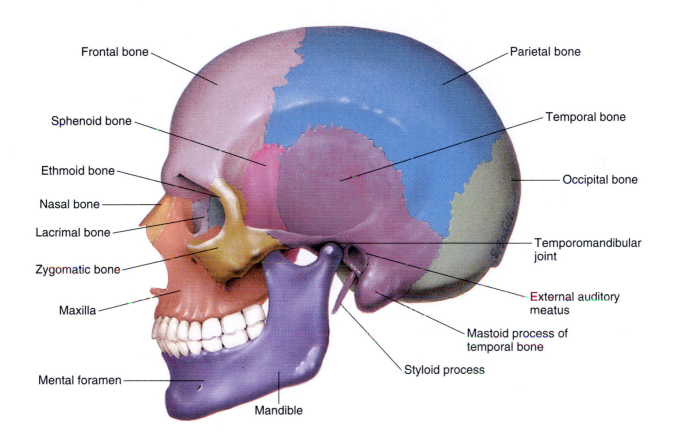

Frontal bone

Sphenoid bone

Ethmoid bone

Nasal bone

Lacrimal bone

Zygomatic bone

Maxilla

Mental foramen

Mandible

Parietal bone

Temporal bone

Occipital bone

Temporomandibular joint

External auditory meatus

Mastoid process of temporal bone

Styloid process

ILLUSTRATION 2   Lateral View of Skull

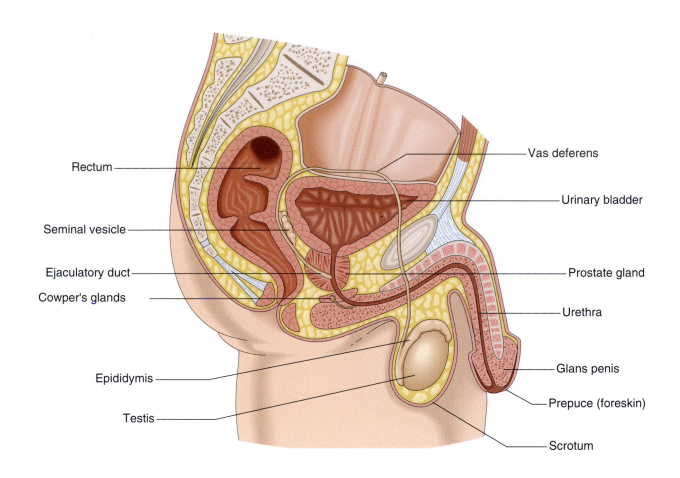

Rectum

Seminal vesicle

Ejaculatory duct

Cowper's glands

Epididymis

Testis

Vas deferens

Urinary bladder

Prostate gland

Urethra

Glans penis

Prepuce (foreskin)

Scrotum

ILLUSTRATION 3   Male Reproductive System

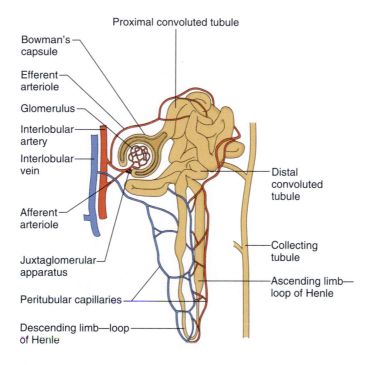

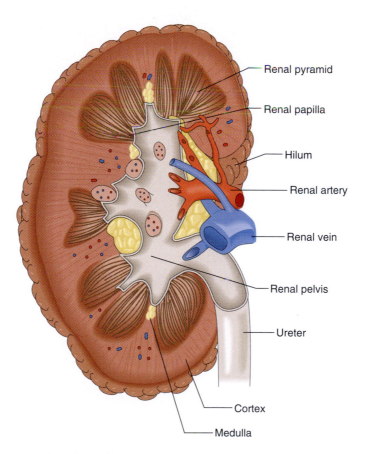

ILLUSTRATION 4   Nephron and Sagittal Section of Kidney

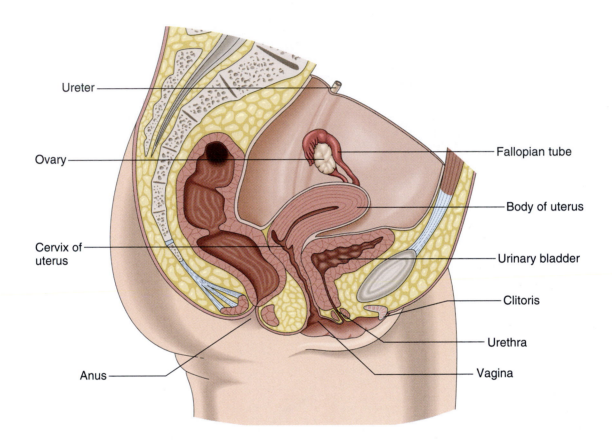

Ureter

Ovary

Cervix of
uterus

Anus

Fallopian tube

Body of uterus

Urinary bladder

Clitoris

Urethra

Vagina

ILLUSTRATION 5   Female Reproductive System

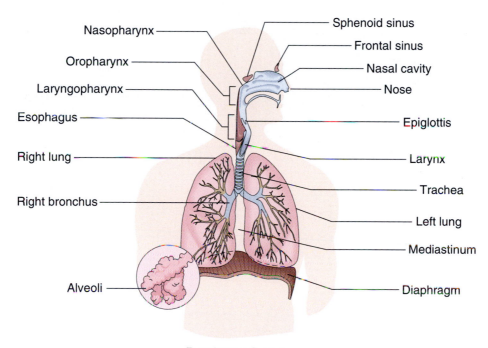

Nasopharynx

Oropharynx

Laryngopharynx

Esophagus

Right lung

Right bronchus

Alveoli

Sphenoid sinus

Frontal sinus

Nasal cavity

Nose

Epiglottis

Larynx

Trachea

Left lung

Mediastinum

Diaphragm

Respiratory System

ILLUSTRATION 6   Respiratory System

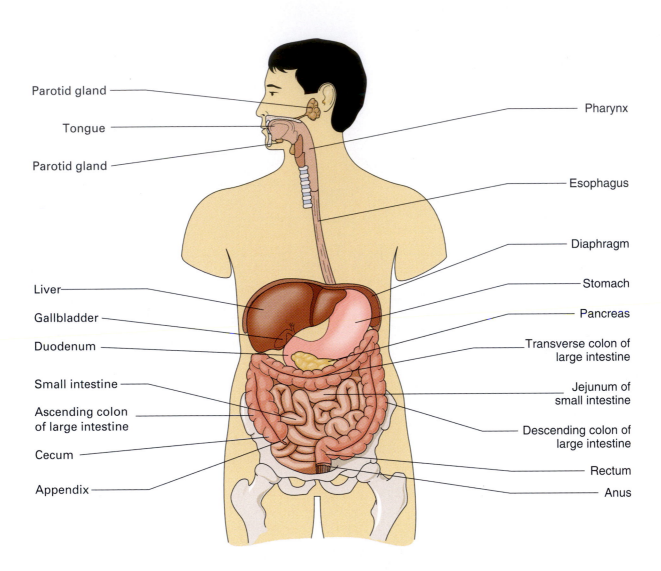

Parotid gland

Tongue

Parotid gland

Pharynx

Esophagus

Diaphragm

Stomach

Pancreas

Liver

Gallbladder

Duodenum

Transverse colon of
large intestine

Small intestine

Jejunum of
small intestine

Ascending colon
of large intestine

Descending colon of
large intestine

Cecum

Rectum

Appendix

Anus

ILLUSTRATION 7   Digestive System

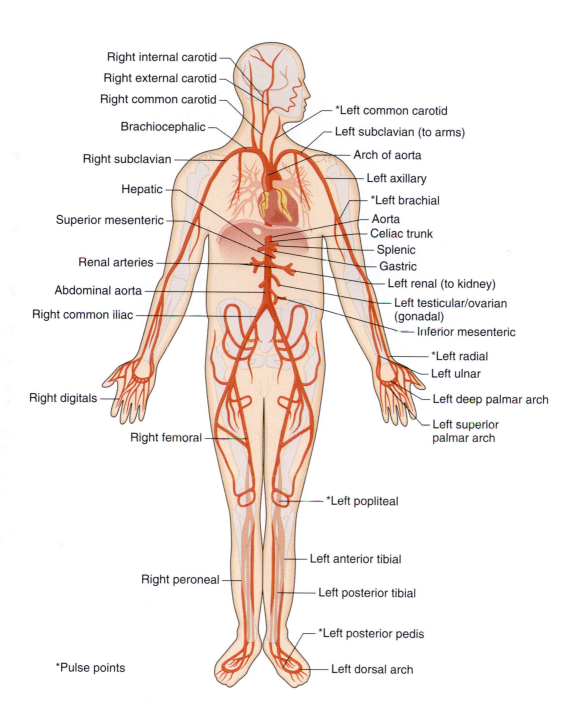

Right internal carotid

Right external carotid

Right common carotid

Brachiocephalic

Right subclavian

Hepatic

Superior mesenteric

Renal arteries

Abdominal aorta

Right common iliac

Right digitals

Right femoral

Right peroneal

*Pulse points

*Left common carotid

Left subclavian (to arms)

Arch of aorta

Left axillary

*Left brachial

Aorta

Celiac trunk

Splenic

Gastric

Left renal (to kidney)

Left testicular/ovarian (gonadal)

Inferior mesenteric

*Left radial

Left ulnar

Left deep palmar arch

Left superior palmar arch

*Left popliteal

Left anterior tibial

Left posterior tibial

*Left posterior pedis

Left dorsal arch

ILLUSTRATION 8   Arterial Distribution

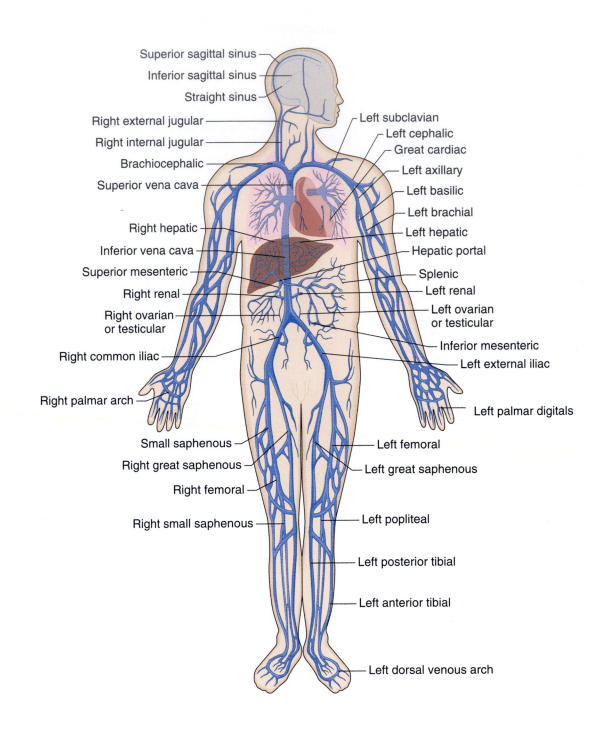

ILLUSTRATION 9 **Venous Distribution**

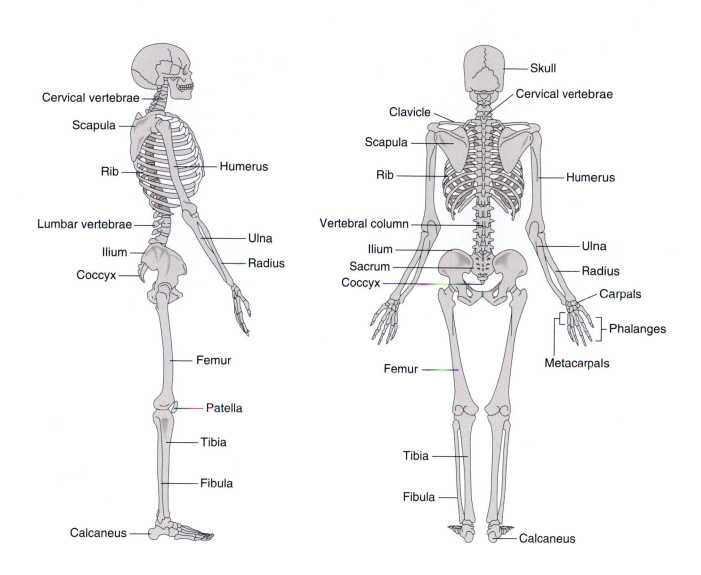

ILLUSTRATION 10   Skeletal System

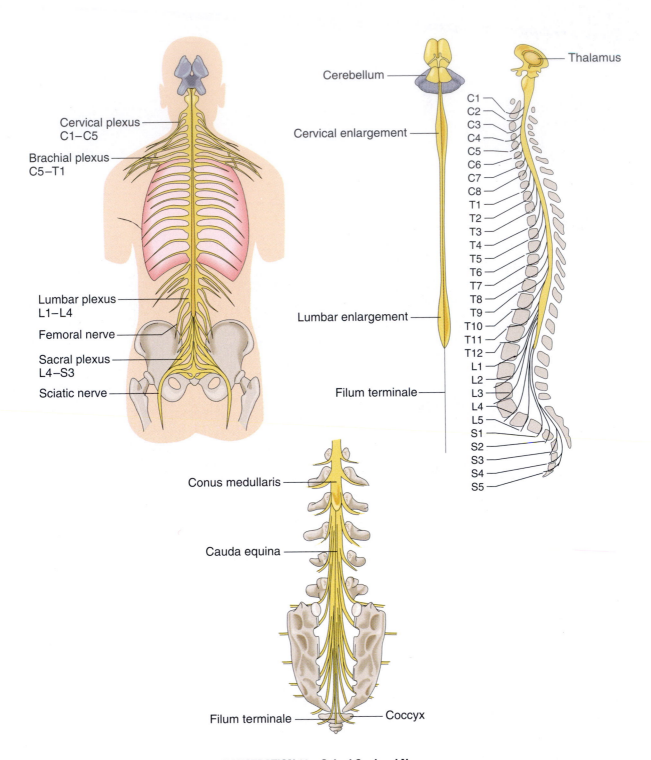

Cervical plexus
C1–C5

Brachial plexus
C5–T1

Lumbar plexus
L1–L4

Femoral nerve

Sacral plexus
L4–S3

Sciatic nerve

Cerebellum

Cervical enlargement

Lumbar enlargement

Filum terminale

Thalamus

C1
C2
C3
C4
C5
C6
C7
C8
T1
T2
T3
T4
T5
T6
T7
T8
T9
T10
T11
T12
L1
L2
L3
L4
L5
S1
S2
S3
S4
S5

Conus medullaris

Cauda equina

Filum terminale

Coccyx

ILLUSTRATION 11   Spinal Cord and Nerves

SECTION I

INTRODUCTION to RADIOGRAPHIC POSITIONING

Introduction to Radiographic Positioning and Procedures

JOANNE S. GREATHOUSE, EdS, RT(R)(ARRT), FASRT

DISCOVERY OF X-RAYS

PATIENT CARE AND MANAGEMENT

BASIC RADIOGRAPHIC EXPOSURE

PRINCIPLES OF RADIATION PROTECTION

GENERAL ANATOMY

POSITIONING TERMINOLOGY

PRINCIPLES OF RADIOGRAPHIC POSITIONING

OBJECTIVES

At the completion of this chapter, the student should be able to:

1. List and discuss patient care considerations relevant to positioning.

2. List the three primary exposure factors.

3. List specific methods of reducing patient radiation exposure.

4. Explain the 10-day rule.

5. List the three primary principles of radiation protection.

6. Define and demonstrate the anatomic position.

7. Define terms related to body planes.

8. Given diagrams, identify body planes.

9. Given topographic landmarks, list the corresponding vertebrae.

10. List and describe the characteristics of each of the four major body types.

11. Given diagrams, identify the body type illustrated.

12. Define and demonstrate terms related to relative body position, body position, and body movement.

13. Define terms related to general positioning.

14. List the three general principles of positioning.

15. List and discuss the six primary elements in radiographic positioning.

DISCOVERY OF X-RAYS

The discovery of x-rays in 1895 by Wilhelm Conrad Roentgen (rĕnt´gĕn) was the beginning of a flurry of activity that sought to explore the potential usefulness of these rays to medicine (Figure 1.1). As early as 1896, x-ray examinations were being used to evaluate a variety of conditions, including a bullet lodged in the skull, a fractured hip, a drainage tube in a lung, and a kidney stone (Figure 1.2).

Perhaps no discovery has so rapidly affected medical practice; indeed, the newly discovered ability to "see through" the human body quickly revolutionized medicine.

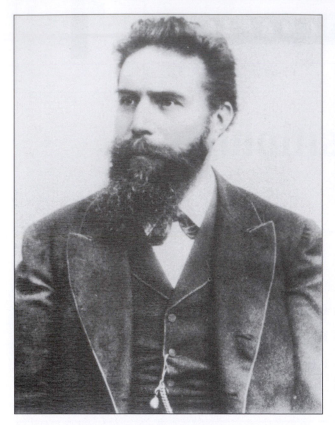

FIGURE 1.1   Wilhelm Conrad Roentgen. (From O. Glasser, Dr. W. C. Roentgen, 2nd edition, 1958. Courtesy of Charles C. Thomas, Publisher, Springfield, Illinois.)

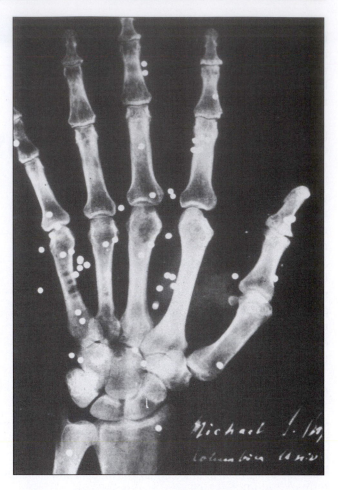

FIGURE 1.2   Early medical radiograph (Courtesy of the American College of Radiology, Reston, VA).

Increasing calls for x-ray consultations gave rise to a new group of medical specialists, known as roentgenologists (rĕnt´´gĕn-ŏl´ō-jĭst) or radiologists (rā-dē-ŏl´ō-jĭst), skilled in the use of the new "rays." Most of these early x-ray specialists performed their own x-ray examinations, a practice that continued into the 1920s and 1930s. Increasing demands on radiologists' time led them to begin training young men and women as apprentices, who were taught to position patients, make x-ray exposures, and develop the "plates." Gradually, the radiologists became increasingly reliant on these radiographers (rā-dē-ŏg´ră-fer) to produce optimal images that provide the maximum information possible. Although the radiologist is the expert in the *interpretation* of images, the radiographer is the expert in the *production* of the images.

Radiography (rā-dē-ŏg´ră-fē) has evolved into a complex specialty encompassing the principles of many related areas: patient care and ethics, radiographic exposure, radiation protection, and anatomy and physiology. The expert radiographer must master each of these subjects in a depth not possible in the introduction to this text. These topics, however, will be briefly addressed with comments related specifically to radiographic positioning and procedures. References are provided at the end of the chapter for major texts in each of the areas.

PATIENT CARE AND MANAGEMENT

The goal of radiography, as for all of medicine, is assistance to the patient in the form of diagnosis, treatment, or support. Although a radiographer's contact with the patient may be somewhat limited in scope, it is intensive for the period of time the patient is in the radiology department. Knowledge of patient care principles from both the physical and psychological standpoints is essential to maximize patient safety and comfort. It is also important for the production of a quality radiographic image because a radiographer who has the trust and cooperation of the patient is better able to position the patient to obtain optimum diagnostic images. Positioning is often difficult and may be seriously compromised without the complete cooperation of the patient.

Each patient should receive a thorough explanation of the procedure and clear, easily understood instructions during the examination. Careful attention to verbal and nonverbal communication will help limit motion on radiographs and reduce the need for repeat exposures.

Initial contact with the patient should include appropriate patient identification and a general assessment of the patient's physical and mental status. It is important to determine the extent to which the patient will be able to understand directions and cooperate during the examination. In cases where the standard examination is not possible, this initial assessment allows the radiographer to plan for appropriate modifications of routine positions or standard technical factors.

The initial contact should also include obtaining a brief history from the patient, which provides the radiographer with valuable information for planning and completing the examination. Any pertinent history should be noted on the requisition or otherwise conveyed to the radiologist to assist in the interpretation of the films.

Aseptic (ā-sĕp´tĭk) **technique** is an area of patient care that is of particular concern to the radiographer. The radiographer must know and apply principles of sterile technique to minimize the transmission of infectious disease. With the increase of serious disease in asymptomatic (ā´´sĭmp-tō-măt´ĭk) patients, particularly drug-resistant tuberculosis, hepatitis B, and human immunodeficiency virus (ĭm´´ū-nō-dĕ-fĭsh´ĕn-sē vī´rŭs) (HIV), the practice of **standard precautions** should be followed.

The simple act of handwashing is the single most important factor in the prevention of transfer of **pathogens** (păth´ō-jĕn). Because the radiographer has physical contact with many pieces of equipment and with many patients, the radiographer should develop the habit of thorough handwashing before beginning work with each patient.

The nature of the health profession requires that practitioners practice ethically, that is, with a sense of duty and right conduct toward others. Radiographers certified by the American Registry of Radiologic Technologists (ARRT) subscribe to the Code of Ethics adopted by the American Society of Radiologic Technologists (ASRT), which requires radiographers to function efficiently and effectively, using only scientifically proven methods. Patients are to be treated with respect and with concern for their rights to privacy and confidentiality. Additionally, the Code of Ethics requires radiographers to provide the physician with information pertinent to the diagnosis and treatment management of the patient but acknowledges that diagnosis is beyond the scope of practice of the radiographer.

BASIC RADIOGRAPHIC EXPOSURE

The best positioning skills will be useless without the selection of appropriate technical factors that make it possible to visualize the image on film. Optimal radiographic quality requires a thorough knowledge of the principles of radiation exposure as well as familiarity with an institution's specific equipment. Manipulation of the three exposure factors—kilovoltage (kV), milliamperage (mA), and time—or appropriate selection of phototiming parameters must be combined with an understanding of the primary image quality factors of density, contrast, recorded detail, and distortion to produce an optimally diagnostic image.

In this text, suggested kVp ranges have been provided for each of the positions/procedures. These are only a guide. The actual kVp selection should be based on the equipment, imaging systems, department protocol, and physician preference at your institution.

Recommendations are also provided for the use of automatic exposure control (AEC), commonly referred to as "phototiming." AECs produce a mid-range diagnostic level density for the structures placed between the ion cell and the x-ray tube. In other words, the art of phototiming is the art of positioning. Whatever is placed over the activated ion cells will be imaged in the middle of the diagnostic range of densities. Thus, a selective determination must be made regarding which AEC cells should be activated and then the anatomical area of interest must be placed over these cells.

The following icon is provided for positions/projections where AEC is an appropriate consideration.

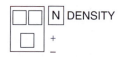

The 3 cells located in the large square represent the location of the ion chambers in the x-ray equipment. In keeping with common practice, the cell(s) which are to be activated for a given position/projection are blackened to indicate they are on. The small box with the N represents the film density control. The "N" represents "normal" density. When special conditions make it desirable to increase or decrease the average density, a "+" or "−", respectively, is used beneath the density control box.

PRINCIPLES OF RADIATION PROTECTION

As a form of electromagnetic radiation, x-rays have the potential to cause harmful effects on living cells. Every effort must be made to protect the patient, operator, and others from unnecessary radiation exposure; the radiographer is bound by the Code of

Ethics to do so. A thorough understanding of the principles of radiation protection is essential to achieving this goal.

Because the developing embryo or fetus is especially sensitive to radiation, women of childbearing age must be asked about the possibility of pregnancy. Many women are unaware of pregnancy in its early stages, so the patient history should include questions about when the last menstrual period occurred. Some facilities prefer that abdominal x-rays of females of reproductive age be done during the first 10 days following the onset of menstruation because it is less likely that a patient would be pregnant at this time (often referred to as the 10-day rule).

Patient radiation exposure can be limited with the use of appropriate exposure factors used in conjunction with appropriate imaging systems, use of appropriate beam-limiting devices (including collimation), proper filtration, and proper immobilization. Attention to minimizing patient radiation exposure must also include gonadal (gō´nădăl) shielding whenever possible without compromising the radiographic examination (Figures 1.3 and 1.4). In this text, an icon is used to identify those situations in which gonadal shields should be used.

 contact shield   shadow shield

Particular care must be taken when radiographing children. Because the rapidly dividing cells of children are more sensitive to radiation than those of adults, the principles of radiation protection warrant even more careful attention in pediatric work.

Radiographers also have a responsibility to protect themselves and others from unnecessary exposure. All radiographers should be familiar with the three primary principles of radiation protection:

1. Keep time of exposure to radiation to a minimum.
2. Maintain the maximum distance possible between the radiation source and the operator.
3. Use protective shielding (e.g., lead aprons and gloves) between the source and radiographer.

Although radiation monitoring devices such as film badges and dosimeters do not afford protection from exposure, they are an essential component of radiation control and should be worn whenever the radiographer is in a radiation area.

An important, but often overlooked, factor in minimizing radiation exposure to both the patient and the radiographer is limiting the number of repeat exposures. It is in the patient's and the radiographer's best interests for the radiographer to position the patient and tube carefully and otherwise work conscientiously

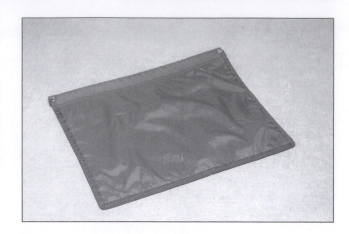

FIGURE 1.3   Contact gonadal shield.

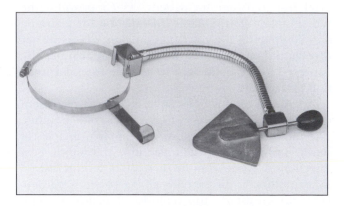

FIGURE 1.4   Shadow gonadal shield (Courtesy of Nuclear Associates, Carle Place, NY).

so that, whenever possible, the first film is adequate and repeat exposures to correct avoidable mistakes are strictly limited.

GENERAL ANATOMY

Radiographic study of the human body is primarily concerned with visualization of internal anatomy and, to a lesser extent, the physiology of the region. Because it is important for the radiographer to have a thorough knowledge of human anatomy and physiology, it is expected that the student will have completed, either before or concurrently with this study of positioning, a course in anatomy and physiology.

Body Planes and Positions

Anatomic Position   When describing any part of the body in relation to other parts, one should begin from the common reference point of **anatomic** (ăn´ă-tŏm´ĭk) **position**. The anatomic position refers to the body being erect, facing forward, feet together, and arms extended with palms turned forward (Figure 1.5).

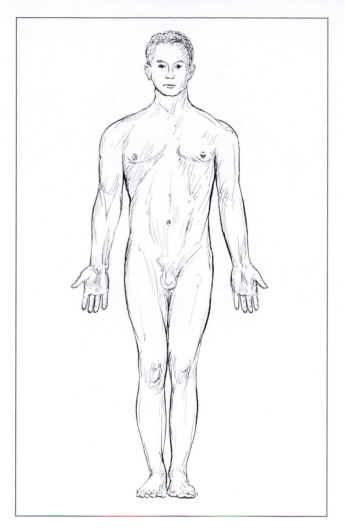

FIGURE 1.5 Anatomic position.

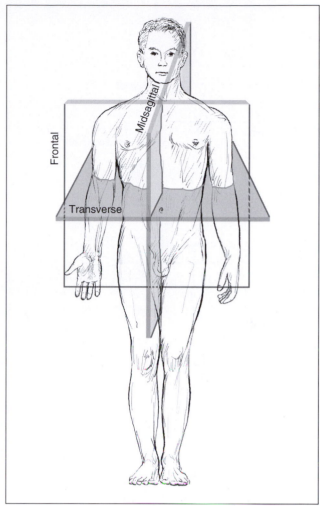

FIGURE 1.6 Planes—frontal view.

Body Planes The use of imaginary planes is helpful to describe central ray locations and to relate one body part to another or to a film orientation.

sagittal (săj´ĭ-tăl) **plane**—plane that passes vertically through the body from front to back; divides the body into left and right portions
midsagittal (median) **plane**—plane that passes vertically through the midline of the body from front to back; divides the body into equal left and right portions (Figure 1.6)
coronal (kŏ-rō´nǎl) (frontal) **plane**—plane that passes vertically through the body from left to right; divides the body into anterior (an-tēr´ē-or) and posterior (pŏs-tē´rē-or) portions
midcoronal plane—plane that passes vertically from right to left through the coronal suture of the skull; divides the body into equal anterior and posterior portions (Figure 1.7)

transverse (horizontal or axial) **plane**—any plane that passes through the body at a right angle to the sagittal or coronal plane
longitudinal plane—plane that passes lengthwise through the body; sagittal and coronal planes are both longitudinal planes

Surface Landmarks In positioning the patient for various procedures, it is necessary to use external surface landmarks as indicators of internal anatomy that cannot be directly visualized. Many of the commonly used landmarks are listed in Table 1.1 (Mills, 1917). Note, however, that the landmarks are accepted averages and can be used only as guidelines. Patients are notoriously unique; variations in anatomic build and pathologic changes may result in differences that must be considered in positioning the patient (Figures 1.8, 1.9, and 1.10).

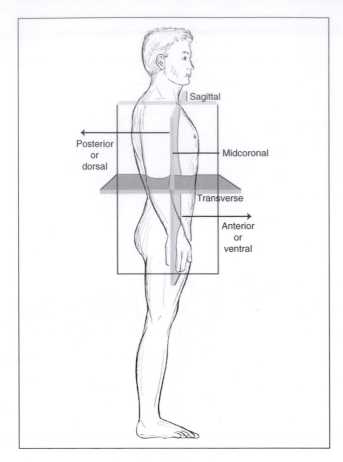

FIGURE 1.7 **Planes—side view.**

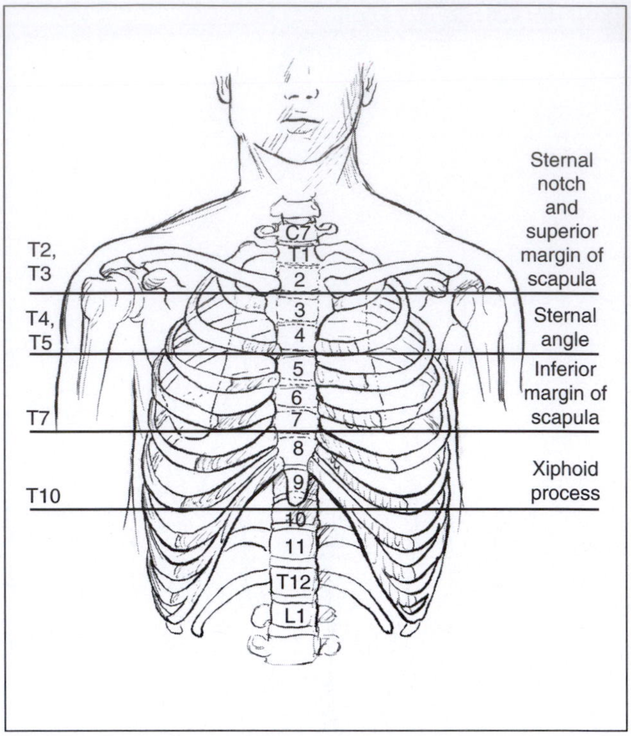

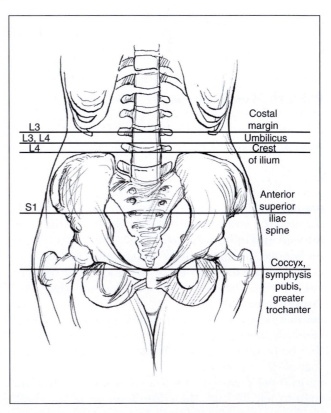

FIGURE 1.9 **Surface landmarks of the thorax.**

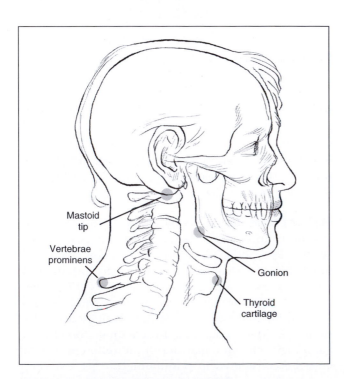

FIGURE 1.8 **Surface landmarks of the head.**

FIGURE 1.10 **Surface landmarks of the pelvis.**

TABLE 1.1 TYPICAL SURFACE LANDMARKS

Corresponding Vertebrae (vĕr´tĕ-brā)	Landmark
C1	Mastoid tip
C2, C3	Gonion (gō´nē-ŏn)
C5	Thyroid cartilage
C7	Vertebra prominences (vĕr´tĕ-brā prŏm´ĭ-nĕns)
T1	Approximately 2 inches superior to sternal (manubrial) notch
T2, T3	Level of sternal (stĕr´nāl) notch Superior margin of scapulae (skap´u-lē)
T4, T5	Level of sternal angle
T7	Level of inferior angle of scapulae
T10	Level of xiphoid (zīf´oyd) tip
L3	Costal margin
L3, L4	Level of umbilicus (ŭm-bĭl´ĭ-kŭs)
L4	Level of most superior aspect of iliac (ĭl´ē-ăk) crest
S1	Level of anterior superior iliac spine
Coccyx (kŏk´sĭks)	Level of pubic (pū´bĭk) symphysis (sĭm´fĭ-sĭs) and greater trochanter (trō-kăn´tĕr)

Body Habitus (hab´ĭ-tus) A knowledge of the general shape and form of the human body, referred to as **body habitus**, is helpful to the radiographer in determining the general location of internal structures. In a classic work, Mills (1917) classified subjects into four major body types. The location and shape of organs within the body vary significantly in the different types.

Sthenic (sthĕn´ĭk)—the "average" body type, which comprises about 50% of the total population. This body type serves as the reference point for others (Figure 1.11).

Hypersthenic (hī´´pĕr-sthĕn´ĭk)—the large body type, which comprises about 5% of the population and is characterized by:

- Massive build
- Broad, deep thorax with more nearly horizontal ribs and shallow thoracic cavity
- Short, wide heart

- Short lungs, broad at base and narrow at apices
- Long abdomen with colon along periphery
- Stomach and gallbladder high and more horizontal with gallbladder away from midline (Figure 1.12).

Asthenic (ăs-thĕn´ĭk)—at the opposite end of the spectrum and comprises about 10% of the population. It is characterized by:

- Extremely slight build
- Narrow, shallow thorax with more vertical ribs and long thoracic cavity
- Long, narrow heart
- Long lungs, broader at top than at base
- Short abdominal cavity
- Stomach and gallbladder low and vertical near midline (Figure 1.13).

Hyposthenic—This habitus is a modification of the more extreme asthenic type and comprises about 35% of the population (Figure 1.14).

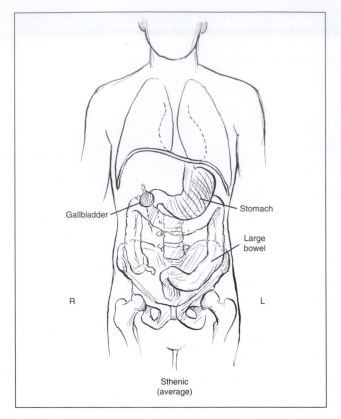

FIGURE 1.11   Sthenic body habitus.

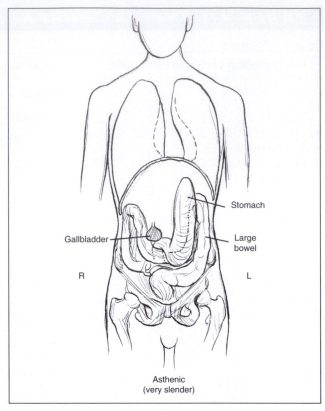

FIGURE 1.13   Asthenic body habitus.

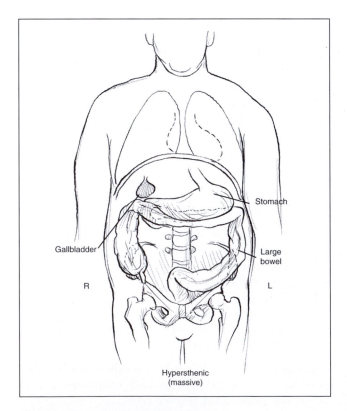

FIGURE 1.12   Hypersthenic body habitus.

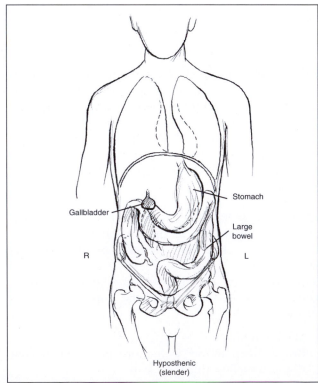

FIGURE 1.14   Hyposthenic body habitus.

POSITIONING TERMINOLOGY

Relative Position

The following terms are routinely used to describe patient positioning. Terms are presented in pairs to facilitate understanding of the relationship between them.

anterior (ventral)—the forward or front part of the body or body part

posterior (dorsal)—the back part of the body or body part (Figure 1.15)

inferior (**caudal** [kawd´ăl] or caudad [kaw´dăd])—part away from the head of the body or, more generally, below some point of reference

superior (cephalic [sĕ-făl´ĭk] or **cephalad** [sĕf´ă-lăd])—part toward the head of the body or, more generally, above some point of reference (Figure 1.16)

lateral (lăt´ĕr-ăl)—away from median plane of body or from middle of a part to right or left

medial (mē´dē-ĕl) (mesial) (mē´zē-ăl)—toward median plane of body or toward middle of a part from right or left (Figure 1.17)

distal (dĭs´tăl)—away from the origin of a part or away from its center or midline

proximal (prŏk´sĭm-ăl)—closer to the origin of a part or closer to its center or midline (Figure 1.18)

plantar (plăn´tăr)—posterior surface (or sole) of foot

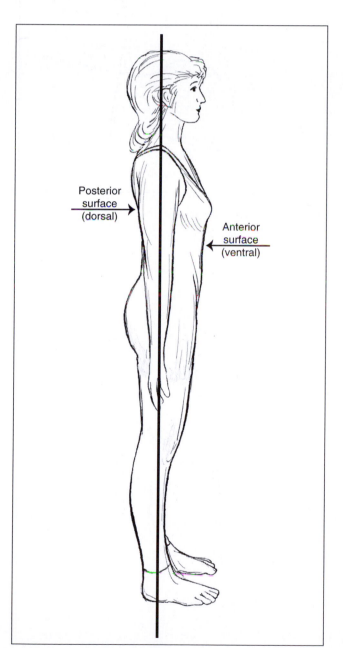

FIGURE 1.15 Anterior/posterior.

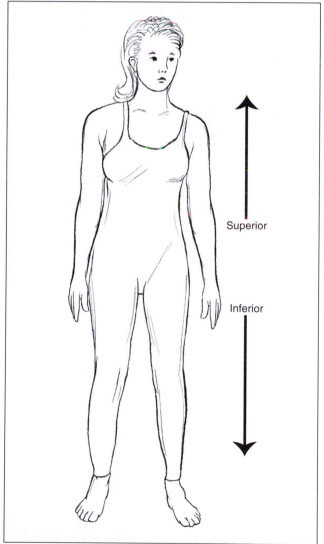

FIGURE 1.16 Inferior/superior.

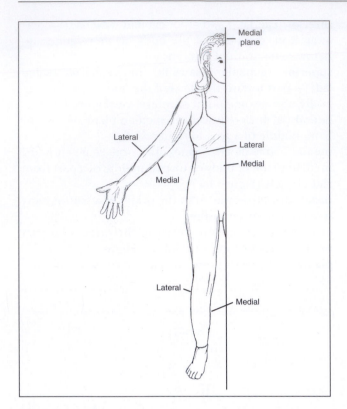

FIGURE 1.17   Lateral/medial.

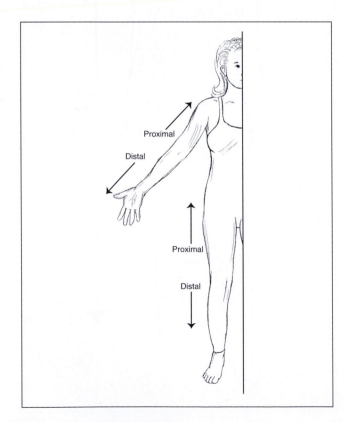

FIGURE 1.18   Distal/proximal.

dorsum (dor´sĕm)—refers to the anterior surface (or top) of foot (Note: Dorsum or dorsal in general refers to the posterior aspect of the body; however, when used in conjunction with the foot, it refers to the anterior part of the foot) (Figure 1.19)

palmar (păl´măr)—the palm of the hand

volar (vō´lăr)—the palm of the hand or the sole of the foot (Figure 1.20)

ipsilateral (ĭp´´sĭ-lăt´ĕr-ăl)—relates to the same side of the body or part

contralateral (kŏn´´tră-lăt´ĕr-ăl)—relates to the opposite side of the body or part (Figure 1.21)

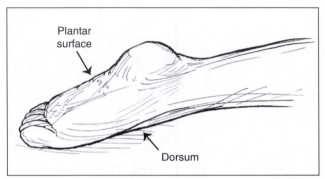

FIGURE 1.19   Plantar/dorsum.

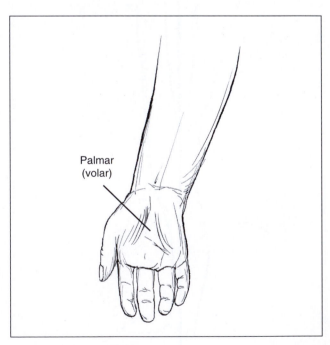

FIGURE 1.20   Palmar/volar.

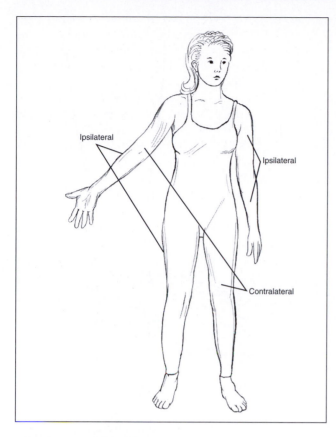

FIGURE 1.21   **Ipsilateral/contralateral.**

Body Positions

The following terms are used to describe the manner in which the patient is placed.

erect—an upright position, standing or sitting
recumbent—any reclining position
prone—lying face down (Figure 1.22)
supine—lying on back; face up (Figure 1.23)

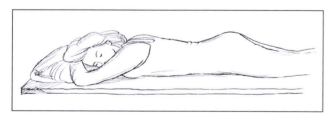

FIGURE 1.22   **Prone/ventral recumbent.**

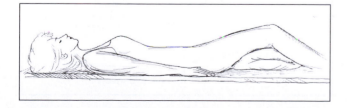

FIGURE 1.23   **Supine/dorsal recumbent.**

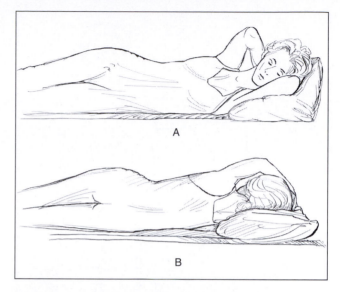

FIGURE 1.24   **(A) Left and (B) right lateral recumbent.**

dorsal recumbent—supine or lying on back
ventral recumbent—prone or lying face down
right lateral recumbent—lying on right side
left lateral recumbent—lying on left side (Figure 1.24)

Body Movement

The following terms are used to describe movement related to the extremities. The terms are presented in pairs to facilitate understanding of relationships.

abduct—to move a part away from the central axis of the body
adduct—to move a part toward the central axis of the body (Figure 1.25)
extend—to straighten a joint; increases the angle between adjacent bones
flex—to bend a joint; decreases the angle between adjacent bones (Figure 1.26)
hyperextend—extreme extension of a joint
hyperflex—extreme flexion of a joint
evert—movement of the foot when the ankle is turned outward
invert—movement of the foot when the ankle is turned inward (Figure 1.27)
pronate—to turn down the palm of the hand
supinate—to turn up the palm of the hand (Figure 1.28)
medial (or **internal**) **rotation**—rotation of a limb toward the midline
lateral (or **external**) **rotation**—rotation of a limb away from the midline (Figure 1.29)

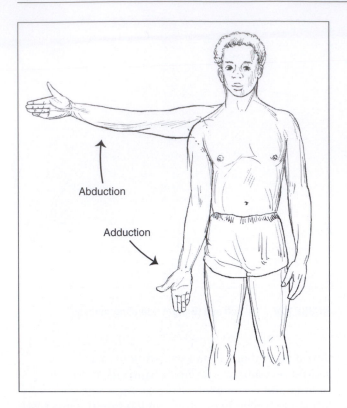

FIGURE 1.25   Abduct/adduct.

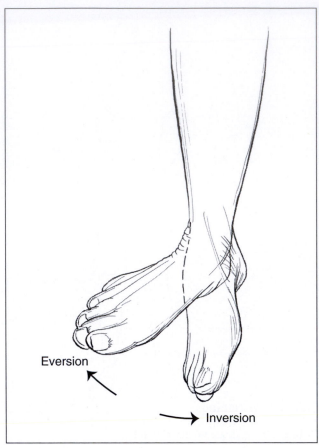

FIGURE 1.27   Evert/invert.

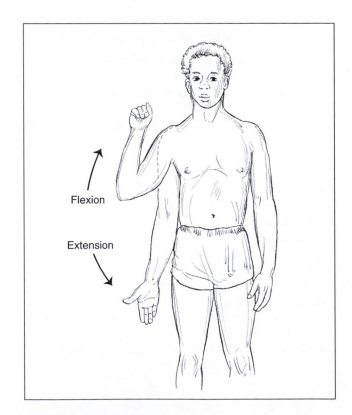

FIGURE 1.26   Extend/flex.

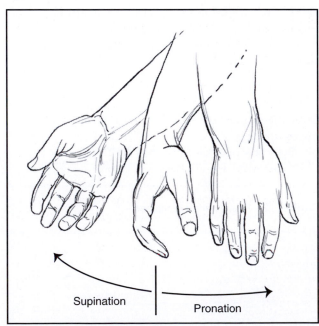

FIGURE 1.28   Pronate/supinate.

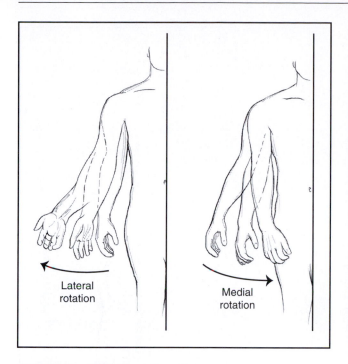

FIGURE 1.29 Medial/lateral rotation.

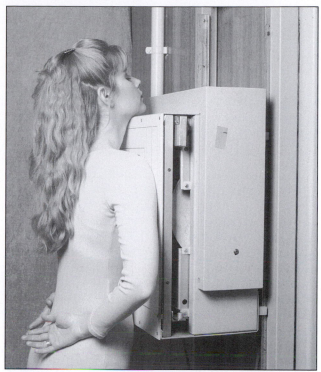

FIGURE 1.30 Projection - PA chest.

General Positioning

The following terms have become standardized within the profession of radiography and are consistent with terminology adopted by the American Registry of Radiologic Technologists (1990).

Projection describes the path of the central ray in the process of recording a body part on an image receptor by indicating the entrance and exit points. The term is restricted to description of the central ray. An example of a projection is the posteroanterior (PA) of the chest. PA signifies that the central ray entered the posterior surface of the patient and exited the anterior surface (Figure 1.30).

View describes the representation of the image from the perspective of the image receptor. View is the opposite of the projection. In the previous example of the PA projection of the chest, an anteroposterior (AP) view would have been produced (Figure 1.31).

Position is the term used to describe the patient's placement when both the entrance and exit points of the central ray are not defined. In a routine chest x-ray, a left lateral is typically obtained; because only one side of the patient is referenced, it is properly called the left lateral position (Figure 1.32). Some procedures have become identified by the individual who developed them and are referred to by a proper name. This text has attempted to limit this type of terminology.

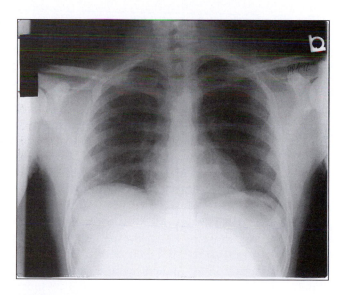

FIGURE 1.31 View - AP chest.

Frontal projections refer to all AP and PA projections.

Lateral positions are named by the side of the patient that is placed closest to the image receptor. In the example of the left lateral chest, the left side of the patient would be closest to the image receptor.

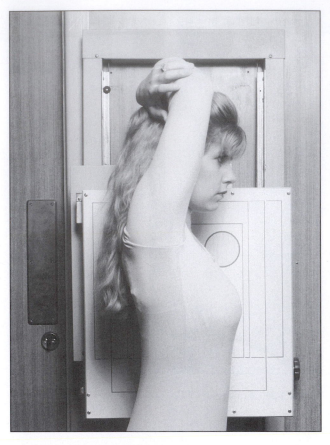

FIGURE 1.32 Position - left lateral chest.

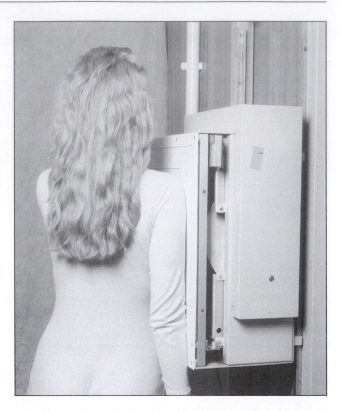

FIGURE 1.33 RAO (right anterior oblique) position.

Oblique (ō-blēk´) positions refer to those in which the patient is rotated somewhere between a frontal and lateral position. Oblique positions are identified by the side closest to the image receptor. For example, in Figure 1.33, the patient is in the right anterior oblique (RAO) position, that is, her right, front surface is closest to the image receptor. The other oblique positions are illustrated in Figures 1.34, 1.35, and 1.36.

Decubitus (dē-kū´bĭ-tŭs) positions, in radiographic positioning, are those in which the patient is recumbent while a radiograph is taken with a horizontal beam. The position is named by the side that is dependent. For example, Figures 1.37 and 1.38 illustrate a left lateral decubitus and a right lateral decubitus, respectively.

Axial positions are those in which the central ray is angled along the longitudinal axis of the body (Figure 1.39).

Tangential (tăn-jĕn´chĕl) positions refer to those in which the central ray skims a body part to demonstrate it in profile, free of superimposition (Figure 1.40).

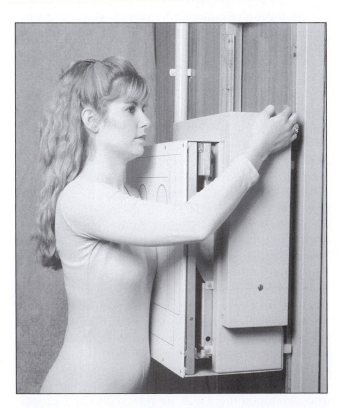

FIGURE 1.34 LAO (left anterior oblique) position.

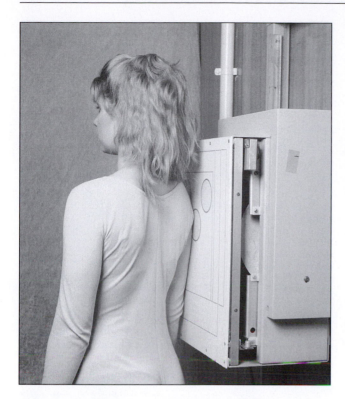

FIGURE 1.35 RPO (right posterior oblique) position.

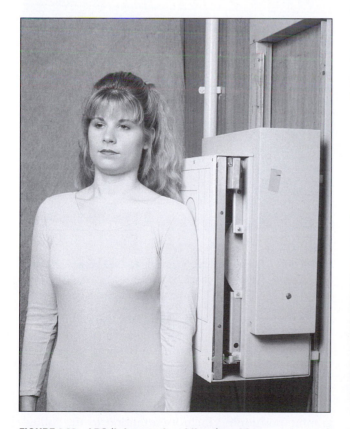

FIGURE 1.36 LPO (left posterior oblique) position.

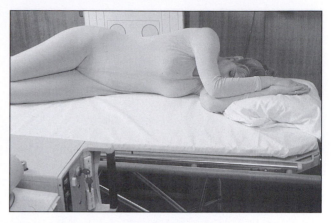

FIGURE 1.37 Left lateral decubitus.

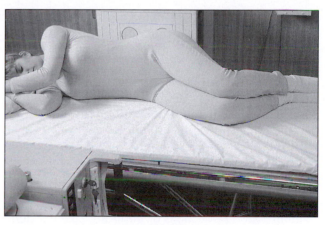

FIGURE 1.38 Right lateral decubitus.

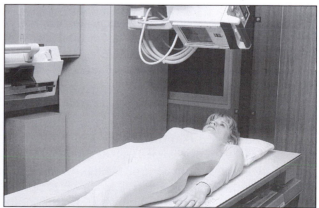

FIGURE 1.39 Axial position.

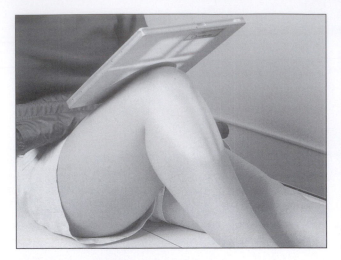

FIGURE 1.40 Tangential position.

PRINCIPLES OF RADIOGRAPHIC POSITIONING

General Positioning Considerations

This text describes both routine and alternative projections and positions for different anatomic parts. Accepted routines vary among institutions; radiographers should be familiar with their department's procedure manual that describes the accepted routine examination for that institution. An understanding of the following principles of positioning will enable radiographers to understand the rationale for certain routines and to be able to adjust appropriately when the routine examination is not possible.

1. As a general rule, an examination requires a minimum of two projections or positions, taken at right angles to one another. (A common exception is the KUB, an examination of the kidneys, ureters, and bladder.) Because the radiograph is a two-dimensional representation of a three-dimensional object, it requires two views to adequately demonstrate position and relationships of internal structures. This is important for three reasons:
   a. To overcome problems of superimposition; a pathologic condition may be overshadowed by an overlying structure as seen in Figure 1.41.
   b. To localize foreign bodies; on the radiograph in Figure 1.42, a foreign body is visualized over the 4th metatarsal as demonstrated on the AP projection. In the lateral position, however, it can be determined that the foreign body is actually closer to the posterior surface of the foot.
   c. To determine alignment of fractured bones; the parts of the femur in Figure 1.43 appear to be reasonably well aligned on the frontal projection; In the lateral position, however, it is clear that there is still significant anterior to posterior displacement.

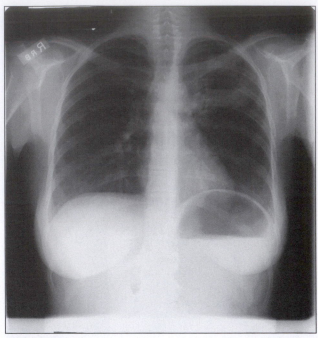

A

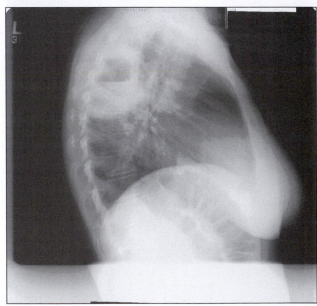

B

FIGURE 1.41 Overlying structures are resolved with (A) PA and (B) lateral chest.

2. Whenever possible, the minimum two radiographs should be a frontal (AP or PA) and a lateral.
3. As a general rule, a minimum of three projections or positions is required when joints are the prime area of interest.

With the above general principles in mind, radiographic positioning includes attention to the following elements.

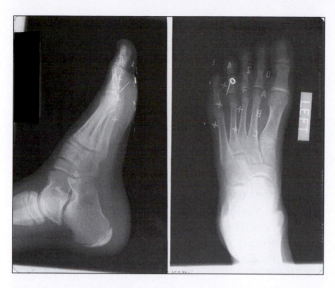

FIGURE 1.42 Foreign body localization is resolved with lateral and AP foot.

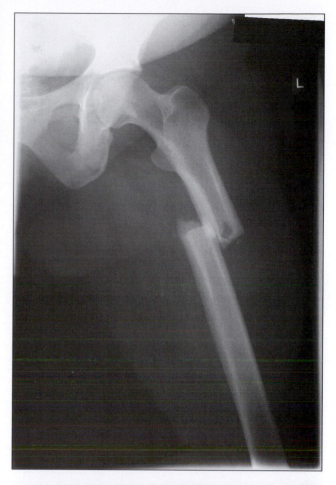

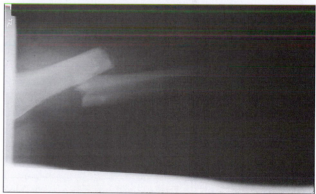

FIGURE 1.43 Fracture alignment is resolved with AP and lateral femur.

1. **Positioning of patient and part**—Both the patient and the specific body part must be correctly positioned. Initial consideration is given to whether the patient is: erect or recumbent, standing or sitting, and in what specific position. Further consideration is then given to the specific body part. For example, a PA projection of the hand would require the patient to be sitting and then the hand to be placed palm down on the cassette.

2. **Alignment of part to film**—As a rule, the image receptor should be placed with its long axis aligned with the long axis of the part. One frequent exception to the alignment along the axis is when a body part needs to be angled from corner to corner of the cassette to include both joints on an examination of a long bone (Figure 1.44).

   When two or more projections are taken on the same film, such as an AP and oblique foot, both should be oriented the same way on the film (Figure 1.45).

3. **Inclusion of relevant anatomy**—The part being radiographed must be correctly placed on the image receptor so that all of the required anatomy is visualized within the collimated borders. This requires the selection of the correct film size, which will be indicated for each procedure throughout the text.

4. **Adjustment of source image-receptor distance (SID)**—Most radiographic procedures are done at 40 or 72 inches (100 or 180 cm) SID. The correct distance, based on all relevant factors, should be selected.

5. **Alignment of tube to image-receptor**—Once the patient and part are correctly positioned and the appropriate SID set, the radiographic tube must be correctly aligned with the image receptor. Although slight variations can be accommodated when doing table-top radiography, work done with a grid or Bucky will be less forgiving of small errors.

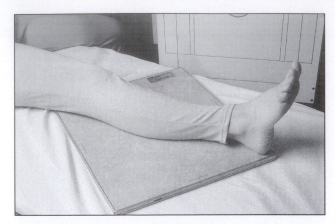

FIGURE 1.44 Lower leg is angled across film to include both joints.

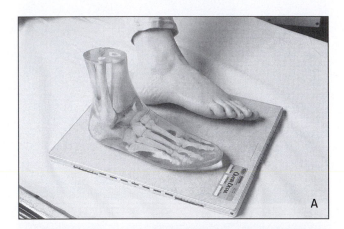

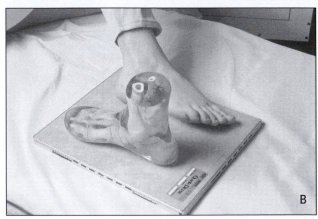

FIGURE 1.45 (A) Correct and (B) incorrect orientation of multiple views on single film.

6. **Placement of patient identification and film markers**—Radiographs must contain identification of the patient, the patient's medical number, the institution, the date, the appropriate side marker (left or right), and the radiographer's initials or marker number. This information is critical not only for

proper film identification but also for legal reasons. Additionally, markers may be required to indicate timed films or films taken in specific positions (e.g., erect versus recumbent). Most of the patient and institutional identification will be displayed on a corner of the film by means of a film identification camera. Throughout this text, an illustration of suggested placement of the identification information will be provided as shown in Figures 1.46 and 1.47.

Organizational Routine

Successful radiography requires attention to a great many details. The successful radiographer will develop a routine that encompasses attention to all of the details in a systematic fashion. The following organizational scheme is suggested to the beginning radiographer, although it should be adapted to both the individual's needs and to the needs of a particular examination.

I. Interpret Requisition (Figure 1.48)
    A. Decide examination to be done.
    B. Check patient's name, age, and history.
    C. Check patient's location and mode of transportation.
II. Prepare Radiographic Room (Figure 1.49)
    A. Clean table; supply fresh linen as appropriate.
    B. Collect appropriate number and type of cassettes.

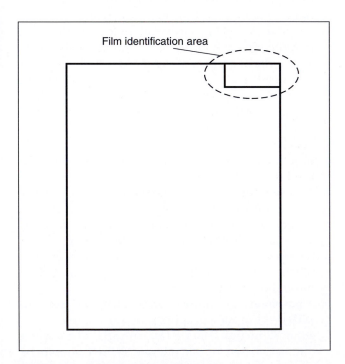

Film identification area

FIGURE 1.46 Film identification blocker.

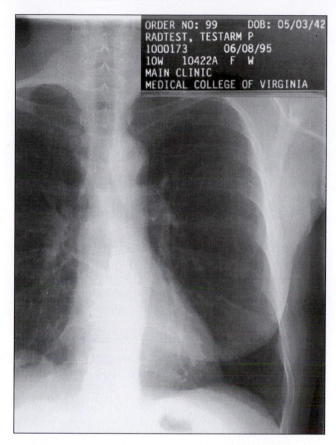

FIGURE 1.47   Radiograph showing patient identification information.

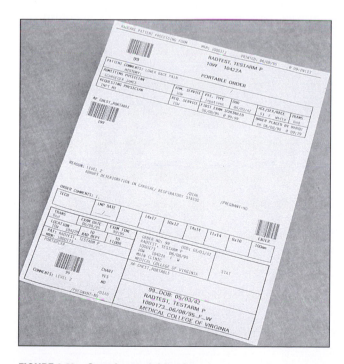

FIGURE 1.48   Sample requisition form.

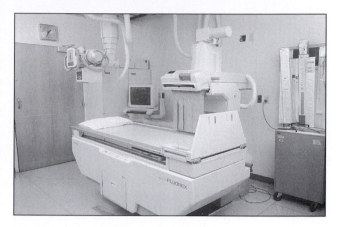

FIGURE 1.49   Radiographic room prepared for procedure.

    C. Collect necessary equipment and supplies (sponges, contrast, etc.).

    D. Place cassette correctly in Bucky tray or on table with correct marker appropriately placed.

    E. Set exposure variables.

III. Identify and Transport Patient (Figure 1.50)

    A. Greet patient; obtain positive identification.

    B. Assess patient for ability to communicate and cooperate.

    C. Provide instructions for disrobing as appropriate.

    D. Transport patient to radiographic room.

    E. Obtain relevant history, including pregnancy status.

    F. Explain procedure.

IV. Perform Examination (Figure 1.51)

    A. Observe standard precautions as appropriate to the patient and the examination.

    B. Assist patient to appropriate initial position; further assess patient for technical considerations.

    C. Position body part.

    D. Position tube for exact central ray alignment.

    E. Collimate; apply gonadal shielding as appropriate.

    F. Make any necessary adjustments at console.

    G. Give necessary breathing instructions; observe patient while making exposure.

    H. While at console, adjust exposure factors for next film as necessary.

    I. Return to patient; exchange cassettes; position for next position.

V. Finish Procedure (Figure 1.52)

    A. Assist patient from room.

    B. Process films.

    C. Wash hands.

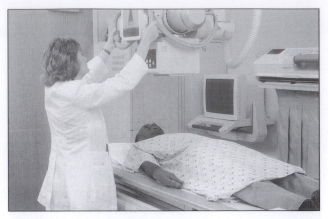

FIGURE 1.51 Radiographer performing radiographic examination.

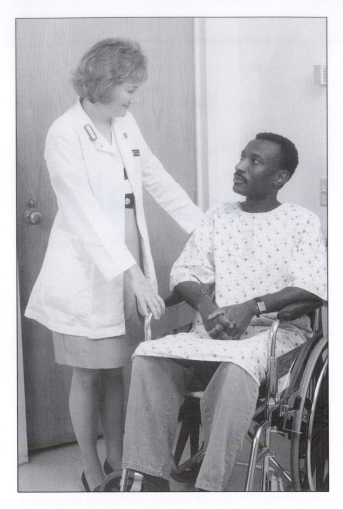

FIGURE 1.50 Greeting patient.

Final Note

One final caution to the student is in order. The material in this text often makes it seem as if there is only one correct way to obtain a radiograph and that this one way is easily accomplished by following the directions in the text. The process is infinitely more involved than it initially seems. In reality, each patient presents a unique challenge. This positioning text describes a place to begin. Throughout your career as a radiographer you will acquire additional knowledge and experience that will help you evolve into a competent radiographer capable of routinely obtaining optimal quality radiographs on even the most difficult and challenging patients.

    D. Analyze films for quality.
    E. Obtain any necessary approvals from supervising radiographer.
VI. Complete Follow-through (Figure 1.53)
    A. Dismiss patient and complete paperwork.
    B. Clean room; return any supplies; dispose of soiled linens.
    C. Wash hands.

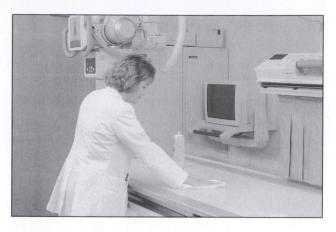

FIGURE 1.53 Cleaning radiographic room after examination completion.

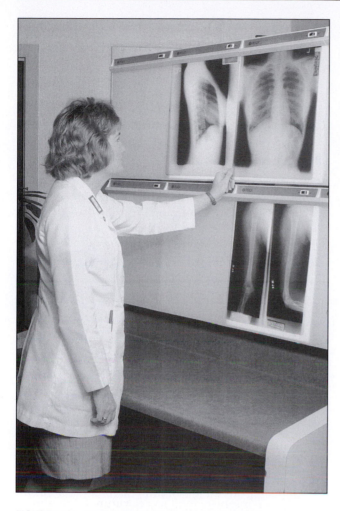

FIGURE 1.52 Radiographer reviewing and analyzing radiographs.

Review Questions

1. Which of the following is an appropriate responsibility of a radiographer prior to performing a radiographic study?

   a. providing an explanation of the procedure to the patient
   b. performing a general assessment of the patient's physical and mental status
   c. obtaining a detailed history from the patient
   d. both a and b
   e. all of the above

2. The 10-day rule calls for x-rays of female patients to be done:

   a. during the first 10 days following the onset of menstruation
   b. during the 10 days immediately before the onset of menstruation
   c. the middle ten days of the menstrual period
   d. within ten days of the date the physician ordered the x-rays

3. At what vertebral level is the sternal angle found?

   a. C1
   b. C7
   c. T1
   d. T4–T5

4. Which of the following is true of the asthenic body type?

   a. colon would be found along abdomen's periphery
   b. stomach is horizontal and away from midline
   c. lungs are long and broader at top than at base
   d. the predominant body type

5. Which of the following is true of the hypersthenic body type?

   a. stomach is vertical and near midline
   b. lungs are short and broad at base
   c. heart is long and narrow
   d. is the predominant body type

6. Anterior refers to the:

   a. front surface of the body
   b. back surface of the body
   c. part away from the head end of the body
   d. part toward the head end of the body

7. Inferior refers to the:

   a. front surface of the body
   b. back surface of the body
   c. part away from the head end of the body
   d. part toward the head end of the body

8. Distal refers to:

   a. away from the head end of the body
   b. toward the head end of the body
   c. away from the origin of a part
   d. toward the origin of a part

9. Which of the following is a recumbent position?

   a. anatomic position
   b. supine
   c. prone
   d. both b and c
   e. all of the above

10. Abduct means to:

    a. move a part toward the central axis of the body
    b. move a part away from the central axis of the body
    c. straighten a joint
    d. bend a joint

11. Medial means away from the median plane of the body.

    a. true
    b. false

12. To extend a joint means to bend it, reducing the angle between adjacent bones.

    a. true
    b. false

13. Obtaining a brief history from the patient before doing a radiographic procedure can benefit both the radiographer and the radiologist.

    a. true
    b. false

14. The midsagittal plane divides the body into

    _____.

15. The _____ plane divides the body into equal anterior and posterior portions.

16. In the right lateral recumbent position, the patient is lying on his _____ side.

17. Oblique positions are those in which the body is

_____

_____.

18. For each of the following anatomic landmarks, list the corresponding vertebra:

    a. xiphoid tip_____
    b. thyroid cartilage_____
    c. mastoid tip_____
    d. anterior superior iliac spine_____
    e. iliac crest_____

19. List the three primary exposure factors.

20. List the three primary principles of radiation protection.

21. List at least three methods of minimizing radiation exposure to the patient during a radiographic study.

22. List the three general principles of positioning.

23. List the six elements of radiographic positioning.

24. To which body habitus group does each of the following belong?

    A.
    B.
    C.

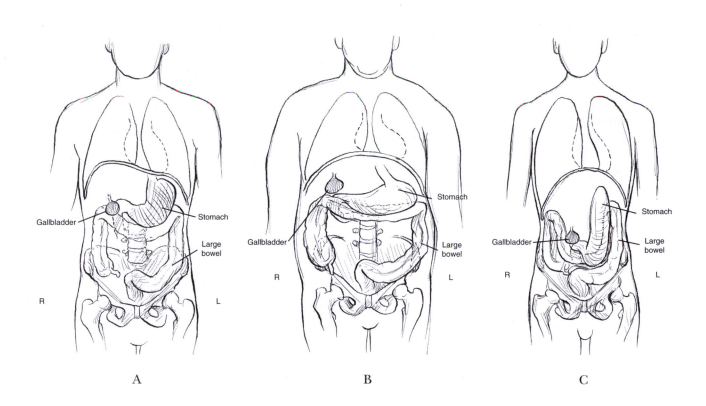

           A   B   C

References and Recommended Reading

Adler, A., & Carlton, R. (Eds.). (1995). *Introduction to radiologic technology and patient care*. Philadelphia: Saunders.

American Registry of Radiologic Technologists. (1995). Conventions specific to the Radiography Examination. St. Paul, MN: Author.

Brecher, R., & Brecher, E. (1969). *The rays: A history of radiology in the United States and Canada*. Baltimore: Williams & Wilkins.

Bushong, S. (1997). *Radiologic science for technologists* (4th ed.). St. Louis: Mosby-Year Book.

Ehrlich, R. A., & McCloskey, E. D. (1993). *Patient care in radiography* (4th ed.). St. Louis: Mosby-Year Book.

Carlton, R., & Adler, A. (1996). *Principles of radiographic exposure* (2nd ed.). Albany, NY: Delmar Publishers.

Cember, H. (1993). *Introduction to health physics* (2nd ed.). New York: Pergamon Press.

Cullinan, A. (1993). *Producing quality radiographs* (2nd ed.). Philadelphia: Lippincott.

Fodor, J., & Malott, J. (1993). *The art and science of medical radiography* (7th ed.). St. Louis: Mosby-Year Book.

Mills, W. R. (1917). The relation of bodily habitus to visceral form, position, tonus, and motility. *American Journal of Radiology, 4*; 155—169.

National Council on Radiation Protection and Measurements. (1977). *Review of NCRP radiation dose limit for embryo and fetus in occupationally exposed women* (Report no. 53). Bethesda, MD: Author.

National Council on Radiation Protection and Measurements. (1977). *Medical exposure of pregnant and potentially pregnant women* (Report no. 54). Bethesda, MD: Author.

National Council on Radiation Protection and Measurements. (1978). *Instrumentation and monitoring methods for radiation protection* (Report no. 57). Bethesda, MD: Author.

National Council on Radiation Protection and Measurements. (1985). *SI units in radiation protection and measurements* (Report no. 82). Bethesda, MD: Author.

National Council on Radiation Protection and Measurements. (1987). *Recommendations on limits for exposure to ionizing radiation* (Report no. 91). Bethesda, MD: Author.

National Council on Radiation Protection and Measurements. (1989). *Radiation protection for medical and allied health personnel* (Report no. 105). Bethesda, MD: Author.

Statkiewicz-Sherrer, M. A., Visconti, P. J., & Ritenour, E. R. (1993). *Radiation protection in medical radiography* (2nd ed.). St. Louis: Mosby-Year Book.

Torres, L. S. (1993). *Basic medical techniques and patient care for radiologic technologists* (4th ed.). Philadelphia: Lippincott.

SECTION II

CHEST
and
ABDOMEN

Chest and Upper Airway

SARAJANE DOTY, MSEd, RT(R)(ARRT)

ANATOMY
Upper Airway
Thoracic Cavity

GENERAL CHEST RADIOGRAPHY
Upright Position
Exposure Factors
Preparation of the Patient

CHEST—ROUTINE POSITIONS/PROJECTIONS
PA
Lateral

CHEST—ALTERNATE POSITIONS/PROJECTIONS
PA (Stretcher/Stool)
Lateral (Stretcher/Stool)

Supine/Semi-upright AP
Lateral Decubitus
Dorsal Decubitus
AP Lordotic
Obliques

UPPER AIRWAY—ROUTINE POSITIONS/PROJECTIONS
AP
Lateral

SPECIAL CONSIDERATIONS
Pediatric Considerations
Selected Pathology
Correlative Imaging

OBJECTIVES

At the completion of this chapter, the student should be able to:

1. List and describe the anatomy of the chest and upper airway.

2. Given drawings and radiographs, locate anatomic structures and landmarks.

3. Explain the rationale for each projection.

4. Explain the patient preparation required for each examination.

5. Describe the positioning used to visualize anatomic structures of the chest and upper airway.

6. List or identify the central ray location and identify the extent of the field necessary for each projection.

7. Explain the protective measures that should be taken during each examination.

8. Recommend the technical factors for producing an acceptable radiograph for each projection.

9. State the patient instructions for each projection.

10. Given radiographs, evaluate positioning and technical factors.

11. Describe modifications of procedures for atypical or impaired patients to better demonstrate the anatomic area of interest.

Anatomy

The study of the respiratory anatomy (Color illustration 6) will be divided into the upper airway, lungs, **mediastinum** (me´´-dē-ăs-tĭ´nŭm) and bony structures. The primary function of the upper airway is to conduct air into the lungs; the primary function of the lungs is the exchange of gases. The bony structures protect the lungs and mediastinum.

UPPER AIRWAY

The upper airway is a conduit that allows air to reach the lungs. It also filters, warms, and moistens the incoming air before reaching the lungs. The upper airway is divided into the **pharynx** (făr´ĭnks), **larynx** (lăr´ĭnks), and **trachea** (trā´kē-ă) (Figure 2.1).

Pharynx

The pharynx has three divisions: **nasopharynx** (nā´´zō-făr´ĭnks), **oropharynx** (or´´ō-făr´ĭnks̄), and **laryngopharynx** (lăr-ĭn´´gō-făr´ĭnks) (Figure 2.2). The nasopharynx serves only as a passage for air and is posterior to the nasal cavity. The oropharynx extends from the soft

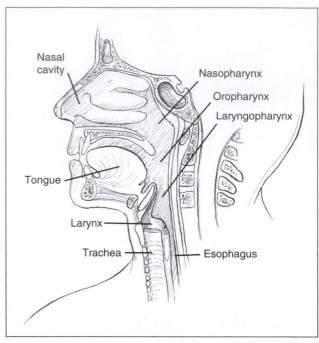

FIGURE 2.2   Lateral view of nasopharynx, oropharynx, and laryngopharynx.

palate to the **epiglottis** (ĕp´´ĭ-glŏt´ĭs) and is posterior to the oral cavity. It serves as the passage for both food and air. The laryngopharynx is posterior to the epiglottis, which also serves as a passage for both food and air.

Larynx

The larynx is made up of three paired and three unpaired laryngeal (lăr-ĭn´jē-ăl) cartilages extending from the level of C4 to C6. The single thyroid cartilage, the largest of all the cartilages, forms the laryngeal prominence, commonly called the "Adam's apple," a frequently used radiographic landmark. The larynx is attached to the hyoid bone superiorly and is continuous with the trachea inferiorly. The two primary functions of the larynx are to prevent food from entering the air passages and permit air through to the lungs. The larynx is also responsible for voice production (Figure 2.3).

Trachea

The trachea, 4 inches (10 to 12 cm) long and 1 inch (2.5 cm) in diameter, is a tubular structure extending from the larynx into the thoracic cavity. It is a highly flexible structure with sixteen to twenty C-shaped tracheal cartilage rings composed of hyline cartilage, which prevents its collapse. The last tracheal cartilage

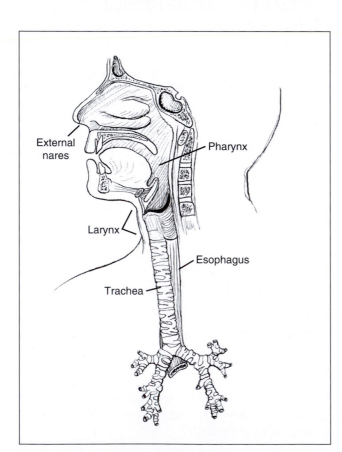

FIGURE 2.1   Lateral view of pharynx, larynx, and trachea.

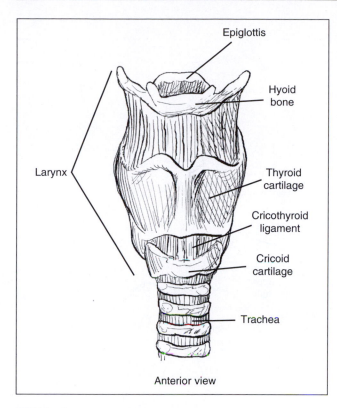

FIGURE 2.3   **Anterior view of larynx.**

has a bony spur of cartilage termed the **carina** (kă-rī′nă) projecting posteriorly into the trachea. At this point, the level of T5, the trachea bifurcates into the two main branches of the bronchi.

THORACIC CAVITY

The thoracic cavity houses the lungs, heart, and mediastinal (mē′′dē-ăs-tī′năl) structures.

Bronchial Tree

At the level of T5, the trachea bifurcates into the right and left primary bronchi. When compared with the left primary bronchus, the right is shorter, wider, and more vertical than the left and is the more common site for inhaled foreign objects. The primary bronchi enter the lungs at the **hilum** (hī′lŭm) where they immediately divide into secondary or **lobar bronchi** (lō′băr brŏng′kī)—three on the right and two on the left. These continue to divide until the terminal **bronchioles** (brŏng′kē-ōl) are reached, which lead to the respiratory structures. The respiratory structures include the respiratory bronchioles where some gases are exchanged, the **alveolar ducts** (ăl-vē′ō-lăr dŭkts), **alveolar sacs** (ăl-vē′ō-lăr săks), and **alveoli** (ăl-vē′ō-lī), where the majority of gases are exchanged. The alve-

oli are clusters of outpouchings along the alveolar ducts with a common opening called the atrium (Figure 2.4).

Mediastinum

The mediastinum is the space that separates the lungs and extends from the sternum anteriorly to the vertebral column posteriorly. Structures of the mediastinum include the heart, great vessels, trachea, esophagus, thoracic duct, and the remains of the thymus (Figure 2.5).

Lungs

The lungs, surrounded by the pleural cavities, lie on each side of the mediastinum. The right lung is divided into the upper, middle, and lower lobes, which are separated by the horizontal and oblique **fissures** (fĭsh′ūrs). The left lung is divided into an upper and lower lobe separated by an oblique fissure. The lungs are enclosed in a pleural cavity on each side of the mediastinum and anchored by various pulmonary vessels and the bronchi, also known as the root of the lung.

The lungs are conical in shape and have an apex, base, three borders, and two surfaces. The apex is a rounded structure that lies above the clavicles. The base is concave and rests on the diaphragm, which separates the thoracic cavity from the abdominal cavity. The three borders of the lung include the inferior border, which in part forms the **costophrenic angle**,

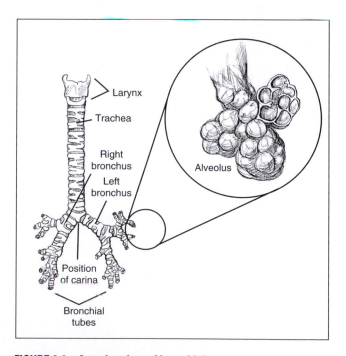

FIGURE 2.4   **Anterior view of bronchial tree.**

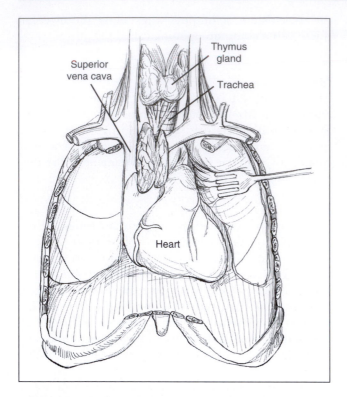

FIGURE 2.5   Mediastinal structures.

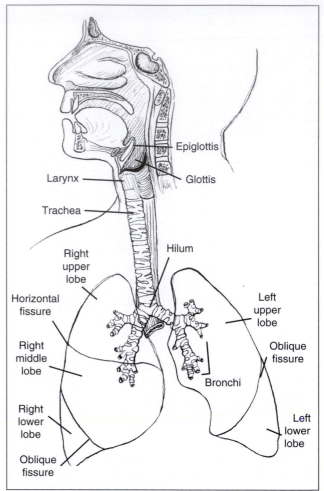

FIGURE 2.6   Anterior view of lungs.

the anterior border, and the cardiac notch. The two surfaces of the lungs are the costal and mediastinal surfaces. The costal surface is the large convex surface that corresponds in shape to the chest cavity. The mediastinal surface is located on the medial side of each lung and is in contact with the mediastinal pleura. It is on this surface that the hilum penetrates the lungs.

As the organs of respiration, the lungs are the mechanism by which oxygen is introduced into the blood and carbon dioxide is removed from it (Figure 2.6).

Pleura

The **pleura** (ploo´rǎ) is a continuous double-walled **serous** (sēr´ŭs) membrane that encases each lung separately and folds around the root of the lungs. The membrane, which adheres to the lungs and dips into each fissure, is termed the pulmonary or visceral pleura. The parietal pleura lines the thoracic cavity

except for the mediastinal structures. To allow the lungs to glide freely over the two surfaces, the pleura produces pleural fluid. This fluid lubricates the slit-like pleural cavity and creates a surface tension that keeps the lungs expanded during respiration.

Diaphragm

The **diaphragm** is the muscular structure that separates the thorax from the abdomen. The superior surface is in contact with the bases of the lungs, and the inferior surface forms the top of the abdominal cavity. The right hemidiaphragm is usually more elevated than the left due to the presence of the liver.

The diaphragm is of great importance radiographically. It expands, and thus is lowered, on inspiration and relaxes, and thus rises, on expiration. The greatest area of lung is visible on full inspiration because of the maximum lowering of the diaphragm.

The costophrenic sinus, or angle, refers to the lower outer corner of each lung where the diaphragm meets the lateral chest wall. It represents the extreme lowermost part of the lungs.

Bony Structures

The bony structures protect the lungs, heart, and mediastinal structures. These structures include the sternum anteriorly, the thoracic vertebrae posteriorly, and the ribs laterally (Figure 2.7). A detailed discussion of these structures is included in Chapters 6 and 8.

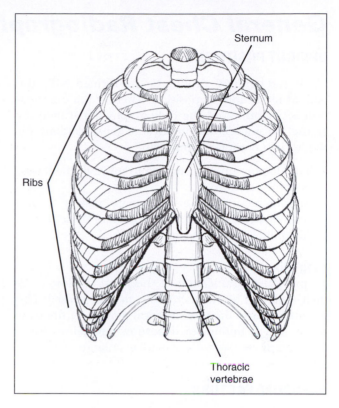

FIGURE 2.7   Bony structures of the thorax.

General Chest Radiography

UPRIGHT POSITION

Chest radiography should be performed with the patient in an upright position, whether the examination is performed in the radiography department or at the bedside. Three important considerations for the upright chest radiograph are:

• The diaphragm is permitted to move to the lowest possible position.
• Engorgement of the pulmonary vessels is prevented, which minimizes distortion of these vessels.
• Air/fluid levels can be demonstrated.

Long SID

To prevent magnification of the heart shadow, a 72-inch (180 cm) or 120-inch (300 cm) SID is used. The longer SID uses the more vertical portion of the x-ray beam, which minimizes distortion and allows for a more accurate diagnosis of cardiac enlargement.

EXPOSURE FACTORS

To ensure proper diagnosis of a chest radiograph, lung markings should be demonstrated throughout the lung field, and a faint shadow of the thoracic vertebrae and ribs will be seen through the heart. Exposure factors should include a kilovoltage peak (kVp) high enough to penetrate the heart while still demonstrating finer lung markings. If the kVp is too high, the finer lung markings will disappear into the surrounding tissue. If the kVp is too low, the finer lung markings will be demonstrated, but the heart will appear very dense and underpenetrated. When using a grid, moving or stationary, a kVp of 100 to 120 should be used. If a nongrid technique is used, as in bedside radiography, a kVp between 75 to 90 should be used. A high milliampere (mA) and short exposure time should be used for chest radiography to prevent motion of the heart.

PREPARATION OF THE PATIENT

If a dedicated chest radiography room is used, the room and the film magazine should be checked to ensure that an ample supply of film is available.

   In addition to having the patient disrobe from the waist up, the patient should be instructed to remove all potential artifacts from the thoracic and neck regions (e.g., necklace or other jewelry). Long hair, especially wet hair, braids, or pony tails, should be pulled to the side. Any patient tubing (e.g., nasogastric tubes, oxygen tubes) that can be moved should also be carefully placed to one side.

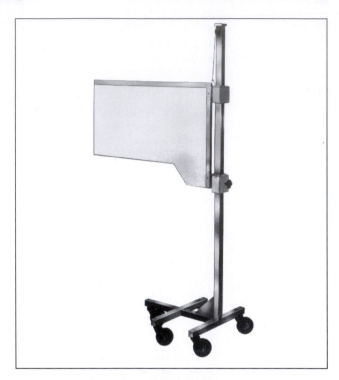

FIGURE 2.8   Mobile pelvic shield (Courtesy of Nuclear Associates, Carle Place, NY).

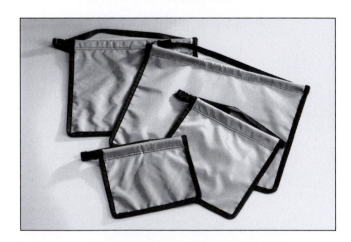

FIGURE 2.9   Lead-impregnated vinyl mini apron (Courtesy of E-Z-EM Company, Westbury, NY).

   To best demonstrate fluid in the lungs, patients must be in the upright, semi-upright, or decubitus position for a minimum of 10 minutes. This allows the fluid in the lungs or the pleural spaces to settle to the lowest level.

   Gonadal shielding for upright chest radiography includes the use of a mobile pelvic shield or lead-impregnated vinyl mini apron placed at waist level. The mobile pelvic shield can be adjusted to accommodate patient height; the lead-impregnated vinyl mini apron comes in a variety of sizes to accommodate patient size (Figures 2.8 and 2.9).

ROUTINE AND ALTERNATIVE POSITIONS/PROJECTIONS

Part	Routine	Page	Alternative	Page
Chest	PA	36	PA (stretcher/stool)	40
			Supine/semi-erect AP	44
			Lateral decubitus	46
			AP lordotic	48
	Lateral	38	Dorsal decubitus (tip: ventral decubitus)	52
			Lateral (stretcher/stool)	42
Upper airway	AP	54		
	Lateral	56		

PA CHEST PROJECTION

Exam Rationale   The PA chest is performed to outline the anatomy of the lungs, heart, great vessels, and mediastinal structures to detect the presence of chest lesions.

Technical Considerations

- Regular screen/film
- Grid
- kVp range: 100–120
- SID: 72 inch (180 cm)

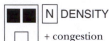

Radiation Protection

AEC (Phototiming)

 N DENSITY

+ congestion
– emphysema

Patient Position   Erect with weight equally distributed on both feet; top of film 1 1/2 to 2 inches (4–5 cm) above shoulders and centered to film T6–T7 (Figure 2.10).

Part Position   Hands low on hips, palms facing outward; shoulders relaxed; scapulae rotated forward; chin elevated.

Central Ray   Perpendicular to the film holder.

Patient Instructions   "Take in a deep breath; let it out. Take in another deep breath and hold it. Don't breathe or move."

Evaluation Criteria (Figures 2.11 and 2.12)

- Sternoclavicular joints should be equidistant from the vertebral column.
- Distance between the vertebral column and the outer margin of the rib cage should be equal on each side.
- Entire apices should be demonstrated 1 inch above the clavicles.
- Both costophrenic angles should be included on the film.
- Scapulae should be rotated outside the lung field.
- Mandible should not be superimposed over the lung field.
- A minimum of ten posterior ribs should be demonstrated.

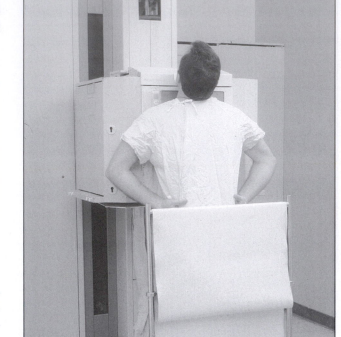

FIGURE 2.10   PA chest.

Tips

1. The film should be turned crosswise for patients with a wide chest.
2. To remove overlapping breast shadows, women with large pendulous breasts should be asked to lift their breasts and pull them to the side holding them in place while leaning forward to the film holder.
3. To demonstrate a pneumothorax, an inhalation and exhalation chest radiograph should be performed. The exhalation chest enhances the pneumothorax.

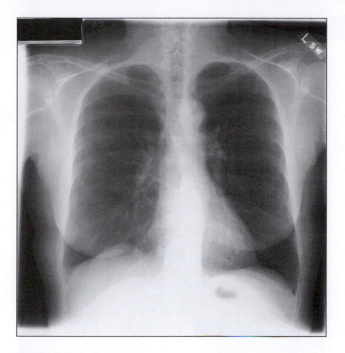

FIGURE 2.11   PA chest.

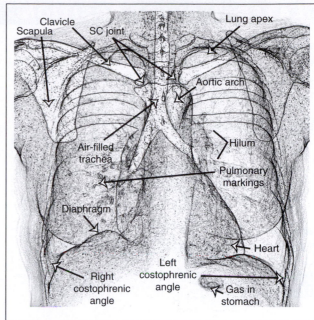

FIGURE 2.12   PA chest.

LATERAL CHEST POSITION

Exam Rationale   The lateral chest demonstrates the anatomy of the lungs, heart, great vessels, and mediastinum structures 90° from the PA to detect the presence of chest lesions.

Technical Considerations

- Regular screen/film
- Grid
- kVp range: 100–120
- SID: 72 inch (180 cm)

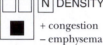

Radiation Protection   AEC (Phototiming)

N DENSITY

+ congestion
– emphysema

Patient Position   Erect; with weight equally distributed on both feet; top of film 1 1/2 to 2 inches (4–5 cm) above shoulders; center x-ray tube to film (T6–T7).

Part Position   Feet, hips, and shoulders in true lateral position; arms raised over the head with each hand grasping opposite elbow (Figure 2.13);
    or
grasp bar positioned in front of and over patient's head underhanded; chin elevated; midcoronal plane centered to the film holder (Figure 2.14).

Central Ray   Perpendicular to the film holder.

Patient Instructions   "Take in a deep breath; let it out. Take in another deep breath and hold it. Don't breathe or move."

Evaluation Criteria (Figures 2.15 and 2.16)

- Posterior aspect of the ribs and lungs should be superimposed.
- Intervertebral joint spaces of the thoracic vertebra should be clearly visible.
- Sternum should be in lateral position.
- Apices and costophrenic angles should be included on the film.
- Hilum should be near the center of the film.
- Midsagittal plane of the patient should be vertical—the patient should not be leaning forward or backward.

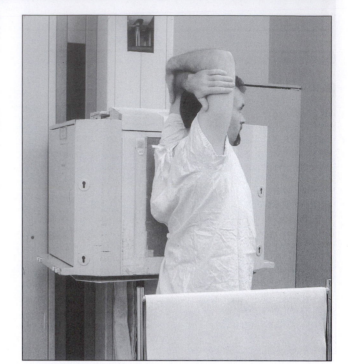

FIGURE 2.13   Lateral chest (arms overhead).

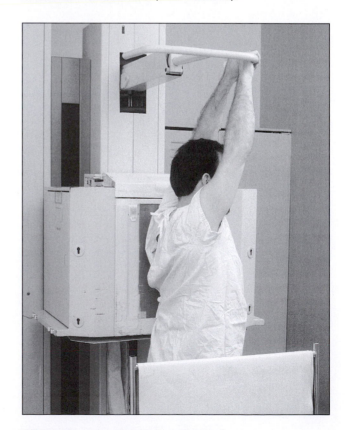

FIGURE 2.14   Lateral chest (grasping bar).

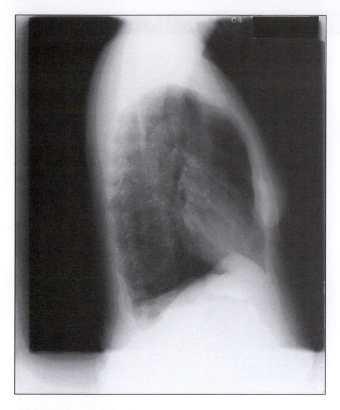

FIGURE 2.15   Lateral chest.

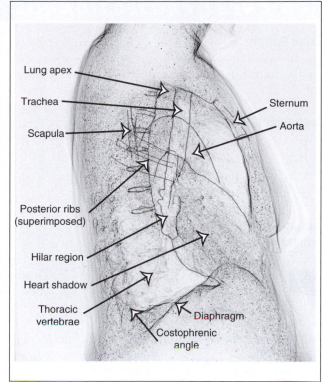

FIGURE 2.16   Lateral chest.

PA CHEST PROJECTION (USING STRETCHER OR STOOL)

Exam Rationale The PA chest is performed to outline the anatomy of the lungs, heart, great vessels, and mediastinum structures to detect the presence of chest lesions.

Technical Considerations

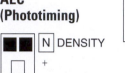

- Regular screen/film
- Grid
- kVp range: 100–120
- SID: 72 inch (180 cm)

Radiation Protection   **AEC (Phototiming)**

   N DENSITY
+
−

Patient Position Erect; weight equally distributed on the ischial tuberosities; legs dangling off side of stretcher; top of film 1 1/2 to 2 inches (4–5 cm) above shoulders centered to T6–T7.

Part Position Hands low on hips, palms facing outward; shoulders relaxed; scapulae rotated forward; chin elevated (Figure 2.17).

Central Ray Perpendicular to the film holder.

Patient Instructions "Take in a deep breath; let it out. Take in another deep breath and hold it. Don't breathe or move."

Evaluation Criteria (Figure 2.18)
Same as for routine PA chest (see page 36).

Tips

1. Lock stool or stretcher in place to prevent movement during the exposure.
2. Center the patient on the stretcher to maintain balance of the stretcher.
3. If the patient is unable to dangle the legs off the stretcher, have him hold the cassette in place (Figure 2.19).

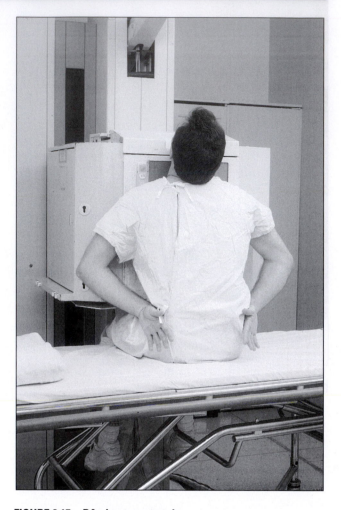

FIGURE 2.17   **PA chest on stretcher.**

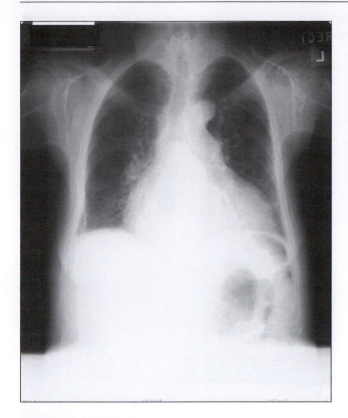

FIGURE 2.18   PA chest.

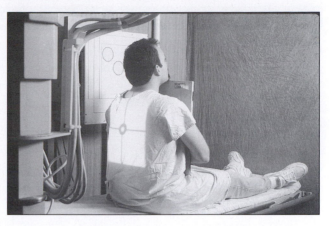

FIGURE 2.19   PA chest on stretcher with patient holding cassette.

LATERAL CHEST POSITION (USING STRETCHER OR STOOL)

Exam Rationale   The lateral chest demonstrates the anatomy of the lungs, heart, and mediastinal structures 90° from the PA to detect the presence of chest lesions for patients unable to stand.

Technical Considerations

- Regular screen/film
- Grid
- kVp range: 100–120
- SID: 72 inch (180 cm)

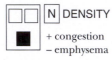

Radiation Protection

AEC (Phototiming)

N DENSITY

+ congestion
– emphysema

Patient Position   Erect; sitting on a stretcher with legs extended or seated upright on a stool with weight equally distributed on the ischial tuberosities; top of film 1 1/2 to 2 inches (4–5 cm) above shoulders centered to T6–T7.

Part Position   Hips and shoulders in true lateral; arms raised over the head with each hand grasping the opposite elbow; or, grasp bar positioned in front of and over patient's head underhanded; chin elevated; midcoronal plane centered to film holder (Figure 2.20).

Central Ray   Perpendicular to the film holder.

Patient Instructions   "Take in a deep breath, let it out. Take in another deep breath and hold it. Don't breathe or move."

Evaluation Criteria (Figure 2.21)
Same as for routine lateral chest.

Tips   If the patient is unable to sit upright without the aid of a support, a wheelchair or stretcher with the head of the stretcher raised should be used. A radiolucent support is placed behind the patient's back to prevent superimposition of the posterior aspect of the chest and the wheelchair or stretcher (Figure 2.22).

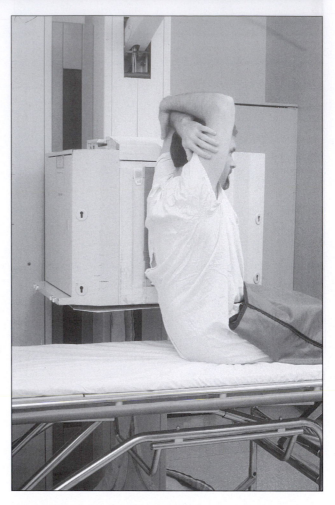

FIGURE 2.20   **Lateral chest on stretcher.**

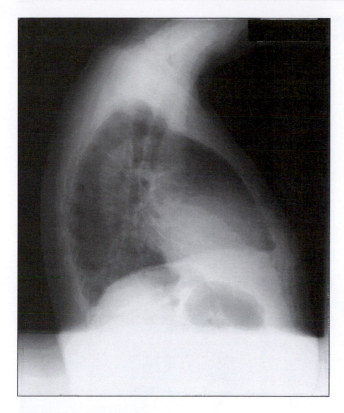

FIGURE 2.21 Lateral chest.

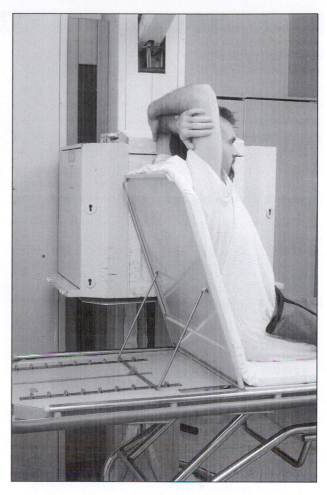

FIGURE 2.22 Lateral chest on stretcher using support.

AP CHEST—SUPINE OR SEMI-ERECT AP PROJECTION

Exam Rationale The AP chest is performed to outline the anatomy of the lungs, heart, great vessels, and mediastinal structures to detect the presence of chest lesions or line placement. This position is performed when the patient is too weak to sit upright or is unable to be placed prone. The AP chest can be performed in the radiography department or as bedside radiography.

Technical Considerations

- Regular screen/film
- Grid
- kVp range: 100–120 (*Note: if grid is not used, the kVp range is 75–90.*)
- SID: Minimum 40 inch (100 cm)

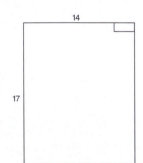

Radiation Protection

AEC (Phototiming)

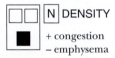

N DENSITY

\+ congestion
\- emphysema

Patient Position Supine or semi-erect on the stretcher or bed; top of film holder 1 1/2 to 2 inches (4–5 cm) above shoulders.

Part Position Hands are pronated and elbows bent and brought out to the side; scapulae are rotated forward away from the lung field; midsagittal plane centered to the film holder (Figures 2.23 and 2.24).

Central Ray Perpendicular to the sternum and centered to the film holder (level of T7 or 3–4 inches (8–10 cm) inferior to suprasternal notch).

Patient Instructions "Take in a deep breath; let it out. Take in another deep breath and hold it. Don't breathe or move."

Evaluation Criteria (Figures 2.25 and 2.26)

- Sternoclavicular joints should be equidistant from the vertebral column.
- Distance between the vertebral column and the outer margin of the rib cage should be equal on each side.
- Clavicles will appear more horizontal and will slightly obscure the apices.

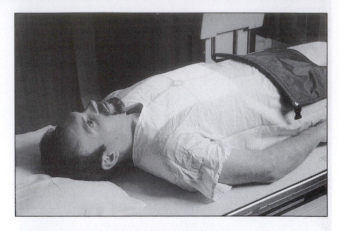

FIGURE 2.23   **AP supine projection chest.**

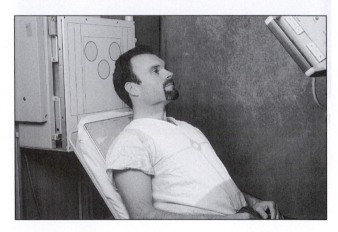

FIGURE 2.24   **AP semi-erect chest.**

- Costophrenic angles should be included on the film.
- Scapula should be rotated outside the lung field.
- Seven to nine posterior ribs should be demonstrated.

Tips

1. To minimize enlargement of the heart in the supine or semi-erect AP chest, use the maximum distance achievable.
2. If possible, the head of the bed or stretcher should be elevated to achieve a semi-erect position.
3. In the supine or semi-erect position, the diaphragm is elevated and full inhalation will be difficult for the patient to obtain.
4. If the patient is on a respirator, make the exposure after the respirator has completed the full inspiration.

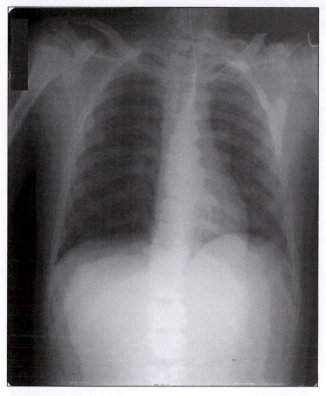

FIGURE 2.25   AP projection chest.

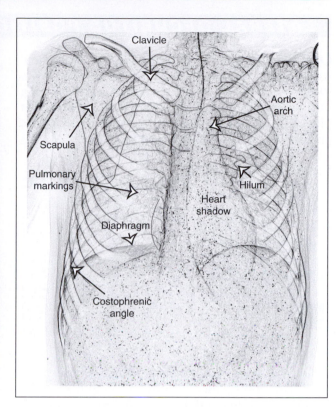

FIGURE 2.26   AP projection chest.

LATERAL DECUBITUS POSITION

Exam Rationale   This position is used to demonstrate small amounts of fluid in the pleural cavity, which would be demonstrated with the patient lying on the affected side, or small amounts of air in the pleural cavity, which would be demonstrated with the patient lying on the unaffected side.

Technical Considerations

- Regular screen/film
- Grid
- kVp range: 100–120
- SID: 72 inch (180 cm)

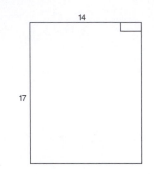

Radiation Protection

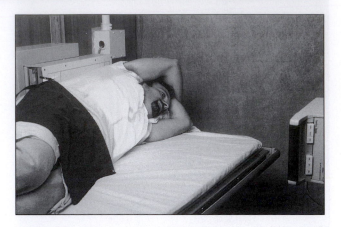

FIGURE 2.27   Left lateral decubitus chest.

Patient Position   Lateral recumbent position; both arms raised over patient's head; ankles and knees on top of one another and the knees flexed for support.

Part Position   Adjust pelvis and shoulders parallel to the film holder; adjust the center of the film holder to the midsagittal plane and place the top of the film 2 inches (5 cm) above the shoulders (Figure 2.27).

Central Ray   Perpendicular to the film holder; center x-ray tube to film (T6–T7).

Patient Instructions   "Take in a deep breath; let it out. Take in another deep breath and hold it. Don't breathe or move."

Evaluation Criteria (Figures 2.28 and 2.29)

- Sternoclavicular joints should be equidistant from the vertebral column.
- Distance between the vertebral column and the outer margin of the rib cage should be equal on each side.

- Apices and both costophrenic angles should be included on the film.
- Affected side must be included on the film.
- Affected side should not be superimposed by the support.
- Patient's arms should not superimpose the upper lung region.

Tips

1. Marker placement is important. A left or right marker can be used but must be placed on the correct side of the patient.
2. If demonstrating fluid levels, the patient should be placed on a radiolucent support to elevate the dependent side enough for the entire side to be demonstrated on the film.

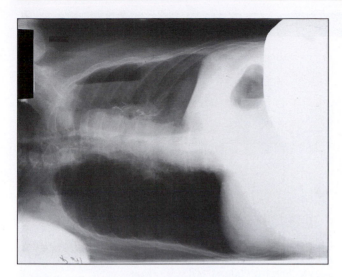

FIGURE 2.28   Lateral decubitus chest.

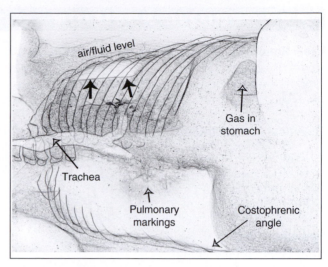

FIGURE 2.29   Lateral decubitus chest.

AP LORDOTIC POSITION

Exam Rationale This position is used to demonstrate the apices free from superimposition of the clavicles or to demonstrate a right middle lobe pneumothorax.

Technical Considerations

- Regular screen/film
- Grid
- kVp range: 100–120
- SID: 72 inch (180 cm)

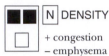

Radiation Protection

AEC (Phototiming)

■ ■ N DENSITY
□ + congestion
   – emphysema

Patient Position Erect; top of the film approximately 3–4 inches (8–10 cm) above the shoulders.

Part Position Standing approximately 1 foot from the film holder, facing forward and leaning back so the top of the shoulder, neck, and head are against the film holder; hands on hips and shoulders rotated forward; midsagittal plane centered to the film holder (Figure 2.30).

Central Ray Perpendicular to the film holder and centered midsternum. (3–4 inches (8–10 cm) inferior to suprasternal notch).

Patient Instructions "Take in a deep breath, let it out. Take in another deep breath and hold it. Don't breathe or move."

Evaluation Criteria (Figures 2.31 and 2.32)

- Clavicles will appear horizontal *above* the apices.
- Sternoclavicular joints should be equidistant from the vertebral column.
- Distance between the vertebral column and the outer margin of the rib cage should be equal on each side.
- Proper exposure factors will demonstrate lung markings throughout the lung field, especially in the apices.
- Ribs will appear distorted with the anterior and posterior ribs somewhat superimposed.

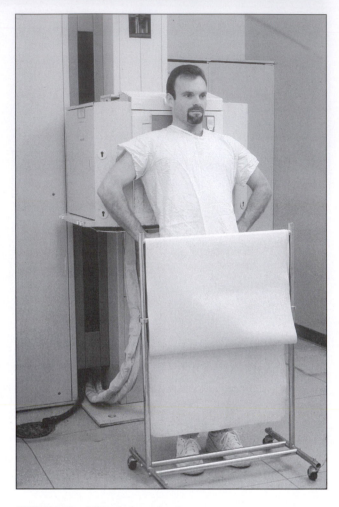

FIGURE 2.30   AP lordotic projection.

Tips

1. Always assist the patient out of this position.
2. A patient who is unable to stand can be placed on a stool and the same procedure followed as for an upright examination.
3. A patient who is unable to be placed in an erect position can lie on a stretcher or x-ray table with the central ray angled 15–20° cephalic to the midsternum.

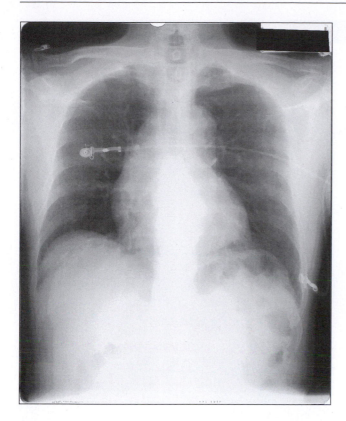

FIGURE 2.31   AP lordotic projection.

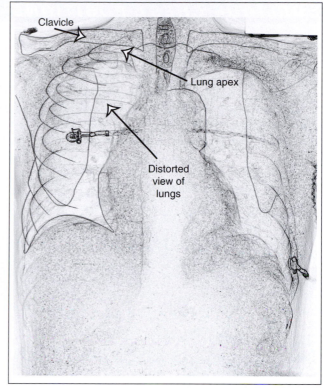

FIGURE 2.32   AP lordotic projection.

OBLIQUE CHEST POSITIONS

Exam Rationale   This position is used to demonstrate the trachea, right and left bronchial trees, heart, and aorta free from superimposition of the vertebral column. Either a right or left oblique position or both may be indicated. The side furthest from the film is demonstrated, so the LAO will demonstrate the right lung and the RAO will demonstrate the left lung.

Technical Considerations

- Regular screen/film
- Grid
- kVp range: 100–120
- SID: 72 inch (180 cm)

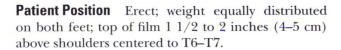

Radiation Protection

AEC (Phototiming)

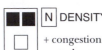 N DENSITY

+ congestion
– emphysema

Patient Position   Erect; weight equally distributed on both feet; top of film 1 1/2 to 2 inches (4–5 cm) above shoulders centered to T6–T7.

Part Position   Rotate patient 45° from the straight PA with either the left (LAO) or right (RAO) shoulder and chest against film holder; the hand closest to the film is on the waist and the opposite hand raised over patient's head resting on the film holder; chin elevated. Patient adjusted so both sides are included (Figure 2.33).

Central Ray   Perpendicular to the film holder.

Patient Instructions   "Take in a deep breath, let it out. Take in another deep breath and hold it. Don't breathe or move."

Evaluation Criteria (Figures 2.34 and 2.35)

- Side furthest from the film holder should be approximately twice the size as the side closest to the film holder.
- Apices and both costophrenic angles should be included on the film.

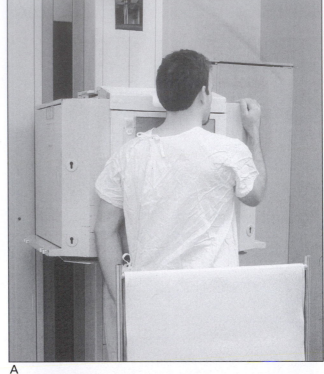

A

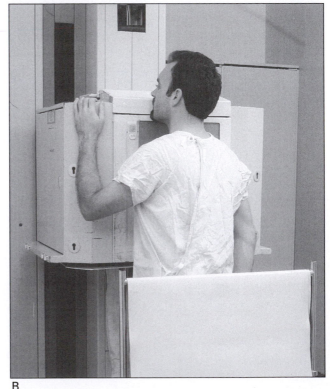

B

FIGURE 2.33   (A) LAO and (B) RAO chest.

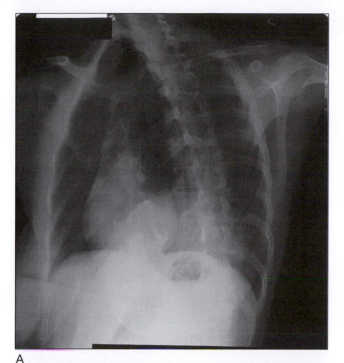

A

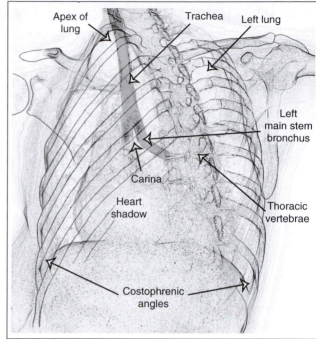

A

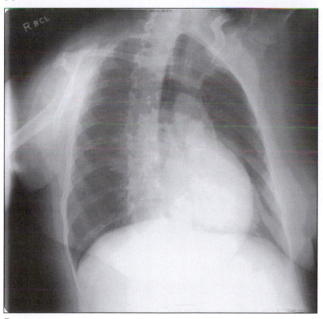

B

FIGURE 2.34   (A) LAO and (B) RAO chest.

B

FIGURE 2.35   (A) LAO and (B) RAO chest.

Tips

1. The degree of rotation may vary according to patient pathology.
2. A 60° LAO may be used to separate the aorta from the thoracic spine.

3. AP obliques can be performed if the patient is unable to stand upright or lie prone. AP obliques demonstrate the side down. The RPO will demonstrate the same structures as the LAO, and the LPO will demonstrate the same structures as the RAO.

DORSAL DECUBITUS POSITION

Exam Rationale The dorsal decubitus radiograph demonstrates fluid levels from the lateral perspective.

Technical Considerations

- Regular screen/film
- Grid
- kVp range: 100–120
- SID: 72 inch (180 cm)

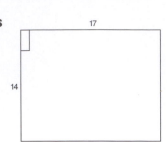

Radiation Protection

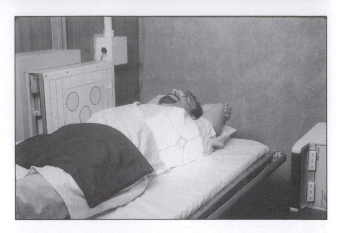

FIGURE 2.36   Dorsal decubitus.

Patient Position Supine on a radiolucent support of 2–3 inches (5–8 cm); knees flexed for patient comfort and support; film holder 1 1/2 to 2 inches (4–5 cm) above the patient's shoulders and centered to the midaxillary line at the level of T6–T7.

Part Position Arms extended over patient's head; film holder adjusted to the midaxillary line (Figure 2.36).

Central Ray Perpendicular to the film holder (x-ray tube must be horizontal to demonstrate air/fluid levels).

Patient Instructions "Take in a deep breath, let it out. Take in another deep breath and hold it. Don't breathe or move."

Evaluation Criteria (Figures 2.37 and 2.38)

- Posterior aspect of the ribs and lungs should be superimposed.
- Intervertebral joint spaces of the thoracic vertebra should be clearly visible.
- Sternum should be in a lateral position.
- Apices and costophrenic angles should be included on the film.
- Hilum should be near the center of the film.
- Anatomy should not be superimposed by the support.

Tip If the patient is unable to lie supine, a ventral decubitus may be done.

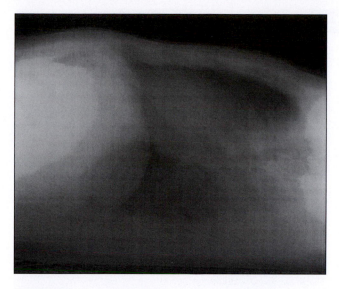

FIGURE 2.37　Dorsal decubitus.

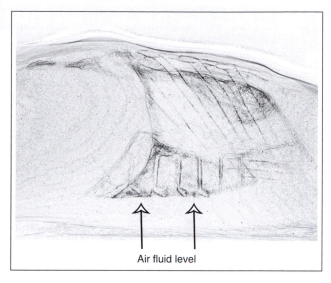

Air fluid level

FIGURE 2.38　Dorsal decubitus.

AP UPPER AIRWAY PROJECTION

Exam Rationale   This position is used to demonstrate the air-filled trachea for pathology or foreign bodies or any lateral shift of the trachea caused by pathology or a radiolucent foreign body.

Technical Considerations

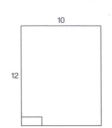

- Regular screen/film
- Grid
- kVp range: 75–85
- SID: 40 inch (100 cm)

Radiation Protection

   Breasts should be shielded.

AEC (Phototiming)

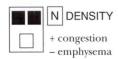 N DENSITY

+ congestion
– emphysema

Patient Position   Erect with back of neck against upright Bucky.

Part Position   Midsagittal plane centered to film holder; chin elevated so it is parallel to floor; arms relaxed at the side (Figure 2.39).

Central Ray   Perpendicular to the film holder; centered to the midsagittal plane and manubrium.

Patient Instructions   "Continue to breathe. Slowly breathe in." (This ensures an air-filled trachea.)

Evaluation Criteria (Figures 2.40 and 2.41)

- Air-filled trachea superimposed over the cervical spine.
- Vertebrae from C3 to T6 should be included.
- Symmetrical appearance between the vertebrae and sternoclavicular joints.
- Appropriate patient identification and anatomic markers must be demonstrated free of superimposition of the structures demonstrated.

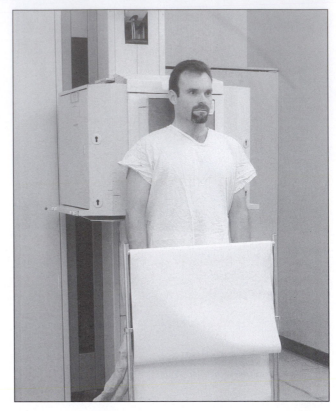

FIGURE 2.39   AP projection for upper airway.

Tip   If the patient is unable to assume an erect position, this can be done in the supine position. The chin must be elevated to place the mandible perpendicular to the film.

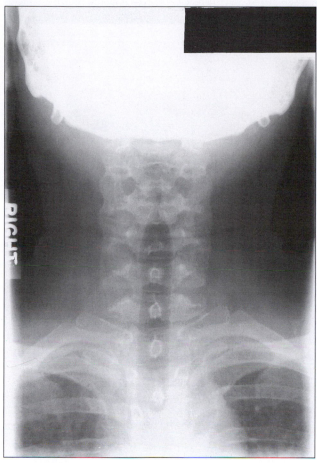

FIGURE 2.40   **AP projection for upper airway.**

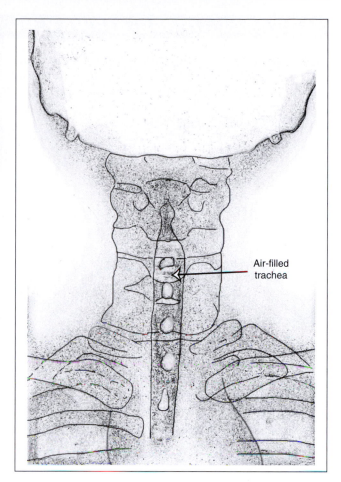

Air-filled trachea

FIGURE 2.41   **AP projection for upper airway.**

LATERAL UPPER AIRWAY POSITION

Exam Rationale This position is used to demonstrate the structures of the upper airway, especially the air-filled trachea for pathology or foreign bodies.

Technical Considerations

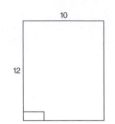

- Regular screen/film
- Grid
- kVp range: 65–70 for upper trachea and area of larynx; 80–85 for lower portion of trachea
- SID: 72 inch (180 cm)

Radiation Protection   AEC (Phototiming)

 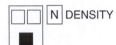 N | DENSITY

Breasts should be shielded.

Patient Position Erect; standing or seated with left side against film holder; adjust top of film holder to the external auditory meatus if the upper trachea and larynx are areas of interest; adjust top of film holder to the level of the gonion (angle of mandible) if the lower trachea is area of interest.

Part Position Chin elevated so it is parallel to floor; arms placed behind patient to draw shoulders posteriorly; midcoronal plane centered to film holder (Figure 2.42).

Central Ray Perpendicular to film holder for upper trachea to C6–C7; for lower trachea T2–T3.

Patient Instructions "Continue to breathe. Slowly breathe in." (This ensures an air-filled trachea.)

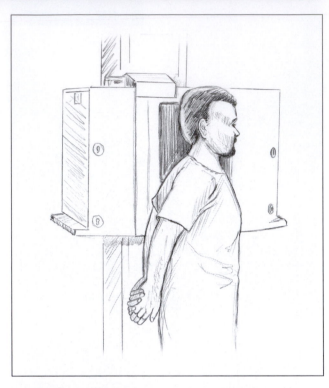

FIGURE 2.42   **Lateral projection for upper airway.**

Evaluation Criteria (Figures 2.43 and 2.44)

- Soft tissue structures of the neck should be demonstrated.
- Upper trachea: demonstrate C1 to T3–T4.
- Lower trachea: demonstrate C5–C6 to T6.
- True lateral position (intervertebral foramen of the thoracic spine should be visible).

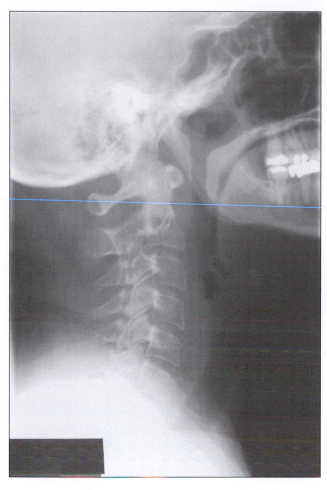

FIGURE 2.43   Lateral projection for upper airway.

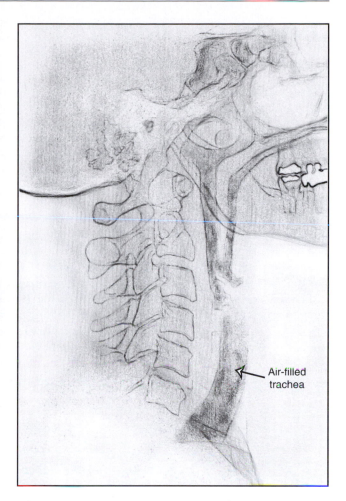

Air-filled
trachea

FIGURE 2.44   Lateral projection for upper airway.

Special Considerations

PEDIATRIC CONSIDERATIONS

Chest radiography for the pediatric patient can be extremely challenging, but quality chest radiographs are important. If the pediatric patient is able to hold his or her head up, the patient can be placed in a Pigg-o-Stat or other immobilization device. The Pigg-o-Stat immobilization device provides the necessary radiolucent restraining device, protective lead shield, markers, and cassette holder (Figure 2.45).

If the pediatric patient is unable to hold his or her head up, then AP and lateral recumbent chest radiographs need to be performed. If a guardian (not pregnant and properly shielded) is available, he or she should hold the patient's arms over the head and the patient's legs should be extended. For the lateral position, have the guardian hold the patient on the left side with the arms over the head and the legs extended. Place a small radiolucent sponge under the patient's head for support and comfort. If a guardian is unavailable, immobilization techniques need to be used. A heavy sandbag can be placed across each arm and the legs for the AP projection. For the lateral projection, position the patient on the left side, place a heavy sandbag over each arm and one across the patient's waist. Place a small radiolucent sponge under the patient's head for support and comfort. For both situations, a protective lead shield is placed across the patient's waist (Figure 2.46).

Pediatric chest radiography should always be performed non-grid using a screen/film combination. The kVp for pediatric chest radiography will vary depending on the patient's age but should range between 65 and 80. The mA should be high and the exposure time low to prevent artifacts from heart motion or patient motion. A minimum 40 inch (100 cm) SID should be used and a longer SID used when possible.

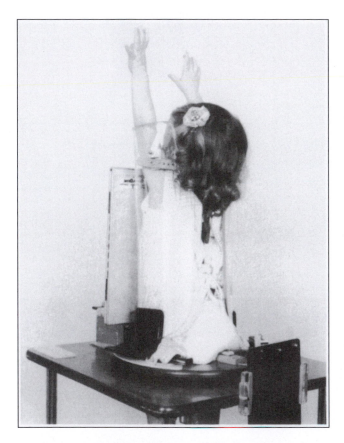

FIGURE 2.45   Pigg-o-Stat (Courtesy of Adler and Carlton, Intoduction to Radiography and Patient Care, Copyright 1994 by W. B. Saunders Company.)

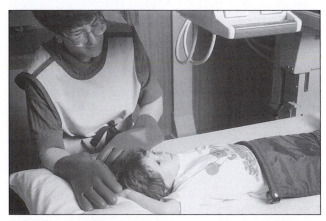

A

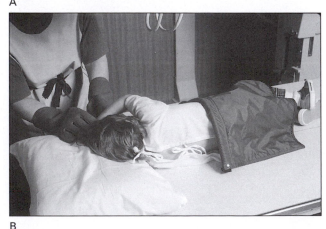

B

FIGURE 2.46   (A) AP and (B) lateral chest-infant.

PATHOLOGY CONSIDERATIONS

Pneumonia

Pneumonia (nŭ-mō´nē-ă) is the sixth leading cause of death in the United States, mainly affecting the very young and the elderly. Pneumonia can be either bacterial or viral and is classified as lobar or bacterial, lobular or bronchopneumonia, or interstitial pneumonia. Lobar or bacterial pneumonia involves the alveoli of an entire lobe and is demonstrated radiographically as a mass of fluid in one or more lobes. Lobular or bronchopneumonia is an inflammation of the bronchi and bronchioles with extension to the alveoli. Radiographically a patchy, irregular mass is demonstrated around the bronchi. Interstitial pneumonia is contracted secondary to other viral infections and is often called viral pneumonia. Because this infection is distributed throughout the lobes, the lungs will have a hazy appearance radiographically (Figure 2.47).

Emphysema

Emphysema (ĕm´´fĭ-sē´mă) is a chronic disease involving the destruction and loss of elasticity of the walls of the alveoli causing enlargement of the alveolar sacs and interference with an exchange of oxygen. Smoking and air pollution are the major causes of emphysema, but there is also a rare hereditary form. Radiographically, emphysema presents with enlarged lungs (barrel chest as seen on the lateral view), loss of lung markings, and, in advanced stages, increased radiographic density indicating a loss of lung tissue and increased trapped air (Figure 2.48).

Pneumothorax

A **pneumothorax** (nū-mō-thō´răks) is the presence of free air in the thoracic cavity caused by trauma, postoperative aspiration, or interstitial lung disease. Radiographically, the pneumothorax is demonstrated by a pleural line indicating that the lung tissue has pulled away from the thoracic wall (Figure 2.49). A loss of lung markings and a loss of radiographic density where the lung tissue collects will also be demonstrated. Because a pneumothorax can cause a shift of the mediastinal structures, it is critical that the patient be properly positioned for the PA or AP chest.

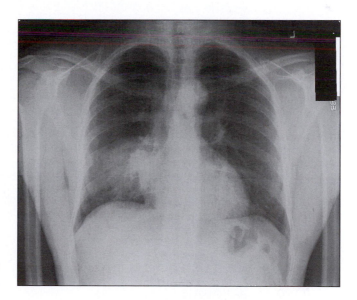

FIGURE 2.47
Pneumonia.

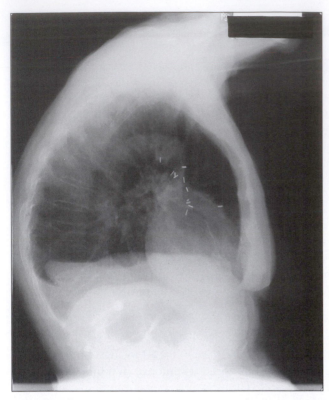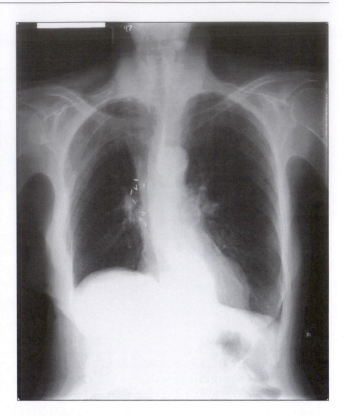

FIGURE 2.48   Emphysema.

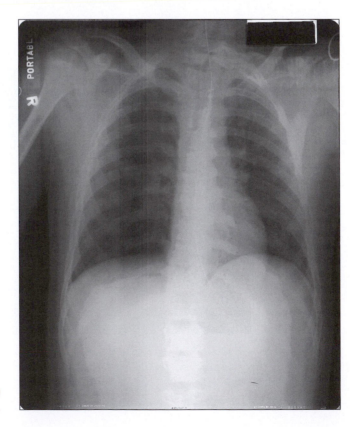

**FIGURE 2.49
Pneumothorax.**

CORRELATIVE IMAGING

Computed Tomography

When a routine chest radiograph demonstrates lesions in either the lung tissue or mediastinal structures or the patient presents with physiologic symptoms but the chest radiograph is read as normal, computed tomography (CT) scanning of the chest is indicated. The CT scan is able to demonstrate normal and abnormal anatomy free from superimposition of overlying structures and is the advanced imaging modality of choice for the chest. The use of contrast media further enhances the delineation of vascular structures and masses that have a vascular supply. By altering the window settings of the CT image, the scale of contrast can be changed to view lung tissue or mediastinal structures. With these capabilities aortic aneurysm, aortic dissections, pulmonary metastases, or subpleural lymph nodes and granulomas are detected (Figure 2.50).

Magnetic Resonance Imaging

Magnetic resonance imaging (MRI) can also be used to diagnose pathology of the chest, but it is not the imaging method of choice. MRI of the chest is difficult due to the low fat content surrounding the structures, which results in poor contrast and artifact problems caused by respiratory, cardiac, and flow motion. These difficulties can be somewhat overcome through scanning techniques but findings are not as specific as in CT scanning (Figure 2.51).

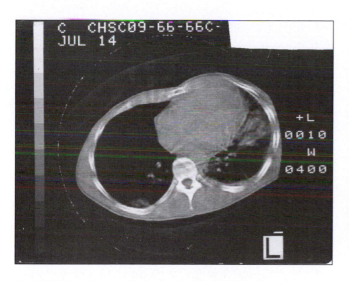

FIGURE 2.50   CT scan of chest with left pleural effusion.

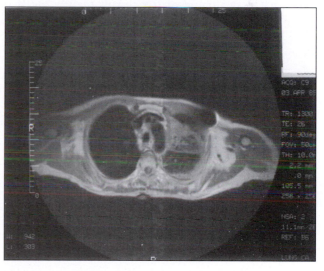

FIGURE 2.51   MRI of chest.

Review Questions

1. What structure serves as the common passageway for both food and air?

   a. nasal passage
   b. esophagus
   c. larynx
   d. pharynx

2. Which of the following is a structure of the mediastinum?

       1. aorta
       2. esophagus
       3. trachea
   a. 1 and 2
   b. 1 and 3
   c. 2 and 3
   d. 1, 2, and 3

3. What is the name of the serous membrane that encloses each lung?

   a. alveolus
   b. hilum
   c. mediastinum
   d. pleura

4. A long SID is used for chest radiography to:

   a. decrease contrast
   b. decrease patient dose
   c. enlarge the heart
   d. minimize distortion

5. When using a grid for chest radiography, which of the following technical considerations is appropriate?

   a. medium kVp and short exposure time
   b. medium kVp and long exposure time
   c. low kVp and short exposure time
   d. high kVp and short exposure time

6. Which of the following positions best demonstrates the left bronchial tree, heart, and aorta?

   a. left anterior oblique
   b. left lateral decubitus
   c. left lateral
   d. right anterior oblique

7. Which of the following will best demonstrate small amounts of pleural effusion?

   a. lateral decubitus
   b. lordotic
   c. PA chest
   d. oblique

8. Which of the following is used to demonstrate small amounts of air in the pleural cavity?

   a. PA
   b. lateral
   c. lateral decubitus/patient lying of affected side
   d. lateral decubitus/patient lying on unaffected side

9. A good lateral chest radiograph will demonstrate the:

   a. apices above the clavicles
   b. heart near the center of the film
   c. posterior ribs nearly superimposed
   d. thoracic vertebrae visible through the heart

10. A properly positioned and exposed PA chest radiograph will demonstrate the:

        1. posterior ribs and thoracic vertebrae through the heart
        2. clavicles above the apices
        3. scapulae rotated off the lung field
    a. 1 and 2
    b. 1 and 3
    c. 2 and 3
    d. 1, 2, and 3

11. The central ray for a PA upright chest should enter at approximately the level of:

    a. T4–T5
    b. T6–T7
    c. T8–T9
    d. T10–T11

12. The central ray for the AP lordotic chest should enter at the:

    a. inferior portion of the scapula
    b. level of the clavicles
    c. midsternum
    d. xiphoid tip

13. A horizontal beam is used to specifically demonstrate:
    1. fluid
    2. free air
    3. pulmonary lesions
    a. 1 and 2
    b. 1 and 3
    c. 2 and 3
    d. 1, 2, and 3

14. To ensure that proper inspiration was achieved on a PA chest radiograph, a minimum of _____ posterior ribs should be demonstrated.
    a. 6
    b. 8
    c. 10
    d. 12

15. The patient's left shoulder is against the film, the body is rotated 45 degrees from the PA, the film is placed 2 inches above the shoulders, and a perpendicular x-ray beam and 72 inch SID utilized. This describes positioning for which of the following?
    a. RAO
    b. LAO
    c. left lateral
    d. left lateral decubitus

16. The AP lordotic chest is used to demonstrate the:
    a. apical areas of the lungs free from superimposition of the clavicles
    b. costophrenic angles
    c. hilar area
    d. mediastinum

17. For chest radiography, kVp should be sufficient to penetrate the heart.
    a. true
    b. false

18. Inclusion of the entire lung field requires visualization of the apices to the costophrenic angles on each side.
    a. true
    b. false

19. Radiographs of the upper airway are sometimes performed to demonstrate foreign bodies in the trachea.
    a. true
    b. false

20. The apex of each lung is the area located _____.

21. High kVp is used for chest radiography to produce a _____ scale of contrast.

22. The AP supine chest is performed on patients too _____.

23. The lateral decubitus chest radiograph uses a _____ x-ray beam.

24. To demonstrate pneumothorax, radiographs should be taken on both _____ and _____.

25. Which primary bronchus is shorter, wider, and more vertical?

26. What is the name of the area where the primary bronchi enter the lungs?

27. What muscular structure separates the thorax from the abdomen?

28. List 3 reasons chest radiographs are preferably performed in the upright position.

29. What are the breathing instructions for a PA upright chest?

30. Identify the following structures.

a.

b.

c.

d.

e.

f.

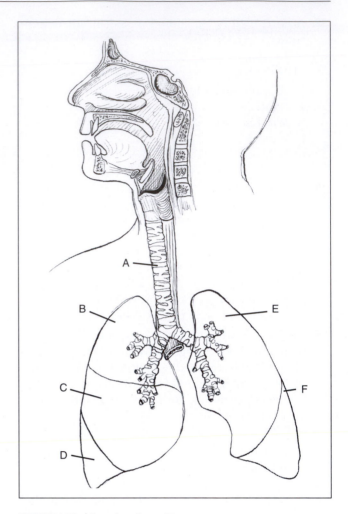

FIGURE 2.52   **Anterior view of lungs.**

References and Recommended Reading

Ballinger, P. W. (1995). *Merrill's atlas of radiographic positions and radiologic procedures.* St. Louis: Mosby-Year Book.

Bontrager, K. L. (1993). *Textbook of radiographic positioning and related anatomy.* St. Louis: Mosby-Year Book.

Carlton, R. R., & McKenna-Adler, A. (1992). *Principles of radiographic imaging: An art and a science.* Albany, NY: Delmar.

Dowd, S. B. (1994). *Practical radiation protection and applied radiobiology.* Philadelphia: Saunders.

Fraser, R. G., & Pare, J. A. P. (1970). *Diagnosis of diseases of the chest: An integrated study based on the abnormal roentgenogram: Vol.I.* Philadelphia: Saunders.

Fraser, R. G., Pare, J. A. P., Pare, P. D., Frase, R. S., Genereux, G. P. (1995). *Diagnosis of diseases of the chest.* Philadelphia: Saunders.

Gedgaudas-McClees, R. K., & Torres, W. E. (1990). *Essentials of body computed tomography.* Philadelphia: Saunders.

Gray, H., & Clemente, C. D. (1985). *Gray's anatomy: 30th American edition.* Philadelphia: Lea & Febiger.

Hall-Craggs, E. C. B. (1985). *Anatomy as a basis for clinical medicine.* Baltimore: Urhan and Schwarzenber.

Hamann, B. (1994). *Disease: Identification, prevention, and control.* St. Louis: Mosby-Year Book.

Lillington, G. A. (1987). *A Diagnostic approach to chest diseases: Differential diagnosis based on roentgenographic patterns.* Baltimore: Williams & Wilkins.

Marieb, E. N. (1992). *Human anatomy and physiology.* Redwood City, CA: Benjamin/Cummings.

Martin, D. E., & Youtsey, J. W. (1988). *Respiratory anatomy and physiology.* St. Louis: Mosby-Year Book.

Seeram, E. (1994). *Computed tomography: Physical principles clinical applications and quality control.* Philadelphia: Saunders.

Thomas, C. L. (Ed.) (1997). *Taber's cyclopedic medical dictionary.* Philadelphia: Davis.

Westbrook, C. (1994). *Handbook of MRI technique.* Cambridge, MA: Blackwell Science.

Abdomen

JEFFREY LEGG, MH, RT(R)(ARRT)

ANATOMY

Divisions of the Abdomen

Abdominal Muscles

Vertebral Column

Abdominal Tissues

Abdominal Organ Systems

Topographic Anatomy

ROUTINE POSITIONS/PROJECTIONS

Supine/KUB

AP Upright

ALTERNATE POSITIONS/PROJECTIONS

Lateral

Lateral Decubitus

ACUTE ABDOMEN SERIES

SPECIAL CONSIDERATIONS

Pediatric Considerations

Common Errors

Selected Pathology

Correlative Imaging

OBJECTIVES

At the completion of this chapter, the student should be able to:

1. List and describe the soft tissue and bony anatomy of the abdomen.

2. Identify the quadrant in which abdominal organs are located.

3. Given drawings and radiographs, locate anatomic structures and landmarks.

4. Explain the rationale for each projection.

5. Explain the patient preparation required for each examination.

6. Describe the positioning used to visualize anatomic structures of the abdomen.

7. List or identify the central ray location and the extent of the field necessary for each projection.

8. Differentiate between the positioning and centering factors for an acute abdomen series and a routine supine and upright abdomen.

9. Explain the protective measures that should be taken for each examination.

10. Recommend the technical factors for producing an acceptable radiograph for each projection.

11. State the patient instructions for each projection.

12. Given radiographs, evaluate positioning and technical factors.

13. Describe modifications of procedures for atypical or impaired patients to better demonstrate the anatomic area of interest.

Anatomy

The **abdominopelvic cavity** is subdivided into the abdominal and pelvic cavities. The abdominopelvic cavity contains many vital organs and body systems, such as the gastrointestinal, genitourinary, and hepatobiliary systems. Most abdominal organs and structures are difficult to visualize because their densities are similar to those of surrounding structures; therefore, contrast media must frequently be used. Contrast media and contrast-enhanced examinations are discussed in subsequent chapters.

DIVISIONS OF THE ABDOMEN

The quadrant system is important for localization of various organs, disease processes, and abdominal pain. The quadrants are formed by passing a line vertically through the vertebral column to the symphysis pubis (this line corresponds with the midsagittal plane) and a second line perpendicular to the first, at the level of the umbilicus (navel). These two lines divide the abdominopelvic cavity into four sections: right upper quadrant (RUQ), left upper quadrant (LUQ), left lower quadrant (LLQ), and right lower quadrant (RLQ) (Figures 3.1 and 3.2).

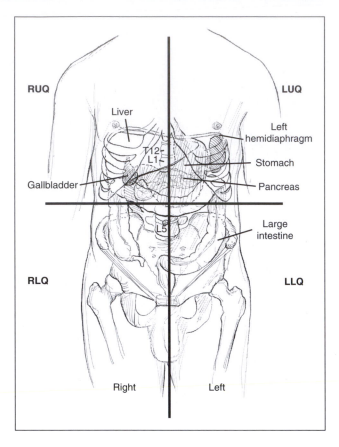

FIGURE 3.2   Abdominal quadrants and organ locations.

The abdomen may also be subdivided into *nine* regions. Use of these divisions allows for more detailed localization of abdominal pain, disease processes, and so forth (Figure 3.3). The nine regions are: right hypochondrium, epigastrium, left hypochondrium, right lumbar, umbilical, left lumbar, right iliac, hypogastrium, and left iliac.

ABDOMINAL MUSCLES

The two primary abdominal muscles important in radiography are the diaphragm and the **psoas muscles** (Figure 3.4).

Diaphragm (dī´ă-frăm)

The diaphragm is a dome-shaped muscle separating the thoracic and abdominopelvic cavities and is the most important of the respiratory muscles. The superior surface is in contact with the bases of the lungs. The concave portion of this muscle faces the abdominal cavity. Due to the presence of the liver, the right

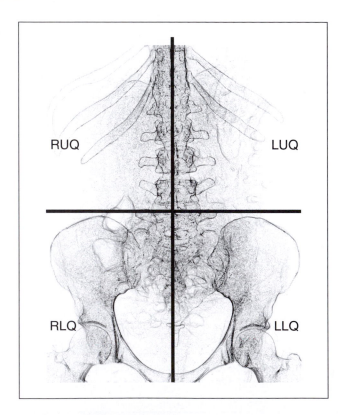

FIGURE 3.1   Abdominal quadrants.

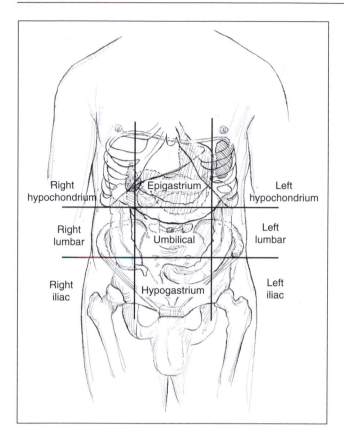

FIGURE 3.3   The nine regions of the abdomen.

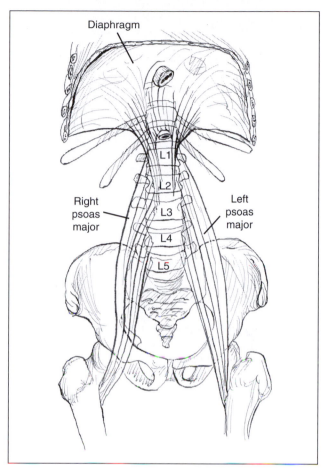

FIGURE 3.4   Abdominal muscles: diaphragm and psoas.

hemidiaphragm is often more superior than the left. The diaphragm expands and thus lowers with inspiration and relaxes and thus rises with expiration. Radiographically, the diaphragm is important because it must remain motionless to avoid blurring (motion unsharpness).

Psoas muscles (sō´ăs)

These two large muscles can be found on both sides of the vertebral column. Psoas muscles attach superiorly to the bodies and transverse processes of the lumbar vertebrae and attach inferiorly to the crest of the ilium. They are visible, radiographically, due to the rich extraperitoneal fat surrounding the muscles. The lateral border of the psoas muscles should be demonstrated on a properly exposed abdomen radiograph.

VERTEBRAL COLUMN

The vertebral column within the abdominopelvic cavity consists of the lumbar vertebrae, sacrum, and coccyx. These bones form the posterior portion of the cavity. The pelvis articulates with the sacrum to form the lower bony portion of the abdominopelvic cavity.

The vertebral column and pelvis are discussed in detail in Chapters 9 and 5, respectively.

ABDOMINAL TISSUES

The abdominal cavity is enclosed by a double layer of **serous** (sēr´ŭs) tissue. Abdominal organs are connected to the abdominal wall and each other by various tissues.

Peritoneum (pĕr´´ĭ-tō-nē´ŭm)

The peritoneum is a serous tissue consisting of two layers covering various organs and structures within the abdominal cavity (Figure 3.5).

Parietal (pă-rī´ĕ-tăl)   This portion of the peritoneum adheres to the abdominopelvic cavity.

Visceral (vĭs´ĕr-ăl)   The inner portion of the peritoneum encapsulates the surface of certain abdominal organs.

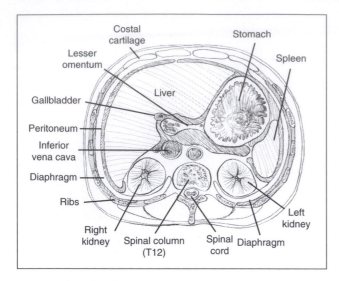

FIGURE 3.5   Abdominal cross section.

Peritoneal cavity   This space between the two perito-neal layers contains a small amount of peritoneal fluid. The fluid keeps the peritoneal layers moist and able to slide freely during respiratory and digestive movements.

Retroperitoneal structures (rĕt´´rō-pĕr´´ĭ-tō-nē´ăl strŭk´shŭrs)   These organs/structures are found *pos-terior* to the peritoneal cavity (e.g., kidneys, aorta, infe-rior vena cava).

Mesentery (mĕs´ĕn-tĕr´´ē)
This portion of the peritoneum attaches most of the small intestines to the posterior abdominal wall.

Omentum (ō-mĕn´tŭm)
This fatty fold of visceral peritoneum hangs from the inferior portion of the stomach, duodenum, and transverse colon. The greater omentum covers most of the small and large intestines.

ABDOMINAL ORGAN SYSTEMS

Gastrointestinal (GI)
Organs in this system include the stomach and the small and large intestines. The GI system is discussed in Chapter 15.

Accessory Digestive Organs
The liver, gallbladder, and pancreas are additional organs that aid in the digestive process. In addition, these organs have other important physiologic roles.

Liver   Situated in the RUQ, the liver is the largest gland in the body. The superior surface of the liver

lies in close proximity to the inferior surface of the diaphragm. The liver is comprised of two large lobes (right and left) and two smaller lobes (quadrate and caudate) (Figure 3.6).

Gallbladder   The pear-shaped gallbladder is found on the inferior surface of the liver. The cystic duct con-nects to the common bile duct, thus forming a path-way to the duodenum (Figure 3.7). The gallbladder stores, concentrates, and secretes bile for digestion.

The liver is involved in the activities of various body systems:

- Forms of bile. The bile acts as an **emulsifier** (ē-mŭl´sĭ-fī-ĕr), a substance that aids in the digestion of fats and fatty foods.
- Converts **glucose** (gloo´kōs) to **glycogen** (glī´kŏ-jĕn) for storage within the liver. At the body's demand, the liver reconverts the substance to glucose.
- Contains **phagocytic** (făg´´ō-sĭt´ĭk) **cells**, which ingest and destroy substances such as bacteria and protozoa.
- Acts as a detoxification organ.

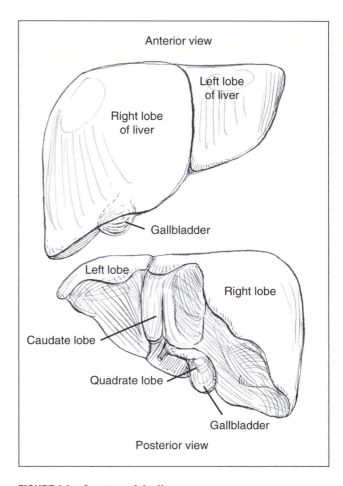

FIGURE 3.6   Anatomy of the liver.

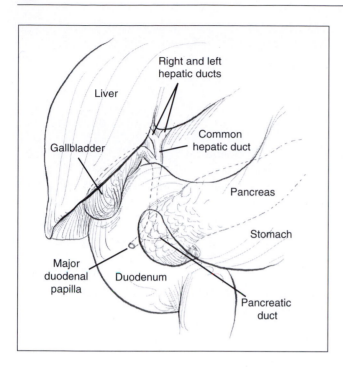

FIGURE 3.7   Anatomy of the gallbladder.

The pancreas has both **endocrine** (ĕn´dō-krĭn) and **exocrine** (ĕks´ō-krĭn) functions. Only the exocrine function is important as an aid to digestion. As an exocrine gland, the pancreas produces pancreatic juice and excretes it *directly* into the duodenum, via the pancreatic duct. The pancreatic juice aids in the digestion of all classes of foods.

Spleen   Found below the diaphragm in the LUQ, the spleen is an organ of the immunologic (im´´ū-nō-lŏj´ĭk) system (Figure 3.9). This organ is responsible for formation of immunologic cells, blood storage, and blood filtration. The spleen stores and discharges red blood cells into circulation and removes bacteria and nonfunctioning red blood cells from the circulatory system.

Genitourinary (GU)

This system is comprised of the kidneys, ureters, urinary bladder, and urethra. The GU system is discussed in Chapter 18.

TOPOGRAPHIC ANATOMY

Various palpable landmarks are vital for accurate positioning and centering of abdominal radiographs. The following landmarks are important aids in positioning the abdomen and for a variety of radiographic examinations (Figures 3.10, 3.11, and 3.12).

Pancreas   The pancreas is a retroperitoneal structure lying horizontally in the abdomen. The organ can be generally divided into a head, body, and tail portions. The head of the pancreas is connected to and nestles within the C̄ loop of the duodenum. The tail of the pancreas is connected to the spleen. The pancreatic duct extends the full length of the organ, from head to tail (Figure 3.8).

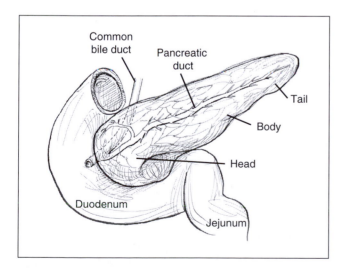

FIGURE 3.8   Anatomy of the pancreas.

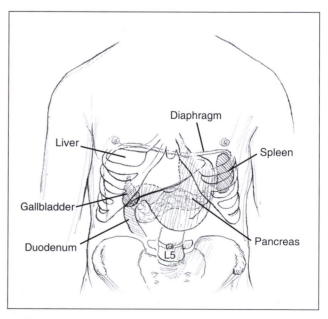

FIGURE 3.9   Location of the spleen.

Iliac Crest

This ridge comprises the curved, superior portions of the iliac bones. The most superior portion of the iliac crest corresponds with the level of the fourth and fifth lumbar vertebrae. The iliac crest is an important topographic landmark and can be palpated through the lateral portion of the abdomen. (Figure 3.10A)

Anterior Superior Iliac Spine (ASIS)

This anterior bony projection is found at the end of the iliac crest. It can be located by palpating and following the iliac crest anteriorly until a bump or projection is felt. (Figure 3.10B)

Symphysis Pubis

This midline structure is formed by the junction of the right and left pubic bones. The most anterior portion of the symphysis pubis can be felt by direct palpation. However, for reasons of patient modesty, the palpation of this landmark should be avoided. Instead, the greater trochanter can be used for determining the level of the symphysis pubis. (Figure 3.10C)

Greater Trochanter

The most palpable portion of this structure lies at approximately the level of the symphysis pubis. This landmark is best used for assessing the location of the symphysis pubis, as compared to direct palpation of the symphysis pubis. (Figure 3.10D)

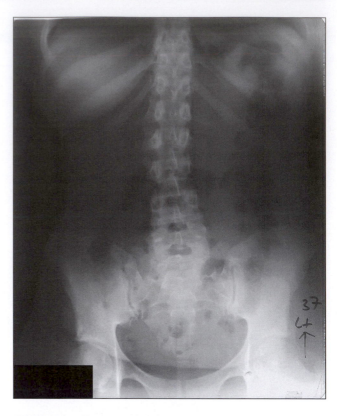

FIGURE 3.11   Topographic landmarks.

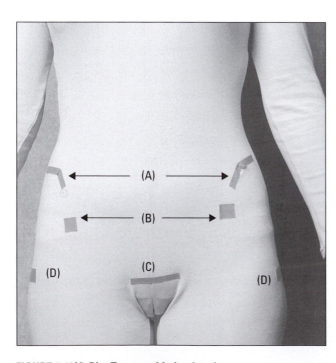

FIGURE 3.10(A-D)   Topographic landmarks.

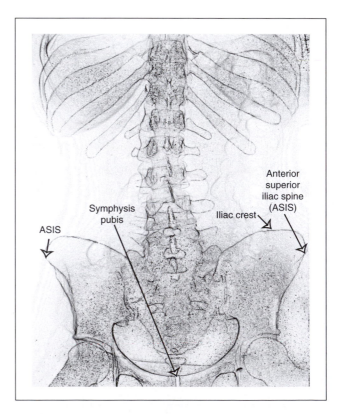

FIGURE 3.12   Topographic landmarks.

ROUTINE AND ALTERNATIVE POSITIONS/PROJECTIONS

Part	Routine	Page	Alternative	Page
Abdomen	Supine/KUB	74		
	AP upright	76	Lateral decubitus	79
	Acute abdomen series	80		
			Lateral	78

Patient Preparation

For abdominal radiography, the patient should disrobe from the waist down and don a patient gown. Any tubing (e.g., nasogastric) should be carefully removed from the radiographic field.

ABDOMEN—SUPINE/KUB (AP) PROJECTION

Exam Rationale　This projection often serves as a scout view for various radiologic exams (e.g., GI, GU). It is valuable for visualizing abdominal masses, calcifications, foreign bodies, and intestinal obstruction. The projection also provides a general survey of the abdominal gas pattern, soft tissue shadows, organ configuration, and skeletal structures.

Technical Considerations

- Regular screen/film
- Grid
- kVp range: 70–80
- SID: 40 inch (100 cm)

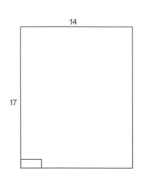

Radiation Protection

 (for males). Females are generally not shielded because the female reproductive organs lie in the area of interest.

AEC (Phototiming)

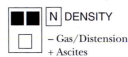 N DENSITY

– Gas/Distension
+ Ascites

Patient Position　Supine on the table.

Part Position　Midsagittal plane of the body is centered to the midline of the table; the shoulders adjusted to lie in the same transverse plane laying at the patient's side, away from the body; the pelvis adjusted so that it is not rotated (distance from anterior superior iliac spine and table top is the same on both sides); the knees may be flexed for patient comfort (Figure 3.13).

Central Ray　Cassette should be positioned so that its lower border is at the level of the greater trochanter (symphysis pubis); central ray perpendicular to midpoint of the film (centered at level of iliac crests).

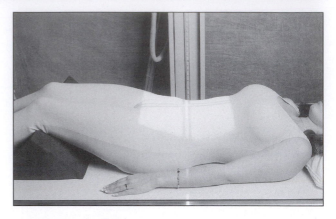

FIGURE 3.13　AP abdomen.

Patient Instructions　"Take in a deep breath, let it out. Don't breathe or move."

Evaluation Criteria (Figures 3.14 and 3.15)

- Pelvis and abdomen should not be rotated as evidenced by:
  —symmetrical iliac alae
  —spinous processes in center of vertebral bodies
- Vertebral column is in center of radiograph.
- A portion of the symphysis pubis must be included at the bottom portion of the radiograph.
- Density should be sufficient to demonstrate bony anatomy of pelvis and soft tissue structures of the abdomen.

Tip　If radiographing a hypersthenic patient, two 14 × 17 cassettes placed crosswise should be used to cover the entire abdominal field.

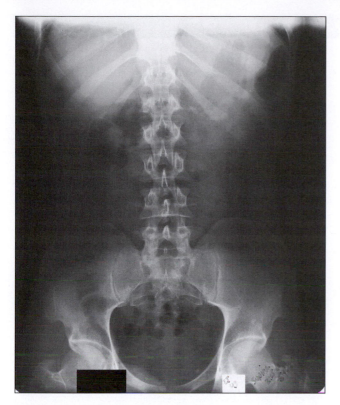

FIGURE 3.14　AP abdomen.

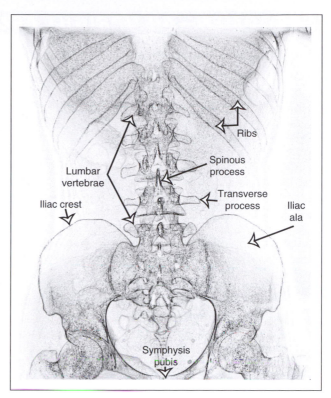

FIGURE 3.15　AP abdomen.

ABDOMEN—AP UPRIGHT PROJECTION

Exam Rationale   This projection is most valuable for demonstrating free intraperitoneal air and air/fluid levels. It is also good for visualization of soft tissue structures, bowel gas patterns, and skeletal structures.

Technical Considerations

- Regular screen/film
- Grid
- kVp range: 75–85
- SID: 40 inch (100 cm)

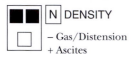

Radiation Protection

    (for males). Females are generally not shielded because the female reproductive organs lie in the area of interest.

AEC (Phototiming)

▊▊ N DENSITY
☐ – Gas/Distension
+ Ascites

Patient Position   Erect with back against Bucky or other film holder (Figure 3.16).

Part Position   The midsagittal plane of the body should be centered to the midline of the upright Bucky or film holder; weight equally distributed on both feet.

Central Ray   To include diaphragm center 2 to 3 inches (5–8 cm) above level of iliac crests; central ray perpendicular to the midpoint of the film.

Patient Instructions   "Take in a deep breath, let it out. Don't breathe or move."

Evaluation Criteria (Figures 3.17 and 3.18)

- Patient should be standing straight as evidenced by spine vertically aligned on radiograph.
- Pelvis and abdomen should not be rotated as evidenced by:
  —symmetrical iliac alae
  —spinous processes in center of vertebral bodies
- Diaphragm should be included at top of radiograph and demonstrate no motion.
- Density should be sufficient to demonstrate bony anatomy of pelvis and soft tissue structures of the abdomen.

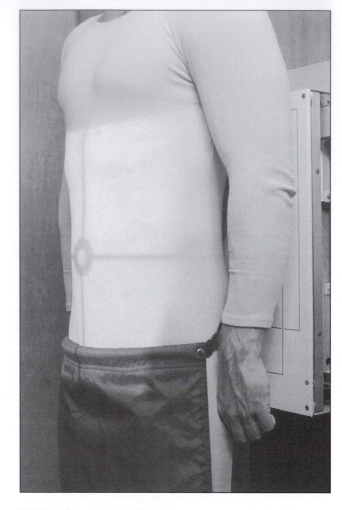

FIGURE 3.16   Upright abdomen.

Tips

1. The patient should be erect a minimum of 5 minutes before exposure.
2. Mark the film as upright with appropriate marker.
3. If a PA or AP chest is performed, centering for the abdomen examination is at the level of the iliac crest.
4. If using a radiographic table, the table may be tilted if the patient has difficulty standing. Compression bands on the chest and legs may also be used for support. The central ray remains horizontal.
5. This projection may be replaced by the left lateral decubitus if the patient has difficulty standing.

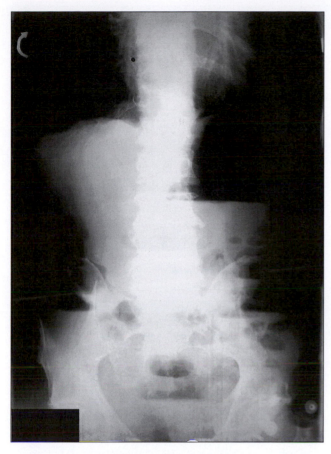

FIGURE 3.17   Upright abdomen.

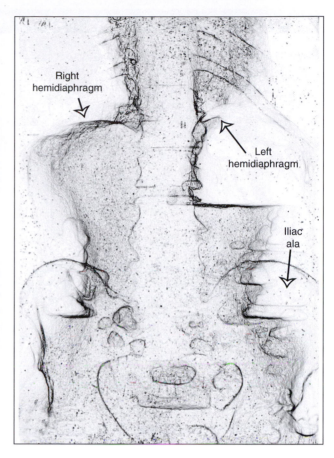

FIGURE 3.18   Upright abdomen.

ABDOMEN—LATERAL POSITION

Exam Rationale   This position is useful for demonstration of calcification of the aorta and blood vessels and **aneurysms**.

Technical Considerations

- Regular screen/film
- Grid
- kVp range: 75–85
- SID: 40 inch (100 cm)

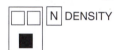

Radiation Protection

   (for males).
Females are generally not shielded because the female reproductive organs lie in the area of interest.

AEC (Phototiming)

☐ ☐ N DENSITY
■

Patient Position   Patient lying on left side (Figure 3.19).

Part Position   Knees may be bent for patient support; arms and elbows moved toward head so that they are not in the area of interest; shoulders and pelvis should be in true lateral position.

Central Ray   Perpendicular to the midpoint of the film at the level of the iliac crests approximately 2 inches (5 cm) anterior to the midaxillary plane.

Patient Instructions   "Take in a deep breath, let it out. Don't breathe or move."

Evaluation Criteria (Figures 3.20 and 3.21)

- Pelvis and lumbar vertebrae are not rotated.
- Density is sufficient to demonstrate soft tissue structures of abdomen.
- Anterior portion of abdomen is demonstrated.

Tip   The centering light should extend to anterior margin of abdomen.

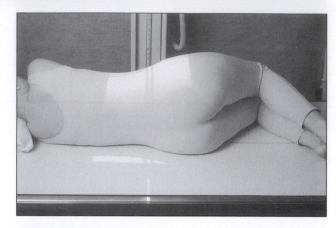

FIGURE 3.19   Lateral abdomen.

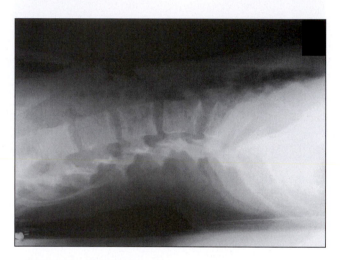

FIGURE 3.20   Lateral abdomen.

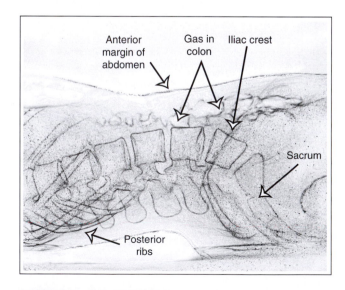

FIGURE 3.21   Lateral abdomen.

ABDOMEN—LATERAL DECUBITUS POSITION

Exam Rationale   This position is useful for demonstrating air/fluid level or free intraperitoneal air in cases of bowel obstruction or perforated **viscus**. It also demonstrates abdominal masses and soft tissue structures of the abdomen.

Technical Considerations

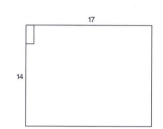

- Regular screen/film
- Grid
- kVp range: 70–80
- SID: 40 inch (100 cm)

Radiation Protection

   (for males). Females are generally not shielded because the female reproductive organs lie in the area of interest.

AEC (Phototiming)

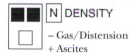 N DENSITY

– Gas/Distension
+ Ascites

Patient Position   Patient lying on left side on top of radiolucent sponge (Figure 3.22).

Part Position   Knees slightly flexed for patient support; arms and elbows moved toward head so that they are not in the area of interest; shoulders and pelvis should be in true lateral position. (If patient is on a radiolucent pad, move the cassette below the level of the pad to include both sides. If both sides cannot be imaged, include the elevated side [in cases of free air] or the dependent side [for fluid visualization]).

Central Ray   Horizontal beam, perpendicular to the midpoint of the film centered 2 to 3 inches (5–8 cm) above level of iliac crests and aligned to midsagittal plane of patient.

Patient Instructions   "Take in a deep breath, let it out. Don't breathe or move."

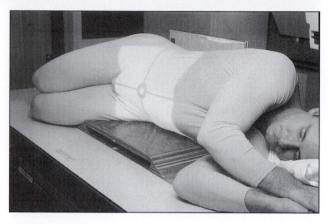

FIGURE 3.22   Left lateral decubitus abdomen.

Evaluation Criteria (Figures 3.23 and 3.24)

- Pelvis and abdomen should not be rotated as evidenced by:
    —symmetrical iliac alae
    —spinous processes in center of vertebral bodies
- Density should be slightly less than for supine abdomen to enable visualization of air/fluid levels and any free intra-abdominal air.
- Diaphragm should be included and demonstrate no motion.

Tips

1. This projection may be performed in either the AP or PA position.
2. Mark the radiograph appropriately to demonstrate the side up.

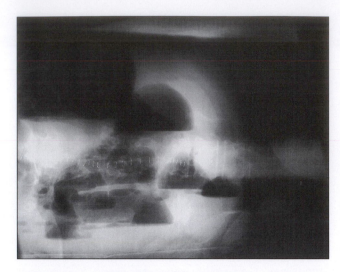

FIGURE 3.23   Left lateral decubitus abdomen.

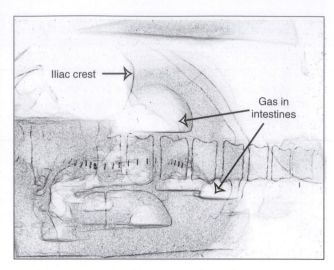

FIGURE 3.24   Left lateral decubitus abdomen.

ACUTE ABDOMEN SERIES

Exam Rationale   A primary indication for an acute abdominal series is abdomen pain. This series includes the following three views with modifications as noted.

1. Supine abdomen: refer to page 74; no modification.
2. Upright abdomen: refer to page 76. The central ray should be at the level of the iliac crests. A por-tion of symphysis pubis should be evident at bottom of film.
3. PA chest: refer to page 36; no modification.

Special Considerations

PEDIATRIC CONSIDERATIONS

When radiographing the abdomen of pediatric patients, the biggest challenge often comes from flailing arms, legs, and movement of the abdomen. Although immobilization may be a time-consuming process and is not always well received by the patient or parents, immobilization of a patient unable or unwilling to cooperate by holding still is highly preferable to repeating radiographs due to motion artifacts.

Infant immobilization is important because abdomen radiographs are often a preliminary film for such examinations as barium enemas, upper GI series, and the like. It is vital that the patient be immobile yet able to assume the necessary positions during the procedure. For a conventional abdomen radiograph, an effective method of immobilization is to mummify the infant. Care should be taken to ensure the arms are not in the area of interest. Sandbags are an additional aid for immobilization. As always, gonadal shielding is critical when radiographing pediatric patients.

COMMON ERRORS

1. Rotated patient—Note the asymmetry of the lumbar vertebrae and the alae of the ilium (Figure 3.25).
2. Artifacts—Note the metallic snaps visible on the lower portion of the radiograph. These artifacts may obscure pertinent anatomy/pathology (Figure 3.26).

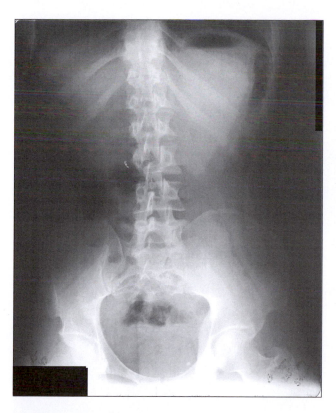

FIGURE 3.25   Common error—rotated patient.

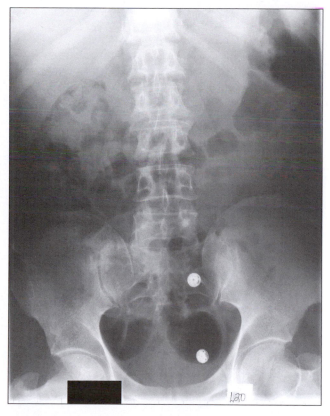

FIGURE 3.26   Common error—radiographic artifacts.

SELECTED PATHOLOGY

Bowel Dilatation

Bowel dilatation may be secondary to either *mechanical* causes (a blockage of the bowel lumen), or **paralytic/adynamic ileus** (păr´´ă-lĭt´ĭk/ā-dĭ-năm´ĭk ĭl´ē-ŭs) resulting from a failure of normal peristalsis. There are a variety of causes of bowel obstruction, including fibrous adhesions from previous surgery, **peritonitis** (pĕr´´ĭ-tō-nī´tĭs), lesions, and **hernias**. Both the large and small bowel are subject to obstruction. Common symptoms include vomiting, abdominal distension, and pain. In cases of small-bowel obstruction (SBO), radiographs, especially erect views, often reveal gas patterns restricted to the small bowel and multiple air/fluid levels (Figure 3.27).

Intraperitoneal (ĭn´´tră-pĕr´´ĭ-tō-nē´ăl) Air

The presence of free air in the peritoneal cavity is usually abnormal. This condition, termed **pneumoperitoneum** (nū´´mō-pĕr-ĭ-tō-nē´ŭm), is often caused by perforation of the GI tract (e.g., rupture of a peptic ulcer, trauma, or carcinoma) and usually necessitates surgical intervention. Visualization of free air on a supine abdominal radiograph is difficult; therefore, it is best demonstrated on erect views. Because the free air rises to the highest point in the abdominal cavity, it accumulates beneath the diaphragm. If the patient is too ill to stand, a left lateral decubitus view can replace the erect abdomen. On this view, the free air will ascend to the patient's right and be visible along the lateral margin of the liver.

Renal Calculi (rē´năl kăl´kū-lī)

These are stones (kidney stones) developing from urine, often containing crystalline materials such as calcium and its salts. Due to the presence of calcium, more than 80% of symptomatic renal calculi are detectable on plain abdominal radiographs. Men tend to develop calculi more often than women. Most calculi are asymptomatic

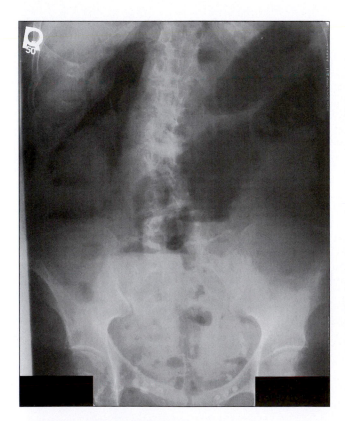

FIGURE 3.27   Abdominal obstruction/dilatation on upright abdomen radiograph.

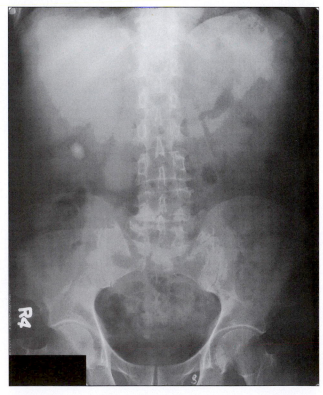

FIGURE 3.28   Renal calculus.

until they are lodged in the ureter. In these cases, renal calculi can cause extreme pain, termed *renal colic* (rē´năl kŏ´lĭk), and obstruct the urinary system. Figure 3.28 shows an example of a calculus in the right kidney.

CORRELATIVE IMAGING

Barium Examinations
Because the soft tissue organs and structures in the abdomen have similar densities, a contrast agent is often used to visualize the GI tract. The most common types of GI imaging are barium enemas and upper GI series; these examinations are discussed in further detail in subsequent chapters.

Endoscopy
Endoscopy is a valuable type of abdominal imaging allowing for direct visualization of the GI tract and abdominal cavity (laparoscopy). An endoscope is a tubular, fiberoptic device that can be introduced into the patient via the mouth, rectum, or abdominal wall. The photographic views provide diagnostic information. In addition, the diagnostic and therapeutic roles of this technique continue to expand. Polyp removal and biopsies are two examples of endoscopy's therapeutic use.

Computed Tomography
An important imaging aid for evaluating the abdomen, CT images the abdomen in cross-section (Figure 3.29). It can demonstrate small differences in tissue density and abdominal organs not normally visible without radiographic contrast. This imaging technique is important for a general survey of the abdomen and has a significant role in evaluation of the GI system. In addition, CT is useful for evaluating retroperitoneal pathology, GI malignancies/metastases, and the abdominal organs. Unlike barium studies and endoscopy, CT is *not* limited to an examination of the surface and contour of the bowel lumen.

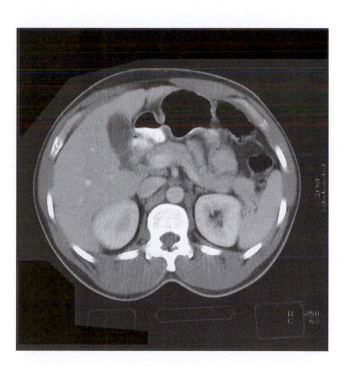

FIGURE 3.29
CT image of abdomen.

Sonography

Sonography is valuable for imaging many organs and structures within the abdominal cavity. For example, sonography has a significant role in hepatic imaging (Figure 3.30) and in gallbladder imaging (Figure 3.31). Sonography is also valuable for imaging the peritoneal space, urinary tract, external male genitalia, prostate, major blood vessels, uterus, and ovaries.

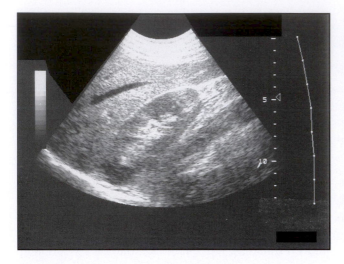

FIGURE 3.30   Sonographic image of the liver.

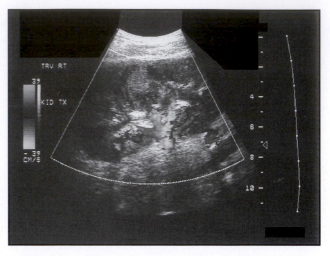

FIGURE 3.31   Sonographic image of the gallbladder.

Review Questions

1. Which of the following is attached, on both sides, to the lumbar vertebra and the crest of the ilium?

   a. diaphragm
   b. duodenum
   c. psoas muscles
   d. symphysis pubis

2. Which portion of the peritoneum adheres to the surface of abdominal organs?

   a. organic
   b. parietal
   c. retroperitoneal
   d. visceral

3. What other palpable structure is located at the level of the symphysis pubis?

   a. anterior superior iliac spine
   b. greater trochanter
   c. iliac crest
   d. obturator foramen

4. Which of the following is a function of the liver?

   1. formation of bile
   2. detoxification
   3. storage/discharge of red blood cells
   4. secretion of urea

   a. 1 only
   b. 1 and 2
   c. 1, 3, and 4
   d. 2, 3, and 4

5. The central ray for a supine abdomen should be directed to:

   a. the iliac crest
   b. one inch superior to the iliac crest
   c. one inch inferior to the iliac crest
   d. the symphysis pubis

6. Which of the following would demonstrate free air in the abdomen?

   1. supine abdomen
   2. upright abdomen
   3. left lateral decubitus abdomen
   4. lateral abdomen

   a. 2 only
   b. 1 and 2
   c. 2 and 3
   d. 2 and 4

7. Which of the following can replace the upright abdomen if the patient is too weak to stand?

   a. supine abdomen
   b. left lateral decubitus abdomen
   c. left lateral abdomen
   d. trendelenburg position abdomen

8. For a supine abdomen examination, the _____ should be seen at the bottom portion of the radiograph.

   a. iliac crest
   b. liver
   c. symphysis pubis
   d. vertebrae

9. Which of the following kVp ranges is most appropriate for abdominal radiography?

   a. 50–60
   b. 60–70
   c. 70–80
   d. 90–100

10. The lateral abdomen is used as an alternate view if a patient cannot stand for an upright abdomen.

    a. true
    b. false

11. When performing an upright or lateral decubitus abdomen, the exposure should be taken immediately after getting the patient into the correct position.

    a. true
    b. false

12. The PA chest for an acute abdomen series is identical to a routine PA chest.

    a. true
    b. false

13. Match the correct abdominal quadrant to the following structures.

_____ a. liver	1. LUQ
_____ b. stomach	2. LLQ
_____ c. appendix	3. RUQ
_____ d. left kidney	4. RLQ
_____ e. gallbladder	

14. To demonstrate the diaphragm on an AP upright abdomen, where should the central ray be in relation to the iliac crests?

15. What is the name of the two-layer serous tissue that covers organs within the abdominal cavity?

16. What is the name of the midline structure formed by the junction of the right and left pubic bones?

17. What are the names of the four quadrants of the abdomen? Where are the imaginary vertical and horizontal lines that are used to create the quadrants located?

18. Most radiographs of the abdomen are taken at what respiratory phase?

19. List the positions/projections for an acute abdomen series.

20. List at least three indications for an acute abdomen series.

References and Recommended Reading

Ballinger, P. W. (Ed.). (1995). *Merrill's atlas of radiographic positions and radiologic procedures* (8th ed., Vol. 2). St. Louis: Mosby-Year Book.

Baker, S. R., & Elkin, M. (1983). *Plain film approach to abdominal calcifications.* Philadelphia: Saunders.

Bell, G. A., & Finlay, D. B. L. (1986). *Basic radiographic positioning and anatomy.* London: Bailliere Tindall.

Bontrager, K. L. (1993). *Textbook of radiographic positioning and related anatomy* (3rd ed.). St. Louis: Mosby Year-Book.

Cartmill, M., Hylander, W. L., & Shafland, J. (1987). *Human structure.* Cambridge, MA: Harvard University Press.

Crouch, J. E. (1985). *Functional human anatomy.* (4th ed.). Philadelphia: Lea & Febiger.

Cullinan, A. M. (1992). *Optimizing radiographic positioning.* Philadelphia: Lippincott.

Eisenberg, R. L., & Dennis, C. A. (1990). *Comprehensive radiographic pathology.* St. Louis: Mosby.

Eisenberg, R. L., Dennis, C. A., & May, C. R. (1989). *Radiographic positioning.* Boston: Little, Brown.

Frick H., Leonhardt, H., & Starck, D. (1991). *Human anatomy 1.* New York: Thieme.

Frick H., Leonhardt, H., & Starck, D. (1991). *Human anatomy 2.* New York: Thieme.

Goldberg, B. B. (Ed.). (1993). *Textbook of abdominal ultrasound.* Baltimore: Williams & Wilkins.

Gough, M. H., Gear, M. W. L., & Darr, A. S. (1986). *Plain x-ray diagnosis of the acute abdomen* (2nd ed.). Oxford: Blackwell Scientific.

Laudicina, P. F. (1989). *Applied pathology for radiographers.* Philadelphia: Saunders.

Lee, J. K. T., Sagel, S. S., & Stanley, R. J. (1989). *Computed body tomography with MRI correlation.* New York: Raven Press.

Mace, J. D., & Kowalczyk, N. (1994). *Radiographic pathology for technologists.* St. Louis: Mosby-Year Book.

Mittelstaedt, C. A. (1987). *Abdominal ultrasound.* New York: Churchill Livingstone.

Sauerbrei, E. E., Nguyen, K. T., & Nolan, R. L. (1992). *Abdominal sonography.* New York: Raven Press.

Swallow, R. A., Naylor, E., Roebuck, E. J., et al. (Eds.). *Clark's positioning in radiography* (11th ed.). London: William Heinemann Medical Books.

Thibodeau, G. A., & Patton, K. T. (1992). *The human body in health and disease.* St. Louis: Mosby-Year Book.

Thomas, C. L. (Ed.). (1997). *Taber's cyclopedic medical dictionary.* (18th ed.). Philadelphia: Davis.

Thomas, F. B. (1983). *Differential diagnosis: Abdominal problems.* New York: Arco.

SECTION

III

LIMBS
and
THORAX

Upper Limb and Shoulder Girdle

MICHAEL PATRICK ADAMS, PhD, RT(R)(ARRT)

HUMERUS—ROUTINE POSITIONS/PROJECTIONS

AP

Lateral

HUMERUS—ALTERNATE POSITIONS/PROJECTIONS

Transthoracic Lateral (Lawrence)

SHOULDER—ROUTINE POSITIONS/PROJECTIONS

AP Internal Rotation

AP External Rotation

AP Neutral Rotation

SHOULDER—ALTERNATE POSITIONS/PROJECTIONS

Transthoracic Lateral

Inferosuperior Axial (Lawrence)

Inferosuperior Axial (West Point)

AP Axial/Coracoid

AP Axial (Lawrence)

Glenoid Cavity (Grashey)

Scapular Y

Intertubercular Groove

SCAPULA—ROUTINE POSITIONS/PROJECTIONS

AP

Lateral

CLAVICLE—ROUTINE POSITIONS/PROJECTIONS

PA

CLAVICLE—ALTERNATE POSITIONS/PROJECTIONS

AP

Tangential (Tarrant)

ACROMIOCLAVICULAR JOINTS—ROUTINE POSITIONS/PROJECTIONS

AP With and Without Weights

SPECIAL CONSIDERATIONS

Trauma Considerations

Pediatric Considerations

Geriatric Considerations

Common Errors

Correlative Imaging

OBJECTIVES

At the completion of this chapter, the student should be able to:

1. List and describe the anatomy of the upper limb and shoulder girdle.

2. Given drawings and radiographs, locate anatomic structures and landmarks.

3. Explain the rationale for each projection.

4. Explain the patient preparation required for each examination.

5. Describe the positioning used to visualize anatomic structures in the upper limb and shoulder girdle.

6. List or identify the central ray location and the extent of the field necessary for each projection.

7. Explain the protective measures that should be taken for each examination.

8. Recommend the technical factors for producing an acceptable radiograph for each projection.

9. State the patient instructions for each projection.

10. Given radiographs, evaluate positioning and technical factors.

11. Describe modifications of procedures for atypical or impaired patients to better demonstrate the anatomic area of interest.

Anatomy

The upper limb and shoulder girdle consist of thirty-two bones ranging in size from some of the smallest bones in the body located in the wrist to one of the longest in the upper arm. In addition to the bones and their processes, the upper limb and shoulder girdle contain a significant number of joints or articulations that are important in radiography (Figure 4.1).

HAND

There are a total of nineteen bones in the hand, including fourteen **phalanges** (fă-lăn´jēz) and five **metacarpals** (mĕt´´ă-kăr´păl). In addition, one or more **sesamoid** (sĕs´ă-moyd) bones commonly lie in the

tendons of the hand, although these are not present in every individual. Occasionally, these sesamoid bones become injured and require imaging by the radiographer (Figure 4.2).

Phalanges

Each finger consists of one metacarpal and several phalanges (singular, phalanx [fāl´ănks]). Phalanges are named according to the finger with which they are associated and whether they are close or distant to the metacarpal. The phalanx most distant from the metacarpal is called the distal phalanx and the one closest is called the proximal phalanx. Fingers two through five also have a middle phalanx. Finger number one, also known as the thumb, has only proximal and distal phalanges (Figure 4.3).

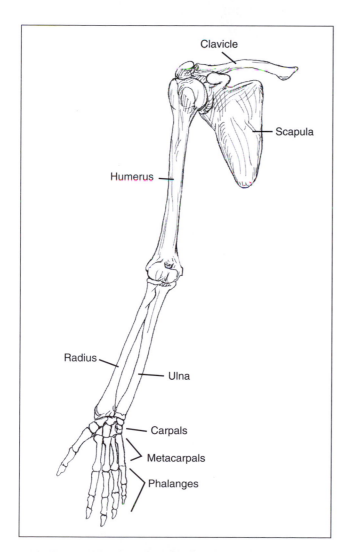

FIGURE 4.1   Upper extremity and shoulder girdle.

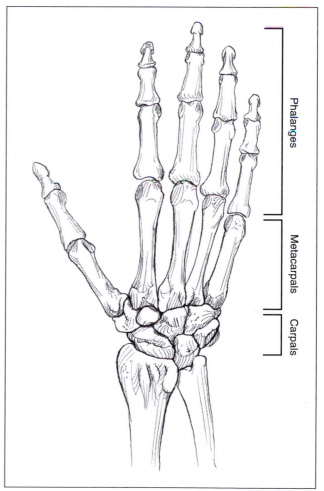

FIGURE 4.2   Basic structure of the hand and wrist.

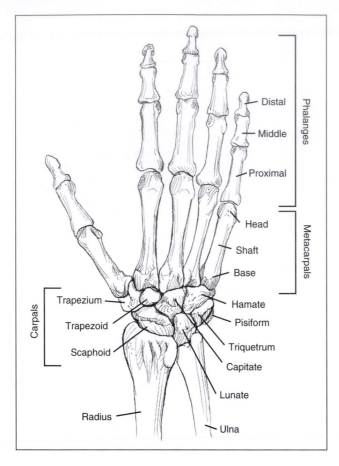

FIGURE 4.3   Detailed structure of the hand.

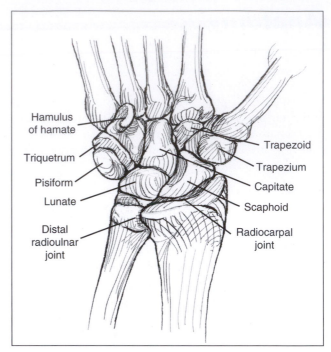

FIGURE 4.4   Detailed structure of the wrist.

Metacarpal

The five metacarpals comprise the palm of the hand. Like the phalanges, metacarpals are numbered, starting with the thumb as number one. Each metacarpal has a head, a shaft, and a base. The rounded, distal head articulates with the proximal phalanx and is commonly known as the knuckle. The base is proximal and articulates with the wrist bones (carpals). Although not very large, the metacarpals and phalanges are classified as long bones.

WRIST

The wrist consists of eight small bones called **carpals** (kăr′păl) and associated joints. The carpals are classified as short bones. The wrist is sometimes referred to as the **carpus** (kăr′pŭs).

Carpals

The carpals are arranged in two transverse rows, referred to as the proximal row (closer to the forearm) and distal row (closer to the metacarpals) (Figure 4.4).

Most of the carpals have two names—a newer, preferred name and an older traditional name. It is recommended that students learn both names because they are commonly interchanged in medical practice. The following memory device may be used to help the student remember the first letter of each carpal, in order, from the proximal to the distal row: <u>S</u>ally <u>L</u>eft <u>T</u>he <u>P</u>arty <u>T</u>o <u>T</u>ake <u>C</u>athy <u>H</u>ome.

Newer (Preferred) Name	Older Name
Proximal row	
scaphoid	navicular
lunate	semilunar
triquetrum	triangular or cuneiform
pisiform	
Distal row	
trapezium	greater multangular
trapezoid	lesser multangular
capitate	os magnum
hamate	unciform

The student may also use the shape of each carpal to assist in memorizing the names. The scaphoid or navicular resembles a boat, the lunate is shaped like a crescent moon, the triquetrum has three articular surfaces, the pisiform is pea shaped, the trapezium and trapezoids are four sided, the capitate is the largest, and the hamate has a hook-shaped region.

Carpal Tunnel

Of special interest is an area of the wrist known as the **carpal tunnel**. With the wrist hyperextended, the carpal tunnel is formed by the anterior aspects of the distal row of carpals forming a shallow concavity. Structures in this region can compress or "pinch" nerves in the wrist, resulting in characteristic symptoms referred to as carpal tunnel syndrome (Figure 4.5).

JOINTS OF THE HAND AND WRIST

Articulations of the hand and wrist are numerous and are important for the diagnosis of diseases such as arthritis and gout. All are classified as diarthroidial or freely movable joints, although some allow substantially more movement than others. Joint names are derived from the particular bones involved in the articulation. The basic joints of the hand and wrist are the interphalangeal (in´´ter-fă-lăn´jē-ăl), metacarpophalangeal (mĕt´´ă-kăr´´pō-fă-lăn´jē-ăl), carpometacarpal (kăr´´pō-mĕt´´ă-kăr´păl), intercarpal (ĭn´´tĕr-kăr´păl), and radiocarpal joints (rā´´dē-ō-kăr´păl).

Interphalangeal joints are found between middle and distal phalanges and between proximal and middle phalanges. These joints are classified as hinge type and their movement is limited to flexion and extension.

Metacarpophalangeal joints are found between each metacarpal and its corresponding proximal phalanx. These joints are classified as ellipsoidal and exhibit slight abduction/adduction movements as well as flexion/extension.

Carpometacarpal joints exist between the distal row of carpals and the metacarpals. The articulation of the trapezium and the first metacarpal allows considerable rotational movement and is one of the few examples of a saddle-type joint in the body. The remaining carpometacarpal joints allow more limited movement and are classified as gliding joints.

Intercarpal joints are found between each of the carpal bones. These gliding-type joints allow a very limited degree of flexion/extension and abduction/adduction.

The radiocarpal joint is found between the proximal row of carpals, primarily the scaphoid and lunate, and the radius bone of the forearm. This is an ellipsoidal-type joint that allows flexion/extension, as well as abduction/adduction (Figure 4.6).

FOREARM

The forearm consists of two long bones, the **radius** (rā´dē-ŭs) and the **ulna** (ŭl´nă). The longest and most central part of each bone is called the shaft. Processes on the ends of the two bones are important to both wrist and elbow radiography.

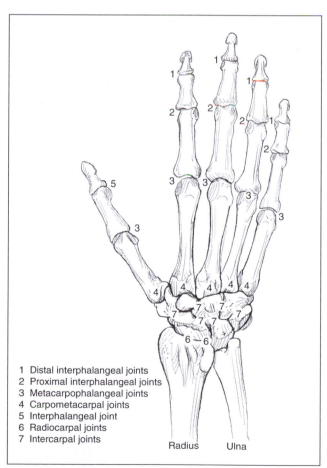

1 Distal interphalangeal joints
2 Proximal interphalangeal joints
3 Metacarpophalangeal joints
4 Carpometacarpal joints
5 Interphalangeal joint
6 Radiocarpal joints
7 Intercarpal joints

Radius   Ulna

FIGURE 4.6   Joints of the hand and wrist.

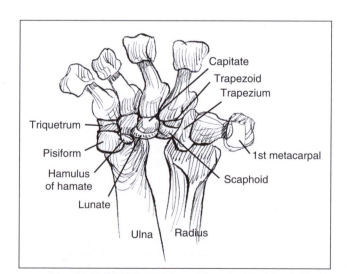

Capitate
Trapezoid
Trapezium

Triquetrum

Pisiform

Hamulus
of hamate

Lunate

Ulna   Radius

1st metacarpal

Scaphoid

FIGURE 4.5   Carpal tunnel.

Distal Forearm

At the distal end of the forearm, the radius is the larger of the two bones and is located on the lateral side. Both the radius and ulna possess a rounded, disk-shaped head and a **styloid** (stī´loyd) **process**. The styloid process of the radius is large and roughened, whereas the ulnar styloid process is small and pointed. The radius and ulna articulate at the ulnar notch to form the distal radioulnar joint, which assists in pronation/supination of the hand (Figure 4.7).

Proximal Forearm (Ulna)

At the proximal end of the forearm the ulna is the larger of the two bones. One of the most prominent and palpable of the ulnar processes is the large, roughened **olecranon** (ō-lĕk´răn-ŏn) **process**. The large, crescent-shaped semilunar or trochlear (trŏk´lē-ăr) notch curves anteriorly to form a pointed, beak-like projection called the **coronoid** (kor´ō-noyd) **process**.

Proximal Forearm (Radius)

Bony markings of the proximal radius include the disk-shaped head, which articulates with the humerus, and a narrow neck just inferior to the head. The head of the radius articulates at a small depression on the ulna known as the radial notch to form the proximal radioulnar joint, which assists in pronation/supination of the hand. Medial and inferior to the neck lies the roughened radial tuberosity (Figure 4.8).

HUMERUS

The **humerus** (hū´mĕr-ŭs) is the longest bone of the upper limb. The long, central portion of the bone is called the shaft.

Distal Humerus

Two rounded, smooth processes on the most inferior portion of the humerus articulate this bone with the forearm to form the elbow joint. The **capitulum** (kă-pĭt´ū-lŭm) or **capitellum** (kăp´´ĭ-tĕl´ŭm) articulates with the head of the radius, and the **trochlea** (trŏk´lē-ă) articulates with the semilunar or trochlear notch of the ulna. Together, the smooth surfaces of the capitulum and trochlea are referred to as the condyle of the humerus.

Epicondyles Above the articulations of the elbow lie two epicondyles, the largest and most easily palpable

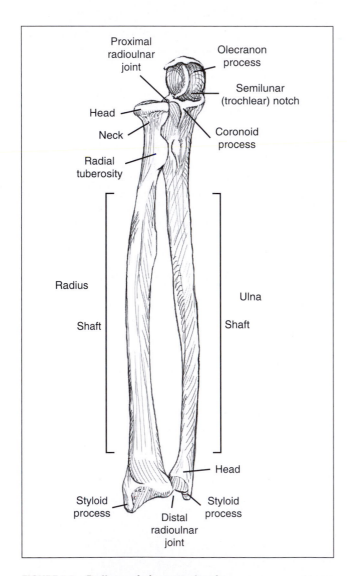

FIGURE 4.7   Radius and ulna, anterior view.

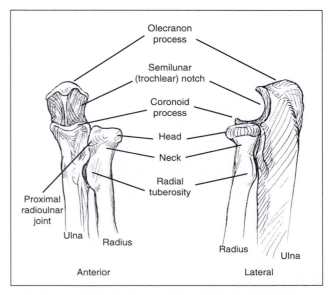

FIGURE 4.8   Proximal radius and ulna, anterior and lateral views.

being the medial **epicondyle** (ĕp-ĭ-kŏn´dĭl), the smaller called the lateral epicondyle (Figure 4.9). An imaginary line drawn between the two epicondyles, known as the epicondylar line/plane, is often used in positioning the elbow and the humerus.

Fossas   The distal humerus contains two shallow depressions or fossas. On the anterior surface, the coronoid fossa receives the coronoid process of the ulna during acute flexion. The posteriorly located olecranon fossa receives the olecranon process of the ulna during extension of the elbow. Normally a thin plate of bone separates the two fossae.

Elbow Joint   The humerus, radius, and ulna combine to form the elbow joint (Figure 4.10). The elbow joint is diarthroidial, with a hinge-type articulation that allows only flexion and extension. Supported by strong ligaments and a tough capsule, this joint is very

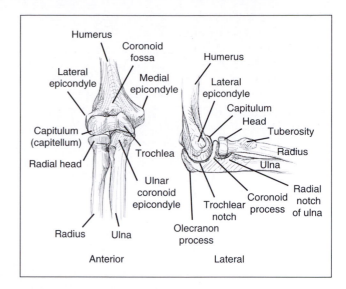

FIGURE 4.10   Elbow joint, anterior and lateral views.

stable. Also surrounding the elbow joint are pads of fat, which can sometimes be visualized radiographically, and several **bursa** or sacs containing joint fluid. These bursa can become inflamed, a condition known as bursitis. One such inflammation is the painful condition called tennis elbow.

Proximal Humerus

The prominent, ball-shaped head of the humerus articulates with the **glenoid** (glē´noyd) **cavity** or fossa of the scapula. Lying obliquely and adjacent to the humeral head is the anatomic neck, which signifies the former site of the epiphyseal plate. Situated laterally to the anatomic neck is a large rough process called the greater **tubercle** (tū´bĕr-kl). A smaller process projecting anteriorly is the lesser tubercle. The intertubercular sulcus (ĭn´´tĕr-tū-ber´kū-lăr sŭl´kŭs) or bicipital (bī-sĭp´ĭ-tăl) groove is a relatively deep fissure lying between the tubercles. Inferior to the tubercles is a narrowing called the surgical neck, a frequent site of fracture (Figure 4.11).

SCAPULA

The **scapula** (skăp´ū-lă) or shoulder blade is one of the largest flat bones in the body. The triangular shape of the bone creates three borders (superior, medial, and lateral) and three angles (superior, inferior, and lateral). The superior border contains a deep indentation called the scapular notch. The lateral angle contains a depression, the glenoid cavity or fossa, which articulates with the humeral head. This articulation is called the glenohumeral joint (Figure 4.12).

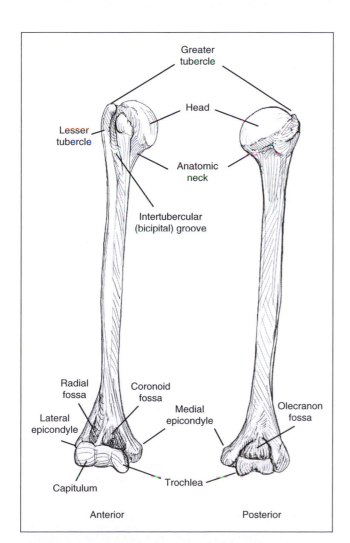

FIGURE 4.9   Humerus, anterior and posterior views.

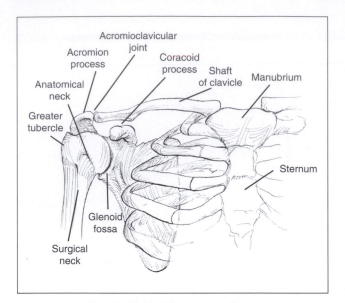

FIGURE 4.11   Proximal humerus, anterior view.

The central portion or body of the scapula contains several large, palpable processes that are important to upper limb radiography. The acromion (ă-krō′mē-ŏn) process lies on the superior aspect of the scapula, projecting posteriorly and superiorly. The lateral end of the acromion process forms an articula-

tion with the clavicle called the acromioclavicular joint. Projecting anteriorly is the coracoid (kor′ă-koyd) process, a frequent landmark for radiographic positioning of the shoulder girdle.

The posterior surface of the scapula contains a large oblique ridge called the scapular spine. Two depressions lie above and below the spine: the supraspinous (soo″′pră-spī′nŭs) fossa and infraspinous (ĭn″′fră-spī′nŭs) fossa, respectively. These fossae and the scapular spine serve as important attachments for shoulder muscles.

CLAVICLE

Although anatomically quite simple, the **clavicle** (klăv′ĭ-kl) or collarbone serves the critical function of attaching the bones of the arm to the axial skeleton. The lateral end, or acromial (ăk-rō′mē-ăl) extremity, articulates with the acromion process of the scapula to form the acromioclavicular joint. The medial end, or sternal extremity, articulates with the sternum to form the sternoclavicular joint. The acromioclavicular and sternoclavicular joints are both diarthroidal, gliding-type joints that allow only limited movement (Figure 4.13).

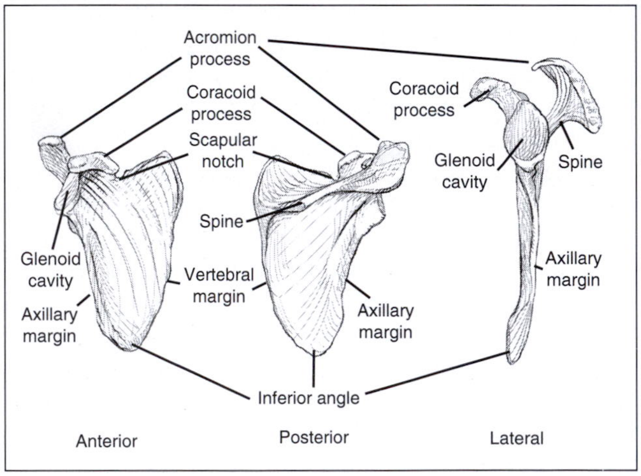

FIGURE 4.12   Scapula, anterior, lateral, and posterior views.

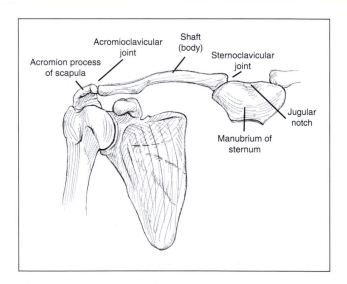

FIGURE 4.13   Clavicle, anterior view.

Shoulder Joint

The shoulder joint, sometimes called the gleno-humeral joint, is a ball-and-socket joint that allows the greatest range of motion of any joint in the body. An articular capsule surrounds the joint; however, it is very thin and does little to restrict movement. A number of tendons and ligaments also surround the joint to lend it considerable stability. Four of these tendons, collectively known as the **rotator cuff**, can tear when the arm is severely circumducted. This type of injury is common in baseball pitchers.

SHOULDER GIRDLE

The shoulder or pectoral girdle consists of the clavicle and the scapula. The shoulder girdle attaches the upper limb to the axial skeleton (Figure 4.14).

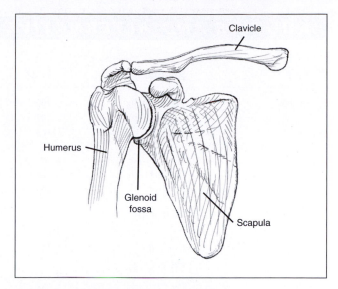

FIGURE 4.14   Shoulder girdle, anterior view.

ROUTINE AND ALTERNATIVE POSITIONS/PROJECTIONS

ROUTINE AND ALTERNATIVE POSITIONS/PROJECTIONS

FINGER (DIGITS 2–5)—PA PROJECTION

Exam Rationale The most common indication for finger examinations is trauma. Joint diseases such as arthritis or gout may also be visualized on finger radiographs. Structures demonstrated on the radiograph include all three phalanges and most or all of the metacarpal of the affected finger.

Technical Considerations

- Extremity screen/film
- Non-grid
- kVp range: 55–60
- SID: 40 inch (100 cm)

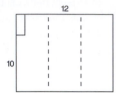

Radiation Protection

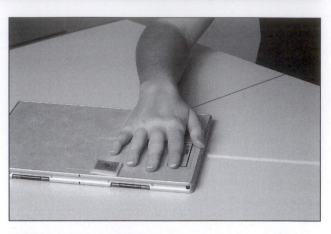

FIGURE 4.15   PA fourth finger.

Patient Position Seated at the end of the radiographic table with all potential artifacts removed from the part (Figure 4.15).

Part Position Pronate the hand and wrist to place them flat on cassette with fingers slightly spread.

Central Ray Perpendicular to the metacarpophalangeal joint of the affected finger.

Patient Instructions "Breathe normally but don't move."

Evaluation Criteria (Figures 4.16 and 4.17)

- Phalanges should not be rotated.
- Distal, middle, and proximal phalanges should be included.
- Distal end of the metacarpal should be included.

Tips

1. This same position of the hand and wrist gives an oblique view of the thumb.
2. Some department protocols require that the entire metacarpal be included.
3. In cases of trauma where a PA would not yield a satisfactory radiograph, the fingers can be radiographed in the AP position.
4. If only the distal end of the finger is affected and it is not necessary to demonstrate the entire metacarpal, the central ray may be directed to the proximal interphalangeal joint.

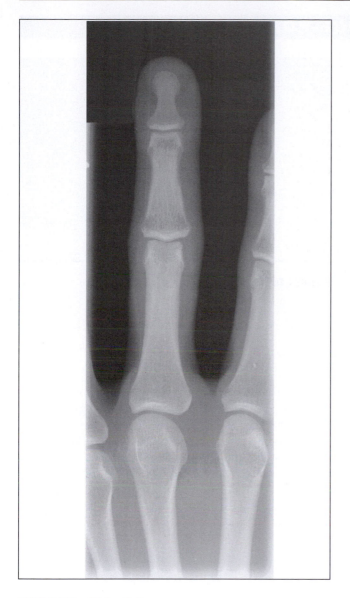

FIGURE 4.16 **PA fourth finger.**

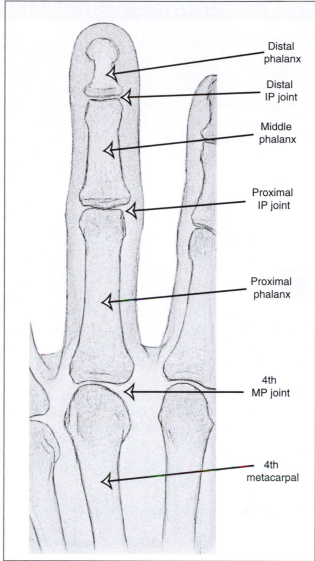

Distal
phalanx

Distal
IP joint

Middle
phalanx

Proximal
IP joint

Proximal
phalanx

4th
MP joint

4th
metacarpal

FIGURE 4.17 **PA fourth finger.**

FINGER (DIGITS 2–5)—OBLIQUE POSITION

Exam Rationale   The oblique is a routine position of the finger that gives a different perspective from the PA, that of a 45° oblique. Structures demonstrated on the radiograph include all three phalanges and most or all of the metacarpal of the affected finger.

Technical Considerations

- Extremity screen/film
- Non-grid
- kVp range: 55–60
- SID: 40 inch (100 cm)

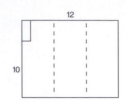

Radiation Protection

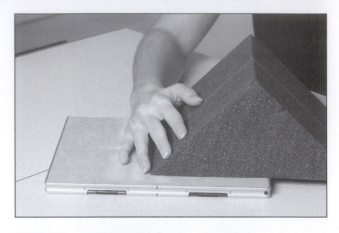

FIGURE 4.18   Oblique fourth finger.

Patient Position   Seated at the end of the radiographic table with all potential artifacts removed from the part (Figure 4.18).

Part Position   Begin with the hand pronated and rotate the finger 45°; fingers should be spread slightly to avoid superimposition with other fingers.

Central Ray   Perpendicular to the metacarpophalangeal joint of the affected finger.

Patient Instructions   "Breathe normally but don't move."

Evaluation Criteria (Figures 4.19 and 4.20)

- Affected finger must not be superimposed on other fingers.
- Distal, middle, and proximal phalanges should be included.
- Distal end of the metacarpal should be visualized.

Tips

1. A 45° foam wedge is helpful in maintaining the finger parallel to the film at the correct angle.
2. For the second finger, a reduced object film distance may be obtained by rotating the digit medially instead of laterally (Figure 4.21).
3. Like the PA finger, if only the distal end of the finger is affected, the central ray may be directed to the proximal interphalangeal joint.

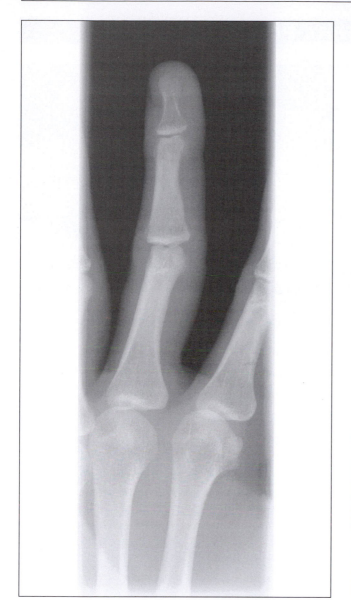

FIGURE 4.19   Oblique fourth finger.

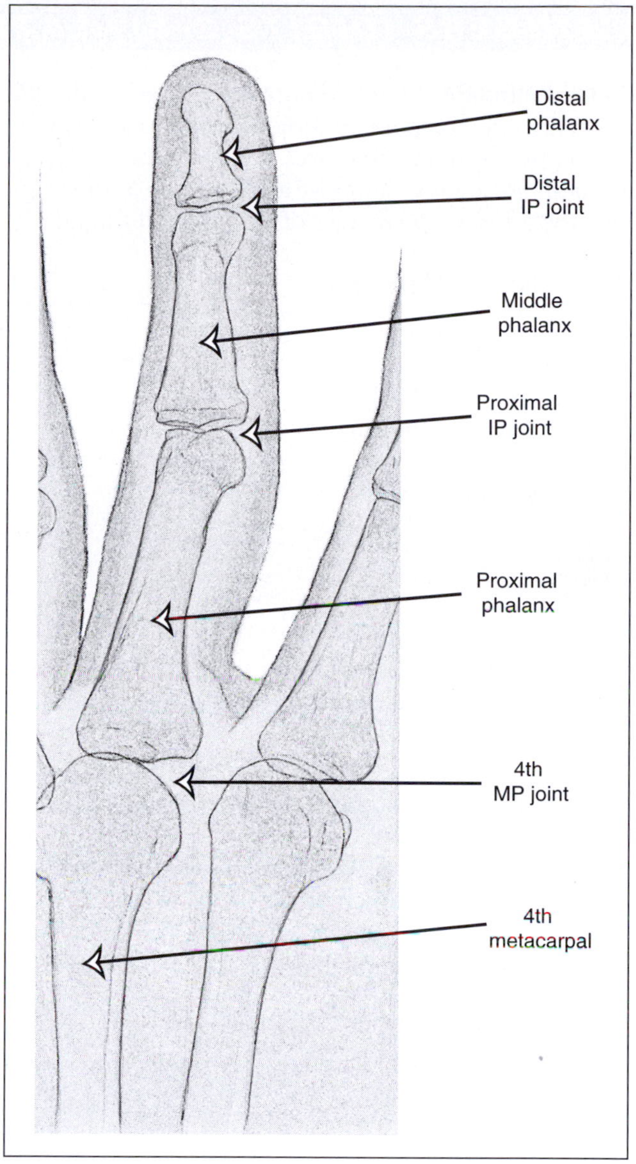

Distal
phalanx

Distal
IP joint

Middle
phalanx

Proximal
IP joint

Proximal
phalanx

4th
MP joint

4th
metacarpal

FIGURE 4.20   Oblique fourth finger.

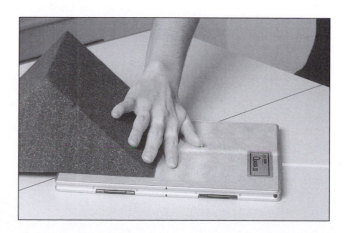

FIGURE 4.21
Oblique second finger (lateral rotation).

FINGERS (DIGITS 2–5)—LATERAL POSITION

Exam Rationale The lateral, taken at 90° to the PA, is used to demonstrate anterior or posterior displacements of the bony structures and to localize foreign bodies. Structures demonstrated on the radiograph include all three phalanges of the affected finger.

Technical Considerations

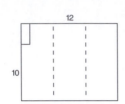

- Extremity screen/film
- Nop-grid
- kVP range: 55–60
- SID: 40 inch (100 cm)

Radiation Protection

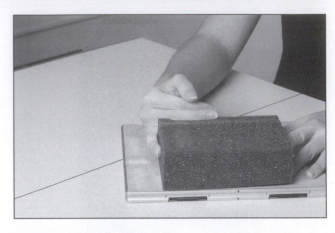

FIGURE 4.22   Lateral fourth finger.

Patient Position Seated at the end of the radiographic table with all potential artifacts removed from the part (Figure 4.22).

Part Position Place the hand at a 90° angle to the film, ulnar side down, with the affected finger in a fully extended lateral position, parallel to the film; flex all remaining fingers.

Central Ray Perpendicular to the proximal interphalangeal joint.

Patient Instructions "Breathe normally but don't move."

Evaluation Criteria (Figures 4.23 and 4.24)

- Phalanx of interest should be seen in profile.
- Distal, middle, and proximal phalanges should be included.
- Metacarpals will not be completely visualized due to superimposition.

Tips

1. Immobilization is highly recommended.
2. For the second finger, a reduced object film distance may be obtained by placing the radial side of the hand closest to the film (Figure 4.25).

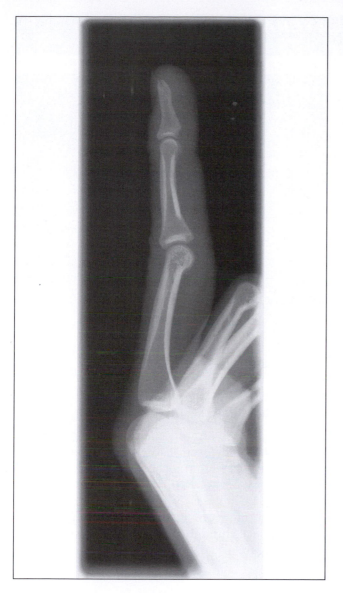

FIGURE 4.23   Lateral fourth finger.

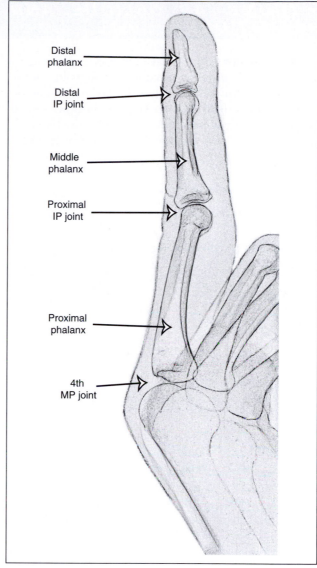

Distal phalanx

Distal IP joint

Middle phalanx

Proximal IP joint

Proximal phalanx

4th MP joint

FIGURE 4.24   Lateral fourth finger.

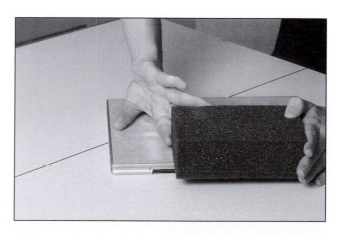

**FIGURE 4.25
Lateral second finger.**

THUMB—AP, OBLIQUE, AND LATERAL PROJECTIONS/POSITIONS

Exam Rationale   The most common indication for thumb examinations is trauma. Although its routine positions are the same as other fingers, the thumb has several unique features that require modifications in positioning. Structures demonstrated on the radiograph include both phalanges and most or all of the first metacarpal.

Technical Considerations

- Extremity screen/film
- Non-grid
- kVp range: 55–60
- SID: 40 inch (100 cm)

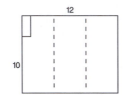

Radiation Protection

Patient Position   Seated at the end of the radiographic table with all potential artifacts removed from the part (Figure 4.26).

Part Position

- AP: rotate the hand internally until the posterior surface of the thumb is flat on the cassette.
- Oblique: pronate the hand and place the hand and thumb flat on the cassette (same as PA hand).
- Lateral: begin with the hand pronated and rotate the thumb toward the radial side until the digit is in a true lateral position.

Central Ray   Perpendicular to the first metacarpophalangeal joint.

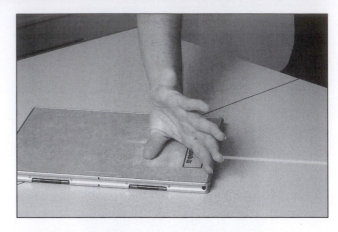

FIGURE 4.26   AP thumb.

Patient Instructions   "Breathe normally but don't move."

Evaluation Criteria (Figures 4.27 and 4.28)

- Distal and proximal phalanges should be included.
- Distal end of the first metacarpal should be visualized.
- Some department protocols require that the entire metacarpal be included.

Tip   When only the tip of the distal phalanx is injured, the PA thumb is sometimes substituted for the AP (Figure 4.29).

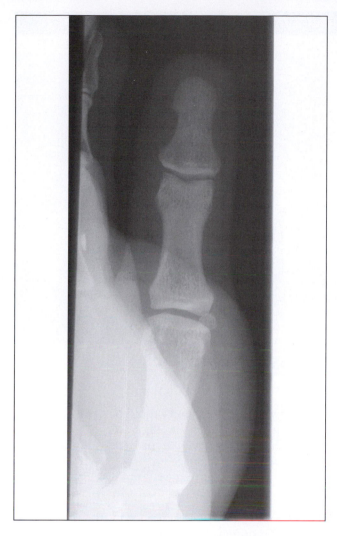

FIGURE 4.27   **AP thumb.**

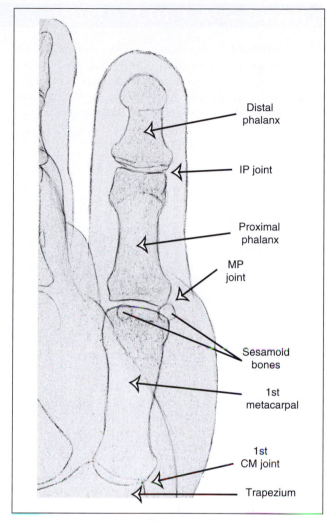

Distal phalanx

IP joint

Proximal phalanx

MP joint

Sesamoid bones

1st metacarpal

1st CM joint

Trapezium

FIGURE 4.28   **AP thumb.**

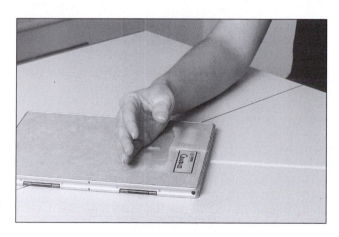

FIGURE 4.29
PA thumb.

HAND—PA PROJECTION

Exam Rationale　The most common indications for hand examinations are trauma and joint diseases such as arthritis or gout. Structures demonstrated on the radiograph include all of the phalanges, the metacarpals, the carpals, and joints of the hand and wrist.

Technical Considerations

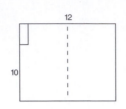

- Extremity screen/film
- Non-grid
- kVp range: 55–60
- SID 40 inch (100 cm)

Radiation Protection

Patient Position　Seated at the end of the radiographic table with all potential artifacts removed from the part (Figure 4.30).

Part Position　Pronate the hand and wrist to place them flat on the cassette with fingers extended and slightly spread.

Central Ray　Perpendicular to the third metacarpophalangeal joint.

Patient Instructions　"Breathe normally but don't move."

Evaluation Criteria (Figures 4.31 and 4.32)

- All phalanges, metacarpals, and carpals should be included.
- Phalanges and metacarpals should not be rotated.

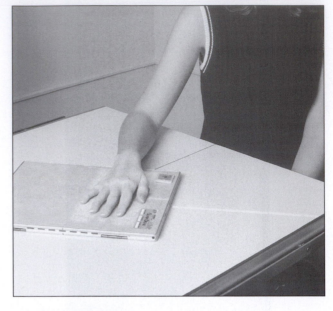

FIGURE 4.30　PA hand.

- Joint spaces of the hand should be open.
- Thumb should be in an oblique view.
- One-half to 1 inch (1–3 cm) of the distal radius/ulna should be visualized.

Tips

1. The part should be immobilized with tape or sandbags if motion is a potential problem.
2. An AP projection may be substituted if the hand cannot be flattened or the fingers extended because the diverging x-ray beam will assist in opening the joint spaces.
3. An AP projection better demonstrates the bases of the metacarpals.

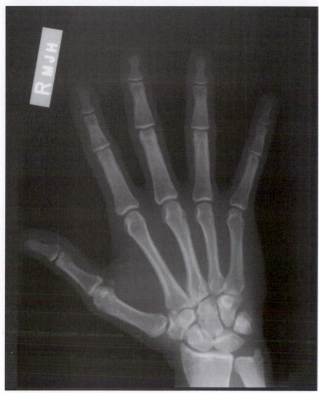

FIGURE 4.31   PA hand.

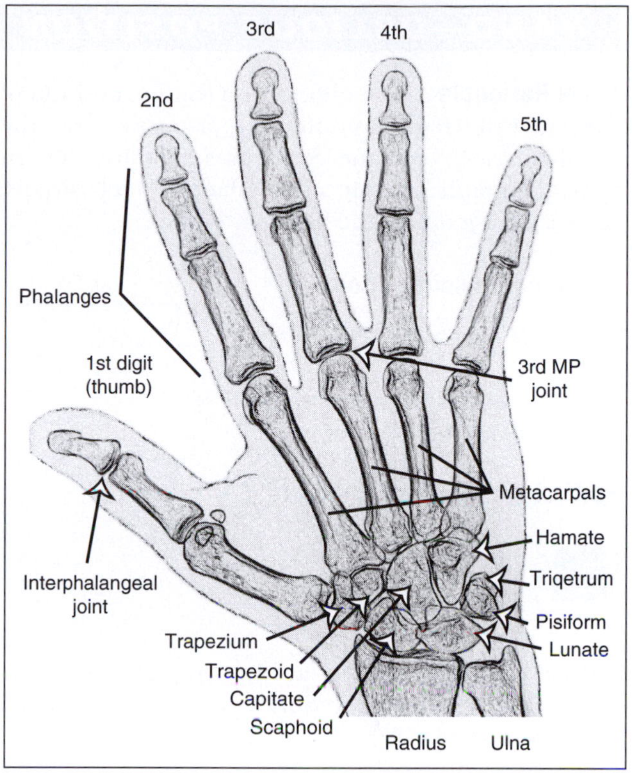

FIGURE 4.32   PA hand.

HAND—OBLIQUE POSITION

Exam Rationale The oblique is a routine position of the hand, which gives a different perspective from the PA, that of a 45° oblique. Structures demonstrated on the radiograph include all phalanges, metacarpals, carpals, and joints of the hand and wrist.

Technical Considerations

- Extremity screen/film
- Non-grid
- kVp range: 55–60
- SID: 40 inch (100 cm)

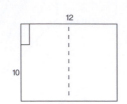

Radiation Protection

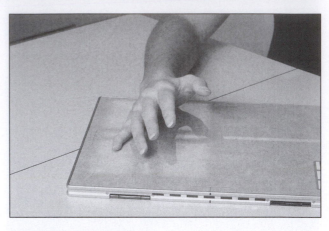

FIGURE 4.33   **Oblique hand.**

Patient Position Seated at the end of the radiographic table with all potential artifacts removed from the part (Figure 4.33).

Part Position Begin with the hand pronated and rotate the radial side of the wrist 45° from the film; keep the fingers parallel to the film and slightly spread to prevent excessive superimposition of bones on the radiograph.

Central Ray Perpendicular to the third metacarpophalangeal joint.

Patient Instructions "Breathe normally but don't move."

Evaluation Criteria (Figures 4.34 and 4.35)

- All phalanges, metacarpals, and carpals should be included.
- Thumb should be in an oblique view.
- One-half to 1 inch(1–3 cm) of the distal radius/ulna should be visualized.
- Little or no overlap of the metacarpals should be evident on the radiograph.

Tip A 45° angle sponge may be used to support the hand and to obtain the correct part angle.

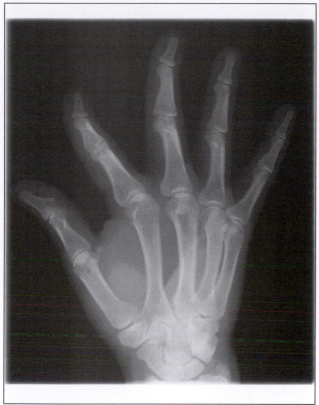

FIGURE 4.34　Oblique hand.

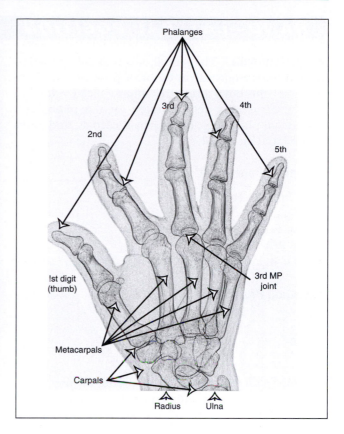

FIGURE 4.35　Oblique hand.

HAND—LATERAL POSITION

Exam Rationale The lateral, taken at 90° to the PA, is used to demonstrate anterior or posterior displacements of the bony structures and to localize foreign bodies. Structures demonstrated on the radiograph include all phalanges, metacarpals, carpals, and joints of the hand and wrist.

Technical Considerations

- Extremity screen/film
- Non-grid
- kVp range: 60–65 (5 more than the PA)
- SID: 40 inch (100 cm)

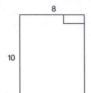

Radiation Protection

Patient Position Seated at the end of the radiographic table with all potential artifacts removed from the part (Figure 4.36).

Part Position Place the hand and wrist at a 90° angle to the film, ulnar side down; fingers should be spread in a fan-like manner; thumb should be projecting away from the palm and parallel to the film.

Central Ray Perpendicular to the second metacarpophalangeal joint.

Patient Instructions "Breathe normally but don't move."

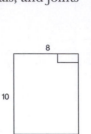

FIGURE 4.36   Lateral hand, fan.

Evaluation Criteria (Figures 4.37 and 4.38)

- Metacarpals should be superimposed on each other.
- Fingers two through five should be seen in profile.
- Carpals and distal radius/ulna should be in true lateral position.
- Thumb should be in PA position.

Tips

1. Patient motion is very common on this position, so immobilization of the part is recommended.
2. Some department protocols require the fingers to be fully extended and superimposed (Figures 4.39 and 4.40).

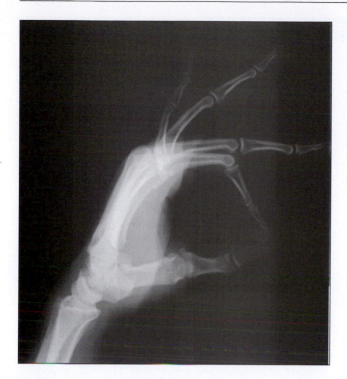

FIGURE 4.37 Lateral hand, fan.

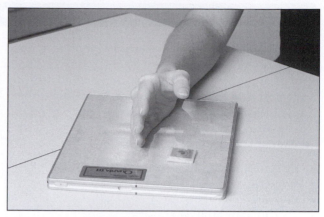

FIGURE 4.39 Lateral hand, extension.

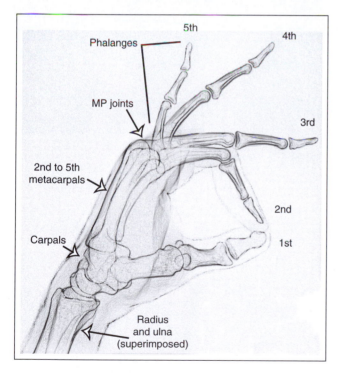

FIGURE 4.38 Lateral hand, fan.

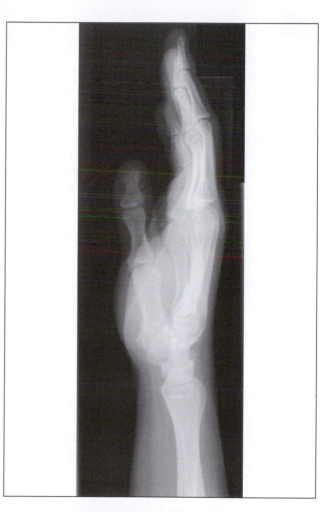

FIGURE 4.40 Lateral hand, extension.

HAND—BALL-CATCHER'S POSITION (NORGAARD METHOD)

Exam Rationale The ball-catcher's position is used to demonstrate early changes in the joints and bony structures of the hand caused by rheumatoid arthritis. The projection includes bilateral AP oblique projections of the hands.

Technical Considerations

- Extremity screen/film
- Non-grid
- kVp range: 55–60
- SID: 40 inch (100 cm)

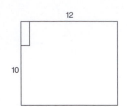

Radiation Protection

Patient Position Seated at the end of the radiographic table with all potential artifacts removed from the part (Figure 4.41).

Part Position With palms facing up, both hands are placed on the cassette and semisupinated at a 45° angle; the fingers should be slightly curled and spread to avoid excess superimposition of bones on the radiograph.

Central Ray Perpendicular to the midpoint of the film.

Patient Instructions "Breathe normally but don't move."

Evaluation Criteria (Figures 4.42 and 4.43)

- All phalanges, metacarpals, and carpals should be included.
- Thumbs should be in an oblique view.
- One-half to 1 inch (1–3 cm) of the distal radius/ulna should be visualized.
- Little or no overlap of the metacarpals should be evident on the radiograph.

Tips

1. Some department protocols require that the fingers be fully extended and parallel to the film to better open up the joint spaces.
2. A 45° angle sponge may be used to support the hands and to obtain the correct part angle.

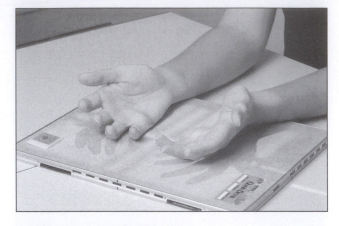

FIGURE 4.41   Norgaard hand.

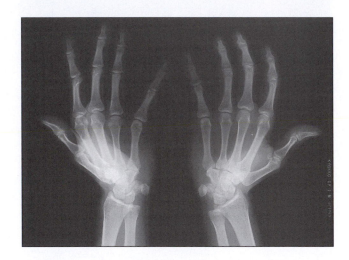

FIGURE 4.42   Norgaard hand.

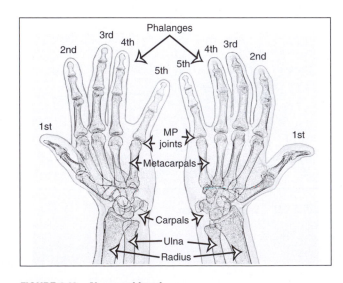

FIGURE 4.43   Norgaard hand.

HAND—AP AXIAL PROJECTION (BREWERTON METHOD)

Exam Rationale   This alternate projection is used to demonstrate bony erosion of the metacarpal heads and phalangeal bases on fingers two through five. Such erosion is a common early finding in rheumatoid arthritis.

Technical Considerations

- Extremity screen/film
- Non-grid
- kVp range: 55–60
- SID: 40 inch (100 cm)

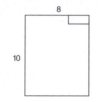

Radiation Protection

Patient Position   Seated at the end of the radiographic table with all potential artifacts removed from the part (Figure 4.44).

Part Position   Begin with the hand supinated with fingers slightly spread and flat on the cassette; flex the metacarpophalangeal joint so that the shafts of the metacarpals form a 45° angle with the cassette.

Central Ray   Directed laterally (toward the thumb) at a 45° angle entering at the third carpometacarpal joint.

Patient Instructions   "Breathe normally but don't move."

Evaluation Criteria (Figures 4.45 and 4.46)

- Metacarpal heads and phalangeal bases on fingers two through five should be clearly demonstrated.
- Wrist should not be flexed.

Tips

1. A 45° angle sponge placed under the doral surface of the metacarpals may assist in positioning.
2. A 30° tube angle may be used to demonstrate occult fractures of the metacarpal bases. The patient is positioned as above except the wrist is dorsiflexed 45° and the central ray enters at the base of the third metacarpal.

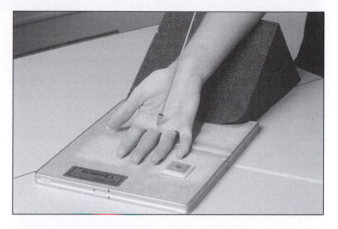

FIGURE 4.44   AP axial hand.

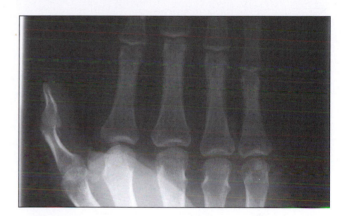

FIGURE 4.45   AP axial hand.

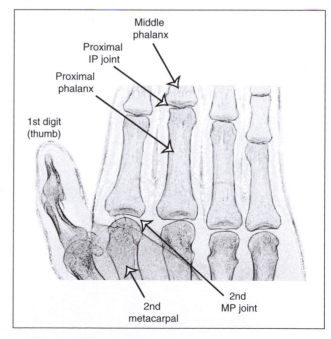

FIGURE 4.46   AP axial hand.

HAND—AP AXIAL PROJECTION (FIRST CARPOMETACARPAL JOINT)

Exam Rationale   This projection is used to demonstrate trauma to the first carpometacarpal joint. Although the resultant image is distorted, the joint space is better demonstrated than on PA hand or AP wrist projections.

Technical Considerations

- Extremity screen/film
- Non-grid
- kVp range: 55–60
- SID: 40 inch (100 cm)

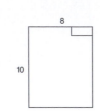

Radiation Protection

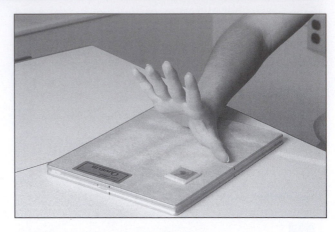

FIGURE 4.47   First carpometacarpal joint.

Patient Position   Seated at the end of the radiographic table with all potential artifacts removed from the part (Figure 4.47).

Part Position   Begin with the hand pronated and flat on the cassette; hyperextend the hand and wrist; rotate the hand to place the thumb parallel to the cassette.

Central Ray   Directed to the first carpometacarpal joint at a 45° angle toward the forearm.

Patient Instructions   "Breathe normally but don't move."

Evaluation Criteria (Figures 4.48 and 4.49)

- First carpometacarpal joint space should be opened.
- Trapezium should be visualized.

Tips

1. Tape or a bandage may assist the patient in obtaining and maintaining adequate hyperextension of the fingers.
2. This position is difficult to obtain because many patients cannot tolerate hyperextension of the hand; it should not be performed when there has been severe trauma.

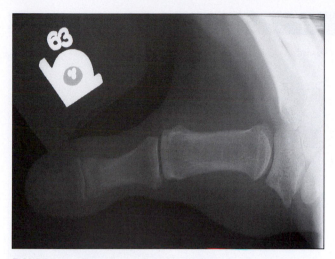

FIGURE 4.48   First carpometacarpal joint.

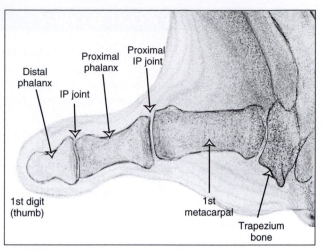

FIGURE 4.49   First carpometacarpal joint.

WRIST—PA PROJECTION

Exam Rationale The most common indication for wrist examinations is trauma. Structures demonstrated on the radiograph include all eight carpals and portions of the proximal metacarpals and distal radius/ulna.

Technical Considerations

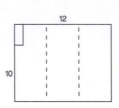

- Crosswise to include three views
- Extremity screen/film
- Non-grid
- kVp range: 55–60
- SID: 40 inch (100 cm)

Radiation Protection

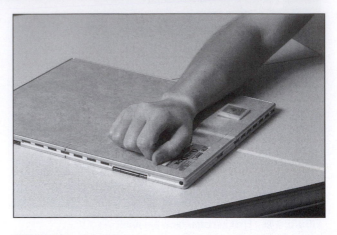

FIGURE 4.50   PA wrist.

Patient Position Seated at the end of the radiographic table with all potential artifacts removed from the part (Figure 4.50).

Part Position Pronate the hand and wrist to place them flat on the cassette; flex the fingers by curling them into a fist, to place the carpals parallel to the film.

Central Ray Perpendicular to the midcarpals.

Patient Instructions "Breathe normally but don't move."

Evaluation Criteria (Figures 4.51 and 4.52)

- All eight carpals should be included.
- One to 2 inches (3–5 cm) distal radius/ulna should be included.

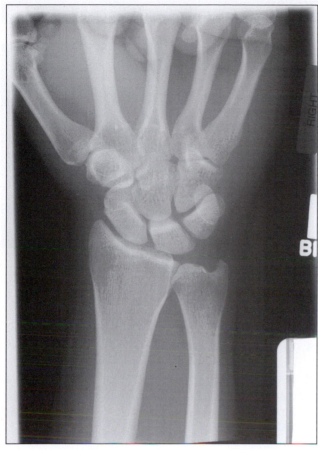

FIGURE 4.51 **PA wrist.**

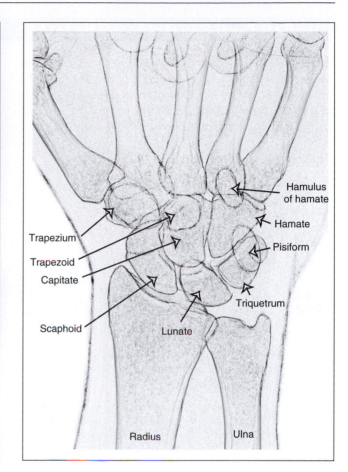

FIGURE 4.52 **PA wrist.**

Hamulus of hamate

Hamate

Trapezium

Pisiform

Trapezoid

Capitate

Scaphoid

Lunate

Triquetrum

Radius

Ulna

WRIST—OBLIQUE POSITION

Exam Rationale   The oblique is a routine position of the wrist, which gives a different perspective from the PA, that of a 45° oblique. Structures demonstrated on the radiograph include all eight carpals and portions of the proximal metacarpals and distal radius/ulna.

Technical Considerations

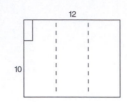

- Extremity screen/film
- Non-grid
- kVp range: 55–60
- SID: 40 inch (100 cm)

Radiation Protection

Patient Position   Seated at the end of the radiographic table with all potential artifacts removed from the part (Figure 4.53).

Part Position   Begin with the hand pronated and rotate the radial side of the wrist 45° from the film; the fingers and wrist are extended.

Central Ray   Perpendicular to the midcarpals.

Patient Instructions   "Breathe normally but don't move."

Evaluation Criteria (Figures 4.54 and 4.55)

- All eight carpals should be included.
- One to 2 inches (3–5 cm) of the metacarpals and distal radius/ulna should be included.
- Scaphoid and trapezium should be well demonstrated.

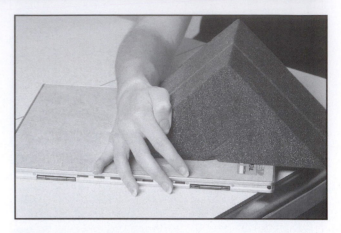

FIGURE 4.53   **PA oblique wrist.**

Tips

1. A 45° angle sponge may be used to support the wrist and to obtain the correct part angle.
2. The less common semisupination oblique position is sometimes taken to better demonstrate the pisiform, hamate, and triquetrum (Figures 4.56 and 4.57).

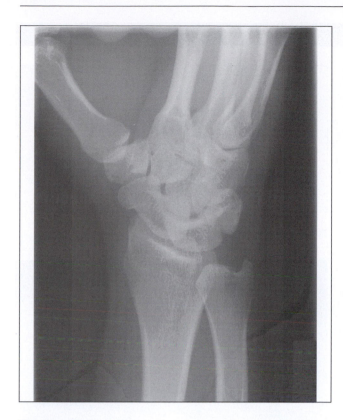

FIGURE 4.54   PA oblique wrist.

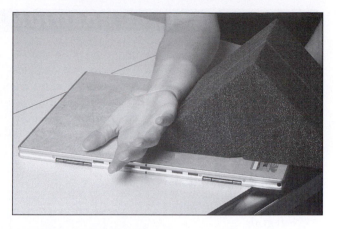

FIGURE 4.56   AP oblique wrist.

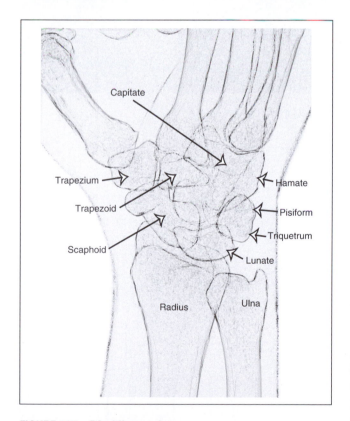

FIGURE 4.55   PA oblique wrist.

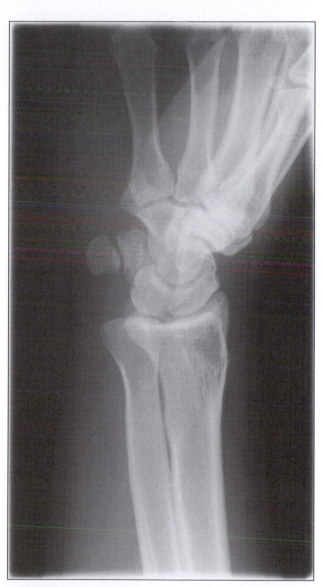

FIGURE 4.57   AP oblique wrist.

WRIST—LATERAL POSITION

Exam Rationale   The lateral, taken at 90° to the PA, is used to demonstrate anterior or posterior displacements of the bony structures. Although all eight carpals are demonstrated on the radiograph, they are substantially superimposed. Also demonstrated are portions of the proximal metacarpals and distal radius/ulna.

Technical Considerations

- Extremity screen/film
- Non-grid
- kVp range: 60–65
- SID: 40 inch (100 cm)

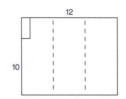

Radiation Protection

Patient Position   Seated at the end of the radiographic table with all potential artifacts removed from the part (Figure 4.58).

Part Position   Extend the fingers and place the hand and wrist at a 90° angle to the film, ulnar side down. The elbow should be flexed 90°.

Central Ray   Perpendicular to the midcarpals.

Patient Instructions   "Breathe normally but don't move."

Evaluation Criteria (Figures 4.59 and 4.60)

- Carpals should be mostly superimposed on each other.
- Distal radius and ulna should be superimposed.
- Scaphoid should be projected anteriorly.

Tip   This position may also be used to demonstrate widening of the wrist joint due to fracture or dislocation by taking two films—one with the wrist in maximum flexion and one with the wrist in hyperextension (Figures 4.61 through 4.64).

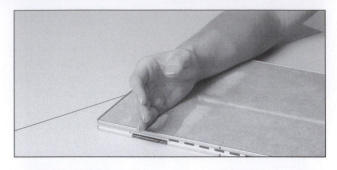

FIGURE 4.58   Lateral wrist.

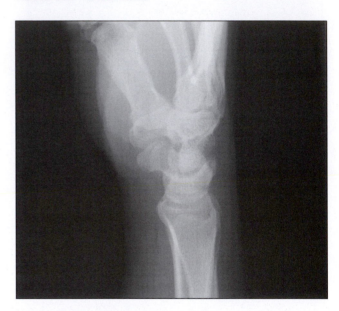

FIGURE 4.59   Lateral wrist.

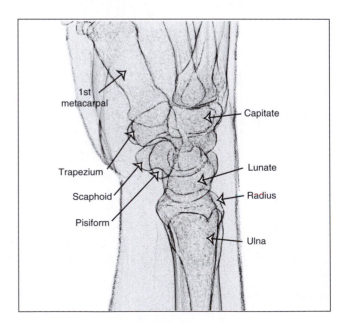

FIGURE 4.60   Lateral wrist.

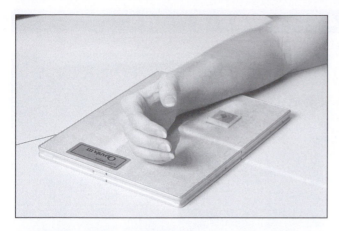

FIGURE 4.61   Lateral wrist, flexion.

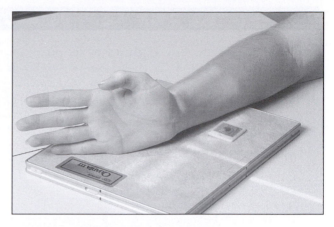

FIGURE 4.63   Lateral wrist, hyperextension.

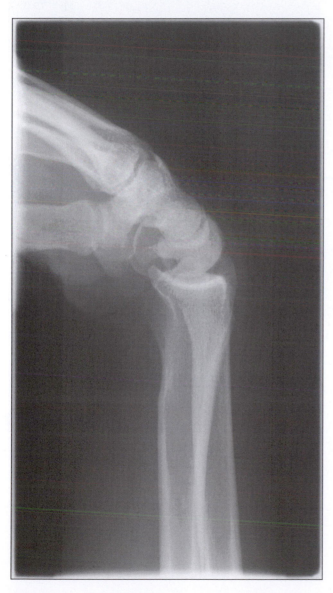

FIGURE 4.62   Lateral wrist, flexion.

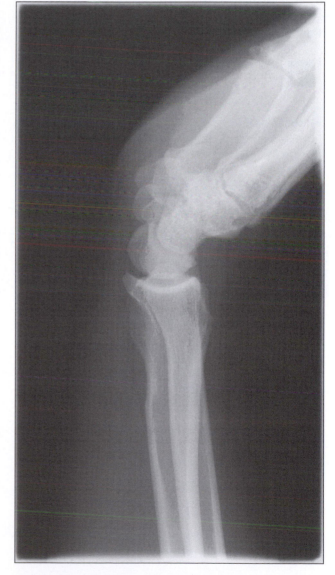

FIGURE 4.64   Lateral wrist, hyperextension.

WRIST—PA AND LATERAL: CASTED VARIATIONS

Exam Rationale Because fractures of the wrist are common, postreduction films are frequently taken with the wrist or forearm in a cast. Generally, only the PA projection and lateral position are necessary.

Technical Considerations

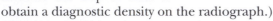
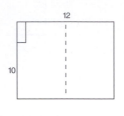

- Extremity screen/film
- Non-grid
- kVp range: 60–65 (Depending on cast type, size, and density, it may be necessary to increase the kVp or mAs to obtain a diagnostic density on the radiograph.)
- SID: 40 inch (100 cm)

Radiation Protection

Patient Position Seated at the end of the radiographic table with all potential artifacts removed from the part.

Part Position

- PA: pronate the hand and wrist to place them flat on the cassette (Figure 4.65).
- Lateral: place the hand and wrist at a 90° angle to the film with the ulnar side down (Figure 4.66).

Central Ray Perpendicular to the midcarpals.

Patient Instructions "Breathe normally but don't move."

Evaluation Criteria (Figures 4.67 and 4.68)

- All eight carpals should be visible through the cast.
- One to 2 inches (3–5 cm)of the proximal metacarpals and distal radius/ulna should be included.

Tips

1. If the patient is supine, it may be necessary to place the film upright and direct the central ray horizontally to the film.
2. Depending on the type of cast, it may be necessary to substitute an AP projection for the PA.

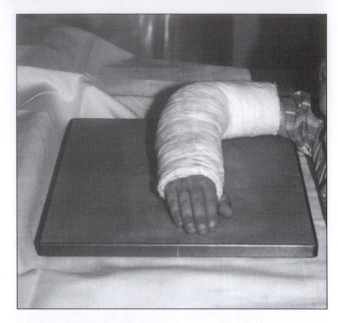

FIGURE 4.65   PA casted wrist.

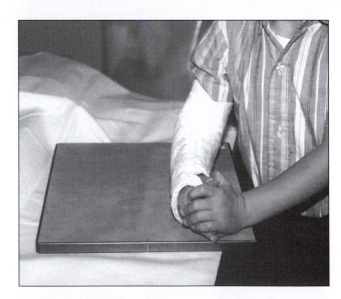

FIGURE 4.68   Casted wrist lateral

3. If the cast does not permit a true PA projection, it is important that the PA and lateral are taken 90° from each other.

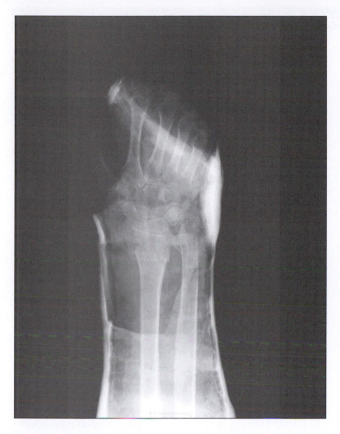

FIGURE 4.66 PA casted wrist.

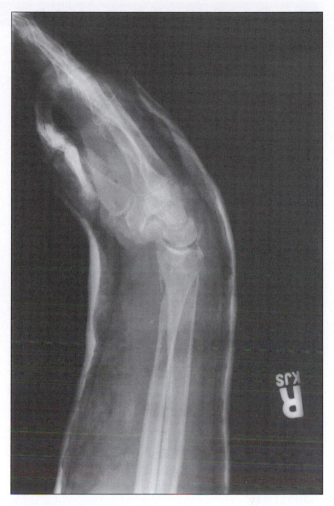

FIGURE 4.67 Casted wrist lateral.

WRIST—ULNAR FLEXION POSITION

Exam Rationale The primary purpose of the ulnar flexion position is to obtain an elongated view of the scaphoid, free from superimposition. The scaphoid is the carpal most frequently fractured. Structures demonstrated on the radiograph include the scaphoid and usually the other carpals and portions of the proximal metacarpals and distal radius/ulna.

Technical Considerations

- Extremity screen/film
- Non-grid
- kVp range: 55–60
- SID: 40 inch (100 cm)

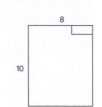

Radiation Protection

Patient Position Seated at the end of the radiographic table with all potential artifacts removed from the part (Figure 4.69).

Part Position Pronate the hand and wrist to place them flat on the cassette, as in a PA hand projection; evert (externally flex) the wrist as much as possible.

Central Ray Directed toward the forearm at a 15° to 20° angle and centered to the scaphoid.

Patient Instructions "Breathe normally but don't move."

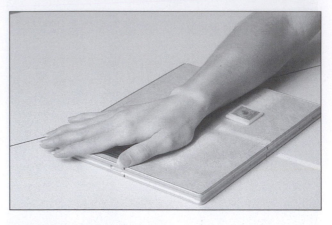

FIGURE 4.69 Ulnar flexion wrist.

Evaluation Criteria (Figures 4.70 and 4.71)

- Scaphoid should be elongated and projected free from superimposition from other carpals.

Tips

1. Ulnar flexion is sometimes called radial deviation.
2. Do not attempt to flex the wrist of patients with severe trauma.
3. Many department protocols require that all carpals, proximal metacarpals, and the distal radius/ulna also be included on the radiograph.
4. Some department protocols use a perpendicular central ray.
5. Some department protocols call for the central ray to be directed to the midcarpal area.

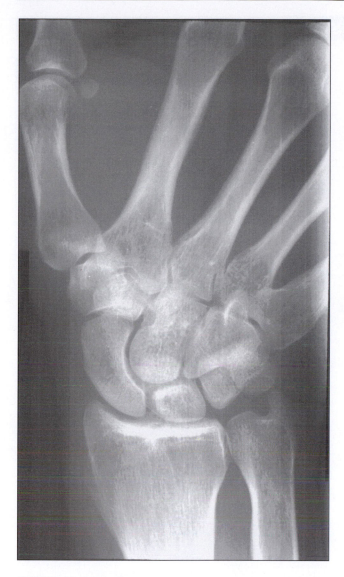

FIGURE 4.70　Ulnar flexion wrist.

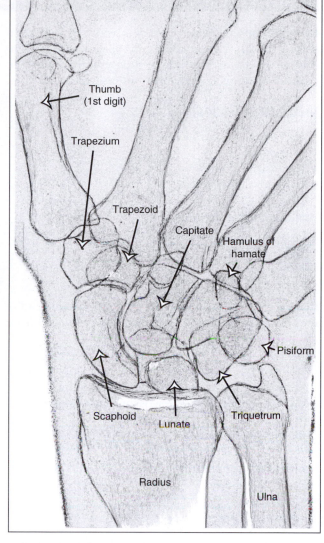

FIGURE 4.71　Ulnar flexion wrist.

WRIST—RADIAL FLEXION POSITION

Exam Rationale The primary purpose of the radial flexion position is to open joint spaces between the carpals on the medial side of the wrist, including the capitate, hamate, triquetrum, and pisiform.

Technical Considerations

- Extremity screen/film
- Non-grid
- kVp range: 55–60
- SID: 40 inch (100 cm)

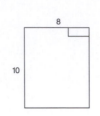

Radiation Protection

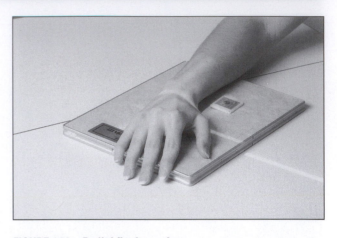

FIGURE 4.72 Radial flexion wrist.

Patient Position Seated at the end of the radiographic table with all potential artifacts removed from the part (Figure 4.72).

Part Position Pronate the hand and wrist to place them flat on the cassette, as in a PA hand projection; invert (flex internally) the wrist as much as possible.

Central Ray Perpendicular to the midcarpals.

Patient Instructions "Breathe normally but don't move."

Evaluation Criteria (Figures 4.73 and 4.74)

- Capitate, hamate, and triquetrum should be well visualized.
- Pisiform remains mostly superimposed on triquetrum.
- Joint spaces of the medial carpals should be opened to a greater degree than is seen on the PA wrist.

Tips

1. Radial flexion is sometimes called ulnar deviation.
2. Do not attempt to flex the wrist of patients with severe trauma.

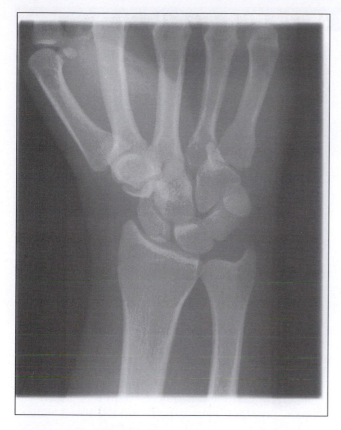

FIGURE 4.73 Radial flexion wrist.

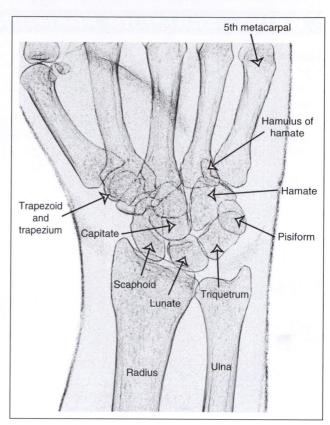

FIGURE 4.74 Radial flexion wrist.

WRIST—SCAPHOID POSITION (STECHER METHOD)

Exam Rationale The primary purpose of this position is to obtain an elongated view of the scaphoid, free from superimposition. The scaphoid is the carpal most frequently fractured. Structures demonstrated on the radiograph include the scaphoid and usually the other carpals and portions of the proximal metacarpals and distal radius/ulna.

Technical Considerations

- Extremity screen/film
- Non-grid
- kVp range: 55–60
- SID: 40 inch (100 cm)

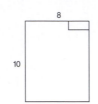

Radiation Protection

Patient Position Seated at the end of the radiographic table with all potential artifacts removed from the part (Figure 4.75).

Part Position Pronate the hand and wrist to place them flat on the cassette. Without allowing forearm to move, evert hand (toward ulnar side) as much as patient can tolerate.

Central Ray Directed toward the forearm at a 20° angle and centered to the scaphoid.

Patient Instructions "Breathe normally but don't move."

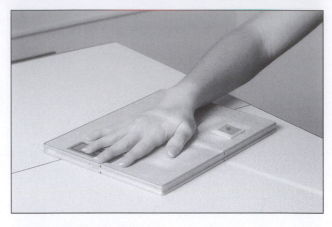

FIGURE 4.75   Scaphoid wrist.

Evaluation Criteria (Figures 4.76 and 4.77)

- Scaphoid should be elongated and projected free from superimposition from other carpals.
- Many department protocols require that all carpals, proximal metacarpals, and the distal radius/ulna also be included on the radiograph.

Tips

1. As originally described by Stecher, the wrist may be placed on a 20° angle sponge and the central ray directed perpendicular.
2. Some department protocols call for the central ray to be placed in the midcarpal area.

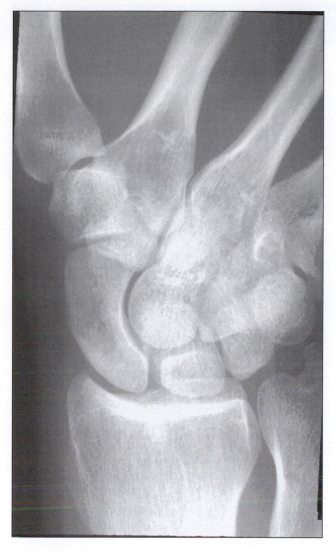

FIGURE 4.76 Scaphoid wrist.

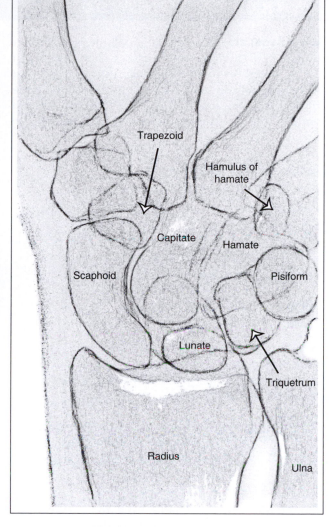

FIGURE 4.77 Scaphoid wrist.

WRIST—PA AXIAL OBLIQUE POSITION (CLEMENTS AND NAKAYAMA METHOD)

Exam Rationale The PA axial oblique is performed primarily to demonstrate fractures of the trapezium or abnormalities of the first carpometacarpal joint. Although the resultant image is distorted, the trapezium and the joint space are freed from the superimposition that is normally present on PA and oblique wrist projections.

Technical Considerations

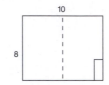

- Extremity screen/film
- Non-grid
- kVp range: 55–60
- SID: 40 inch (100 cm)

Radiation Protection

Patient Position Seated at the end of the radiographic table with all potential artifacts removed from the part (Figure 4.78).

Part Position Begin with the hand pronated and rotate the radial side of the wrist 45° from the film; place the hand in ulnar flexion, if patient condition permits.

Central Ray Directed away from the forearm at a 45° angle and centered to the trapezium.

Patient Instructions "Breathe normally but don't move."

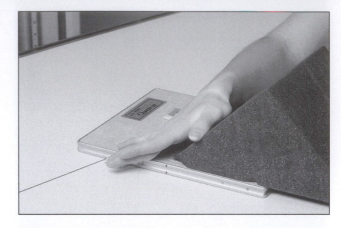

FIGURE 4.78   PA axial wrist.

Evaluation Criteria (Figures 4.79 and 4.80)

- Trapezium should be mostly free of superimposition.
- First carpometacarpal joint should be open.

Tips

1. A 45° angle sponge may be used to support the wrist and to obtain the correct part angle.
2. Some department protocols call for the central ray to be directed to the midcarpal area.
3. When performed to demonstrate arthritis, both wrists may be included on a single 10 × 12 inch (25 × 30 cm) film for comparison.

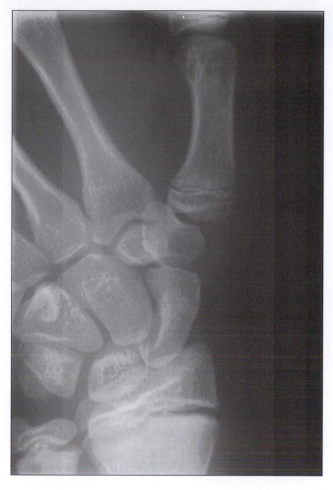

FIGURE 4.79   PA axial wrist.

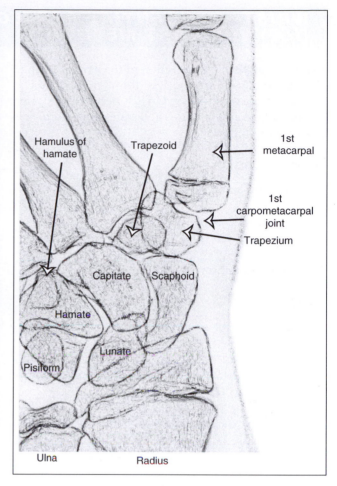

FIGURE 4.80   PA axial wrist.

WRIST—TANGENTIAL PROJECTION: CARPAL CANAL (GAYNOR-HART METHOD)

Exam Rationale   This position of the wrist is taken to visualize the palmar aspect of the carpals known as the carpal canal or tunnel. Carpals best demonstrated on the radiograph include the scaphoid, pisiform, trapezium, and hamate.

Technical Considerations

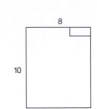

- Extremity screen/film
- Non-grid
- kVp range: 60–65
- SID: 40 inch (100 cm)

Radiation Protection

Patient Position   Seated at the end of the radiographic table with all potential artifacts removed from the part (Figure 4.81).

Part Position   Begin with the hand pronated and flat on the cassette, hyperextending the wrist as much as possible; patient should/may hold hand back.

Central Ray   Directed to the midcarpals at a 25–30° angle toward the forearm.

Patient Instructions   "Breathe normally but don't move."

Evaluation Criteria (Figures 4.82 and 4.83)

- Concave arch of the carpal canal should be clearly demonstrated.
- Scaphoid, pisiform, trapezium, and the hamulus of the hamate should be visualized.

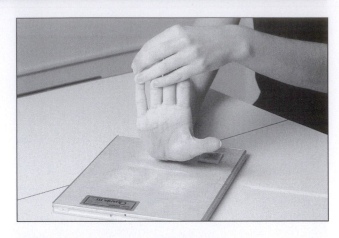

FIGURE 4.81   Tangential: carpal canal.

Tips

1. Tape or a bandage may assist the patient in obtaining and maintaining this hyperextension.
2. This position is difficult to obtain because many patients cannot tolerate hyperextension of the hand. The following variations are sometimes performed:
   - Place the fingers at a 75° angle to the film and angle the tube 40°.
   - A superoinferior projection may also be substituted. With the patient standing and the palmar surface of the hand on the cassette, the central ray is angled according to the amount of hyperextension obtained to maintain an approximate 45° angle between the palmar surface of the hand and the central ray (Figures 4.84 and 4.85).

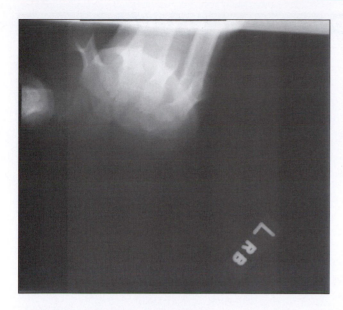

FIGURE 4.82   Tangential: carpal canal.

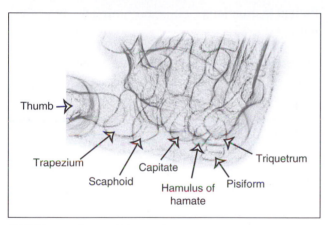

FIGURE 4.83   Tangential: carpal canal.

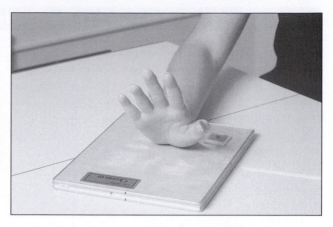

FIGURE 4.84   Tangential: carpal canal variation (75° tube angle).

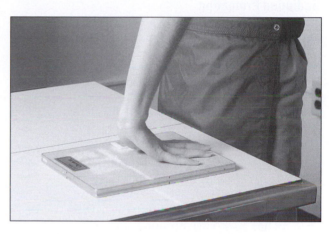

FIGURE 4.85   Tangential: carpal canal variation (superoinferior projection).

WRIST—TANGENTIAL POSITION: CARPAL BRIDGE

Exam Rationale　This position of the wrist is taken specifically to demonstrate dislocations or fractures in the area known as the carpal bridge. Carpals best demonstrated on the radiograph include the scaphoid, lunate, trapezium, and triquetrum.

Technical Considerations

- Extremity screen/film
- Non-grid
- kVp range: 60–65 (5 more than the PA)
- SID: 40 inch (100 cm)

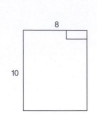

Radiation Protection

Patient Position　Upright with all potential artifacts removed from the part (Figure 4.86).

Part Position　Hyperflex the wrist by placing the dorsal surface of the hand flat on the cassette (palm upward) with the forearm perpendicular to the film.

Central Ray　Directed to the midcarpals, entering 1 to 2 inches (3–5 cm) proximal to the wrist at a 45° angle.

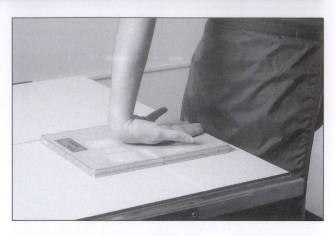

FIGURE 4.86　**Tangential: carpal bridge.**

Patient Instructions　"Breathe normally but don't move."

Evaluation Criteria (Figures 4.87 and 4.88)

- Concave arch of the carpal canal should be clearly demonstrated.
- Scaphoid, lunate, trapezium, and triquetrum should be visualized.

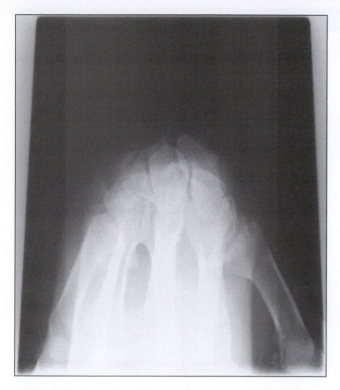

FIGURE 4.87   Tangential: carpal bridge.

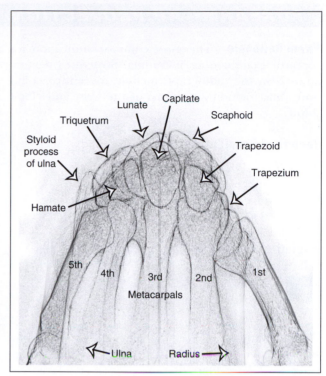

FIGURE 4.88   Tangential: carpal bridge.

FOREARM—AP PROJECTION

Exam Rationale   The most common indication for forearm examinations is trauma. Structures demonstrated on the radiograph include the entire radius and ulna, including portions of the wrist and elbow joints.

Technical Considerations

- Extremity screen/film
- Non-grid
- kVp range: 60–65
- SID: 40 inch (100 cm)

Radiation Protection

Patient Position   Seated at the end of the radiographic table with all potential artifacts removed from the part (Figure 4.89).

Part Position   With the hand supinated, center the long axis of the forearm to the film and attempt to get both the wrist and elbow flat on the cassette; the entire upper limb from the shoulder to the hand should lie in the same horizontal plane, parallel to the cassette.

Central Ray   Perpendicular to the mid-forearm.

Patient Instructions   "Breathe normally but don't move."

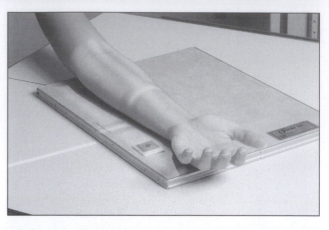

FIGURE 4.89   AP forearm.

Evaluation Criteria (Figures 4.90 and 4.91)

- Both wrist and elbow joints should be included.
- Radius and ulna should have only slight superimposition at both the proximal and distal ends.

Tips

1. The PA projection is never performed because the radius and ulna cross over each other.
2. If both elbow and wrist joints cannot be demonstrated on a single film, a separate AP of one joint should be done.

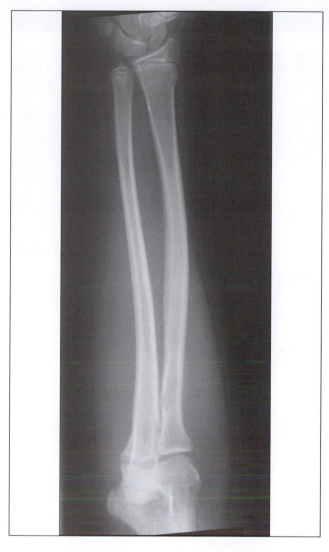

FIGURE 4.90 **AP forearm.**

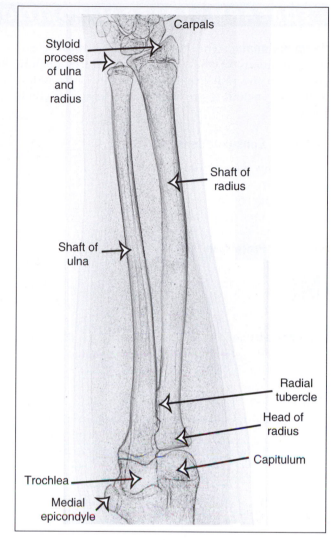

FIGURE 4.91 **AP forearm.**

FOREARM—LATERAL POSITION

Exam Rationale   The lateral is the second of two basic positions of the forearm. Structures demonstrated on the radiograph include the entire radius and ulna, including portions of the wrist and elbow joints.

Technical Considerations

- Extremity screen/film
- Non-grid
- kVp range: 60–65
- SID: 40 inch (100 cm)

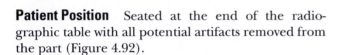

Radiation Protection

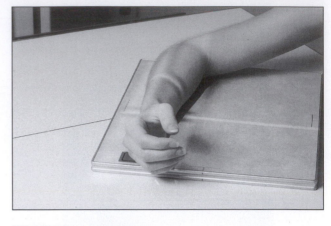

FIGURE 4.92   Lateral forearm.

Patient Position   Seated at the end of the radiographic table with all potential artifacts removed from the part (Figure 4.92).

Part Position   Flex the elbow 90° and place the hand, wrist, and elbow in a true lateral position, resting on the ulnar surface; the patient may need to lean forward to place the entire upper limb in the same plane.

Central Ray   Perpendicular to the mid-forearm.

Patient Instructions   "Breathe normally but don't move."

Evaluation Criteria (Figures 4.93 and 4.94)

- Radius and ulna should be mostly superimposed.
- Both wrist and elbow joints should be included.

Tip   If both elbow and wrist joints cannot be demonstrated on a single film, a separate lateral of one joint should be done.

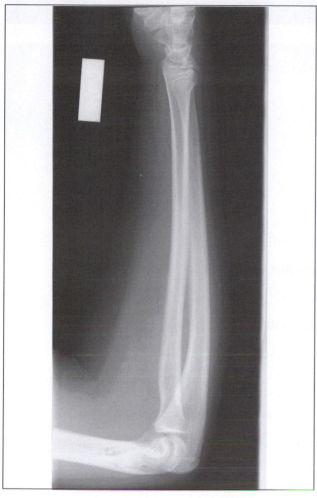

FIGURE 4.93   **Lateral forearm.**

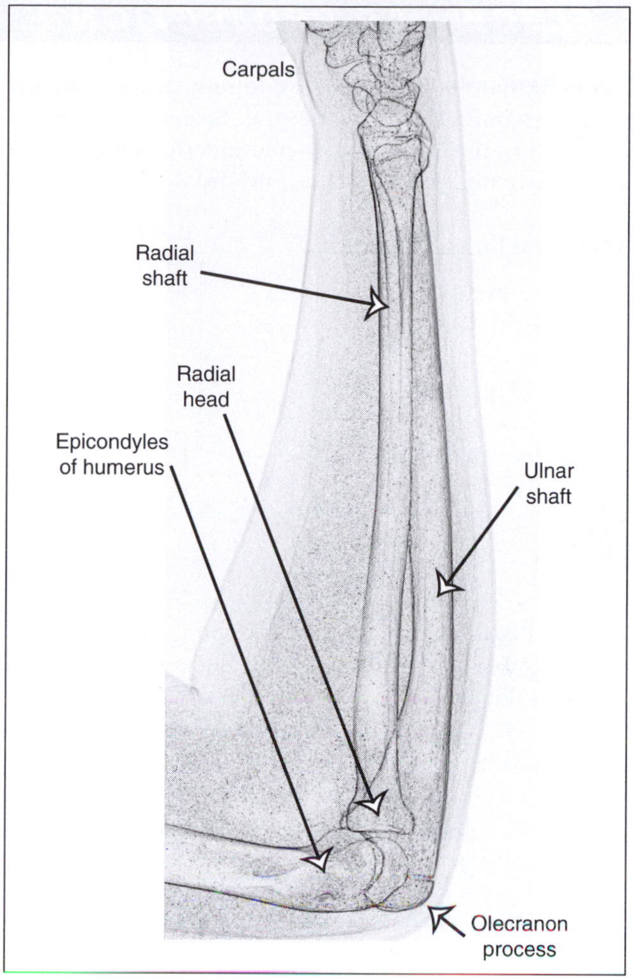

Carpals

Radial
shaft

Radial
head

Epicondyles
of humerus

Ulnar
shaft

Olecranon
process

FIGURE 4.94   **Lateral forearm.**

ELBOW—AP PROJECTION

Exam Rationale The most common indication for elbow examinations is trauma. Structures demonstrated on the radiograph include the elbow joint space, proximal radius/ulna, and distal humerus.

Technical Considerations

- Extremity screen/film
- Non-grid
- kVp range: 65–70
- SID: 40 inch (100 cm)

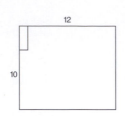

Radiation Protection

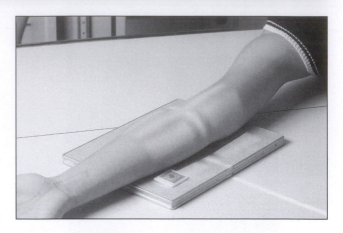

FIGURE 4.95   AP elbow.

Patient Position Seated at the end of the radiographic table with all potential artifacts removed from the part (Figure 4.95).

Part Position Place both the humerus and forearm flat on the film, parallel to the cassette; with the hand supinated, fully extend the elbow and place the epicondylar line parallel to the film.

Central Ray Perpendicular to the elbow joint.

Patient Instructions "Breathe normally but don't move."

Evaluation Criteria (Figures 4.96 and 4.97)

- Joint space should be open and centered to the film.
- Radius and ulna should be slightly superimposed near the radial tuberosity.
- Epicondyles should not be rotated.

Tip For patients who are unable to fully extend their arm, the trauma AP projection should be substituted (see page 148).

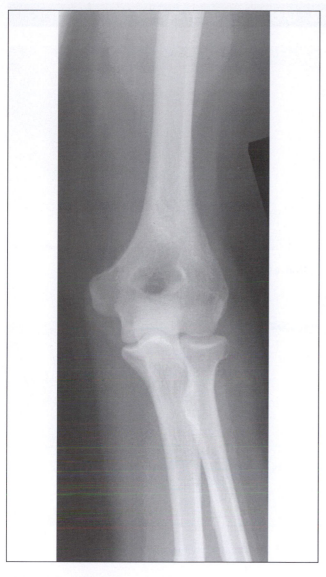

FIGURE 4.96   AP elbow.

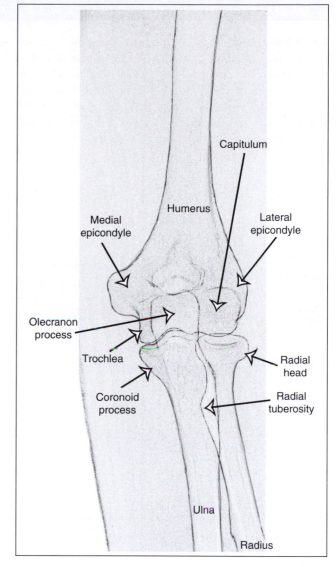

FIGURE 4.97   AP elbow.

Humerus

Medial epicondyle

Capitulum

Lateral epicondyle

Olecranon process

Trochlea

Radial head

Coronoid process

Radial tuberosity

Ulna

Radius

ELBOW—MEDIAL AND LATERAL OBLIQUE POSITIONS

Exam Rationale Although the obliques demonstrate anatomy similar to what is demonstrated on the AP, they are essential to better visualize certain specific structures. The medial (internal) oblique demonstrates the coronoid process in profile, whereas the lateral (external) oblique demonstrates the radial tuberosity, head, and neck free of superimposition.

Technical Considerations

- Extremity screen/film
- Non-grid
- kVp range: 65–70
- SID: 40 inch (100 cm)

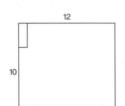

Radiation Protection

Patient Position Seated at the end of the radiographic table with all potential artifacts removed from the part.

Part Position Place both the humerus and forearm flat on film, parallel to the cassette; with the hand supinated, fully extend the elbow.

- Medial (internal) oblique: pronate the hand until the elbow joint is rotated *medially* 45° (Figure 4.98).
- Lateral (external) oblique: supinate the hand until the elbow joint is rotated *laterally* 45° (Figure 4.99).

Central Ray Perpendicular to the elbow joint.

Patient Instructions "Breathe normally but don't move."

Evaluation Criteria (Figures 4.100 through 4.103)

- Internal oblique: radius and ulna should be substantially superimposed with the coronoid process visualized in profile.
- External oblique: radius and ulna should be free from superimposition of each other with the radial tuberosity, head, and neck clearly demonstrated.

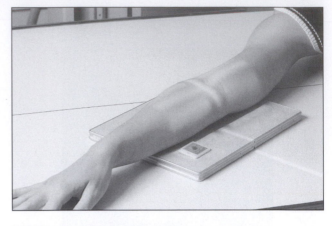

FIGURE 4.98   Internal oblique elbow.

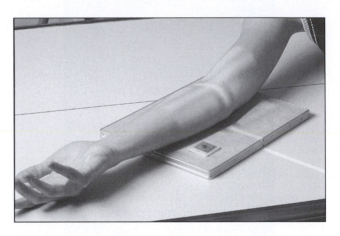

FIGURE 4.99   External oblique elbow.

Tip In cases of acute injury, trauma obliques should be substituted (see page 152).

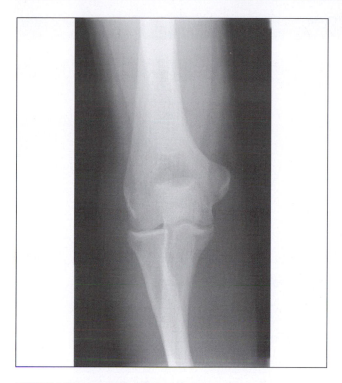

FIGURE 4.100   Internal oblique elbow.

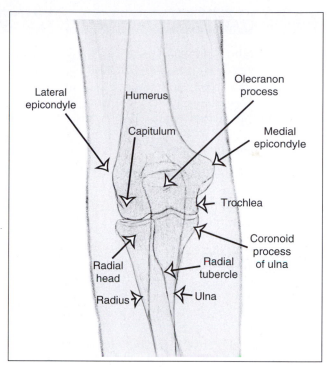

FIGURE 4.102   Internal oblique elbow.

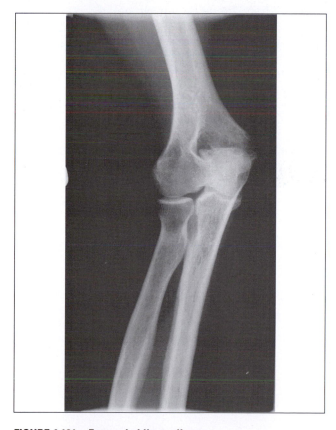

FIGURE 4.101   External oblique elbow.

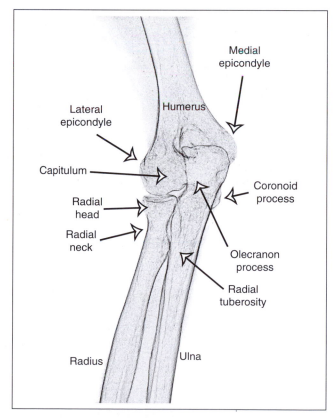

FIGURE 4.103   External oblique elbow.

ELBOW—LATERAL POSITION

Exam Rationale The lateral is a routine position of the elbow that demonstrates the elbow joint space, proximal radius/ulna, and distal humerus. Of the routine elbow positions, the lateral gives the best visualization of the olecranon process.

Technical Considerations

- Extremity screen/film
- Non-grid
- kVp range: 65–70
- SID: 40 inch (100 cm)

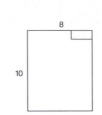

Radiation Protection

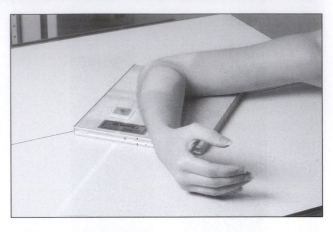

FIGURE 4.104   Lateral elbow.

Patient Position Seated at the end of the radiographic table with all potential artifacts removed from the part (Figure 4.104).

Part Position Place both the humerus and forearm flat on film, parallel to the cassette; flex the elbow 90°, placing the hand, wrist, and elbow in a true lateral position with the epicondylar line perpendicular to the film.

Central Ray Perpendicular to the elbow joint.

Patient Instructions "Breathe normally but don't move."

Evaluation Criteria (Figures 4.105 and 4.106)

- Humerus and radius/ulna should form a 90° angle.
- Epicondyles should be superimposed.

Tip It is essential that the elbow be flexed 90° because this gives the best visualization of fat pads, which offer clues to possible elbow fractures.

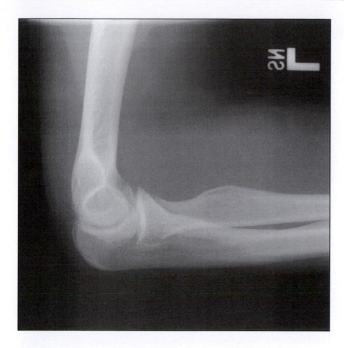

FIGURE 4.105 Lateral elbow.

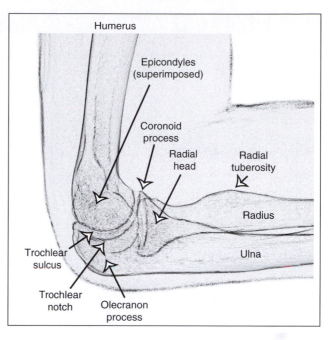

FIGURE 4.106 Lateral elbow.

ELBOW—TRAUMA AP PROJECTIONS: PARTIAL FLEXION

Exam Rationale   These positions are used when injuries to the elbow do not allow the patient to fully extend the elbow joint for the routine AP. Structures demonstrated on the radiograph include the elbow joint space, proximal radius/ulna, and distal humerus.

Technical Considerations

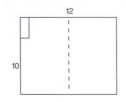

- Extremity screen/film
- Non-grid
- kVp range: 65–70
- SID: 40 inch (100 cm)

Radiation Protection

Patient Position   Seated at the end of the radiographic table with all potential artifacts removed from the part.

Part Position   The elbow is maintained in whatever degree of flexion comfortable for the patient.

- First AP: place the elbow so that the forearm is parallel to the cassette (Figure 4.107).
- Second AP: place the elbow so that the humerus is parallel to the cassette (Figure 4.108).

Central Ray   Perpendicular to the elbow joint.

Patient Instructions   "Breathe normally but don't move."

Evaluation Criteria (Figures 4.109 through 4.112)

- Rotation of the epicondyles is minimal.
- Structures of the proximal radius/ulna should be best visualized on the AP with the forearm parallel to the film.
- Structures of the distal humerus should be best visualized on the AP with the humerus parallel to the film.

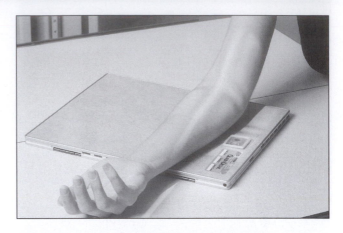

FIGURE 4.107   Trauma AP elbow, partial flexion.

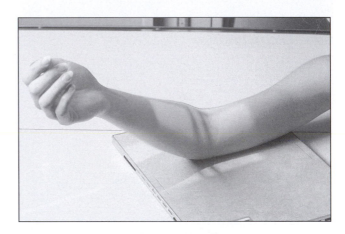

FIGURE 4.108   Trauma AP elbow, partial flexion.

Tip   Trauma AP radiographs demonstrate similar structures as the routine AP; however, their radiographic appearance will be more distorted.

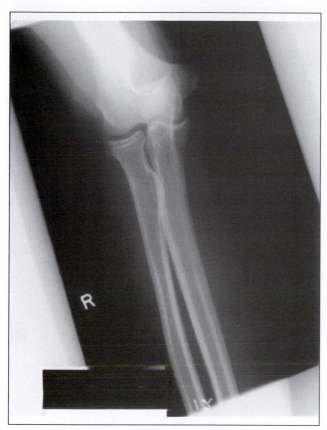

FIGURE 4.109   Trauma AP elbow, partial flexion.

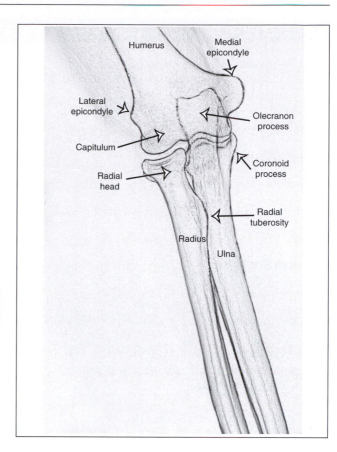

FIGURE 4.111   Trauma AP elbow, partial flexion.

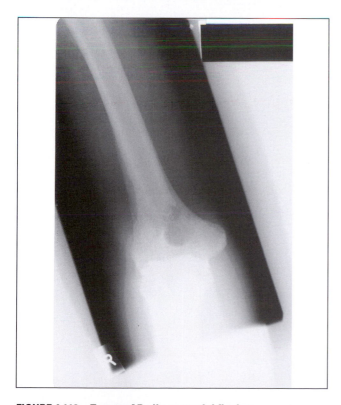

FIGURE 4.110   Trauma AP elbow, partial flexion.

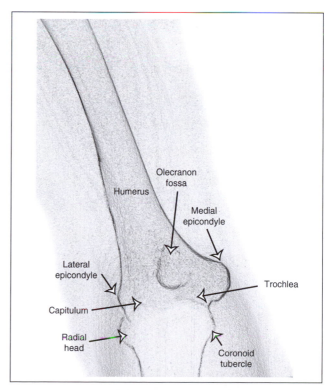

FIGURE 4.112   Trauma AP elbow, partial flexion.

ELBOW—ACUTE FLEXION POSITION

Exam Rationale This position is used primarily to demonstrate injuries to the olecranon process. Structures demonstrated on the radiograph include the olecranon process, proximal radius/ulna, and humeral epicondyles.

Technical Considerations

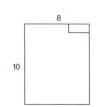

- Extremity screen/film
- Non-grid
- kVp range: 65–70
- SID: 40 inch (100 cm)

Radiation Protection

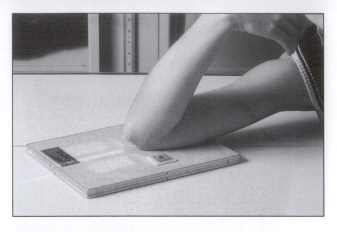

FIGURE 4.113   Acute flexion elbow.

Patient Position Seated at the end of the radiographic table with all potential artifacts removed from the part (Figure 4.113).

Part Position Rest the posterior surface of the humerus on the cassette so that the humerus is parallel to the film; flex the elbow as much as possible; the epicondylar plane line should be parallel to the film.

Central Ray Perpendicular to the film and centered to the epicondyles.

Patient Instructions "Breathe normally but don't move."

Evaluation Criteria (Figures 4.114 and 4.115)

- Distal humerus and proximal radius/ulna should be superimposed.
- Epicondyles and olecranon process should be visualized in profile.

Tip Some department protocols call for 15° to 25° tube angulation toward the shoulder.

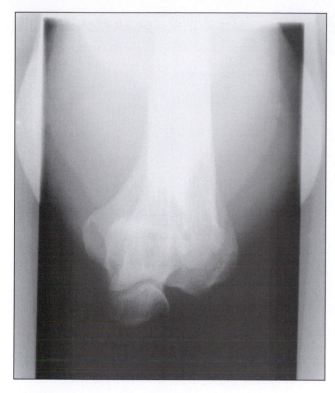

FIGURE 4.114   Acute flexion elbow.

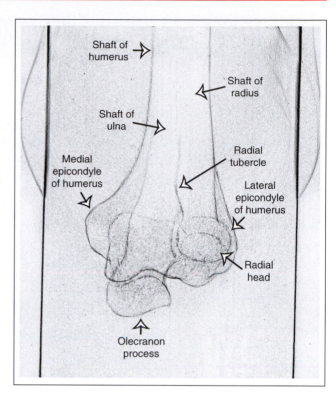

FIGURE 4.115   Acute flexion elbow.

ELBOW—RADIAL HEAD/CORONOID PROCESS POSITIONS (COYLE METHOD)

Exam Rationale These positions are used when injuries to the elbow do not allow the patient to extend the elbow joint for routine obliques. With the central ray angled toward the shoulder, the coronoid process is demonstrated in profile. With the central ray angled away from the shoulder, the radial tuberosity, head, and neck are demonstrated relatively free of superimposition.

Technical Considerations

- Extremity screen/film
- Non-grid
- kVp range: 65–70
- SID: 40 inch (100 cm)

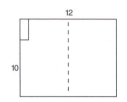

Radiation Protection

Patient Position Seated at the end of the radiographic table with all potential artifacts removed from the part.

Part Position The elbow is maintained in whatever degree of flexion is comfortable for the patient, usually 80° to 90°; rest the medial surface of the forearm and humerus on the cassette and place the epicondylar plane as close to perpendicular as possible.

Central Ray Directed to the joint space at a 45° angle.

- *Toward* the shoulder to demonstrate the radial head (Figure 4.116).
- *Away* from the shoulder to demonstrate the coronoid process (Figure 4.117).

Patient Instructions "Breathe normally but don't move."

Evaluation Criteria (Figures 4.118 through 4.121)

- With central ray *toward* the shoulder, the radius and ulna should be substantially superimposed with the coronoid process visualized in profile.
- With central ray *away* from the shoulder, the radius and ulna should be free from superimposition with the radial tuberosity, head, and neck clearly demonstrated.

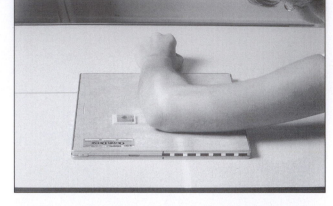

FIGURE 4.116 Trauma oblique elbow, for radial head.

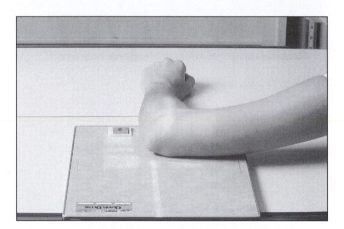

FIGURE 4.117 Trauma oblique elbow, for coronoid process.

Tips

1. These obliques are sometimes called the Coyle trauma positions.
2. Oblique trauma radiographs demonstrate the same structures as routine obliques; however, the radiographic appearance of the structures is more distorted due to the tube angulation.

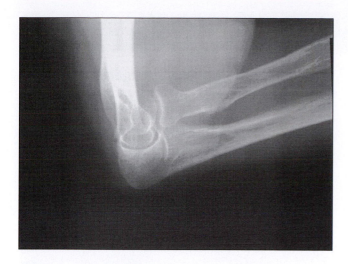

FIGURE 4.118   Trauma oblique elbow, for radial head.

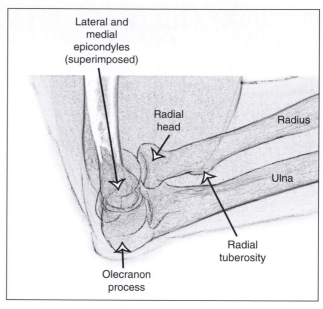

FIGURE 4.120   Trauma oblique elbow, for radial head.

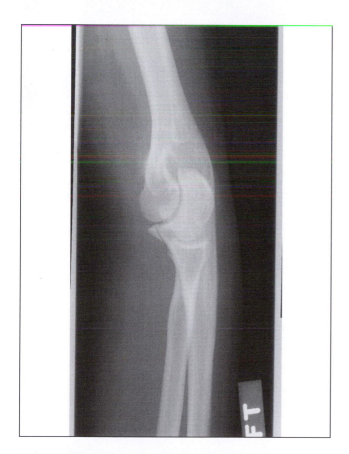

FIGURE 4.119   Trauma oblique elbow, for coronoid process.

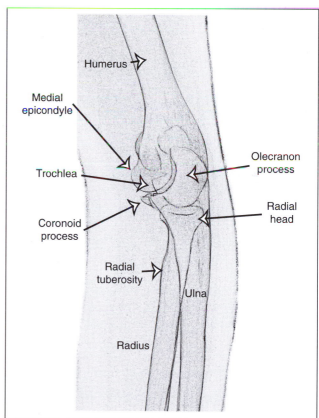

FIGURE 4.121   Trauma oblique elbow, for coronoid process.

ELBOW—RADIAL HEAD/LATEROMEDIAL ROTATION PROJECTIONS

Exam Rationale   These lateral positions of the radial head are taken primarily to demonstrate trauma to this region. Fractures of the radial head are often occult and special means are required to visualize them.

Technical Considerations

- Extremity screen/film
- Non-grid
- kVp range: 65–70
- SID: 40 inch (100 cm)

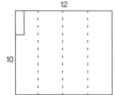

Radiation Protection

Patient Position   Seated at the end of the radiographic table with all potential artifacts removed from the part.

Part Position   Place the forearm and humerus flat on film, parallel to the cassette; flex the elbow 90° into a true lateral position with the epicondylar line perpendicular to the film. Four films are taken varying the position of the hand as follows:

1. Hand supinated as much as possible (Figure 4.122).
2. Hand in true lateral (Figure 4.123).
3. Hand pronated with palm flat on table (Figure 4.124).
4. Hand internally rotated with the thumb side of the hand resting on the table (Figure 4.125).

Central Ray   Perpendicular to the elbow joint.

Patient Instructions   "Breathe normally but don't move."

Evaluation Criteria (Figures 4.126 through 4.129)

- Humerus and radius/ulna should form a 90° angle.
- Epicondyles should be superimposed.
- Radial head should be seen in profile.
- Position of the radial tuberosity should vary between views.

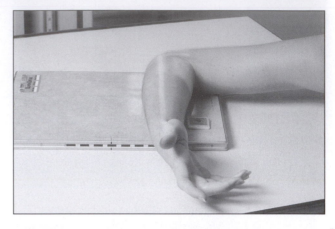

FIGURE 4.122   Radial head: hand supinated.

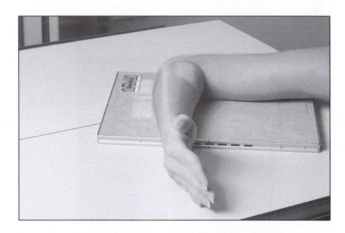

FIGURE 4.123   Radial head: hand in lateral position.

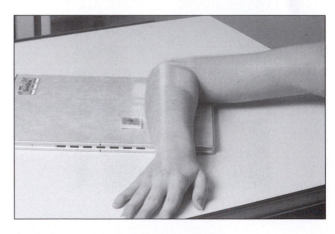

FIGURE 4.124   Radial head: hand pronated.

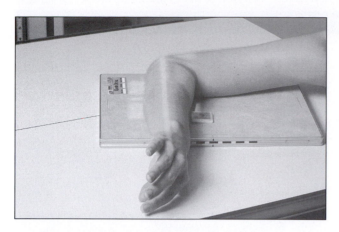

FIGURE 4.125   Radial head: hand internally rotated.

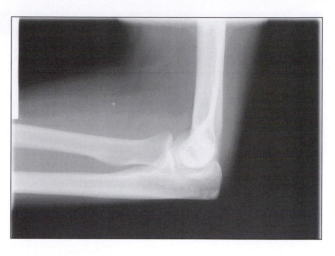

FIGURE 4.128   Radial head: hand pronated.

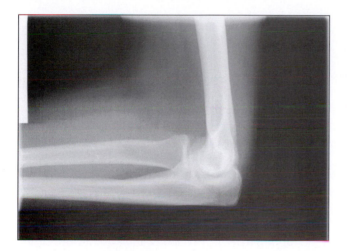

FIGURE 4.126   Radial head: hand supinated.

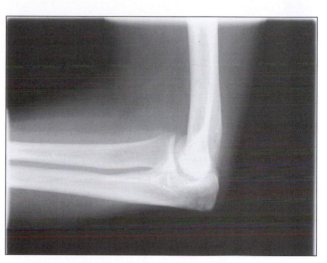

FIGURE 4.129   Radial head: hand internally rotated.

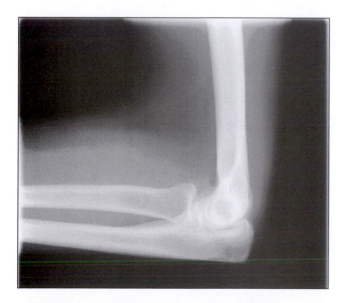

FIGURE 4.127   Radial head: hand in lateral position.

HUMERUS—AP PROJECTION

Exam Rationale   The most common indication for humerus examinations is trauma. Bony tumors and cysts are occasionally visualized on long bones such as the humerus. Structures demonstrated on the radiograph include the entire humerus and a portion of the elbow and shoulder joints.

Technical Considerations

- Screen/film
- Grid
- kVp range: 70–80
- SID: 40 inch (100 cm)

Radiation Protection

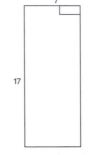

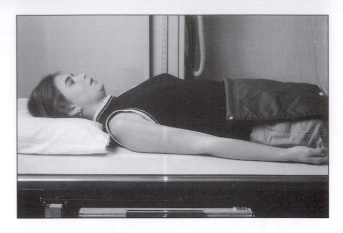

FIGURE 4.130   AP humerus.

Patient Position   Supine or upright, depending on patient condition, with the posterior surface of the body against the cassette; all potential artifacts removed from the part (Figure 4.130).

Part Position   Fully extend the elbow and place the epicondylar line parallel to the film; align the long axis of the humerus to the long axis of the film, being certain to include 1/2 to 1 inch (1–3 cm) of both joints; the patient may be turned slightly toward the affected side to reduce object-film distance.

Central Ray   Perpendicular to the midshaft.

Patient Instructions   "Breathe normally but don't move."

Evaluation Criteria (Figures 4.131 and 4.132)

- Both elbow and shoulder joints should be included.
- Greater tubercle should be demonstrated in profile on the lateral aspect of the humerus.

Tips

1. For parts measuring less than 12 cm, this projection can be done without a grid.
2. If acute trauma is evident or suspected, the AP is taken in whatever position the arm is presented. Do not attempt to rotate the arm of a patient with injuries to the humerus.
3. If both elbow and shoulder joints cannot be demonstrated on a single film, a separate AP of one joint should be done.
4. Some department protocols allow follow-up radiographs to include only the joint closest to the site of injury.

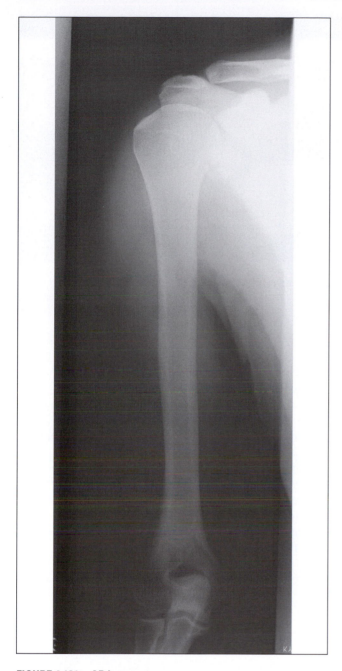

FIGURE 4.131   AP humerus.

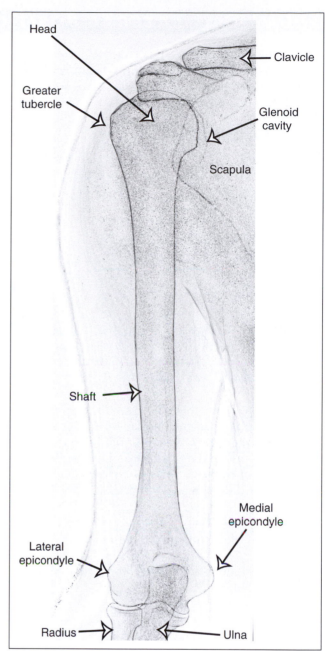

FIGURE 4.132   AP humerus.

HUMERUS—LATERAL POSITION

Exam Rationale   The lateral is one of two routine positions of the humerus. Structures demonstrated on the radiograph include the entire humerus and a portion of the elbow and shoulder joints.

Technical Considerations

- Screen/film
- Grid
- kVp range: 70–80
- SID: 40 inch (100 cm)

Radiation Protection

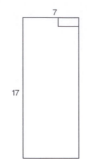

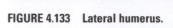

FIGURE 4.133   Lateral humerus.

Patient Position   Supine or upright, depending on patient condition, with the posterior surface of the body against the cassette; all potential artifacts removed from the part (Figure 4.133).

Part Position   Flex the elbow and rotate the arm medially to place the epicondylar line perpendicular to the film; align the long axis of the humerus to the long axis of the film, being certain to include 1/2 to 1 inch of both joints; the patient may be turned slightly toward the affected side to reduce object-film distance.

Central Ray   Perpendicular to the midshaft.

Patient Instructions   "Breathe normally but don't move."

Evaluation Criteria (Figures 4.134 and 4.135)

- Both elbow and shoulder joints should be included.
- Epicondyles should be superimposed.
- Lesser tubercle should be demonstrated in profile on the medial aspect of the humerus.

Tips

1. For parts measuring less than 12 cm, this projection can be done without a grid.
2. If acute trauma is evident or suspected, the trauma lateral or transthoracic lateral should be substituted. Do not attempt to rotate the arm of a patient with injuries to the humerus.
3. If both elbow and shoulder joints cannot be demonstrated on a single film, a separate lateral of one joint should be done.
4. Some department protocols allow follow-up radiographs to include only the joint closest to the site of injury.

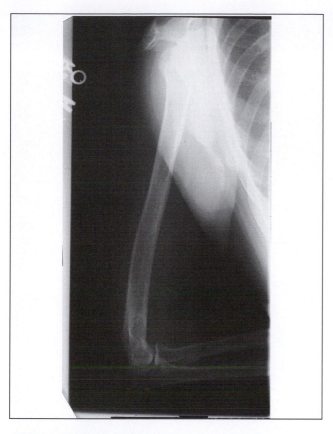

FIGURE 4.134   Lateral humerus.

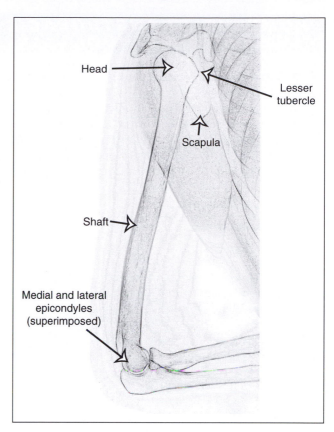

FIGURE 4.135   Lateral humerus.

HUMERUS—TRANSTHORACIC LATERAL POSITION (LAWRENCE METHOD)

Exam Rationale The transthoracic lateral is an alternate position taken primarily in cases of acute trauma to the upper arm or shoulder or when the patient is otherwise unable to rotate the arm. Structures demonstrated on the radiograph include the head and shaft of the humerus in a lateral perspective, superimposed on rib and lung anatomy.

Technical Considerations

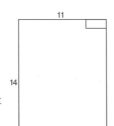

- Screen/film
- Grid
- kVp range: 70–80
- SID: 40 inch (100 cm)
- Long exposure time (see Patient Instructions below)

Radiation Protection

AEC (Phototiming)

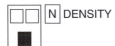 N DENSITY

Patient Position Upright with affected arm against film holder; all potential artifacts removed from the part (Figure 4.136).

Part Position The affected arm is maintained in a neutral position; the top of the film should be placed 1 inch (3 cm) above the top of the affected shoulder; the opposite arm is raised over the head, elevating the unaffected shoulder as much as possible.

Central Ray Horizontal and perpendicular to the film, directed to exit at the midshaft of the affected humerus.

Patient Instructions "Breathe normally but don't move." The patient is allowed to continue normal breathing during the exposure because this will blur thorax shadows, which frequently obscure bony detail.

Evaluation Criteria (Figures 4.137 and 4.138)

- Proximal two-thirds of the humerus and the relationship of the humeral head to the glenohumeral joint should be demonstrated.

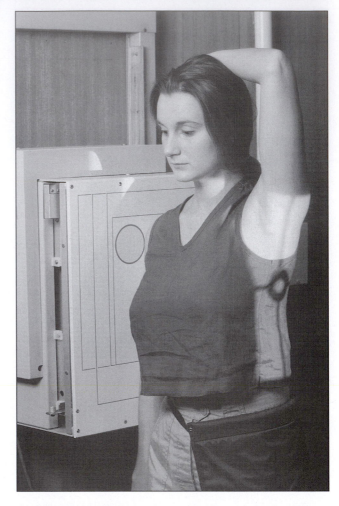

FIGURE 4.136 Trauma lateral humerus.

Tips

1. For parts measuring less than 12 cm, this projection can be done without a grid.
2. Although the collimator light appears very small on the unaffected side, the beam diverges as it travels through the patient. This causes many radiographers to open the collimator too wide for this position. It is best to set the size of the collimator opening to slightly smaller than 11 × 14 inches (28 × 36 cm) before positioning the patient.
3. If only the shoulder is affected, a 10 × 12 inch (25 × 30 cm) film may be substituted and the central ray raised accordingly.

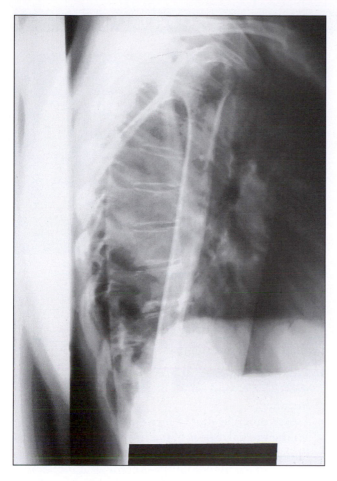

FIGURE 4.137   Trauma lateral humerus.

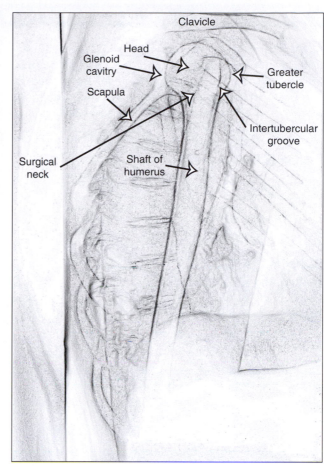

FIGURE 4.138   Trauma lateral humerus.

4. A 15° cephalad angle can be used to prevent super-imposition of the shoulders if the patient is unable to raise the unaffected arm high over the head.

5. An exposure time of at least 2 seconds is needed to accommodate the breathing technique.

6. This projection may be done in the supine position or with the patient seated in a wheelchair.

SHOULDER—AP PROJECTION: INTERNAL ROTATION

Exam Rationale　Indications for shoulder examinations are numerous and include fracture, dislocation, bursitis, tendon or ligament damage, bony tumors, and cysts. Structures demonstrated on the radiograph include the proximal humerus and most of the clavicle and scapula.

Technical Considerations

- Regular screen/film
- Grid:
- kVp range: 70–80
- SID: 40 inch (100 cm)

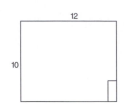

Radiation Protection　AEC (Phototiming)

 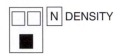 N DENSITY

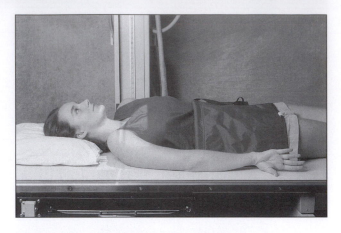

FIGURE 4.139　**AP shoulder, internal rotation.**

Patient Position　Supine or upright, depending on patient condition, with the posterior surface of the body against the cassette; all potential artifacts removed from the part (Figure 4.139).

Part Position　Place the affected arm by the patient's side with the back of the hand resting on the thigh to place the intercondylar line perpendicular to the film.

Central Ray　Perpendicular to the coracoid process.

Patient Instructions　"Take in a breath and hold it. Don't breathe or move."

Evaluation Criteria (Figures 4.140 and 4.141)

- Proximal humerus, at least the distal two-thirds of the clavicle, and most of the scapula should be included.
- Lesser tubercle should be demonstrated in profile on the medial aspect of the humerus.
- Humeral head should be slightly more superimposed on the glenoid fossa as compared to the neutral position.

Tip　The internal rotation should never be done if acute trauma is evident or suspected.

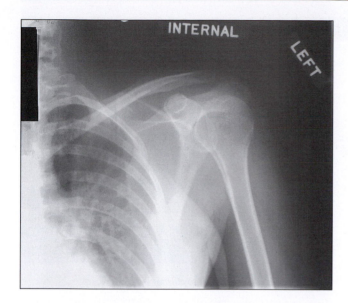

FIGURE 4.140   AP shoulder, internal rotation.

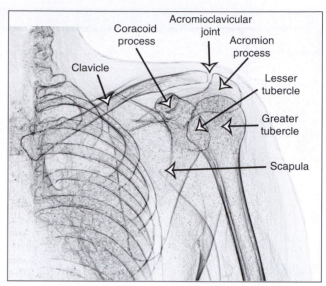

FIGURE 4.141   AP shoulder, internal rotation.

SHOULDER—AP PROJECTION: EXTERNAL ROTATION

Exam Rationale Indications for shoulder examinations are numerous and include fracture, dislocation, bursitis, tendon or ligament damage, bony tumors, and cysts. Structures demonstrated on the radiograph include the proximal humerus and most of the clavicle and scapula.

Technical Considerations

- Regular screen/film
- Grid:
- kVp range: 70–80
- SID: 40 inch (100 cm)

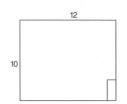

Radiation	AEC
Protection	**(Phototiming)**

 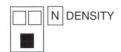 N DENSITY

Patient Position Supine or upright, depending on patient condition, with the posterior surface of the body against the cassette; all potential artifacts removed from the part (Figure 4.142).

Part Position Place the affected arm by the patient's side with the hand supinated to place the intercondylar line parallel to the film.

Central Ray Perpendicular to the coracoid process.

Patient Instructions "Take in a breath and hold it. Don't breathe or move."

Evaluation Criteria (Figures 4.143 and 4.144)

- Proximal humerus, at least the distal two-thirds of the clavicle, and most of the scapula should be demonstrated.
- Greater tubercle should be demonstrated in profile on the lateral aspect of the humerus.
- Humeral head should be slightly superimposed on the glenoid fossa.

Tip The external rotation should never be done if acute trauma is evident or suspected.

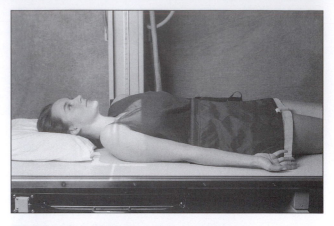

FIGURE 4.142   AP shoulder, external rotation.

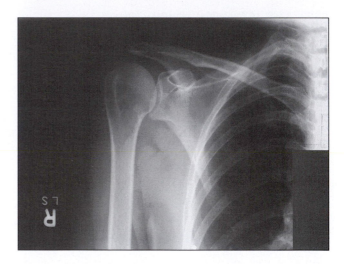

FIGURE 4.143   AP shoulder, external rotation.

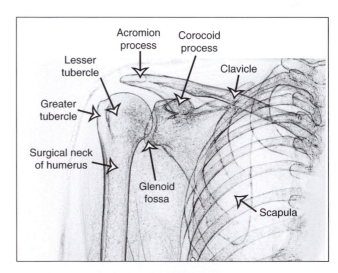

FIGURE 4.144   AP shoulder, external rotation.

SHOULDER—AP PROJECTION: NEUTRAL ROTATION

Exam Rationale   Indications for shoulder examinations are numerous and include fracture, dislocation, bursitis, tendon or ligament damage, bony tumors, and cysts. Structures demonstrated on the radiograph include the proximal humerus and most of the clavicle and scapula.

Technical Considerations

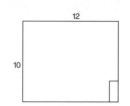

- Regular screen/film
- Grid:
- kVp range: 70–80
- SID: 40 inch (100 cm)

Radiation   AEC
Protection   (Phototiming)

 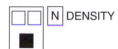

Patient Position   Supine or upright, depending on patient condition, with the posterior surface of the body against the cassette; all potential artifacts removed from the part (Figure 4.145).

Part Position   Place the affected arm by the patient's side with the palm resting on the thigh.

Central Ray   Perpendicular to the coracoid process.

Patient Instructions   "Take in a breath and hold it. Don't breathe or move."

Evaluation Criteria (Figures 4.146 and 4.147)

- Proximal humerus, at least the distal two-thirds of the clavicle, and most of the scapula should be demonstrated.
- Humeral head should be slightly superimposed on the glenoid fossa.
- Neither the greater nor lesser tubercle should appear in profile.

Tip   The neutral position is generally used with trauma patients because the arm should not be rotated in cases of acute injury.

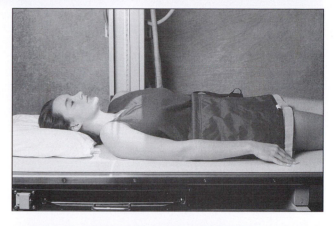

FIGURE 4.145   **AP shoulder, neutral rotation.**

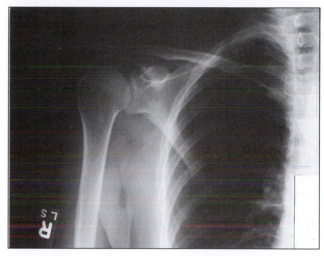

FIGURE 4.146   **AP shoulder, neutral rotation.**

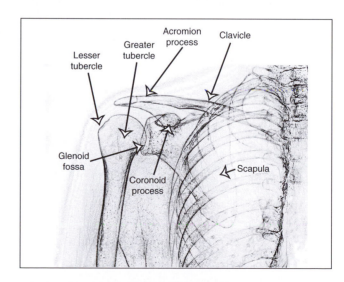

FIGURE 4.147   **AP shoulder, neutral rotation.**

SHOULDER—INFEROSUPERIOR AXIAL PROJECTION (LAWRENCE METHOD)

Exam Rationale The inferosuperior axial projection is used primarily to obtain a lateral view of the proximal humerus and its relationship to the glenoid fossa. Structures demonstrated on the radiograph include the glenoid fossa and the proximal humerus.

Technical Considerations

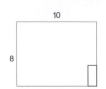

- Regular screen/film
- Grid or non-grid
- kVp range: 70–80
- SID: 40 inch (100 cm)

Radiation Protection

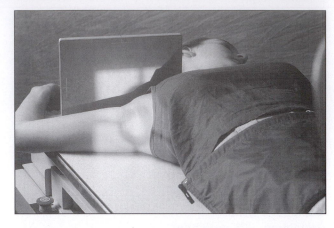

FIGURE 4.148   Inferosuperior, axial shoulder: Lawrence method.

Patient Position Supine with all potential artifacts removed from the part (Figure 4.148).

Part Position Place the cassette perpendicular to the table, as close to neck as possible; adduct the affected arm 90° from the body; turn the patient's head away from the affected shoulder; a nonopaque sponge may be placed under the affected shoulder to center the part to the film.

Central Ray Horizontal, directed through the axilla to exit at the acromioclavicular joint at the midpoint of film.

Patient Instructions "Take in a breath and hold it. Don't breathe or move."

Evaluation Criteria (Figures 4.149 and 4.150)

- Lesser tubercle should be visualized in profile superiorly.
- Glenohumeral joint should be clearly demonstrated.

Tips

1. A similar radiograph may be obtained with a superoinferior axial projection.
2. It is desirable to keep the beam as close to perpendicular to the film as possible; however, a 15° to 20° medial angulation may be necessary to align the tube, part, and film accurately.

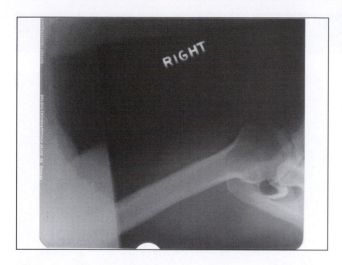

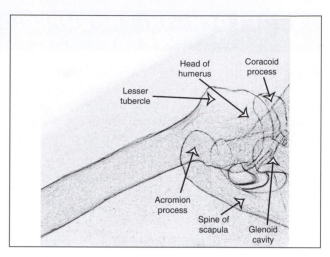

FIGURE 4.149 Inferosuperior, axial shoulder: Lawrence method.

FIGURE 4.150 Inferosuperior, axial shoulder: Lawrence method.

SHOULDER—INFEROSUPERIOR AXIAL PROJECTION (WEST POINT METHOD)

Exam Rationale The inferosuperior axial projection is used primarily to obtain a lateral view of the proximal humerus and its relationship to the glenoid fossa. Structures demonstrated on the radiograph include the glenoid fossa and the proximal humerus.

Technical Considerations

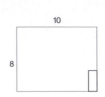

- Regular screen/film
- Grid or non-grid
- kVp range: 70–80
- SID: 40 inch (100 cm)

Radiation Protection

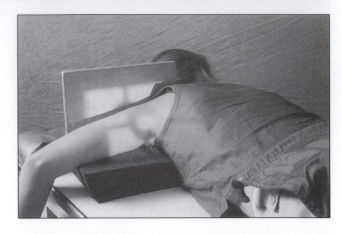

FIGURE 4.151   Inferosuperior, axial shoulder: West Point method.

Patient Position Prone with all potential artifacts removed from the part (Figure 4.151).

Part Position Place the cassette perpendicular to the table, as close to neck as possible; adduct the affected arm 90° from the body; turn the patient's head away from the affected shoulder; a nonopaque sponge may be placed under the affected shoulder to center the part to the film.

Central Ray Angled 25° up from horizontal and 25° medially, directed to exit at the acromioclavicular joint at the midpoint of film.

Patient Instructions "Take in a breath and hold it. Don't breathe or move."

Evaluation Criteria (Figures 4.152 and 4.153)

- Lesser tubercle should be visualized in profile superiorly.
- Coracoid process should not be superimposed on the humeral head.
- Glenohumeral joint should be clearly demonstrated.

Tip If the patient cannot assume a prone position, the Clements modification may be performed. The patient is placed in a lateral position with the affected side up. The affected arm is placed 90° from the body. The central ray is directed horizontally and may be angled 5° to 15° medially for patients who cannot adduct the arm 90° (Figure 4.154).

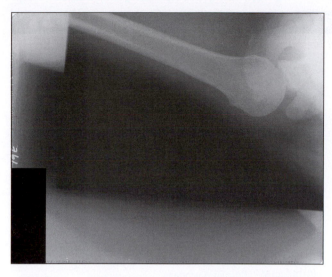

FIGURE 4.152 Inferosuperior, axial shoulder: West Point method.

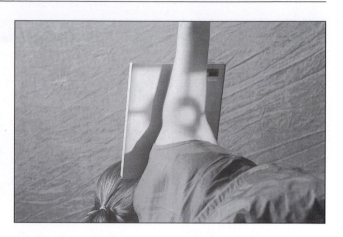

FIGURE 4.154 Superoinferior, axial shoulder.

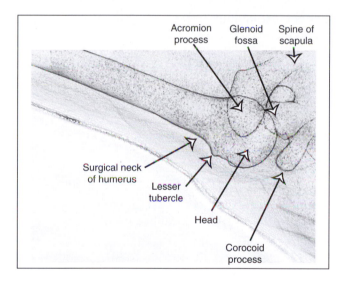

FIGURE 4.153 Inferosuperior, axial shoulder: West Point method.

SHOULDER—AP AXIAL PROJECTION: CORACOID PROCESS

Exam Rationale   This alternate projection is used to demonstrate the coracoid process. Because this anatomic structure projects anteriorly it is not well demonstrated on conventional AP projections of the shoulder.

Technical Considerations

- Regular screen/film
- Grid:
- kVp range: 70–80
- SID: 40 inch (100 cm)

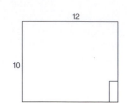

Radiation Protection   **AEC (Phototiming)**

 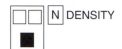 N DENSITY

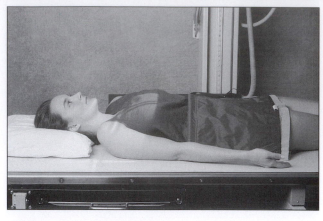

FIGURE 4.155   Coracoid process.

Patient Position   Supine or upright, depending on patient condition, with the posterior surface of the body against the cassette; all potential artifacts removed from the part (Figure 4.155).

Part Position   Place the arm by the patient's side with the hand supinated and resting on the table; patient may be turned slightly toward the affected side to reduce object film distance.

Central Ray   Angled 30° cephalad and directed to the coracoid process.

Patient Instructions   "Take in a breath and hold it. Don't breathe or move."

Evaluation Criteria (Figures 4.156 and 4.157)

- Coracoid process should appear elongated and slightly superimposed on the distal clavicle.
- Proximal humerus and the distal one-third of the clavicle should be demonstrated.

Tip   The tube angle varies according to patient size. Larger patients may require a 45° tube angle to elongate the coracoid process, whereas small patients may require as little as 15° tube angulation.

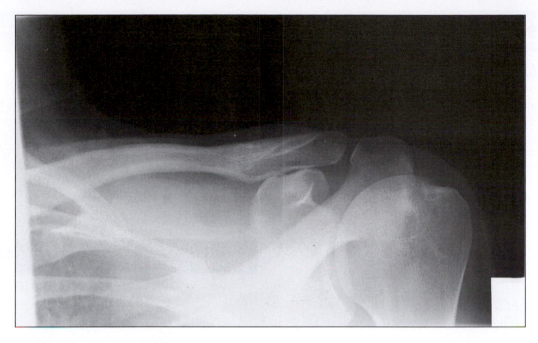

FIGURE 4.156   **Coracoid process.**

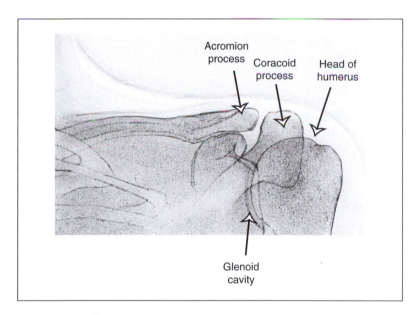

FIGURE 4.157   **Coracoid process.**

SHOULDER—GLENOID CAVITY POSITION (GRASHEY METHOD)

Exam Rationale   The Grashey position is an alternate view of the shoulder that is taken primarily to demonstrate possible dislocations of the head of the humerus. Structures demonstrated on the radiograph include the proximal humerus, a portion of the clavicle and scapula, and the glenoid fossa free from superimposition from the humeral head.

Technical Considerations

- Regular screen/film
- Grid:
- kVp range: 70–80
- SID: 40 inch (100 cm)

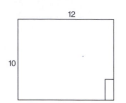

Radiation Protection

AEC (Phototiming)

 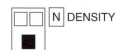 N DENSITY

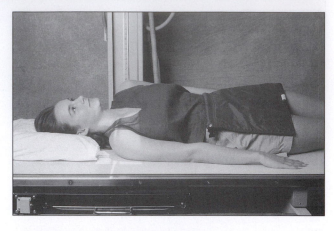

FIGURE 4.158   Shoulder, glenoid cavity.

Patient Position   Supine or upright, depending on patient condition, with the posterior surface of the body against the cassette; all potential artifacts removed from the part (Figure 4.158).

Part Position   Place the affected arm by the patient's side in a neutral position or rest the forearm on the chest; turn patient 35° to 45° toward the affected side to place the scapula parallel to the film (LPO for injuries to the left side and RPO for injuries to the right side).

Central Ray   Perpendicular to the glenohumeral joint space, 1 to 2 inches lateral to the coracoid process.

Patient Instructions   "Take in a breath and hold it. Don't breathe or move."

Evaluation Criteria (Figures 4.159 and 4.160)

- Glenoid fossa should be visualized free from superimposition of the humeral head.

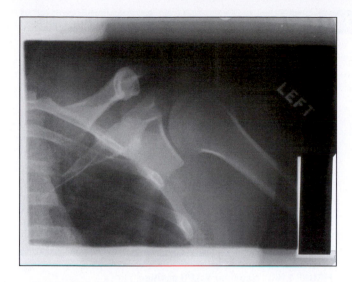

FIGURE 4.159   Shoulder, glenoid cavity.

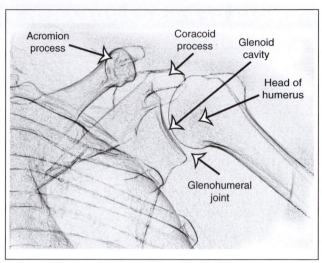

FIGURE 4.160   Shoulder, glenoid cavity.

SHOULDER—SCAPULAR Y POSITION

Exam Rationale   The scapular Y is an alternate view of the shoulder used primarily with trauma patients to demonstrate possible dislocations of the head of the humerus. Structures demonstrated on the radiograph include the glenoid cavity, humeral head, and most of the scapula.

Technical Considerations

- Regular screen/film
- Grid:
- kVp range: 70–80
- SID: 40 inch (100 cm)

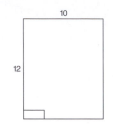

Radiation Protection

AEC (Phototiming)

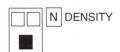

N DENSITY

Patient Position   Supine or upright, depending on patient condition, with the posterior surface of the body against the cassette; all potential artifacts removed from the part (Figure 4.161).

Part Position   Place the affected arm by the patient's side in a neutral position; turn the patient 30° away from the affected side (LPO for injuries to the right side and RPO for injuries to the left side).

Central Ray   Perpendicular to the glenohumeral joint, 2 to 3 inches below the acromion process.

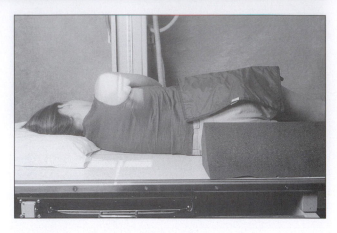

FIGURE 4.161   Scapular Y, LPO position.

Patient Instructions   "Take in a breath and hold it. Don't breathe or move."

Evaluation Criteria (Figures 4.162 and 4.163)

- Scapula should be in truly lateral position, free from rib superimposition.
- Shaft of the humerus should be superimposed on the body of the scapula.

Tip   If patient condition allows, anterior obliques may be done upright to achieve less object-film distance. With the patient facing the film, rotate the patient into a 60° anterior oblique (30° from lateral). The RAO is used for injuries to the right side, and the LAO for injuries to the left side (Figure 4.164).

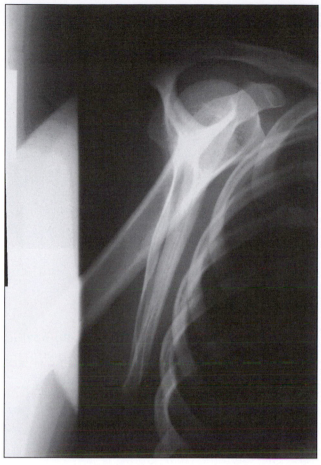

FIGURE 4.162   Scapular Y.

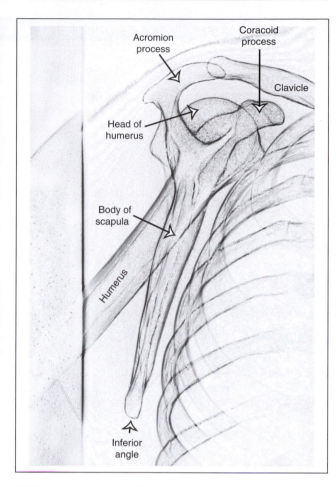

FIGURE 4.163   Scapular Y.

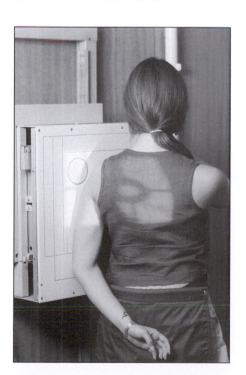

FIGURE 4.164
Scapular Y, LAO position.

SHOULDER—INTERTUBERCULAR GROOVE POSITION

Exam Rationale This alternate position is performed to examine the intertubercular groove that lies on the anterior surface of the humerus between the greater and lesser tubercles.

Technical Considerations

- Regular screen/film
- Grid or non-grid
- kVp range: 70–80
- SID: 40 inch (100 cm)

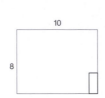

Radiation Protection

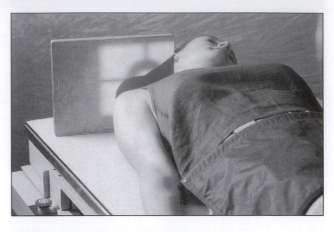

FIGURE 4.165 Intertubercular groove.

Patient Position Supine with all potential artifacts removed from the part (Figure 4.165).

Part Position Place the affected arm by the patient's side with the palm up; turn the patient's head away from the affected shoulder and place the cassette perpendicular on the table, as close to neck as possible; a nonopaque sponge may be placed under the affected shoulder to align the tube, part, and film accurately.

Central Ray Directed through the intertubercular groove, angled 15° posterior to the long axis of the humeral shaft.

Patient Instructions "Take in a breath and hold it. Don't breathe or move."

Evaluation Criteria (Figures 4.166 and 4.167)

- Intertubercular groove should be visualized in profile superiorly.

Tip The intertubercular groove is also called the bicipital groove.

FIGURE 4.166 Intertubercular groove.

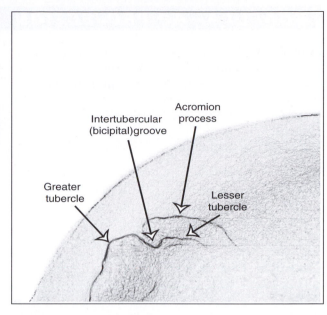

FIGURE 4.167 Intertubercular groove.

SCAPULA—AP PROJECTION

Exam Rationale   The most common indication for scapula examinations is trauma. Structures demonstrated on the radiograph include the scapular body, acromion process, glenoid fossa, and the scapular spine, mostly superimposed on the ribs and lungs.

Technical Considerations

- Regular screen/film
- Grid:
- kVp range: 70–80
- SID: 40 inch (100 cm)

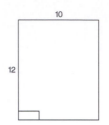

Radiation Protection

AEC (Phototiming)

 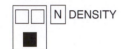 N DENSITY

Patient Position   Supine or upright, depending on patient condition, with the posterior surface of the body against the cassette; all potential artifacts removed from the part (Figure 4.168).

Part Position   With the elbow flexed, adduct the arm 90° from the body to place the scapula in better contact with the table; the top of the film is placed 1 to 2 inches above the acromion process.

Central Ray   Perpendicular to the midscapula, 1 to 2 inches inferior to the coracoid process.

Patient Instructions   "Breathe normally but don't move." The patient is allowed to continue normal breathing during the exposure because this will blur thorax shadows, which frequently obscure bony detail.

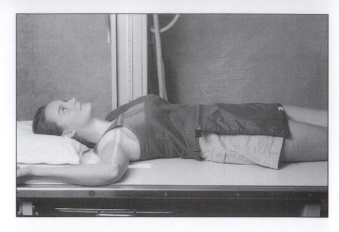

FIGURE 4.168   AP scapula.

Evaluation Criteria (Figures 4.169 and 4.170)

- Entire scapula must be included.
- Most of the scapula should be superimposed over the lung and ribs.
- Lateral border of the scapula should be mostly free from superimposing rib and lung anatomy.

Tip   In cases of acute trauma, the arm is kept in a neutral position and the patient may be turned slightly toward the affected side to place the scapula flat on the table.

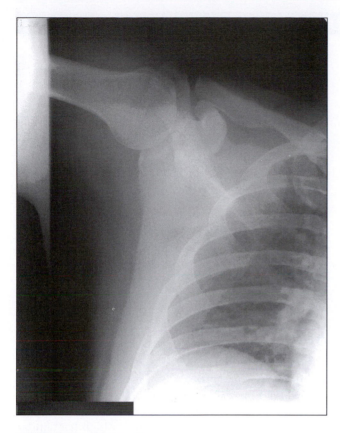

FIGURE 4.169 AP scapula.

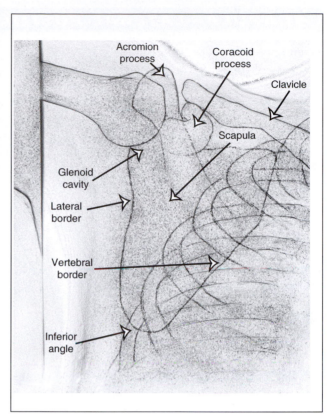

FIGURE 4.170 AP scapula.

SCAPULA—LATERAL POSITION

Exam Rationale   The lateral is one of two routine positions of the scapula. Structures demonstrated on the radiograph include the coracoid process, acromion process, and the body of the scapula in a lateral perspective, free from superimposing rib and lung anatomy.

Technical Considerations

- Regular screen/film
- Grid:
- kVp range: 70–80
- SID: 40 inch (100 cm)

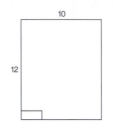

Radiation Protection

AEC (Phototiming)

   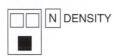 N DENSITY

Patient Position   Recumbent or upright, depending on patient condition; all potential artifacts removed from the part (Figure 4.171).

Part Position   Start from the supine position and have the patient reach across the chest and grasp the unaffected shoulder; rotate the patient 30° away from the affected side (LPO for injuries to the right side and RPO for injuries to the left side); adjust the patient's obliquity to place the scapula perpendicular to the film; the top of the film is placed 1 to 2 inches above the acromion process.

Central Ray   Perpendicular to the midscapula, 1 to 2 inches inferior to the coracoid process.

Patient Instructions   "Take in a breath and hold it. Don't breathe or move."

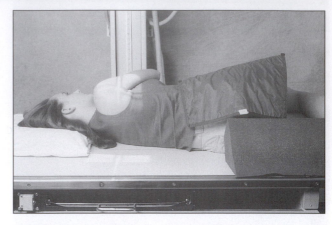

FIGURE 4.171   Lateral scapula, LPO position.

Evaluation Criteria (Figures 4.172 and 4.173)

- Entire scapula should be demonstrated free of superimposition from ribs.
- Coracoid process should be projected anteriorly.
- Acromion process should be projected posteriorly.
- Unlike the scapular Y projection, which has similar positioning, the shaft of the humerus should *not* be superimposed on the body of the scapula on the lateral scapula radiograph.

Tip   If patient condition allows, anterior obliques may be done on the upright to achieve less object-film distance. With the patient facing the film, rotate the patient into a 60° oblique (30° from lateral). The RAO is used for injuries to the right side, and the LAO for injuries to the left side (Figure 4.174).

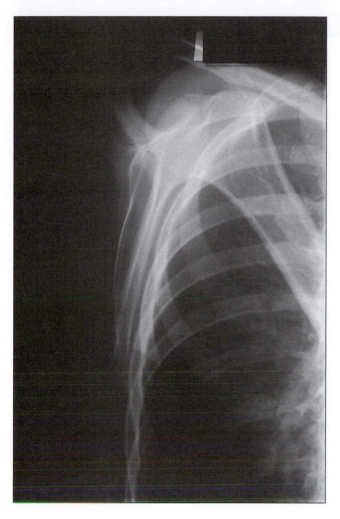

FIGURE 4.172   **Lateral scapula.**

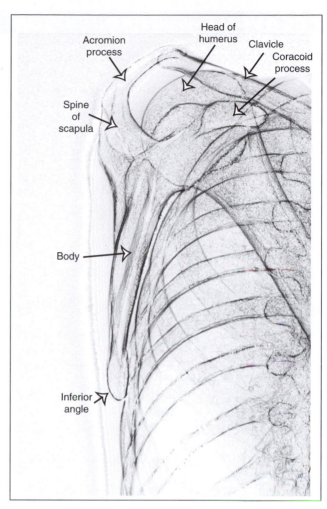

Acromion process

Head of humerus

Clavicle

Coracoid process

Spine of scapula

Body

Inferior angle

FIGURE 4.173   **Lateral scapula.**

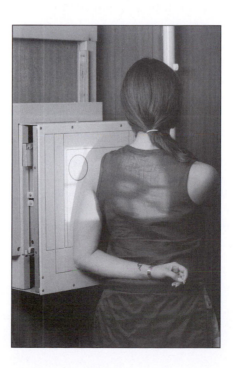

FIGURE 4.174
Lateral scapula, LAO position.

CLAVICLE—PA PROJECTION

Exam Rationale The most common indication for clavicle examinations is trauma. Structures demonstrated on the radiograph include the entire clavicle, including the acromioclavicular and sternoclavicular joints.

Technical Considerations

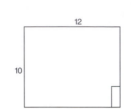

- Regular screen/film
- Grid:
- kVp range: 70–80
- SID: 40 inch (100 cm)

Radiation Protection
AEC (Phototiming)

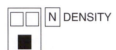 N DENSITY

Patient Position Prone or upright, depending on patient condition, with the anterior surface of the body facing the cassette; all potential artifacts, including radiopaque pillows, removed from the part (Figure 4.175).

Part Position Place the affected arm by the patient's side in a neutral position.

Central Ray Perpendicular to the midclavicle.

Patient Instructions "Take in a breath and hold it. Don't breathe or move."

Evaluation Criteria (Figures 4.176 and 4.177)

- Both acromioclavicular and sternoclavicular joints should be demonstrated.
- Proximal one-third of clavicle will be superimposed on thorax shadows.

Tip The PA axial projection is sometimes used to project more of the clavicle off the thorax shadows. The tube angle for a PA axial varies from 10° to 30° caudal, depending on department protocol and the size of the patient. Thinner patients require a larger tube angle.

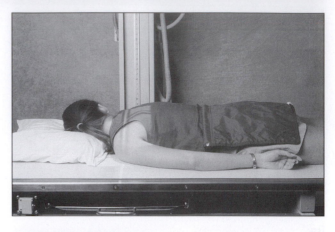

FIGURE 4.175   PA clavicle.

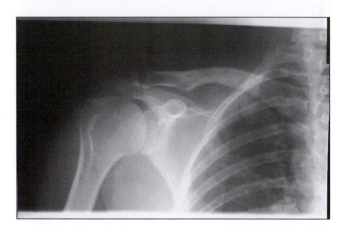

FIGURE 4.176   PA clavicle.

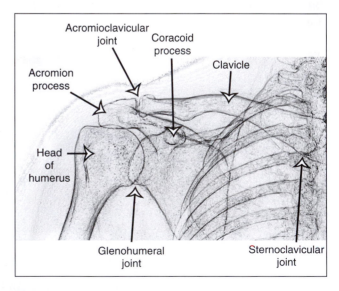

FIGURE 4.177   PA clavicle.

CLAVICLE—AP AXIAL PROJECTION

Exam Rationale The most common indication for clavicle examinations is trauma. The AP clavicle is performed when the patient cannot be placed into a prone position. Although the AP clavicle demonstrates the same structures as the PA, the AP results in more magnification of the structures of interest.

Technical Considerations

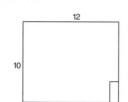

- Regular screen/film
- Grid:
- kVp range: 70–80
- SID: 40 inch (100 cm)

Radiation Protection

Patient Position Supine or upright, depending on patient condition, with the posterior surface of the body against the cassette; all potential artifacts, including radiopaque pillows, removed from the part (Figure 4.178).

Part Position Place the affected arm by the patient's side in a neutral position.

Central Ray Directed to the midclavicle at a 15° to 25° cephalad angle.

Patient Instructions "Take in a breath and hold it. Don't breathe or move."

Evaluation Criteria (Figures 4.179 and 4.180)

- Acromioclavicular and sternoclavicular joints should both be demonstrated.
- Clavicle may be superimposed on thorax shadows, depending on degree of tube angle.

Tips

1. Tube angle varies from 10° to 30° depending on department protocol and the size of the patient. Thinner patients require a larger tube angle.
2. Greater tube angles project the clavicle away from rib and thorax superimposition, although these angles also create more image distortion.

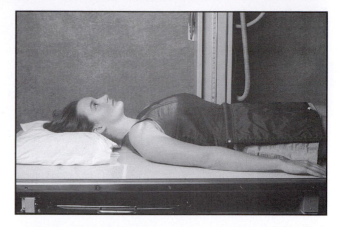

FIGURE 4.178 AP clavicle.

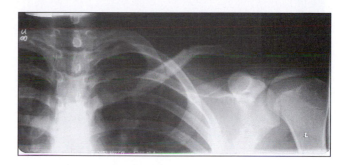

FIGURE 4.179 AP clavicle.

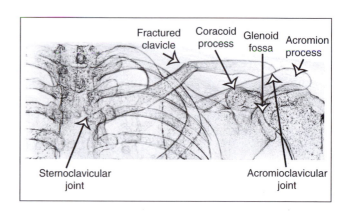

FIGURE 4.180 AP clavicle.

CLAVICLE—TANGENTIAL POSITION (TARRANT METHOD)

Exam Rationale The tangential position is used primarily for patients who cannot assume positions required for conventional AP or PA radiographs. The tangential position demonstrates the entire clavicle, although the bone will appear distorted due to large object-film distance.

Technical Considerations

- Regular screen/film
- Grid:
- kVp range: 70–80
- SID: 40 inch (100 cm)

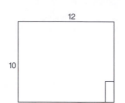

Radiation Protection

Patient Position Seated at the end of the radiographic table with all potential artifacts removed from the part (Figure 4.181).

Part Position Place the cassette on the patient's lap and have the patient bend forward slightly.

Central Ray Directed at a 15° to 30° anterior angle exiting at the midclavicle.

Patient Instructions "Take in a breath and let it out. Don't breathe or move."

Evaluation Criteria (Figures 4.182 and 4.183)

- Both acromioclavicular and sternoclavicular joints should be demonstrated.
- Proximal one-third of clavicle will be superimposed on thorax shadows.

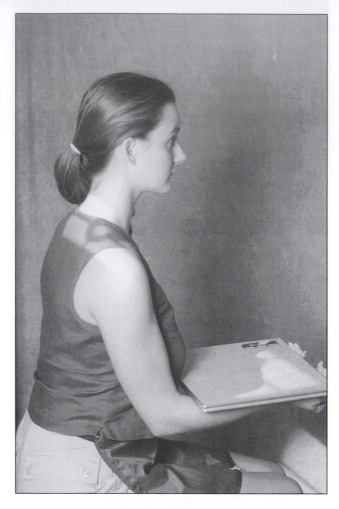

FIGURE 4.181   Clavicle: Tarrant method.

Tip A lead apron should be placed in the lap of male patients, under the cassette, to reduce gonadal dose.

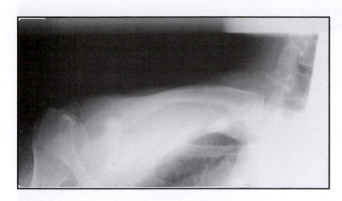

FIGURE 4.182   Clavicle: Tarrant method.

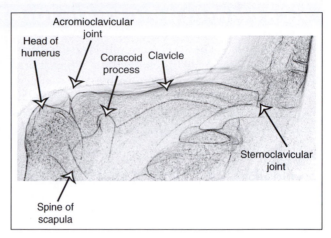

FIGURE 4.183   Clavicle: Tarrant method.

ACROMIOCLAVICULAR JOINTS—AP PROJECTION

Exam Rationale The AP acromioclavicular joint projection is taken to demonstrate dislocations. Because dislocations are often subtle, a complete series includes both right and left acromioclavicular joints for comparison. To demonstrate small dislocations, the joint must be stressed by the use of weights.

Technical Considerations

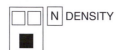

- Regular screen/film
- Grid
- kVp range: 70–80
- SID: 40 or 72 inch (100 or 180 cm)

Radiation Protection

AEC (Phototiming)

Patient Position Upright with arms placed by the patient's sides (Figure 4.184).

Part Position

- Bilateral film *without* stress or weights.
- Bilateral film *with* the patient holding a 10- to 15-lb weight in each hand; weights must be equal and the arms relaxed for the weight to stress the joint.

Central Ray Perpendicular to the midpoint between the acromioclavicular joints, centered 1 to 2 inches above the jugular notch.

Patient Instructions "Take in a deep breath, let it all out. Don't breathe or move."

Evaluation Criteria (Figures 4.185 and 4.186)

- Acromioclavicular joint space should be well demonstrated.
- Rotation, as observed by symmetry of the sternoclavicular joints, should not be evident.

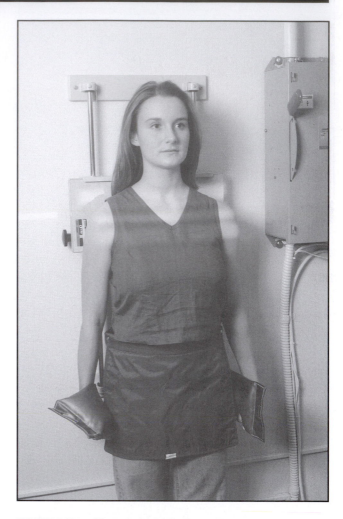

FIGURE 4.184   AP acromioclavicular joints.

Tips

1. Technical factors require some reduction in mAs from an AP shoulder to demonstrate the soft tissue of the acromioclavicular joint.
2. Breathing is suspended after expiration because this usually depresses the shoulders.
3. Whenever possible, these films should be done with the patient in an upright position. If the patient cannot stand, the films may be taken with the patient supine. To stress the joints, the arms must be gently pulled down.

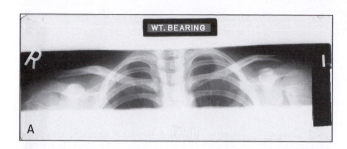

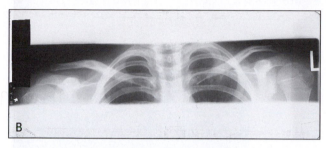

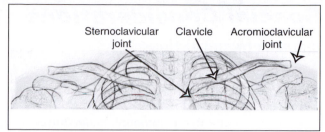

FIGURE 4.186   AP acromioclavicular joints.

FIGURE 4.185A and B   AP acromioclavicular joints. (A) With weights. (B) Without weights.

Special Considerations

TRAUMA CONSIDERATIONS

Fractures and dislocations are the most common indications for upper limb radiography. A transverse fracture of the distal radius, called a **Colles fracture**, is very common when a patient tries to break a fall by extending the arm (Figure 4.187).

Another fracture that commonly occurs during falls is a radial head fracture. Because of its impacted nature, this fracture is often difficult to visualize radiographically (Figure 4.188).

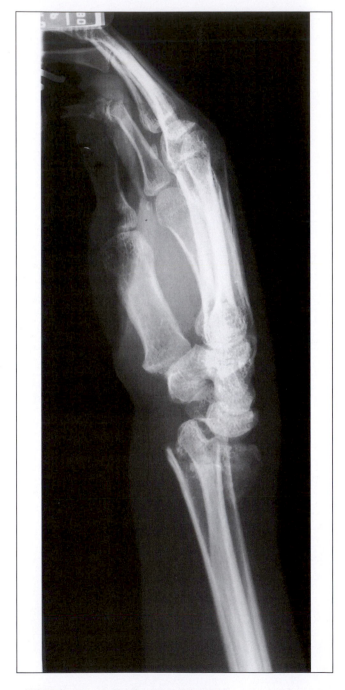

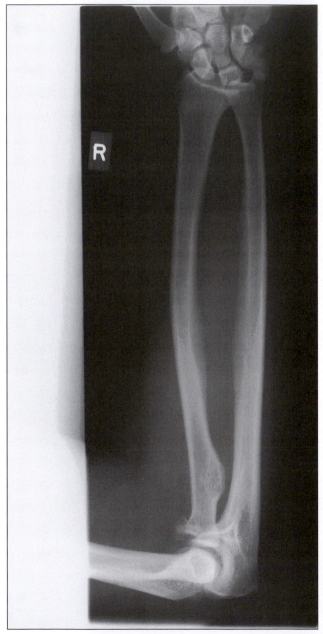

FIGURE 4.187   Colles fracture of the wrist.

FIGURE 4.188   Radial head fracture.

The most common carpal fractured is the scaphoid. The angle of the scaphoid and superimposition from other carpals necessitates special views of this bone (Figure 4.189).

Although the shoulder joint is surrounded by ligaments and tendons that make it very stable, dislocation of the humeral head from the glenoid fossa is relatively common. Normally, acute trauma is necessary to cause this condition; however, some patients have normally weak tendons and ligaments in this area and tend to dislocate with very little stress on the joint (Figure 4.190).

PEDIATRIC CONSIDERATIONS

Pediatric patients require special handling in the radiography department. Good images of the extremities nearly always require some form of immobilization for infants and young children. Sandbags are usually effective in immobilizing extremities (Figure 4.191).

Radiographs of children appear different, depending on their age. The size and shape of the epiphyses can give important clues as to the developmental age of a child. The epiphyseal lines can sometimes be confused with fracture lines and bilateral, comparison views are many times required (Figures 4.192 and 4.193).

GERIATRIC CONSIDERATIONS

Many diseases limit the mobility of geriatric patients. **Rheumatoid arthritis** is a relatively common inflammatory disease of the joints that can cause severe deformity as well as limit flexibility. Assisting patients to slowly ease into position usually yields the best results (Figure 4.194).

Osteoarthritis is a progressive, degenerative disease primarily caused by wear-and-tear at joints. In response to increased stress, the body creates additional bone tissue which, in the most severe cases, can lead to complete fusion of joints (Figure 4.195).

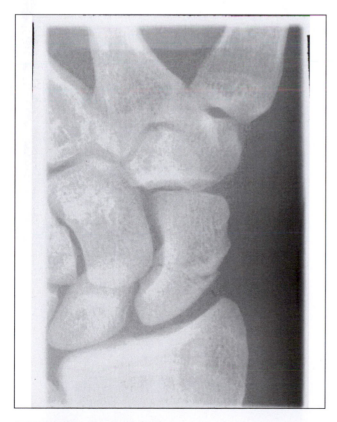

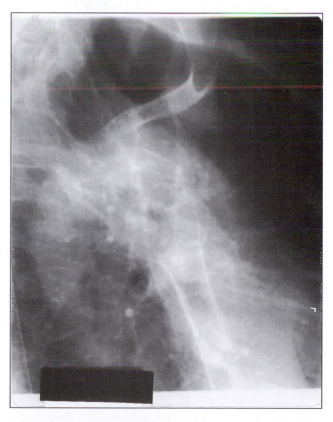

FIGURE 4.189   Scaphoid fracture.   FIGURE 4.190   Shoulder dislocation as shown on transthoracic.

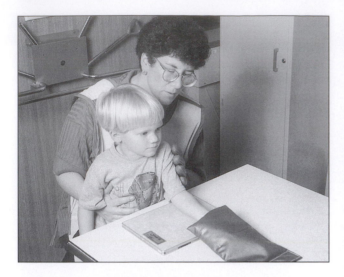

FIGURE 4.191   Pediatric immobilization.

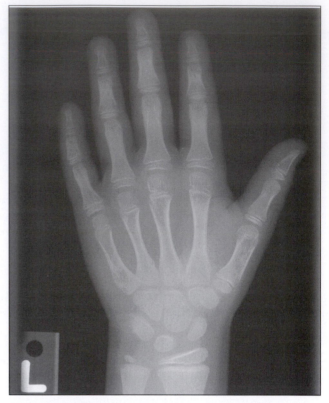

FIGURE 4.193   Hand: 8-year-old.

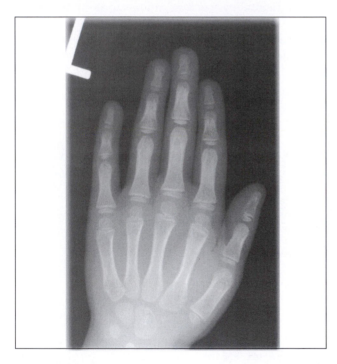

FIGURE 4.192   Hand: 4-year-old.

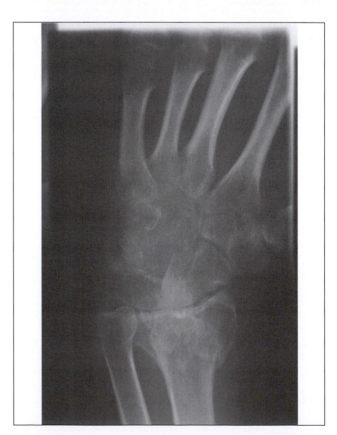

FIGURE 4.194   Rheumatoid arthritis of the hand.

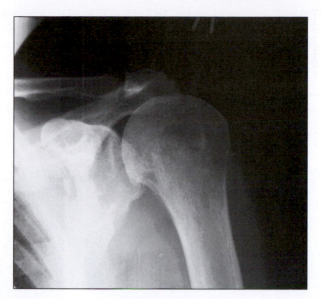

FIGURE 4.195
Osteoarthritis of the shoulder.

COMMON ERRORS

Certain positioning errors occur repetitively in radiology departments. One such error is the failure to use the correct 45° angle for an oblique hand. This is easily recognized by the overlapping of the metacarpals (Figure 4.196).

Failure to remove artifacts from the body part being radiographed is one of the most common reasons for repeat radiographs. In most cases this can be easily avoided by checking the patient's clothing and otherwise removing potential artifacts from the area (Figure 4.197).

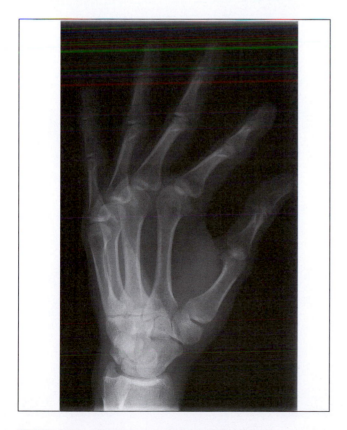

FIGURE 4.196 Wrong part angle for an oblique hand.

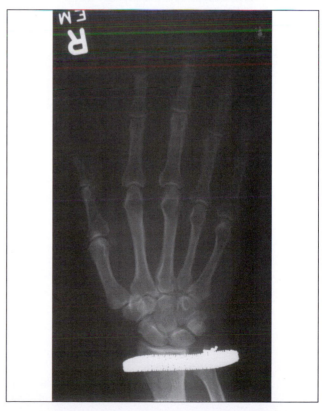

FIGURE 4.197 Failure to remove artifacts from radiograph.

Although all the anatomy appears to be included on the radiograph, a lateral elbow should be taken with the elbow flexed at exactly 90° if the surrounding soft tissue and fat pads are to be visualized optimally (Figure 4.198).

Because the hand and wrist are taken as PA projections, the beginning student radiographer sometimes makes the embarrassing error of taking the AP forearm with the hand pronated. This is immediately recognized by the radius and ulna crossing over at approximately midfilm (Figure 4.199).

The lateral scapula projection is commonly repeated because the scapula overlies the ribs on the radiograph. The correct patient angle for this projection requires experienced judgment on the part of the radiographer (Figure 4.200).

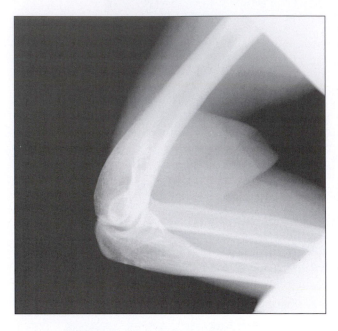

FIGURE 4.198   **Failure to flex the elbow 90˚.**

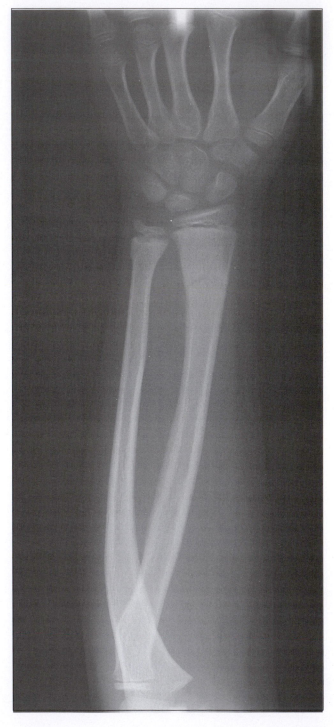

FIGURE 4.199
PA forearm taken instead of AP.

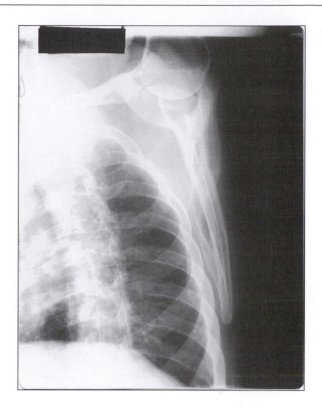

FIGURE 4.200
Scapula superimposed on ribs on the lateral position.

CORRELATIVE IMAGING

Bone can be imaged by a number of modalities. Nuclear medicine has the advantage of showing the physiology of bone. Certain diseases have physiologic defects long before they show up anatomically on radiographs (Figure 4.201).

Diseases of joints, ligaments, and tendons can rarely be demonstrated directly through radiography. MRI can be used to visualize structures such as those involved in rotator cuff injury (Figure 4.202).

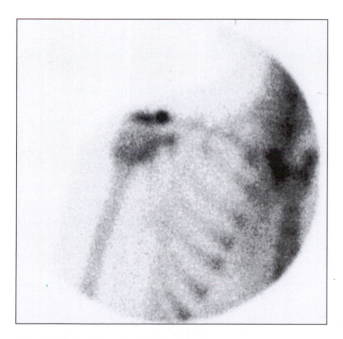

FIGURE 4.201   Bone scan illustrating tumor.

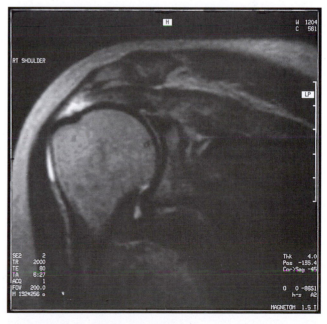

FIGURE 4.202   MRI of rotator cuff tear.

Review Questions

1. Each metacarpal consists of
   a. proximal, middle, and distal phalanges
   b. proximal and distal phalanges
   c. head and base
   d. head, shaft, and base
   e. head, middle phalanx, and base

2. The glenohumeral joint is also called the:
   a. wrist
   b. elbow
   c. shoulder
   d. acromioclavicular joint

3. The routine PA projection of the hand yields what perspective of the thumb?
   a. AP
   b. PA
   c. oblique
   d. lateral

4. The ball catcher's projection of the hands is used to demonstrate which of the following?
   a. fractures of the phalanges
   b. fractures of the metacarpals
   c. fractures of the carpals
   d. changes in bones and joints of the hand secondary to rheumatoid arthritis

5. The central ray for a PA hand enters at the:
   a. proximal interphalangeal joint
   b. distal interphalangeal joint
   c. metacarpophalangeal joint
   d. carpophalangeal joint

6. Although the PA oblique is more common when examining the wrist, the AP oblique is sometimes necessary because it better demonstrates:
   1. scaphoid
   2. trapezium
   3. hamate
   4. pisiform
   a. 1 and 2
   b. 1 and 3
   c. 3 and 4
   d. 2, 3, and 4
   e. 1, 2, 3, and 4

7. On the AP projection of the elbow, the hand should be:
   a. pronated
   b. supinated
   c. in a neutral position
   d. either a or b

8. Which projection of the elbow demonstrates the head and neck of the radius free of superimposition?
   a. AP
   b. lateral
   c. medial oblique
   d. lateral oblique
   e. either c or d

9. For a lateral elbow, the arm should be flexed so that the forearm and humerus form an angle of _____ degrees.
   a. 45
   b. 60
   c. 90
   d. 180

10. For the medial (internal) oblique elbow, the hand should be:
    a. pronated
    b. supinated
    c. rotated 45° medially
    d. rotated 45° laterally

11. The forearm is never radiographed in the PA projection because:
    a. it is too uncomfortable for the patient
    b. the radius and ulna cross over one another
    c. it could be dangerous for someone with severe trauma
    d. the patient receives more radiation

12. The lesser tubercle of the humerus is best demonstrated on the:
    a. AP projection of the shoulder with internal rotation
    b. AP projection of the shoulder with external rotation
    c. transthoracic lateral position of the shoulder

13. Which projection of the shoulder best demonstrates the proximal humerus in relationship to the glenoid fossa?

    a. AP with internal rotation
    b. AP with external rotation
    c. transthoracic lateral
    d. AP axial

14. The scapular Y position is taken with the patient in the supine position, rotated _____ degrees away from the affected side.

    a. 10
    b. 20
    c. 30
    d. 45

15. Which of the following could be safely performed on a patient with a shoulder dislocation?

    a. AP shoulder with neutral rotation
    b. scapular Y position
    c. transthoracic shoulder
    d. a and c only
    e. all of the above

16. For which position of the shoulder is the back of the hand placed on the lateral surface of the thigh?

    a. internal rotation
    b. neutral rotation
    c. external rotation
    d. transthoracic

17. The Grashey position of the shoulder is sometimes requested to better demonstrate what anatomical structure?

    a. coracoid process
    b. glenoid fossa
    c. lesser tubercle
    d. greater tubercle

18. The central ray for a lateral scapula should be directed to:

    a. 1–2 inches superior to coracoid process
    b. 1–2 inches inferior to coracoid process
    c. to the coracoid process

19. What is the tube angle for the AP projection of the clavicle?

    a. 10–15° caudal
    b. 10–15° cephalad
    c. 15–25° caudal
    d. 15–25° cephalad

20. At the proximal end of the forearm, the ulna is the larger of the 2 bones.

    a. true
    b. false

21. The styloid process of the radius is larger than the styloid process of the ulna.

    a. true
    b. false

22. The semilunar notch is on the humerus.

    a. true
    b. false

23. The capitulum articulates with the 2nd metacarpal.

    a. true
    b. false

24. The supraspinatous fossa lies on the posterior surface of the scapula.

    a. true
    b. false

25. The PA and lateral forearm should include both the wrist and elbow joints.

    a. true
    b. false

26. For the AP projection of the humerus, the epicondylar plane should be parallel to the film.

    a. true
    b. false

27. On a PA projection of the clavicle, both the acromioclavicular and sternoclavicular joints should be demonstrated.

    a. true
    b. false

28. When performing a PA axial clavicle, thinner patients require a greater tube angle than larger patients.

    a. true
    b. false

29. The preferred method for radiographing the acromioclavicular joints is in the supine position.

    a. true
    b. false

30. Fingers two through five each consists of _____(number) phalanges.

31. The olecranon process is located on the _____ (proximal or distal) end of the _____.

32. The head of the humerus articulates with the _____ of the scapula.

33. A frequent landmark in positioning of the shoulder girdle, the _____ process extends anteriorly from the scapula.

34. The lateral end of the clavicle is called the _____ extremity and the medial end is called the _____ extremity.

35. For an oblique projection of the hand, it should be rotated _____ degrees.

36. When performing the AP projection of the scapula, the arm on the affected side should be _____.

37. To accommodate the breathing technique on a transthoracic lateral humerus, the exposure time should be at least _____.

38. The primary purpose of the _____ flexion position is to obtain an elongated view of the scaphoid, free of superimposition.

39. The ulnar flexion position of the scaphoid utilizes a central ray angulation of _____ degrees.

40. The primary purpose of the radial flexion position is to open the joint spaces between the carpals on the _____ side of the wrist.

41. What group of bones comprise the palm of the hand?

42. What is the name of the joint found between a metacarpal and its corresponding phalanx?

43. What two bones comprise the forearm?

44. What three bones combine to form the elbow joint?

45. List the carpals, in order from medial to lateral side. (Remember anatomic position.)
    a. Proximal:

    b. Distal:

46. For each of the following body parts, list the routine positions/projections required at your clinical facility.
    a. Hand

    b. Wrist

    c. Forearm

    d. Elbow

    e. Humerus

    f. Shoulder

    g. Scapula

    h. Clavicle

47. Describe how routine positioning would vary for the following types of patients.
    a. hand exam for a patient with arthritis who cannot flatten the hand for a PA projection

    b. elbow exam for a patient with cast on the elbow

c. humerus exam for a patient with bone protruding through the skin

d. shoulder exam for a patient who is unconscious and has an obvious dislocation

c. scapular Y

d. grashey of the shoulder

e. transthoracic lateral humerus

48. Special positions/projections are often required to demonstrate specific structures or for certain patients. Explain why the following might be done.

a. tangential wrist

b. acute flexion position of the elbow

References and Recommended Reading

Ballinger, P. W. (1991). *Merrill's atlas of radiographic positions and radiologic procedures* (8th ed., Vol. 2). St. Louis: Mosby-Year Book.

Bontrager, K. L. (1993). *Textbook of radiographic positioning and related anatomy* (3rd ed.). St. Louis: Mosby-Year Book.

Clements, R., & Nakayama, H. (1981). Radiography of the polyarthritic hands and wrists. *Radiologic Technology, 53,* 203–217.

Clements, R. W. (1979). Adaptation of the technique for radiography of the glenohumeral joint in the lateral position. *Radiologic Technology, 51,* 305–312.

Coyle, G. (1980). Unit 7: Radiographing immobile trauma patients. In *Special angled views of joints—elbow, knee, ankle.* Denver: Multi-media Publishing.

Marieb, E. N. (1995). *Human anatomy and physiology* (3rd ed.). Redwood City, CA: Benjamin/Cummings.

McInnes, J. (1973). *Clark's positioning in radiography* (9th ed., Vol. 1). Chicago: Year Book.

Meschan, I. (1975). *An atlas of anatomy basic to radiology.* Philadelphia: Lea & Febiger.

Norgaard, F. (1965). Earliest roentgenological changes in polyarthritis of the rheumatoid type: Rheumatoid arthritis. *Radiology, 85,* 325–329.

Stecher, W. R. (1937). Roentgenography of the carpal navicular bone, *American Journal of Roentgenology, 37,* 704–705.

Lower Limb and Pelvis

JOANNE S. GREATHOUSE, EdS, RT(R)(ARRT), FASRT

MICHAEL MADDEN, PhD, RT(R)(ARRT)

INTERCONDYLOID FOSSA—ROUTINE POSITION/PROJECTION

PA Axial (Holmblad)

INTERCONDYLOID FOSSA—ALTERNATIVE POSITIONS/PROJECTIONS

PA Axial (Camp-Coventry)

AP Axial (Beclere)

FEMUR—ROUTINE POSITIONS/PROJECTIONS

AP

Lateral

FEMUR—ALTERNATE POSITION/PROJECTION

Translateral

PELVIS—ROUTINE POSITION/PROJECTION

AP

PELVIS—ALTERNATE POSITION/PROJECTION

AP Axial (Taylor)

HIP—ROUTINE POSITIONS/PROJECTIONS

AP

Lateral (Frog Lateral)

HIP—ALTERNATE POSITIONS/PROJECTIONS

Bilateral (Modified Cleaves)

Superoinferior (Danelius-Miller)

Superoinferior (Clements-Nakayama)

SACROILIAC JOINTS—ROUTINE POSITIONS/PROJECTIONS

AP Axial

AP Oblique

SPECIAL CONSIDERATIONS

Pediatric Considerations

Geriatric Considerations

Common Errors

Selected Pathology

Correlative Imaging

OBJECTIVES

At the completion of this chapter, the student should be able to:

1. List and describe the bony anatomy of the lower limb and pelvis.

2. Given drawings and radiographs, locate anatomic structures and landmarks.

3. Explain the rationale for each projection.

4. Explain the patient preparation required for each examination.

5. Describe the positioning used to visualize anatomic structures in the lower limb and pelvis.

6. List or identify the central ray location and identify the extent of field necessary for each projection.

7. Explain the protective measures that should be taken for each projection.

8. Recommend the technical factors for producing an acceptable radiograph for each projection.

9. State the patient instructions for each projection.

10. Given radiographs, evaluate positioning and technical factors for radiographs of the lower limb and pelvis.

11. Describe modifications for procedures for atypical or impaired patients to better demonstrate the anatomic area of interest.

Anatomy

The anatomic study of the lower limb and the pelvis will be divided into eight major regions: foot, ankle joint, lower leg, knee joint, thigh, pelvic girdle, hip joint, and pelvis (Figure 5.1). The primary functions of the bony anatomic structures of the lower limb and pelvis are to provide weight-bearing support for the rest of the body and to enable the body to move during walking, running, and so forth.

FOOT

The foot is made up of twenty-six bones, subdivided into three groups: the toes or phalanges; the instep or metatarsals; and the ankle or tarsals (Figures 5.2, 5.3, and 5.4).

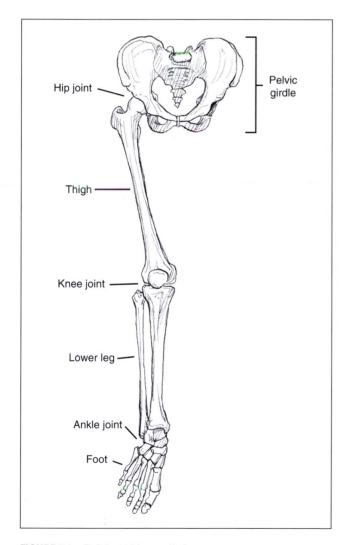

FIGURE 5.1   Pelvis and lower limb.

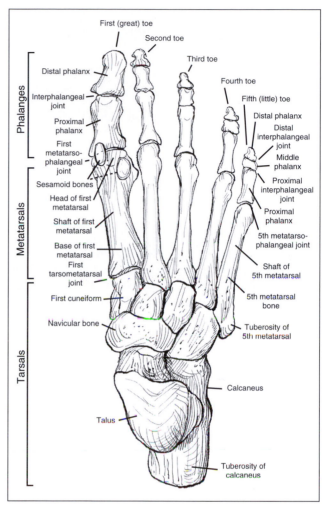

FIGURE 5.2   Foot, superior aspect.

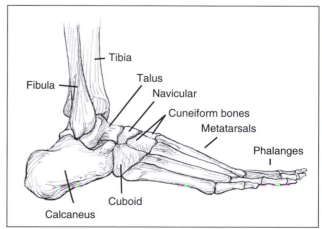

FIGURE 5.3   Foot, lateral aspect.

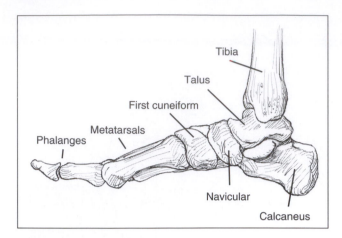

FIGURE 5.4 **Foot, medial aspect.**

Phalanges (fă-lăn´jēz)

The phalanges are commonly referred to as the bones of the toes. The first digit or great toe has two phalanges: a proximal phalanx (fāl´ănks) and a distal phalanx. Toes two through five each consists of three phalanges: proximal phalanx, middle phalanx, and distal phalanx. Altogether, there are fourteen phalanges in each foot.

Interphalangeal Joints (ĭn´´tĕr-fă-lăn´jē-ăl)
Often abbreviated as IP joints, the joints between the phalanges are classified as diarthrodial hinge-type joints capable of flexion and extension movements. The articulation between the phalanges of the great toe is called the interphalangeal joint of the first toe. The articulations in toes two through five are described by the number of the toe and as either proximal (between the proximal and middle phalanx) or distal (between the middle and distal phalanx).

Metatarsals (mĕt´´ă-tăr´săl)

The five bones of the instep are numbered similarly to the digits, with the first metatarsal being most medial or at the base of the big toe and the fifth the most lateral or at the base of the little toe. The first metatarsal is the largest, the second is the longest, and the fifth has a tuberosity on its proximal end, which can easily be palpated on the lateral side of the foot. Each metatarsal has three basic parts:

- Head—The rounded, distal end that is slightly larger than the shaft and articulates with the proximal phalanx. When standing, these structures support 50% of the body's weight.
- Base—The rounded, proximal end that articulates with the bones of the proximal foot or tarsals.
- Shaft—The long, slender portion of the bone connecting the articular regions.

Metatarsophalangeal Joints
Commonly abbreviated as MP joints, these are the articulations between the five proximal phalanges and the five metatarsals. The metatarsophalangeal joints are classified as the modified condyloid type of diarthrodial joint and are capable of flexion, extension, abduction, and adduction movements.

Sesamoids
These small, detached bones are commonly located in tendons within a variety of regions of the body including the foot. In the foot, two sesamoid bones can often be found just inferior to or on the plantar surface of the head of the first metatarsal.

Tarsals (tăr´săl)

The seven bones of the ankle and proximal foot include the calcaneus, talus, cuboid, navicular, and three cuneiforms. The names and order may be more easily remembered with a mnemonic device:

Come (calcaneus)
To (talus)
Cuba (cuboid)
(the)
Next (navicular)
Three Christmases (three cuneiforms)

Calcaneus (kăl-kā´nē-ŭs)
Also referred to as the os calcis, this is the largest tarsal bone and is found within the heel of the foot (Figure 5.5). The calcaneus articulates anteriorly with the cuboid and superiorly with the talus. The bone has the following features.

Tuberosity This most posterior aspect of the bone is located closest to the ground. In the anatomic position, 25% of the body's weight is supported at each calcaneal tuberosity, or, together, they support 50% of the body's weight.

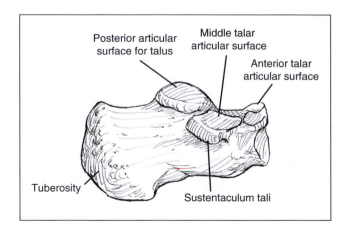

FIGURE 5.5 **Calcaneus, medial aspect.**

Sustentaculum Tali (sŭs´´tĕn-tăk´ū-lŭm tā´lī) This bony projection on the upper, medial aspect creates a "shelf" to hold the head of the talus. On the superior aspect of the bone are several articular facets for the talus: posterior, middle, and anterior.

Calcaneal Sulcus This depression or groove is found between the posterior and middle talar articular facets.

Talus (tā´lŭs) Also referred to as the astragalus or the ankle bone, the talus is the most superior tarsal bone and is generally located above the anterior calcaneus and below the lower leg. The trochlea is the most superior surface of the talus, which articulates with the lower leg. The talus articulates with four bones: tibia, fibula, calcaneus, and navicular (Figure 5.6).

Cuboid (kū´boyd) The cuboid bone is located on the lateral aspect of the foot between the calcaneus and the bases of the fourth and fifth metatarsals.

Navicular (nă-vĭk´ū-lăr) This boat-shaped bone is located on the medial side of the foot between the talus and the three cuneiforms. The navicular bone articulates with five bones: the talus, cuboid, and three cuneiforms.

Three Cuneiforms (kū-nē´ĭ-fōrm) These wedge-shaped bones are located on the medial aspect of the foot. The first cuneiform is the most medial; the second is intermediate; and the third cuneiform is the most laterally located, adjacent to the cuboid bone. All three

cuneiforms articulate with the navicular bone posteriorly and the bases of the metatarsals anteriorly.

Ossification

The development of the bones of the foot is often used to clinically evaluate bone growth as compared to age and has been characterized as follows:

Phalanges—two ossification centers: body, begins at tenth fetal week; base, begins at 4 to 10 years and joins at 18 years.

First metatarsal—two ossification centers: body, begins at ninth fetal week; base, begins at 3 years, and joins at 18 to 20 years.

Second through fifth metatarsals—two ossification centers: body, begins at ninth fetal week; head, begins at 5 to 8 years and joins at 18 to 20 years.

Calcaneus—two ossification centers: body, appears during sixth fetal month; heel, begins in tenth year and joins at puberty.

Talus—one ossification center: appears at seventh fetal month.

Cuboid—one ossification center: appears at ninth fetal month.

Navicular—one ossification center: appears at fourth year.

First cuneiform—one ossification center: appears at third year.

Second cuneiform—one ossification center: appears at fourth year.

Third cuneiform—one ossification center: appears at first year.

Tarsometatarsal and Intertarsal Joints Both the tarsometatarsal joints, between the distal tarsals and the proximal metatarsals, and the intertarsal joints, between tarsals, are classified as diarthrodial gliding-type joints. Although the gliding type of joint is capable of only sliding movements, the combination of these joints results in inversion and eversion movements of the foot.

Arches of the Foot The bones of the foot form two arches: longitudinal, anterior to posterior, and transverse, medial to lateral (Figure 5.7). The longitudinal arches can be further divided into the medial and lateral, the medial being the higher and more important arch because it bears most of the weight. Both arches provide strong weight support and "shock absorption" for the body during movements such as walking, running, or jumping. In the clinical condition of flat feet or pes planus, the medial longitudinal arch is nonexistent due to misalignment of the bones on the medial side of the foot.

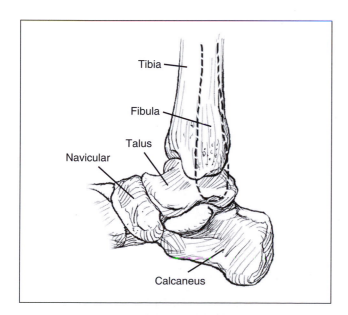

FIGURE 5.6   Talar articulations, medial aspect.

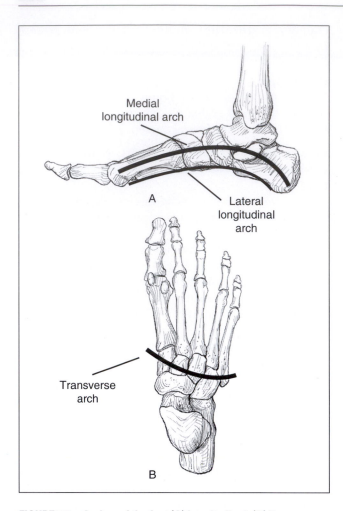

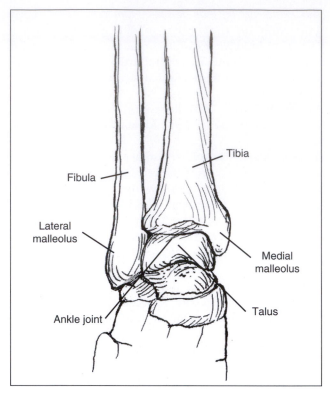

FIGURE 5.8   Ankle, anterior.

FIGURE 5.7   Arches of the foot (A) Longitudinal, (B) Transverse.

ANKLE JOINT

This joint, also called the talocrural joint, is formed where the superior bone of the foot, the talus, articulates with the bones of the lower leg, the tibia and fibula (Figures 5.8 and 5.9).

The distal ends of the tibia and fibula create a socket or a mortise for the trochlea of the talus. The mortise is formed by the distal ends of the fibula (**lateral malleolus**) and the tibia (**medial malleolus**), which extend downward on either side of the trochlea. Most of the weight is transmitted from the tibia to the talus and the malleoli grip the trochlea so there is little lateral movement. The joint is considered a diarthrodial, hinge-type joint with flexion (dorsiflexion) and extension (plantar flexion) movements only. The movement of the foot in inversion and eversion, often attributed to the ankle, is actually a synergistic movement of the joints within the foot, especially the intertarsal joints.

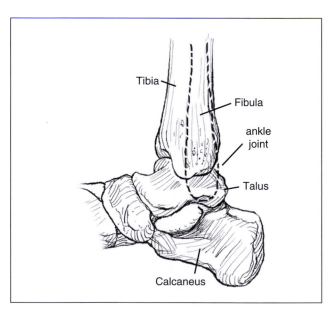

FIGURE 5.9   Ankle, medial.

LOWER LEG

The lower leg has two, slender bones extending from the knee to the ankle (Figures 5.10 and 5.11).

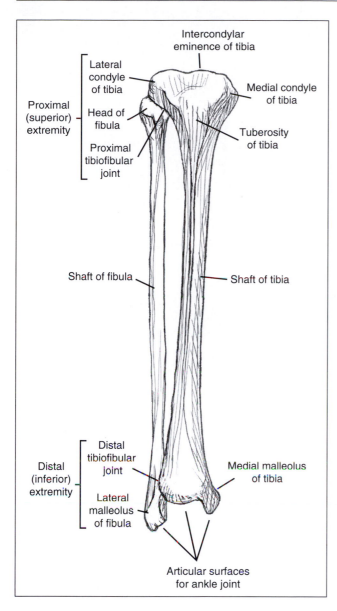

FIGURE 5.10   Lower leg, anterior.

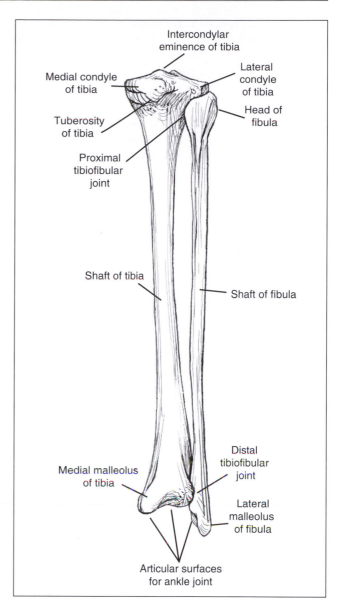

FIGURE 5.11   Lower leg, posterior.

Tibia (tĭb´ē-ă)

Commonly called the shin bone, the tibia is the second longest bone in the body. In the leg, the tibia is larger and more medially located than the fibula and bears most of the body's weight. The tibia is anatomically divided into three regions: the distal (inferior) extremity, the shaft, and the proximal (superior) extremity.

Distal Extremity   The medial malleolus is the most inferior process and forms the medial wall of the ankle joint. Medial to the malleolus, the smooth concave articular surface for the talus is located on the inferior end of the tibia.

Shaft   This portion of the bone has a sharp anterior border or crest and is commonly referred to as the shin.

Proximal Extremity   The most superior portion of the tibia that forms the lower aspect of the knee joint. At the most superior edge of the anterior border extending upward from the shaft is a roughened area of bone called the **tibial tuberosity**, which is the site of attachment for the patella tendon. Slightly above the tuberosity, the oblique line is formed as the crest continues in a more lateral direction. As part of the knee joint, the expanded superior end forms the medial and lateral **condyles** and an articular facet for the head of the fibula. On the superior end of the tibia, an **intercondylar eminence** formed by two tubercles is located between the condyles and the anterior and posterior intercondylar fossae.

Fibula (fĭb´ū-lă)

Commonly called the calf bone, the more slender bone located more laterally in the leg. Similar to the tibia, the fibula is also anatomically divided into three regions: the distal extremity, shaft, and proximal extremity.

Distal Extremity   The lateral malleolus extends most inferiorly in the leg, approximately one-half inch below the medial malleolus, to form the lateral wall of the ankle joint.

Proximal Extremity   The expanded region, or the head, articulates with the tibia. The most superior portion of this articular surface forms the apex or styloid process.

Tibiofibular Joints   The distal tibiofibular joint is an amphiarthrodial syndesmosis type of joint capable of only slight movement up and down (Figure 5.12). By comparison, the proximal tibiofibular joint, located between the head of the fibula and the posterior aspect of the lateral condyle of the tibia, is a diarthrodial gliding type of joint capable of up and down movements (Figure 5.13).

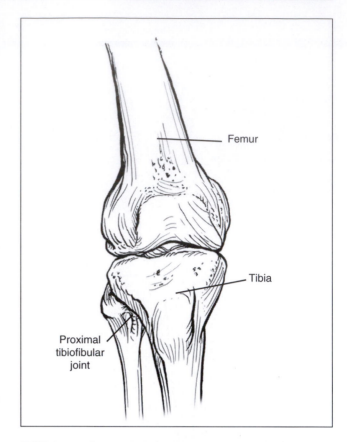

FIGURE 5.13   Proximal tibiofibular joint.

KNEE JOINT

The largest joint in the body, the knee, is located primarily between the distal femur and the tibia and is also called the tibiofemoral joint (Figures 5.14 and 5.15). The knee is considered a diarthrodial special hinge type of joint allowing flexion and extension and gliding and rotational movements when the leg is partially flexed. Although the patella does not articulate with the tibia, it does articulate with the distal femur, creating the patellofemoral joint, and is considered part of the knee joint.

Patella

The largest of the sesamoid bones, the patella has an irregular diameter of about 2 inches (Figure 5.16). It is generally described as a flat bone, roughly oval in shape, which is "upside down" in the knee. The superior border, the base, and the anterior rough convex surface are the sites of attachment for the large quadriceps femoris muscle of the thigh. Inferiorly, the ligamentum patella attaches to the apex and extends downward to the tibial tuberosity.

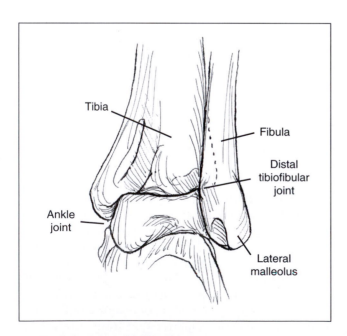

FIGURE 5.12   Distal tibiofibular joint.

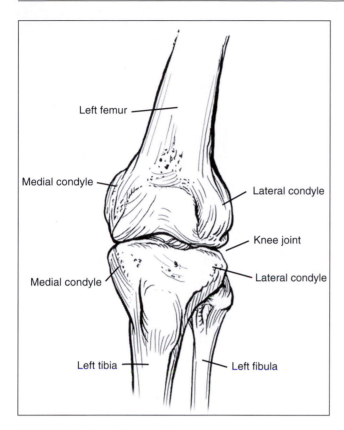

FIGURE 5.14   Knee joint, anterior.

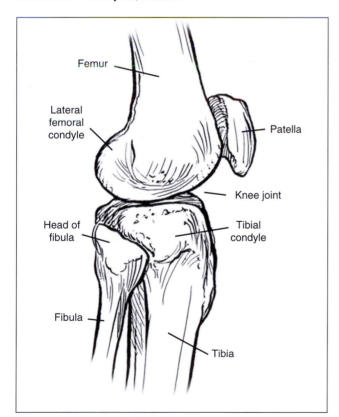

FIGURE 5.15   Knee joint, lateral.

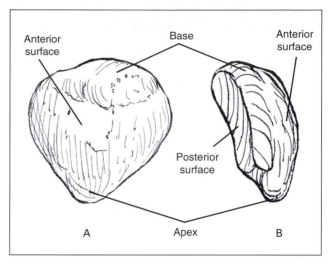

FIGURE 5.16   Patella: (A) anterior, (B) lateral.

In general terms, the patella is often described as a bone embedded in the back of the tendinous insertion of the quadriceps femoris muscle that is located 1/2 inch above the knee joint. On the posterior aspect of the patella, smooth articular surfaces for the medial and lateral condyles of the femur are evident with the lateral surface being slightly larger.

Distal Extremity of Femur

On the posterior aspect of the femur (Figure 5.17), the medial and lateral condyles can be easily seen with the intervening **intercondylar fossa** or notch. In the anatomic position, the shaft of the femur is angled medially approximately 10°. To partially compensate for this angulation, the medial condyle extends more inferiorly than the lateral condyle. If a line were drawn across the most inferior aspect of the condyles, the line would be approximately 5° to 7° from perpendicular to the shaft of the femur. The roughened areas of the bone just superior to the condyles, the medial and lateral **epicondyles**, provide a major site of attachment for muscles to the distal femur and are easily palpated above the knee.

Patellofemoral Joint   The posterior surface of the patella articulates with the patellar surface (intercondylar surface or trochlear groove) on the distal femur (Figure 5.18). This joint is considered a diarthrodial saddle type of joint due to the shape and relationship between the femur and patella capable of sliding movements up and down. Although both the medial and lateral portions of the patellar surface articulate with the patella, the lateral surface is slightly higher in this view.

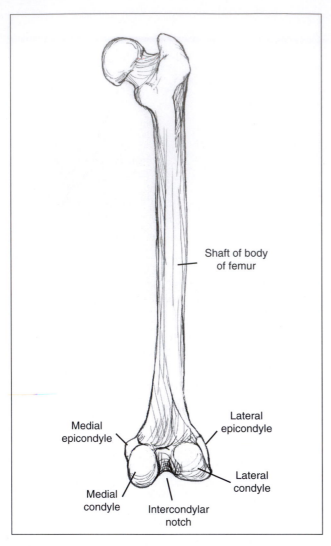

FIGURE 5.17   Femur, posterior.

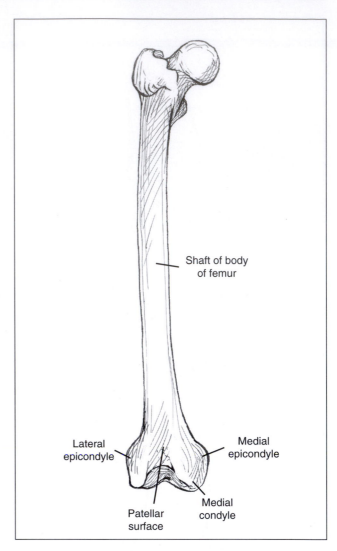

FIGURE 5.18   Femur, anterior.

Ligaments

All the ligaments of the knee joint contribute to its mobility and stability (Figures 5.19 and 5.20).

Tibial or Medial Collateral Ligament   These ligaments extend across the knee joint from the medial condyle of the femur to the medial condyle and body of the tibia. Their primary functions are to prevent lateral bending and to limit extension and lateral rotation.

Fibular or Lateral Collateral Ligament   These ligaments extend from the distal femur to the head of the fibula.

Anterior Cruciate (kroo´shē-āt)   This round ligament extends from the anterior tibial intercondylar eminence to the posterior lateral femoral condyle and crosses other cruciate ligaments in the knee joint. The

primary functions are to prevent anterior slipping of tibia on femur and to limit extension and lateral rotation.

Posterior Cruciate   This round ligament extends from the posterior end of lateral meniscus to the anterior medial femoral condyle and crosses other cruciate ligaments in the knee joint. The primary functions are to prevent posterior slipping of tibia on femur and to limit extension and lateral rotation.

Medial Meniscus (mĕn-ĭs´kŭs)   This crescent-shaped or oval ligament is located on the superior aspect of the medial tibial condyle. It acts as a cushion for the bones of the knee and deepens the medial tibial condyle.

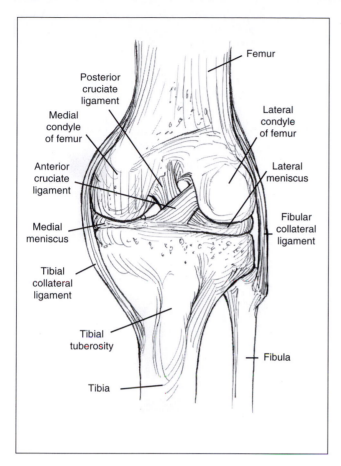

FIGURE 5.19   Ligaments of the knee, anterior.

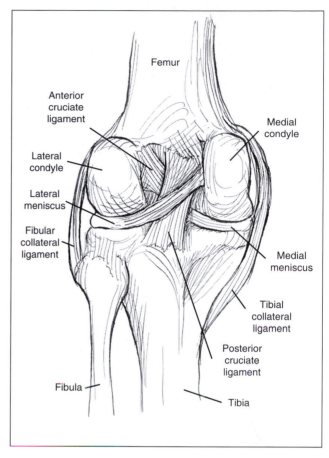

FIGURE 5.20   Ligaments of the knee, posterior.

Lateral Meniscus   This circular ligament is located on the superior aspect of the lateral tibial condyle. It acts as a cushion for the bones of the knee and deepens lateral tibial condyle.

Trauma

The knee is frequently a site of injury in contact sports such as football and basketball. Most commonly, a strong force is applied to the lateral aspect of the knee, which separates the medial tibial and femoral condyles. This force often results in lesions of the tibial collateral ligament creating a "loose-knee" capable of lateral movement. Also, the medial meniscus may be torn or loosened from its sites of attachment, frequently referred to as a torn or floating cartilage, causing the knee joint to jam or lock up.

Synovial Membrane

The synovial membrane in the knee joint is the largest and most extensive in the body. The synovial-lined joint space within the knee can easily be subdivided into three joints: two joints located medially and later-

ally between the condyles of the femur and the tibia and the patellofemoral joint. Furthermore, the joint space is continuous with many of the surrounding bursae (Figure 5.21).

THIGH

The thigh is comprised of one large bone, the femur, surrounded on all sides by musculature extending from the hip to the knee (Figures 5.22 and 5.23).

Femur

This longest, strongest, and heaviest bone in the body is located in the region of the thigh. It can be subdivided into three parts: proximal extremity, shaft, and distal extremity. The latter was previously described in the region of the knee and will be omitted from this description.

Shaft   The long slender portion of the bone, or body, with the posteriorly situated roughened area, the linea aspera, delineated by medial and lateral lips.

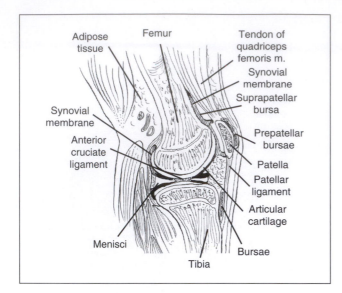

FIGURE 5.21   Knee joint.

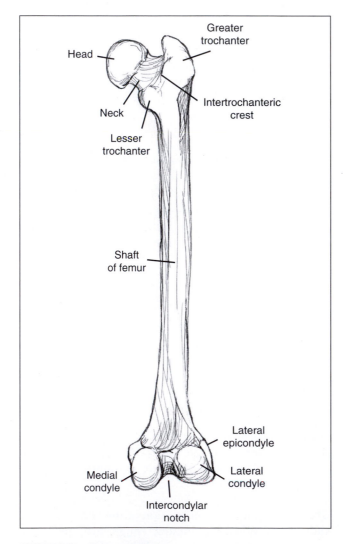

FIGURE 5.22   Femur, posterior.

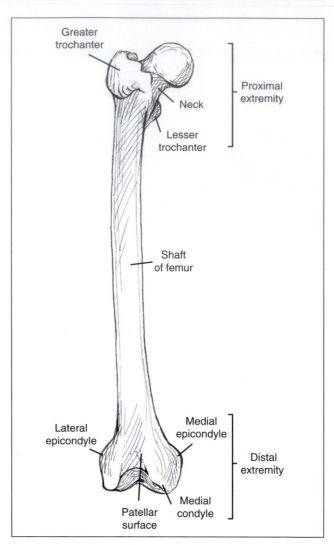

FIGURE 5.23   Femur, anterior.

Proximal Extremity   The greater **trochanter** appears much like an extension of the shaft and is located on the superior, lateral aspect. By comparison, the lesser trochanter is an expansion of bone more inferiorly located on the posterior, medial aspect. On the posterior view, a ridge of bone extends between the greater and lesser trochanters, the intertrochanteric crest. Adjacent to the trochanters, the narrowed region of the neck extends toward the rounded head. The angle between the shaft and the neck averages 120° to 125° but is greater in children and less in females.

PELVIC GIRDLE

The innominate, or hip bone, is a large, irregular-shaped bone with a centrally located socket, the acetabulum, for articulation with the head of the femur (Figures 5.24 and 5.25). The pelvic girdle is divided

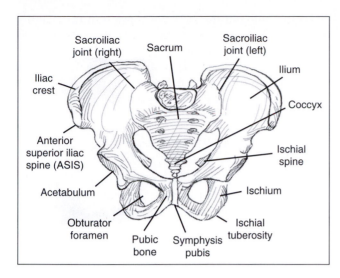

FIGURE 5.24   Pelvis, anterior.

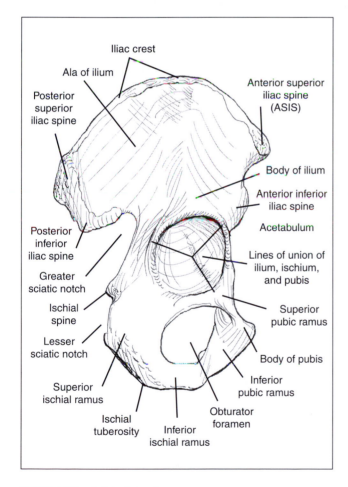

FIGURE 5.25   Pelvis, lateral.

into three parts, which are connected by cartilage in the young and fused in the adult: ilium, pubis, and ischium.

Ilium (ĭl´ē-ŭm)

The ilium forms the upper part of the pelvic girdle. The most superior edge, the iliac crest, can be easily palpated along the lateral side. If the iliac crest is followed anteriorly, the termination, the anterior superior iliac spine (ASIS), can also be felt on the anterior aspect of the hip. Below the superior spine, a second less prominent spine, anterior inferior iliac spine, also extends from the anterior margin of the ilium. Similarly, on the posterior ilium, the iliac crest terminates at the posterior superior iliac spine and the posterior inferior iliac spine extends more inferiorly. Inferiorly, the central wing-shaped region of the ilium, the ala, is located above the projection and forms part of the superior **acetabulum**.

Pubis (pū´bĭs)

The pubis forms the lower anterior part of the pelvic girdle and meets the opposite pubis to form the **symphysis pubis** joint. The pubis consists of the body, the inferior ramus, and the superior ramus, which forms the anterior part of the acetabulum.

Ischium (ĭs´kē-ŭm)

This lower posterior part of the pelvic girdle forms the most inferior portion of the pelvic girdle. It has an enlarged roughened area, the ischial tuberosity, which is the bony structure the body rests on in the seated position. Extending anteriorly from the tuberosity, the inferior ischial ramus joins the inferior pubic ramus, and, together, they form the lower boundary of the obturator foramen. Above the tuberosity, the ischial spine projects posteriorly, forming the lesser sciatic notch, and, with the ilium, the greater sciatic notch.

HIP JOINT

This diarthrodial, ball and socket type of joint is located between the proximal extremity of the femur and the pelvic girdle (Figure 5.26). The joint is capable of a wide range of movements including flexion, extension, abduction, adduction, lateral rotation, and medial rotation.

Alignment of Joint

Due to the shape of the femur and the pelvic girdle, the hip joint is not truly vertical (Figure 5.27). In the anatomic position, the shaft of the femur is from 5° to 15° medial from vertical. Typically, a short woman with a wide pelvis will measure closer to 15°, whereas a tall man with a narrow pelvis will be closer to 5°. The neck and head of the femur are perpendicular to the midpoint between the anterior superior iliac spine of

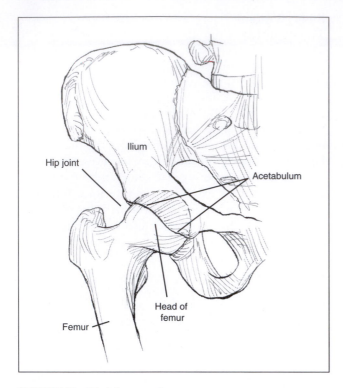

FIGURE 5.26   Hip joint, anterior.

the hip bone and the superior margin of the symphysis pubis. As compared to the shaft of the femur, the average angulation of the head and neck is 125° but may vary from 110° to 135° depending on the width of the pelvis and the length of the legs. Also, the head and neck of the femur are angled 15° to 20° degrees anteriorly (Figure 5.28).

PELVIS

The term pelvis, meaning basin, is used to describe the irregularly shaped opening created by the two hip bones, the sacrum, and the coccyx (Figure 5.29). The opening within the pelvis is often separated into greater and lesser segments, sometimes referred to as the true and false pelvis, by an oblique plane at the pelvic inlet. The pelvis transmits the weight of the upper body to the lower limbs and forms the lower part of the abdominal cavity.

Pelvic Inlet
This is a flat plane extending from the sacral promontory to the superior border of the pubic symphysis and the middle of the pelvic brim.

Greater Pelvis
The pelvic space, also called the false pelvis, above the pelvic inlet. The space is irregular in shape with the boundaries being formed posteriorly by the lower

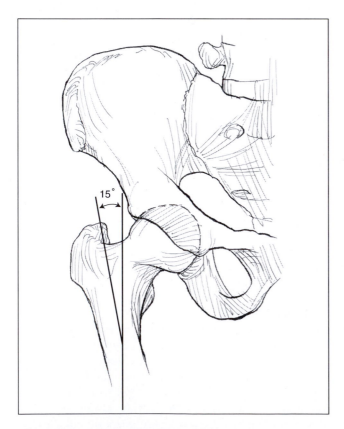

FIGURE 5.27   Hip joint variance from vertical.

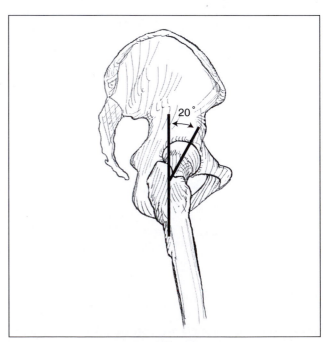

FIGURE 5.28   Anterior angulation of femur.

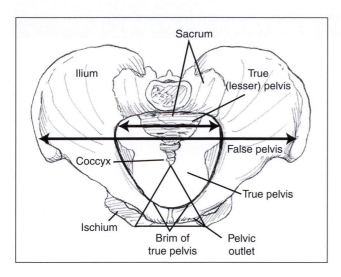

FIGURE 5.29 Pelvis.

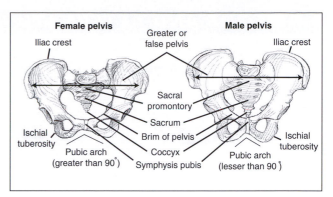

FIGURE 5.30 Comparison of female and male pelvis.

lumbar vertebrae and laterally by the alae or wings of the ilia. Anteriorly there is little bony wall due to the downward slope of the plane.

Pelvic Outlet
Irregularly shaped, it does not form a flat plane. Anteroposteriorly, it is located between the tip of the coccyx and the inferior border of the symphysis pubis. Transversely, the plane extends between the ischial tuberosities.

Lesser Pelvis
Also referred to as the true pelvis, it is the short, curved pelvic space located within the bony pelvis between the pelvic inlet and outlet. The size and shape of this space is of great importance in birthing because the baby passes through this space in vaginal deliveries.

Classifications of the Pelvis
The pelvis is the distinctive skeletal feature markedly different between men and women (Figure 5.30). The male pelvis is typically narrower, whereas the female pelvis is wider and the alae or wings of the ilia are more open. Less obviously, the subpubic arch or angle, situated below the symphysis pubis between the inferior pubic rami, can also be used to determine the sex of the pelvis. In the male pelvis, this region is more angular, on the order of 50° to 60° as compared to 80° to 85° in the female pelvis.

Sacroiliac (sā´´krō-ĭl´ē-ăk) Joints
Slightly movable amphiarthrodial syndesmosis type of joints, the sacroiliac or SI joints are located between

the auricular surfaces of the wedge-shaped sacrum and ilium (Figure 5.31). The joint is broad and irregularly shaped but can generally be described as the concave edge of the sacrum fitting into the corresponding convex surface of the ilium. The irregular joint is obliquely situated, and the interlocking structure significantly increases the strength of the joint.

Symphysis Pubis (sĭm´fĭ-sĭs pū´bĭs)
The cartilaginous joint where the pubic bones meet each other in the median plane is classified as amphiarthrodial symphysis type. The thick articular cartilage between the pubic bones is held in place by surrounding ligaments and is generally larger in women than in men. Movement is very limited but separation or rotation are demonstrated during childbirth and in situations of pelvic trauma.

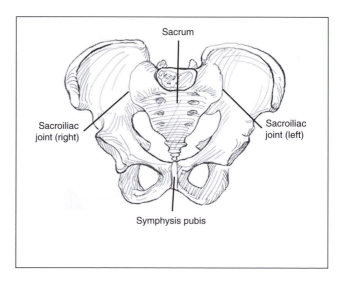

FIGURE 5.31 Sacroiliac joints.

ROUTINE AND ALTERNATIVE POSITIONS/PROJECTIONS

ROUTINE AND ALTERNATIVE POSITIONS/PROJECTIONS

TOES—AP (DORSOPLANTAR) PROJECTION

Exam Rationale The most common indication for examination of the toe(s) is trauma. Structures demonstrated on the AP projection include the phalanges, the interphalangeal joints, and the distal ends of the metatarsals; the metatarsophalangeal joints are not well visualized.

Technical Considerations

- Extremity screen/film
- Non-grid
- kVp range: 55–60
- SID: 40 inch (100 cm)

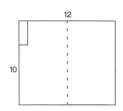

Radiation Protection

Patient Position Seated on the table with the knee flexed; all potential artifacts, including shoe and sock, removed from the part (Figure 5.32).

Part Position Place the foot flat on the cassette with the toes centered to the unexposed portion of the cassette.

Central Ray Perpendicular to the second metatarsophalangeal joint.

Patient Instructions "Breathe normally but don't move."

Evaluation Criteria (Figures 5.33 and 5.34)

- Phalanges should not be rotated; toes should be slightly separated from each other; and distal ends of the metatarsals should be included.

Tips

1. To open joint spaces, angle central ray 15° posteriorly.
2. Many department protocols require that, on initial examination, the entire foot be demonstrated on the AP projection; this can be done on half a 10 × 12 (25 × 30 cm) with the oblique and lateral of only the toe on the other half of the cassette.

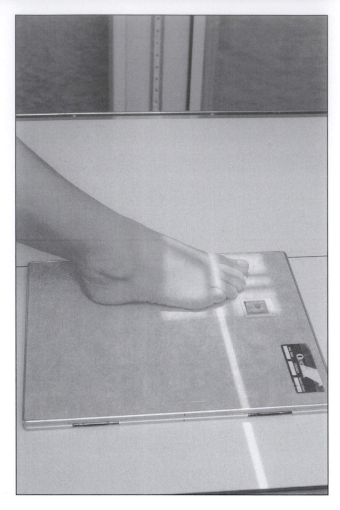

FIGURE 5.32   **AP toes.**

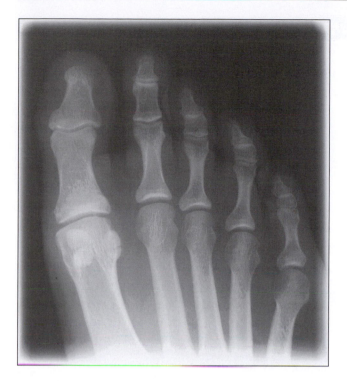

FIGURE 5.33   AP toes.

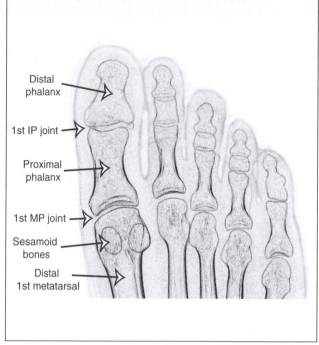

Distal
phalanx

1st IP joint

Proximal
phalanx

1st MP joint

Sesamoid
bones

Distal
1st metatarsal

FIGURE 5.34   AP toes.

TOES—OBLIQUE DORSOPLANTAR POSITION

Exam Rationale   The oblique is a routine position of the toes that gives a different perspective than that of the AP. Structures demonstrated on the radiograph include the phalanges, the interphalangeal joints, and the distal ends of the metatarsals.

Technical Considerations

- Extremity screen/film
- Non-grid
- kVp range: 55–60
- SID: 40 inch (100 cm)

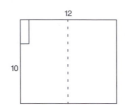

Radiation Protection

Patient Position   Seated on the table with the knee flexed; all potential artifacts, including shoe and sock, removed from the part (Figure 5.35).

Part Position   Place the foot flat on the cassette with the toes centered to the unexposed portion of the cassette; rotate the foot internally 30°.

Central Ray   Perpendicular to the third metatarsophalangeal joint.

Patient Instructions   "Breathe normally but don't move."

Evaluation Criteria (Figures 5.36 and 5.37)

- All phalanges of the digit should be seen; toes should be slightly separated from each other.
- Obliquity of the toes should be evident; interphalangeal and second through fifth metatarsophalangeal joint spaces should be open; first metatarsophalangeal joint space is not always open.
- Distal ends of the metatarsals should be included.

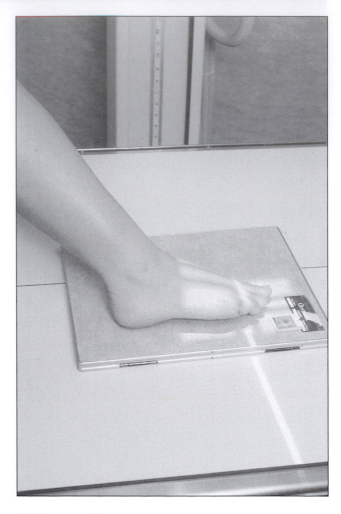

FIGURE 5.35   Oblique toes.

Tip   Some department protocols call for a 45° rotation of the foot.

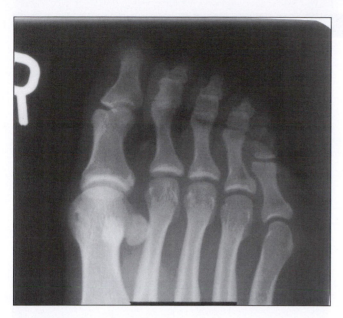

FIGURE 5.36 Oblique toes.

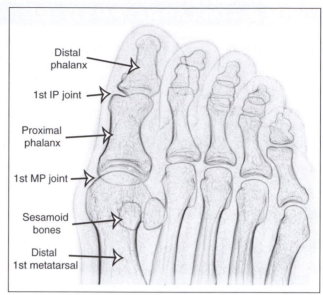

FIGURE 5.37 Oblique toes.

TOES—LATERAL POSITION

Exam Rationale   This projection provides a lateral view of the affected toe free of superimposition from other phalanges. Structures demonstrated on the radiograph include the phalanges and interphalangeal joints of the affected toe.

Technical Considerations

- Extremity screen/film
- Non-grid
- kVp range: 55–60
- SID: 40 inch (100 cm)

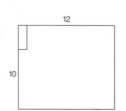

Radiation Protection

Patient Position   Lateral recumbent position; potential artifacts, including shoe and sock, removed from the part.

Part Position   Center the toes to the unexposed portion of the cassette; rest the foot on its medial surface for toes one, two, and three; on the lateral surface for toes four and five; use a strip of gauze to gently pull the affected toe forward or backward from the other toes to prevent superimposition.

Central Ray   For toe one, perpendicular to the interphalangeal joint (Figure 5.38); for toes two through five, perpendicular to the proximal interphalangeal joint of the affected toe (Figure 5.39).

Patient Instructions   "Breathe normally but don't move."

Evaluation Criteria (Figures 5.40 and 5.41)

- Phalanx of interest should be seen in profile.
- Phalanx of interest should be seen without superimposition of the other toes; when complete separation is not possible, the proximal phalanx should be visualized through the superimposed structures.
- Interphalangeal and metatarsophalangeal joint spaces should be open.

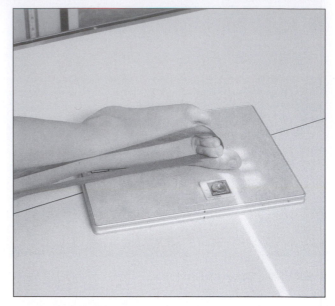

FIGURE 5.38   Lateral great toe.

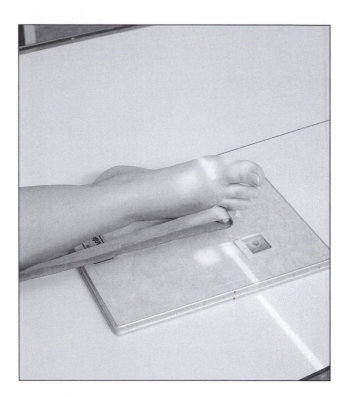

FIGURE 5.39   Lateral toes (2–5).

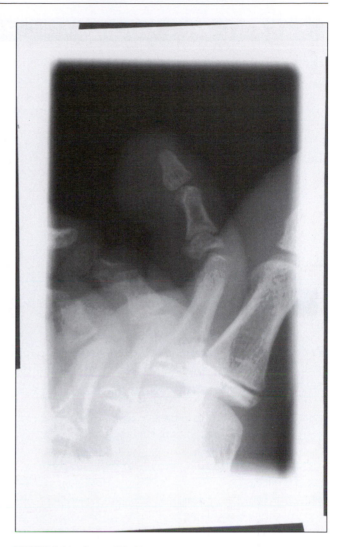

FIGURE 5.41   Lateral 2nd toe.

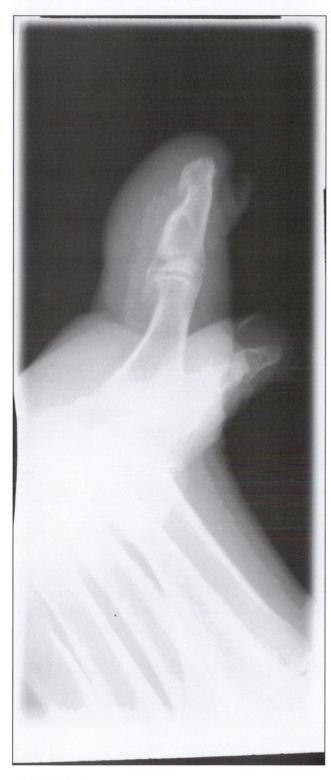

FIGURE 5.40   Lateral great toe.

SESAMOIDS—TANGENTIAL POSITION (LEWIS METHOD)

Exam Rationale   The most common indication for an examination of the sesamoids is possible fracture. Structures demonstrated on the radiograph include a profile view of the sesamoids and the metatarsal heads.

Technical Considerations

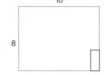

- Extremity screen/film
- Non-grid
- kVp range: 55–60
- SID: 40 inch (100 cm)

Radiation Protection

Patient Position   Prone on the table; all potential artifacts, including shoe and sock, removed from the part (Figure 5.42).

Part Position   With the toes centered to the cassette, rest the foot on the plantar surface of the great toe; dorsiflex the foot until the ball of the foot is perpendicular to the cassette.

Central Ray   Perpendicular and tangential to the second metatarsophalangeal joint.

Patient Instructions   "Breathe normally but don't move."

Evaluation Criteria (Figures 5.43 and 5.44)

- Sesamoids should be projected free of superimposition by the metatarsal heads.
- Metatarsal heads should be visualized.

Tip   If the patient is unable to assume the prone position, Holly described an alternative with the patient in the supine position; with the patient seated

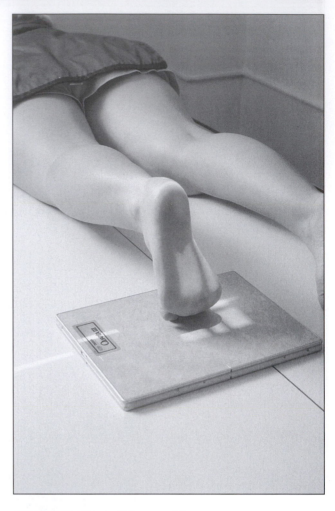

FIGURE 5.42   Tangential sesamoids.

and the knee extended, center the heel to the cassette and adjust the foot so its medial border is perpendicular to the cassette and the plantar surface is at an angle of 75°; the patient uses gauze to place/maintain the toes in flexed position; the central ray is directed perpendicular to the head of the first metatarsal (Figures 5.45 and 5.45a).

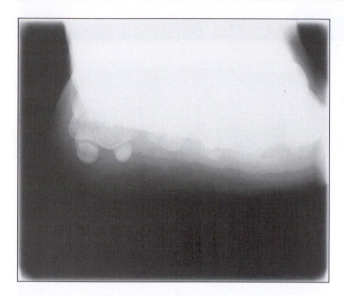

FIGURE 5.43　Tangential sesamoids.

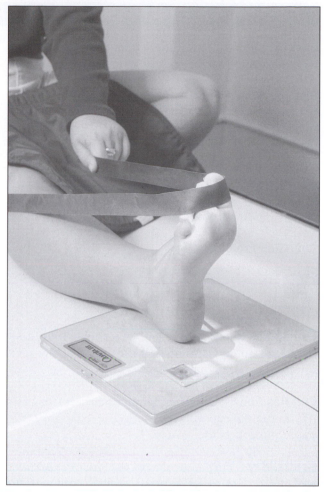

FIGURE 5.45　Alternative sesamoid position (Holly).

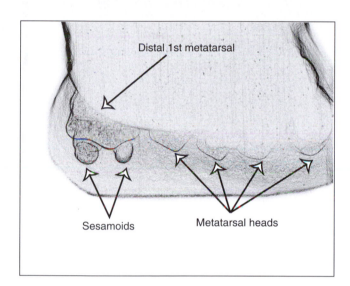

Distal 1st metatarsal

Sesamoids

Metatarsal heads

FIGURE 5.44　Tangential sesamoids.

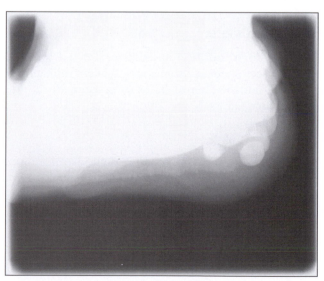

FIGURE 5.45a　Tangential sesamoids (Holly).

FOOT—AP (DORSOPLANTAR) PROJECTION

Exam Rationale The most common indication for an examination of the foot is trauma. The AP projection provides a general survey of the bones of the foot, including demonstration of the phalanges, the metatarsals, and the tarsals anterior to the talus.

Technical Considerations

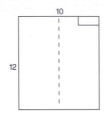

- Extremity screen/film
- Non-grid
- kVp range: 55–60
- SID: 40 inch (100 cm)

Radiation Protection

Patient Position Seated on the table with knee flexed; all potential artifacts, including shoe and sock, removed from the part.

Part Position Place the plantar surface of the foot flat on the cassette with the foot centered to the unexposed portion of the cassette.

Central Ray Perpendicular to the base of the third metatarsal (Figure 5.46), or 10° cephalic angle to the base of the third metatarsal (Figure 5.47).

Patient Instructions "Breathe normally but don't move."

Evaluation Criteria (Figure 5.48)

- Foot should not be rotated as evidenced by equal space between midshafts of adjacent metatarsals (2–4) and overlap of bases of second, third, and fourth metatarsals.

Tips

1. Use of central ray angulation demonstrates more open metatarsophalangeal joints (Figures 5.49 and 5.49a).
2. Use of a compensating filter is helpful in achieving consistent density throughout the foot.

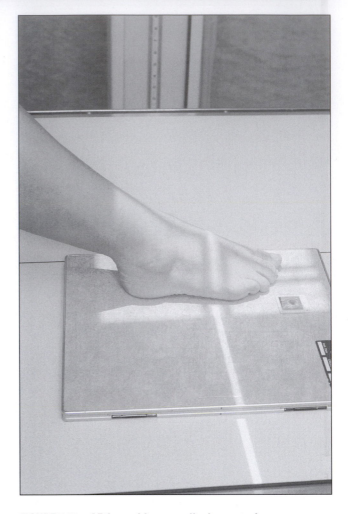

FIGURE 5.46   AP foot with perpendicular central ray.

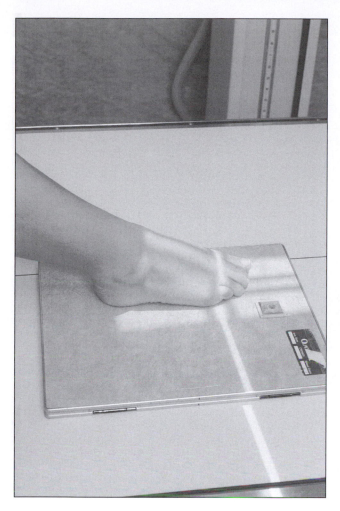

FIGURE 5.47 AP foot with 10° cephalic angulation.

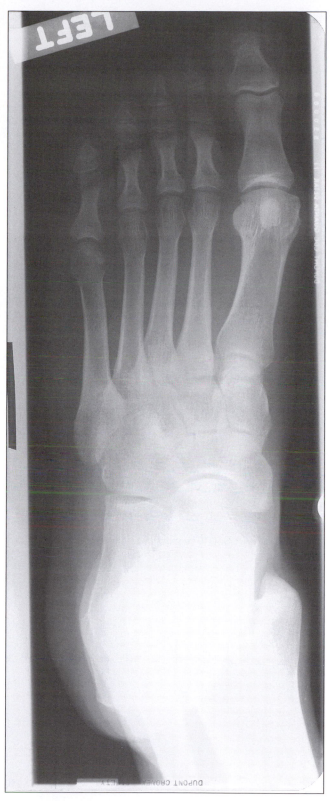

FIGURE 5.48 AP foot (perpendicular central ray).

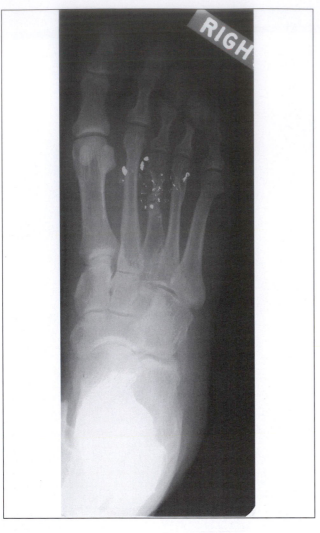

FIGURE 5.49   AP foot (10° cephalic angulation).

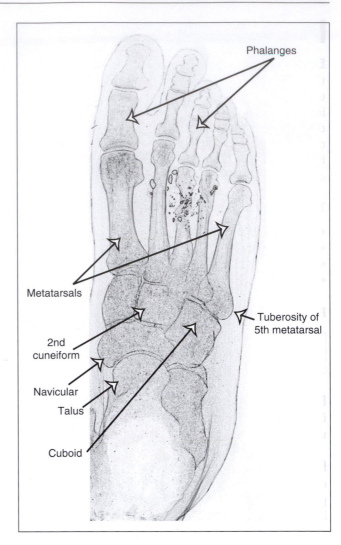

FIGURE 5.49A   AP foot.

FOOT—OBLIQUE POSITION

Exam Rationale The oblique is a routine position of the foot that gives a different perspective than that of the AP. Structures demonstrated on the radiograph include the phalanges; metatarsals; sinus tarsi; and the following interspaces: between the cuboid and the calcaneus, between the cuboid and the fourth and fifth metatarsals, between the cuboid and the lateral cuneiform, and between the talus and the scaphoid.

Technical Considerations

- Extremity screen/film
- Non-grid
- kVp range: 55–60
- SID: 40 inch (100 cm)

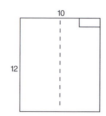

Radiation Protection

Patient Position Seated on the table with the knee flexed; all potential artifacts, including shoe and sock, removed from the part (Figure 5.50).

Part Position Place the plantar surface of the foot on the cassette with the foot centered to the unexposed portion of the cassette; rotate the foot medially 30°.

Central Ray Perpendicular to the base of the third metatarsal.

Patient Instructions "Breathe normally but don't move."

Evaluation Criteria (Figures 5.51 and 5.52)

- Third to fifth metatarsal bases should be free of superimposition; bases of the first and second metatarsals should be superimposed.
- Sinus tarsi should be visualized.
- Tuberosity of the fifth metatarsal should be visualized
- Equal amount of space should exist between shafts of the second through fifth metatarsals.

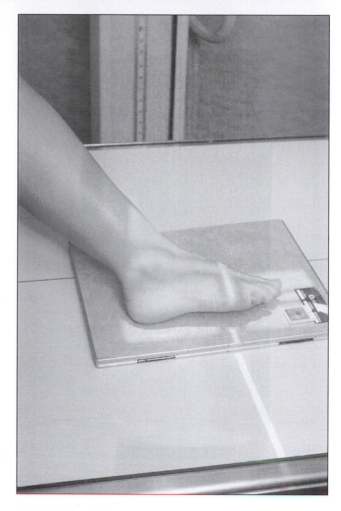

FIGURE 5.50 Oblique foot.

Tip The foot can be rotated laterally 30° to better demonstrate the interspace between the first and second metatarsals and between the medial and intermediate cuneiform (Figures 5.53 and 5.54).

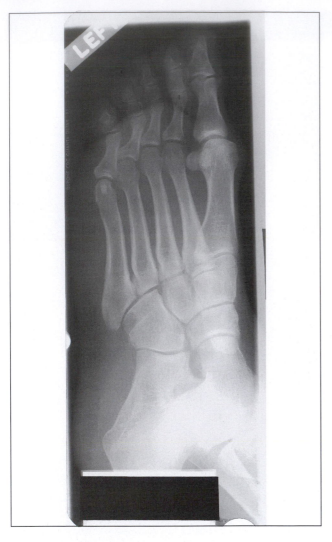

FIGURE 5.51   Oblique foot.

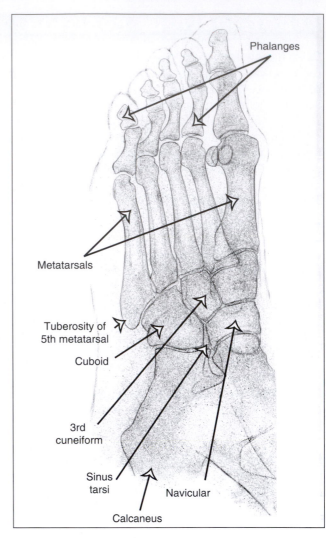

FIGURE 5.52   Oblique foot.

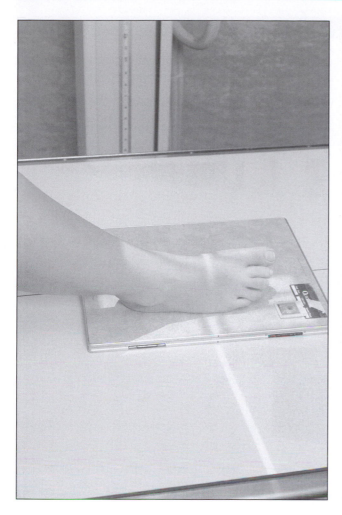

FIGURE 5.53   Oblique foot (rotated laterally).

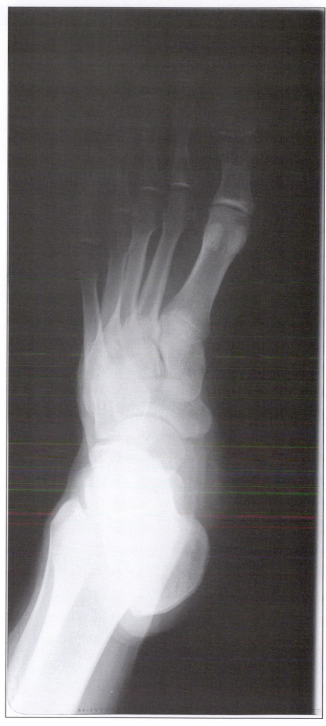

FIGURE 5.54   Oblique foot (rotated laterally).

FOOT—LATERAL POSITION

Exam Rationale The lateral, taken at 90° from the AP, is used to demonstrate anterior/posterior displacements of bony structures and to localize foreign bodies. Structures demonstrated on the radiograph include the foot in profile, the ankle joint, and the distal ends of the tibia and fibula.

Technical Considerations

- Extremity screen/film
- Non-grid
- kVp range: 55–60
- SID: 40 inch (100 cm)

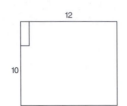

Radiation Protection

Patient Position Lateral recumbent on the affected side with the unaffected leg behind the affected leg; all potential artifacts, including shoe and sock, removed from the part (Figure 5.55).

Part Position Rest the lateral surface on the cassette with the foot centered to the cassette; dorsiflex the foot and adjust it so the plantar surface is perpendicular to the cassette.

Central Ray Perpendicular to the middle of the foot.

Patient Instructions "Breathe normally but don't move."

Evaluation Criteria (Figures 5.56 and 5.57)

- Metatarsals should be nearly superimposed on each other.
- Should include the distal tibia and fibula with the fibula slightly overlapping the posterior tibia.
- Tibiotalar joint should be visualized.

Tips

1. Placing a support under the knee may be helpful in maintaining the foot in a true lateral position.
2. If patient condition permits, the patient can be placed in the lateral recumbent position on the unaf-

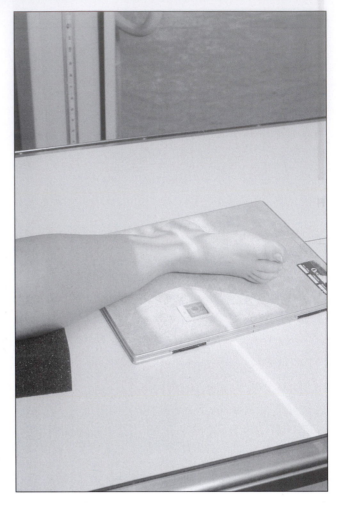

FIGURE 5.55   Lateral foot.

fected side; the foot should rest on its medial surface (lateromedial) and should be adjusted so the plantar surface is perpendicular to the cassette. This provides a truer lateral view of the foot, ankle joint, and distal tibia and fibula (Figures 5.58 and 5.59).

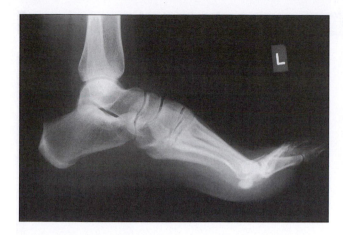

FIGURE 5.56   Lateral foot.

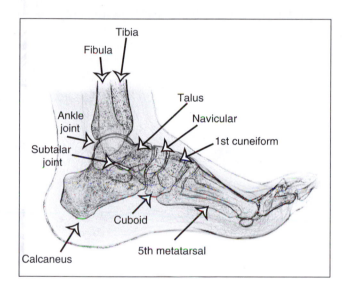

Tibia
Fibula
Talus
Ankle joint
Navicular
Subtalar joint
1st cuneiform
Cuboid
Calcaneus
5th metatarsal

FIGURE 5.57   Lateral foot.

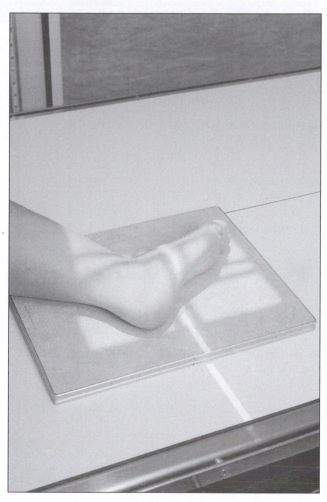

FIGURE 5.58   Lateromedial foot.

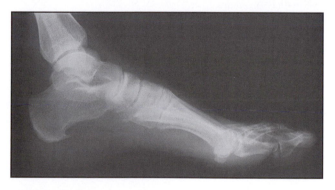

FIGURE 5.59   Lateromedial foot.

FOOT—AP WEIGHT-BEARING PROJECTION

Exam Rationale This position is used to demonstrate a weight-bearing, axial projection of all the bones of the foot, projected free from the distal lower leg.

Technical Considerations

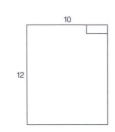

- Extremity screen/film
- Non-grid
- kVp range: 55–60
- SID: 40 inch (100 cm)

Radiation Protection

Patient Position Standing, all potential artifacts, including shoe and sock, removed from the part.

Part Position Place the plantar surface of the foot flat, centering the foot to the cassette:

- Exposure 1: unaffected foot should be approximately 12 inches (30 cm) behind the affected foot.
- Exposure 2: unaffected foot should be approximately 12 inches (30 cm) ahead of the affected foot.

Both exposures are made using a single cassette, superimposing the two images of the foot.

Central Ray

- Exposure 1: 15° posterior angulation to the scaphoid (Figure 5.60).
- Exposure 2: 25° anterior angulation to the posterior ankle so that it exits at the level of the lateral malleolus (Figure 5.61).

Patient Instructions "Breathe normally but don't move."

Evaluation Criteria (Figures 5.62 and 5.63)

- Foot should not be rotated, as evidenced by an equal amount of space between the midshafts of the adjacent metatarsals (2–4) and overlap of the bases of the second, third, and fourth metatarsals.
- All tarsals should be seen.

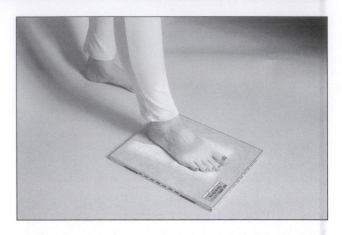

FIGURE 5.60 AP weight-bearing foot (15° posterior angulation).

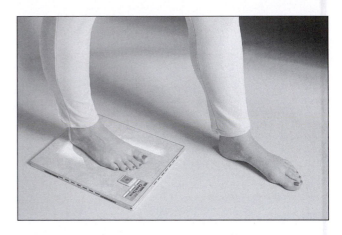

FIGURE 5.61 AP weight-bearing foot (25° anterior angulation).

Tip Care must be taken that the patient carefully maintains the position of the affected foot while moving the unaffected leg between the first and second exposures.

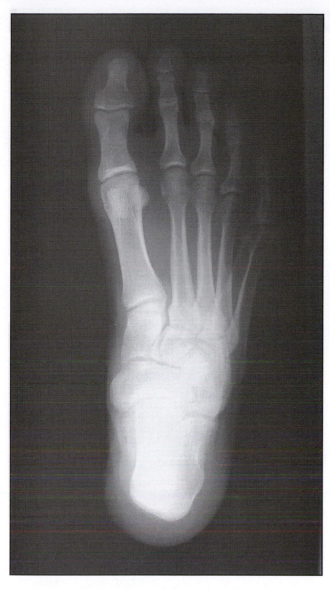

FIGURE 5.62   AP weight-bearing foot.

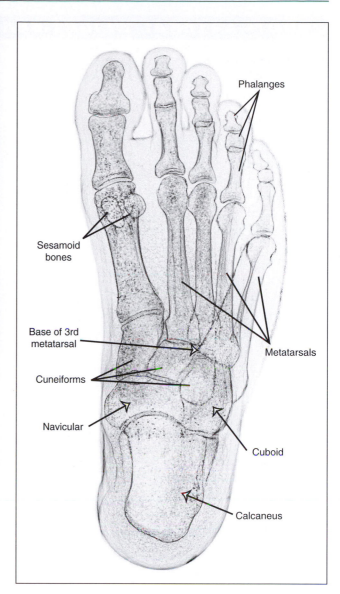

FIGURE 5.63   AP weight-bearing foot.

FOOT—LATERAL WEIGHT-BEARING POSITION

Exam Rationale   This projection is used to demonstrate the structural status of the longitudinal arch. Both sides are examined for comparison.

Technical Considerations

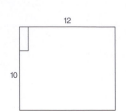

- Extremity screen/film
- Non-grid
- kVp range: 55–60
- SID: 40 inch (100 cm)

Radiation Protection

Patient Position   Standing; all potential artifacts, including shoes and socks, removed (Figure 5.64).

Part Position   The feet should be flat in a natural position with the weight equally distributed on the feet, one on each side of the cassette.

Central Ray   Perpendicular (horizontal) to a point just above the base of the fifth metatarsal.

Patient Instructions   "Breathe normally but don't move."

Evaluation Criteria (Figures 5.65 and 5.66)

- Plantar surfaces of the metatarsal heads should be superimposed.
- Should include the entire foot and the distal tibia and fibula, with the fibula overlapping the posterior tibia.

Tip   It may be necessary to have the patient stand on a step stool or other low bench to raise the feet to tube level.

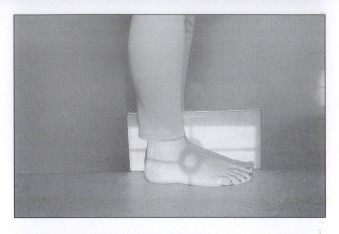

FIGURE 5.64   Lateral weight-bearing foot.

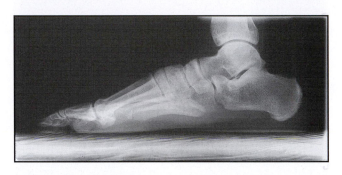

FIGURE 5.65   Lateral weight-bearing foot.

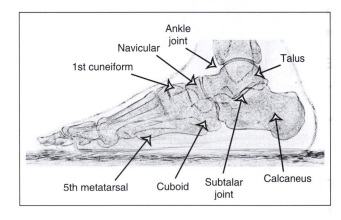

FIGURE 5.66   Lateral weight-bearing foot.

CALCANEUS—AXIAL (PLANTODORSAL)

Exam Rationale   The most common indication for an examination of the heel is trauma. Structures demonstrated on the radiograph include the entire calcaneus and the talocalcaneal joint.

Technical Considerations

- Extremity screen/film
- Non-grid
- kVp range: 55–60
- SID: 40 inch (100 cm)

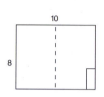

Radiation Protection

Patient Position   Seated on the table with the knee extended; all potential artifacts, including shoe and sock, removed from the part (Figure 5.67).

Part Position   With the heel centered to the unexposed portion of the cassette, adjust the foot so it is not rotated and dorsiflex the foot until the plantar surface is perpendicular to the cassette.

Central Ray   40° cephalic angle to the midpoint of the plantar surface of the foot at the level of the base of the third metatarsal.

Patient Instructions   "Breathe normally but don't move."

Evaluation Criteria (Figures 5.68 and 5.69)

- All of the calcaneus and the talocalcaneal joint should be visualized.
- Calcaneus should not be rotated as evidenced by the first and fifth metatarsals not being visible on either side of the foot.

Tips

1. A gauze strip may be placed around the ball of the foot and held by the patient to assist in adjusting/

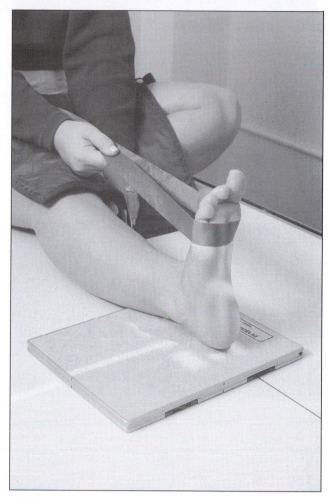

FIGURE 5.67   **Axial calcaneus.**

maintaining the plantar surface perpendicular to the film.

2. The density should be appropriate to visualize the talocalcaneal joint without "burning out" the tuberosity of the calcaneus.

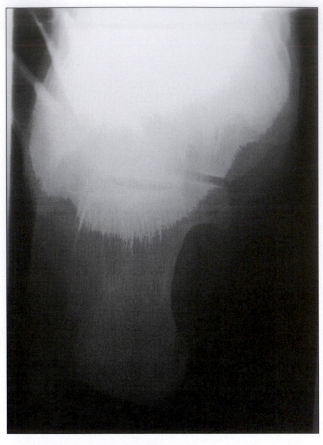

FIGURE 5.68   Axial calcaneus.

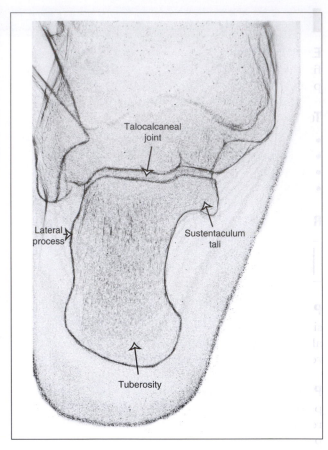

FIGURE 5.69   Axial calcaneus.

CALCANEUS—LATERAL POSITION

Exam Rationale   The lateral shows the heel in profile and is used to demonstrate anterior/posterior displacements of bony pieces.

Technical Considerations

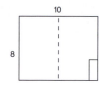

- Extremity screen/film
- Non-grid
- kVp range: 55–60
- SID: 40 inch (100 cm)

Radiation Protection

Patient Position   Lateral recumbent on the affected side with the unaffected leg behind the affected leg; all potential artifacts, including shoe and sock, removed from the part (Figure 5.70).

Part Position   With the heel centered to the unexposed portion of the cassette, dorsiflex the foot and rest its lateral surface on the cassette; adjust so the plantar surface is perpendicular to the cassette.

Central Ray   Perpendicular to the midportion of the calcaneus (about 1 to 1 1/2 inches [3–4 cm] distal to the medial malleolus).

Patient Instructions   "Breathe normally but don't move."

Evaluation Criteria (Figures 5.71 and 5.72)

- Calcaneus should not be rotated.
- Sinus tarsi should be visualized.
- Ankle joint and adjacent tarsals should be included.

Tip   Placing a support under the knee may be helpful in maintaining the foot in true lateral position.

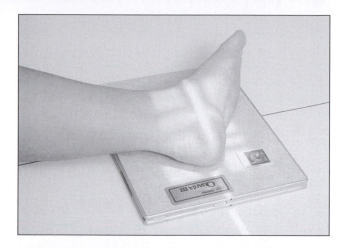

FIGURE 5.70   Lateral calcaneus.

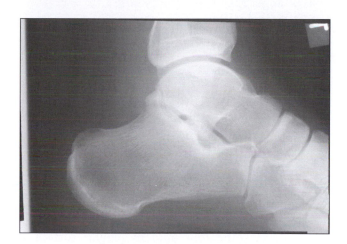

FIGURE 5.71   Lateral calcaneus.

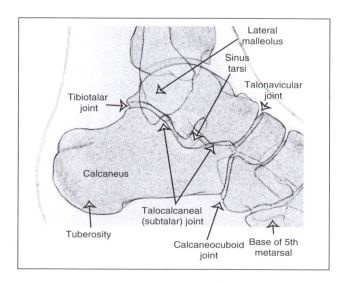

FIGURE 5.72   Lateral calcaneus.

SUBTALAR JOINT—LATEROMEDIAL PROJECTION (BRODEN METHOD)

Exam Rationale An examination of the subtalar joint is indicated when joint involvement is suspected in cases of comminuted fractures. Structures demonstrated on the radiograph include the calcaneus and the talocalcaneus joint. The 40° angle best demonstrates the posterior articular facet of the calcaneus and the 10° angle the anterior articular facet; the articulation between the talus and sustentaculum is best demonstrated on one of the two intermediate angulations.

Technical Considerations

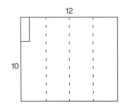

- Extremity screen/film
- Non-grid
- kVp range: 55–60
- SID: 40 inch (100 cm)23

Radiation Protection

Patient Position Seated on the table with the knee extended; all potential artifacts, including shoe and sock, removed from the part (Figure 5.73).

Part Position With the heel positioned approximately 1 inch (3 cm) above the lower end of the cassette, dorsiflex the foot until its plantar surface is perpendicular to the cassette; with the ankle maintained at the right angle flexion, rotate the leg and foot medially approximately 45°.

Central Ray Directed to a point approximately 1 inch (3 cm) superoanteriorly to the lateral malleolus; four exposures are made with the central ray angled cephalad at 40°, 30°, 20° and 10°.

Patient Instructions "Breathe normally but don't move."

Evaluation Criteria (Figures 5.74 through 5.78)

- All of the calcaneus and talocalcaneal joint should be visualized.

Tip A gauze strip may be placed around the ball of the foot to assist in adjusting/maintaining the plantar surface perpendicular to the film.

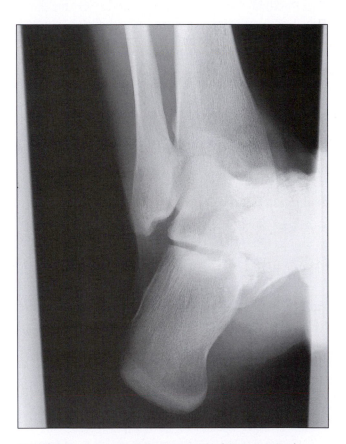

FIGURE 5.73 Lateromedial subtalar joint (40° angulation).

FIGURE 5.74 Lateromedial subtalar joint (40° angulation).

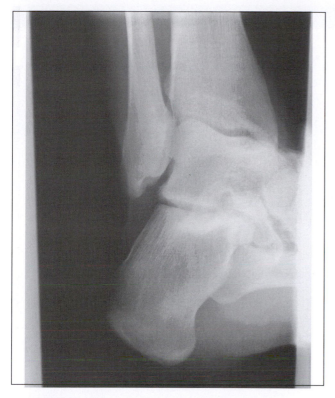

FIGURE 5.75 Lateromedial subtalar joint (30° angulation).

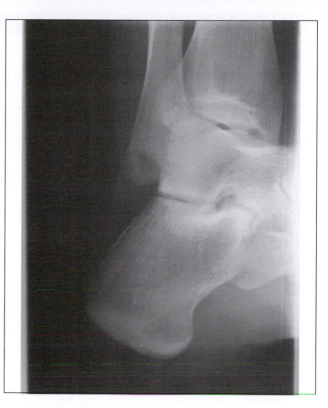

FIGURE 5.77 Lateromedial subtalar joint (10° angulation).

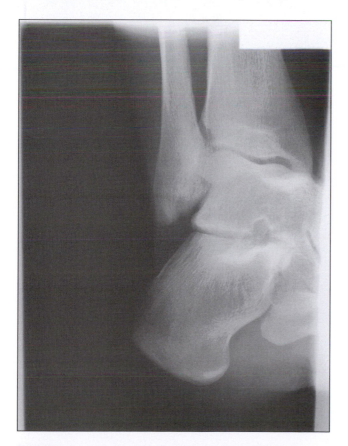

FIGURE 5.76 Lateromedial subtalar joint (20° angulation).

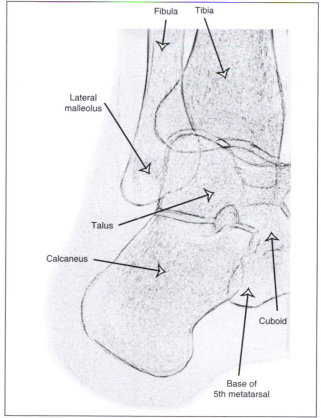

FIGURE 5.78 Lateromedial subtalar joint.

ANKLE—AP PROJECTION

Exam Rationale The most common indication for an examination of the ankle is trauma. Structures demonstrated on the AP projection include the distal tibia and fibula and the proximal portion of the talus.

Technical Considerations

- Extremity screen/film
- Non-grid
- kVp range: 55–60
- SID: 40 inch (100 cm)

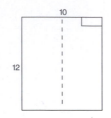

Radiation Protection

Patient Position Seated on the table with the knee extended; all potential artifacts, including shoe and sock, removed from the part (Figure 5.79).

Part Position Dorsiflex the foot so its plantar surface is perpendicular to the cassette; center the ankle to the unexposed portion of the cassette and adjust the foot so the ankle is in true AP position (intermalleolar plane will *not* be parallel with the film's surface).

Central Ray Perpendicular midway between the malleoli.

Patient Instructions "Breathe normally but don't move."

Evaluation Criteria (Figures 5.80 and 5.81)

- Visualization of both the lateral and medial malleoli with moderate overlapping at the distal tibiofibular articulation.
- Visualization of the tibiotalar joint space with the medial tibiotalar articulation free of overlap.

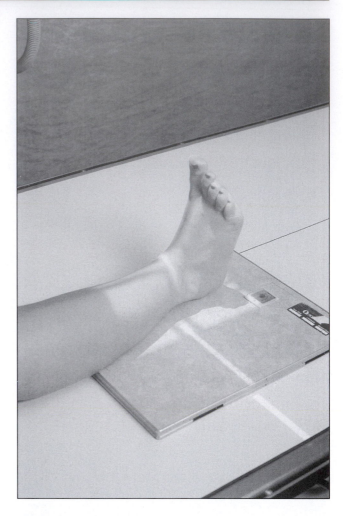

FIGURE 5.79   AP ankle.

Tip To visualize more of the tibia and fibula, position the ankle closer to the lower edge of the cassette; if the ankle joint is involved, the central ray should be directed through the ankle joint to prevent distortion of the joint space.

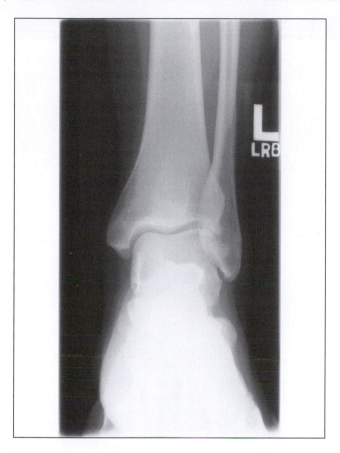

FIGURE 5.80 **AP ankle.**

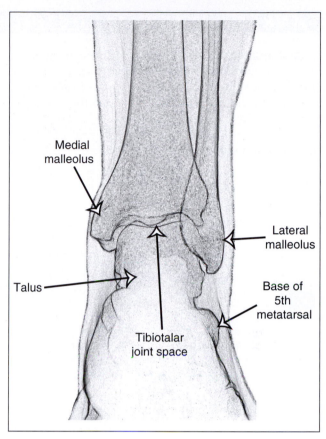

FIGURE 5.81 **AP ankle.**

ANKLE—(INTERNAL) OBLIQUE POSITION

Exam Rationale   The oblique is a routine position of the ankle that gives a different perspective than that of the AP. Structures demonstrated on the radiograph include the distal tibia and fibula and the tibiotalar joint.

Technical Considerations

- Extremity screen/film
- Non-grid
- kVp range: 55–60
- SID: 40 inch (100 cm)

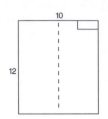

Radiation Protection

Patient Position   Seated on the table with the knee extended; all potential artifacts, including shoe and sock, removed from the part (Figure 5.82).

Part Position   Adjust the long axis of the ankle parallel with the long axis of the cassette and center the ankle to the unexposed portion of the cassette; rotate the entire leg and foot 45° and dorsiflex the foot to place its plantar surface perpendicular to the cassette.

Central Ray   Perpendicular midway between the malleoli.

Patient Instructions   "Breathe normally but don't move."

Evaluation Criteria (Figures 5.83 and 5.84)

- Distal tibia and fibula should be somewhat overlapped.

Tip   To visualize more of the tibia and fibula, position the ankle closer to the lower edge of the cassette; if the ankle joint is involved, the central ray should be directed through the ankle joint to prevent distortion of the joint space.

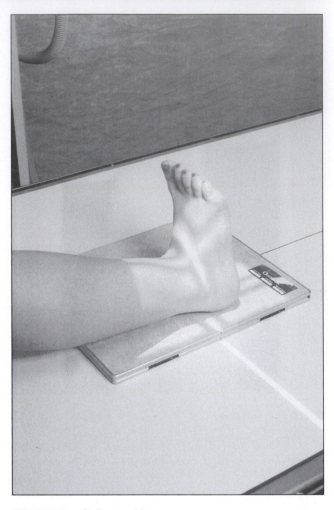

FIGURE 5.82   Oblique ankle.

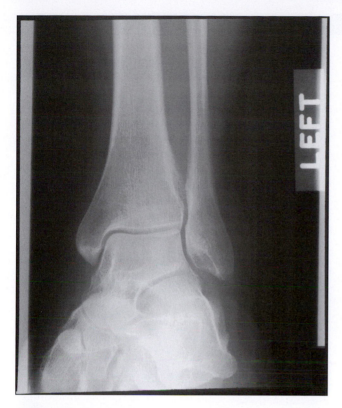

FIGURE 5.83   Oblique ankle.

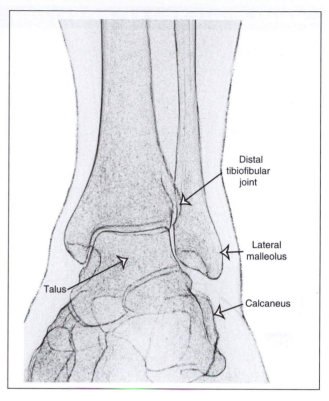

FIGURE 5.84   Oblique ankle.

ANKLE—LATERAL POSITION

Exam Rationale   The lateral, taken at 90° from the AP, is used to demonstrate anterior/posterior displacements of bony structures and to localize foreign bodies. Structures demonstrated on the radiograph include the distal tibia and fibula, the ankle joint, and the proximal tarsals.

Technical Considerations

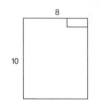

- Extremity screen/film
- Non-grid
- kVp range: 55–60
- SID: 40 inch (100 cm)

Radiation Protection

Patient Position   Lateral recumbent on the affected side with the unaffected leg behind the affected leg; all potential artifacts, including shoe and sock, removed from the part (Figure 5.85).

Part Position   Rest the lateral surface on the cassette and adjust so the longitudinal axis of the leg is parallel with the longitudinal axis of the cassette and the ankle is centered to the cassette; dorsiflex the foot to a right angle and adjust so its plantar surface is perpendicular to the cassette to place the intermalleolar plane perpendicular to the film.

Central Ray   Perpendicular to the medial malleolus.

Patient Instructions   "Breathe normally but don't move."

Evaluation Criteria (Figures 5.86 and 5.87)

- Fibula should be overlapped by the posterior tibia.

Tips

1. Placing a support under the knee may be helpful in maintaining the foot in a true lateral position.
2. To visualize more of the tibia and fibula, position the ankle closer to the lower edge of the cassette; if

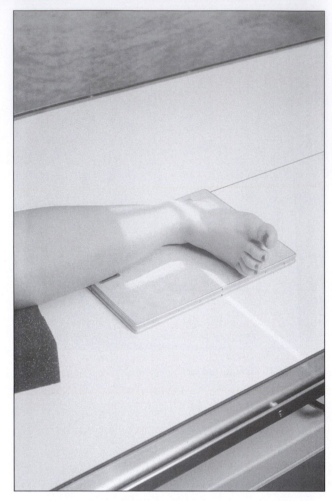

FIGURE 5.85   Lateral ankle.

the ankle joint is involved, the central ray should be directed through the ankle to prevent distortion of the joint space.
3. If patient condition permits, the patient can be placed in the lateral recumbent position on the unaffected side; the foot should rest on its medial surface (lateromedial) and should be adjusted so the plantar surface is perpendicular to the cassette. This provides a truer lateral view of the ankle joint and the distal tibia and fibula (Figures 5.88 and 5.89).

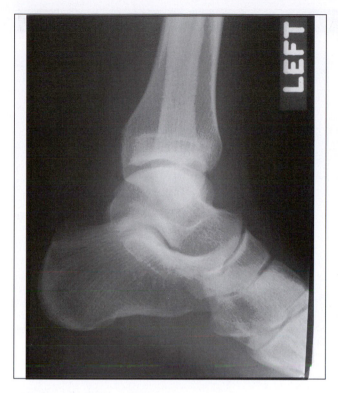

FIGURE 5.86 Lateral ankle.

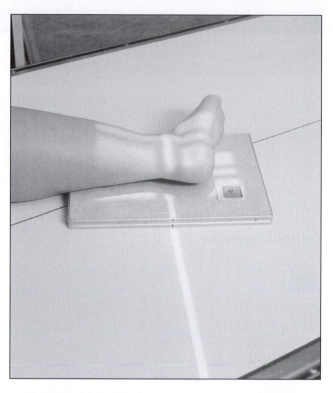

FIGURE 5.88 Lateromedial ankle.

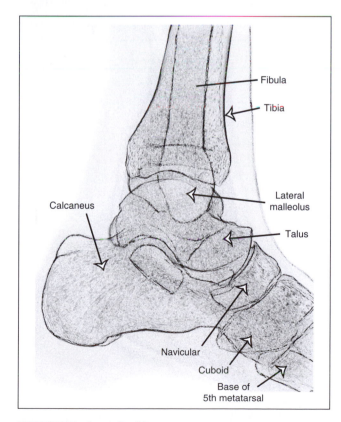

Fibula

Tibia

Lateral
malleolus

Talus

Calcaneus

Navicular

Cuboid

Base of
5th metatarsal

FIGURE 5.87 Lateral ankle.

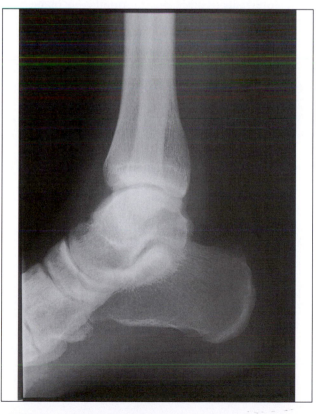

FIGURE 5.89 Lateromedial ankle.

ANKLE—AP MORTISE PROJECTION

Exam Rationale   This projection is an alternative view of the ankle that demonstrates the mortise joint free of superimposition of the talus or distal tibia and fibula.

Technical Considerations

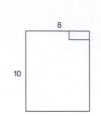

- Extremity screen/film
- Non-grid
- kVp range: 55–60
- SID: 40 inch (100 cm)

Radiation Protection

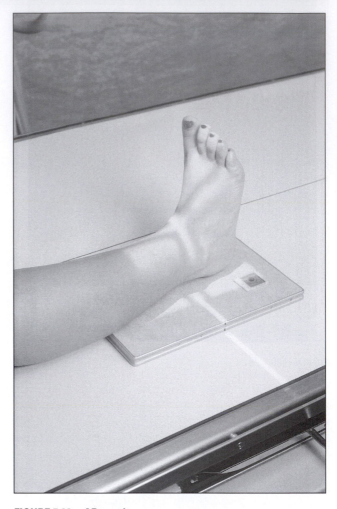

FIGURE 5.90   **AP mortise.**

Patient Position   Seated on the table with the knee extended; all potential artifacts, including shoe and sock, removed from the part (Figure 5.90).

Part Position   Center the ankle to the cassette and adjust the long axis of the ankle parallel with the long axis of the cassette; rotate the entire leg and foot 15° to 20° internally to place the intermalleolar plane parallel with the surface of the film; dorsiflex the foot to place its plantar surface perpendicular to the cassette.

Central Ray   Perpendicular midway between the malleoli.

Patient Instructions   "Breathe normally but don't move."

Evaluation Criteria (Figures 5.91 and 5.92)

- Mortise joint should be projected free of both the tibia and fibula.

Tip   This view should supplement, not replace, a routine oblique projection of the ankle.

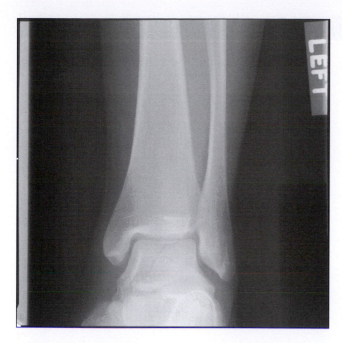

FIGURE 5.91   AP mortise.

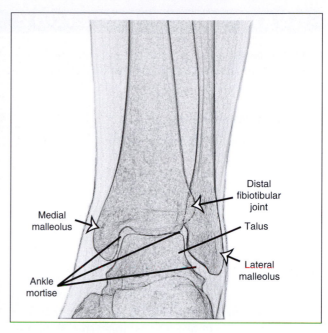

FIGURE 5.92   AP mortise.

ANKLE—AP STRESS STUDY

Exam Rationale The most common indication for a stress study of the ankle is trauma resulting in a possible tear of ligaments.

Technical Considerations

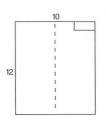

- Extremity screen/film
- Non-grid
- kVp range: 55–60
- SID: 40 inch (100 cm)

Radiation Protection

Patient Position Seated on the table with the knee extended; all potential artifacts, including shoe and sock, removed from the part.

Part Position With the ankle in the AP position, the foot is:

- Exposure 1: inverted as much as possible (Figure 5.93).
- Exposure 2: everted as much as possible (Figure 5.94).

Central Ray Perpendicular midway between the malleoli.

Patient Instructions "Breathe normally but don't move."

Evaluation Criteria (Figures 5.95 through 5.98)

- Should include the distal tibia and fibula and talus.

Tips

1. If patient condition permits, a strip of gauze around the ball of the foot may be held by the patient and used to invert/evert the foot and maintain its position for the exposure.
2. For recent or very painful injuries, a local anesthetic may be required; placing and maintaining the foot in position is done by a physician or other health care personnel.

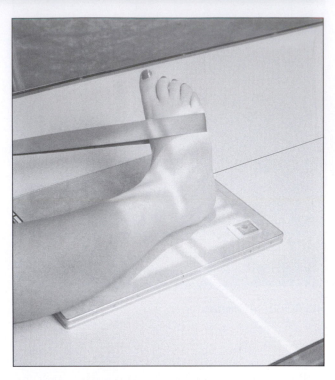

FIGURE 5.93   AP ankle with inversion stress.

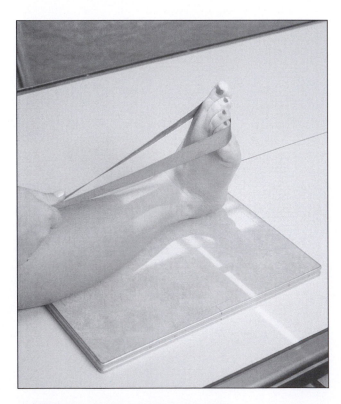

FIGURE 5.94   AP ankle with eversion stress.

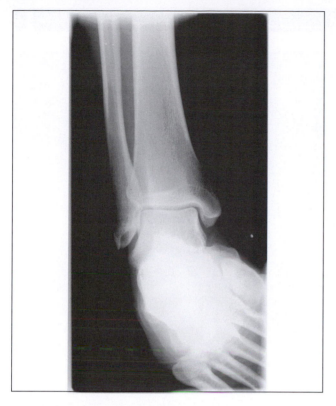

FIGURE 5.95   AP ankle with inversion stress.

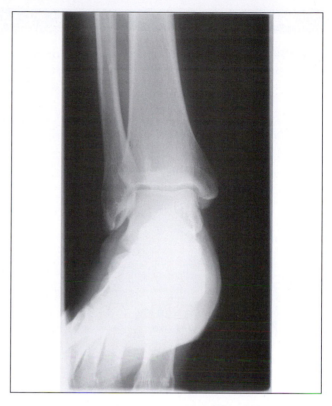

FIGURE 5.97   AP ankle with eversion stress.

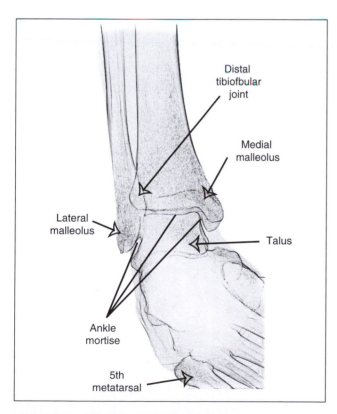

Distal
tibiofbular
joint

Medial
malleolus

Lateral
malleolus

Talus

Ankle
mortise

5th
metatarsal

FIGURE 5.96   AP ankle with inversion stress.

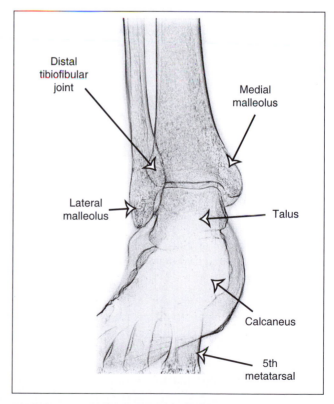

Distal
tibiofibular
joint

Medial
malleolus

Lateral
malleolus

Talus

Calcaneus

5th
metatarsal

FIGURE 5.98   AP ankle with eversion stress.

LOWER LEG—AP PROJECTION

Exam Rationale　The most common indication for an examination of the lower leg is trauma. Structures demonstrated on the radiograph include the tibia, fibula, and adjacent joints.

Technical Considerations

- Extremity screen/film
- Non-grid
- kVp range: 55–60
- SID: 40 inch (100 cm)

Radiation Protection

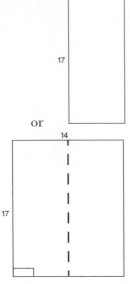

Patient Position　Seated on the table with the knee extended; all potential artifacts, including shoe and sock, removed from the knee down (Figure 5.99).

Part Position　Center the leg to the cassette and adjust it into the AP position; dorsiflex the foot so it is perpendicular to the cassette.

Central Ray　Perpendicular to the midpoint of the leg.

Patient Instructions　"Breathe normally but don't move."

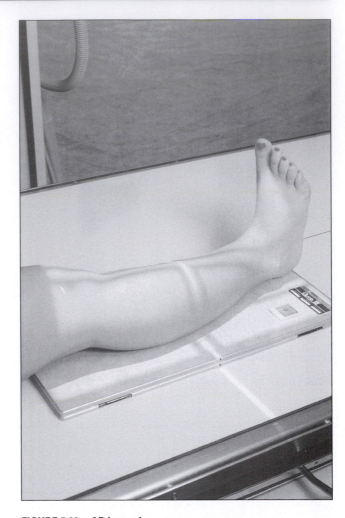

FIGURE 5.99　AP lower leg.

Evaluation Criteria (Figures 5.100 and 5.101)

- Both the ankle and knee joints should be included; if necessary, a separate AP of one joint may be needed.
- Ankle and knee joints should be in true AP position.
- Tibia and fibula should be slightly overlapped at both the proximal and distal ends.

Tips

1. It may be necessary to invert the foot slightly to adjust the leg into the true AP position, but care must be taken to not rotate the entire leg.
2. It is important, on initial examination, to include both joints; some departmental protocols may permit follow-up examinations that include only the joint nearest the site of injury.
3. If the leg is too long to include both joints, the leg may be positioned diagonally on a 14 × 17 (36 × 43 cm) for each view.

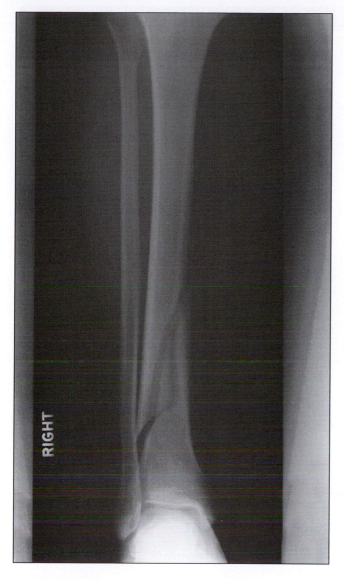

FIGURE 5.100　**AP lower leg.**

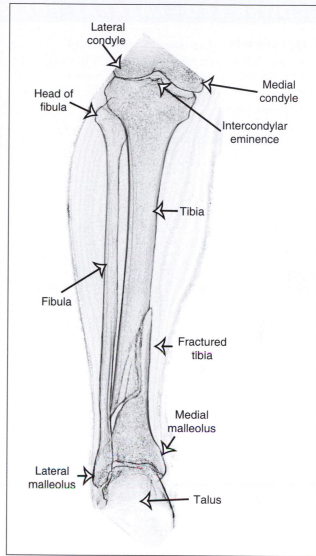

FIGURE 5.101　**AP lower leg.**

LOWER LEG—LATERAL POSITION

Exam Rationale   The lateral, taken at 90° degrees from the AP, is used to demonstrate anterior/posterior displacements of bony structures. Structures demonstrated on the radiograph include the tibia, fibula, and adjacent joints.

Technical Considerations

- Extremity screen/film
- Non-grid
- kVp range: 55–60
- SID: 40 inch (100 cm)

Radiation Protection

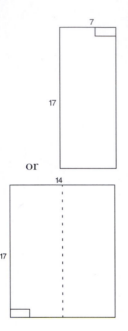

Patient Position   Lateral recumbent on the affected side with the unaffected leg behind the affected leg; all potential artifacts, including shoe and sock, removed from the knee down (Figure 5.102).

Part Position   Dorsiflex the foot and rest the lateral surface of the leg on the cassette so the leg is centered to the cassette and the longitudinal axis of the leg is parallel with the longitudinal axis of the cassette; adjust the rotation of the leg so the patella is perpendicular to the cassette.

Central Ray   Perpendicular to the midpoint of the leg.

Patient Instructions   "Breathe normally but don't move."

Evaluation Criteria (Figures 5.103 and 5.104)

- Both the ankle and knee joints should be included.
- There should be slight separation of the shafts of the tibia and fibula except at the proximal and distal ends.
- Proximally, there will be some overlap of the fibula and tibia.
- Distally, the fibula should overlap posterior tibia.

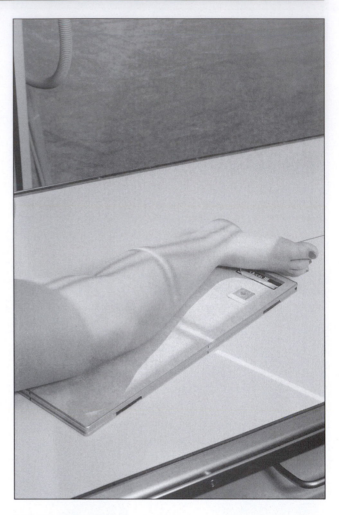

FIGURE 5.102   Lateral lower leg.

Tips

1. If patient condition does not permit turning the patient, a cross-table projection may be taken; the affected leg should be carefully lifted so that a firm support can be placed beneath it; the cassette is placed on the medial surface of the leg and the central ray directed from the lateral side (Figure 5.105).

2. It is important, on initial examination, to include both joints; some departmental protocols may permit follow-up examinations that include only the joint nearest the site of injury.

3. If the leg is too long to include both joints, it may be positioned diagonally on a 14 × 17 (36 × 43 cm) for each view.

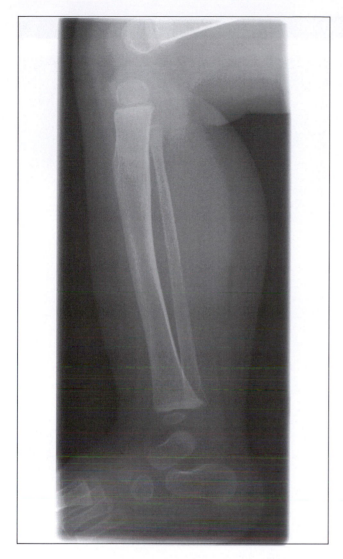

FIGURE 5.103 Lateral lower leg.

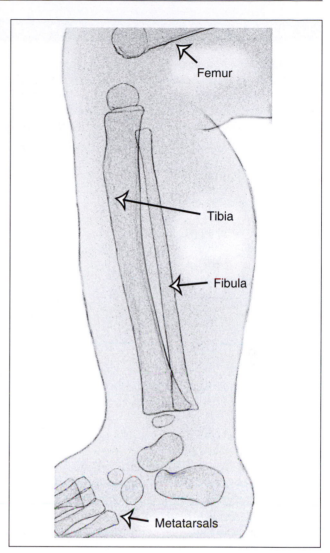

FIGURE 5.104 Lateral lower leg.

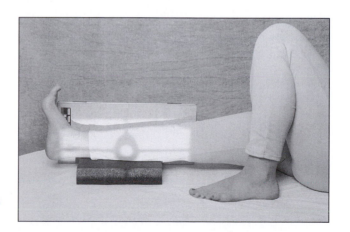

FIGURE 5.105
Cross-table lateral lower leg.

LOWER LEG—OBLIQUE POSITION

Exam Rationale   The oblique is an alternative position of the leg that is occasionally requested to demonstrate the tibiofibular articulations. Structures demonstrated on the radiograph include both the ankle and knee joints and the shafts of the tibia and fibula.

Technical Considerations

- Extremity screen/film
- Non-grid
- kVp range: 55–60
- SID: 40 inch (100 cm)

Radiation Protection

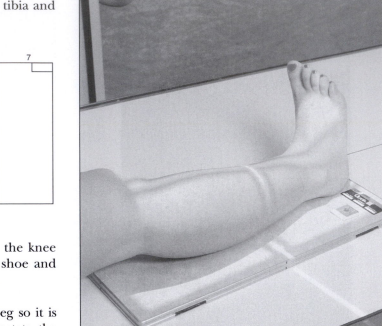

FIGURE 5.106   Oblique lower leg.

Patient Position   Seated on the table with the knee extended; all potential artifacts, including shoe and sock, removed from the part (Figure 5.106).

Part Position   Adjust the long axis of the leg so it is parallel with the long axis of the cassette; rotate the entire leg and foot 45° medially and dorsiflex the foot to place its plantar surface perpendicular to the cassette.

Central Ray   Perpendicular to the midpoint of the leg.

Patient Instructions   "Breathe normally but don't move."

Evaluation Criteria (Figures 5.107 and 5.108)

- Both the ankle and knee joints should be included.
- Proximal and distal tibiofibular articulations should be visualized.
- Should demonstrate maximum space between the tibia and fibula.

Tip   Occasionally, a 45° external oblique may be requested; this will yield a radiograph that shows complete overlap of the tibia and fibula (Figures 5.109 and 5.110).

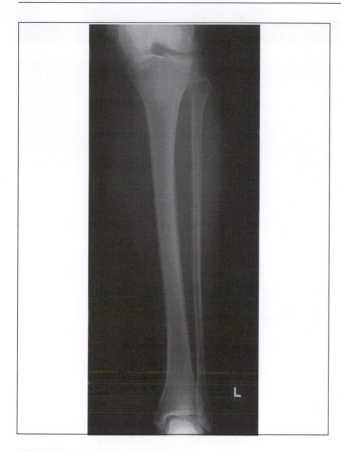

FIGURE 5.107   Oblique lower leg.

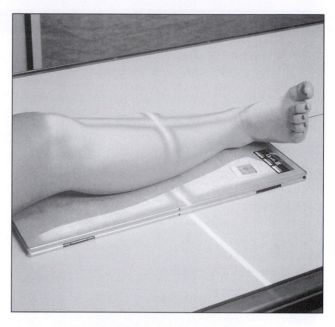

FIGURE 5.109   External oblique lower leg.

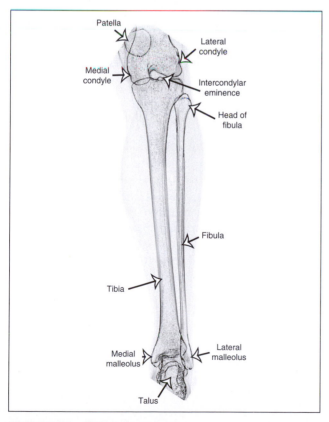

Patella

Lateral condyle

Medial condyle

Intercondylar eminence

Head of fibula

Fibula

Tibia

Medial malleolus

Lateral malleolus

Talus

FIGURE 5.108   Oblique lower leg.

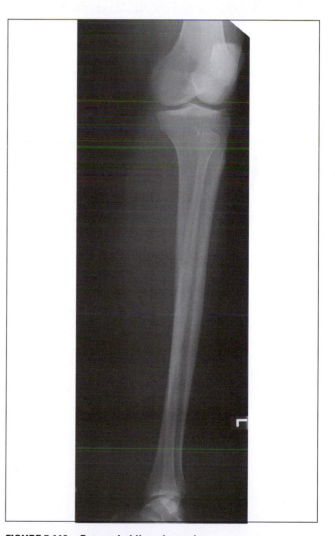

FIGURE 5.110   External oblique lower leg.

KNEE—AP PROJECTION

Exam Rationale   Radiographic examination of the knee is commonly indicated in cases of trauma or degenerative joint disease. Structures demonstrated include the knee joint, the proximal tibia and fibula, and the distal femur.

Technical Considerations

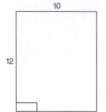

- Regular screen/film
- Grid
- kVp range: 60–70
- SID: 40 inch (100 cm)

Radiation   AEC
Protection   (Phototiming)

      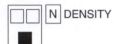 N DENSITY

Patient Position   Seated or supine on the table with the knee extended; all potential artifacts from the distal femur down removed (Figure 5.111).

Part Position   Center the knee joint (1/2 inch distal to patellar apex) to the midline of the table and adjust the knee so the interepicondylar plane is parallel to the surface of the film; the patella will lie slightly to the medial side of the knee.

Central Ray   One-half inch (1 cm) distal to the patellar apex at a 5° cephalic angle.

Patient Instructions   "Breathe normally but don't move."

Evaluation Criteria (Figures 5.112 and 5.113)

- Femur and tibia should be seen without rotation.
- Femorotibial joint space should be open.
- The head of the fibula will be slightly overlapped by the proximal tibia.
- Patella should be completely superimposed over the femur.
- In the normal knee, the femorotibial joint space should be equal on both sides.

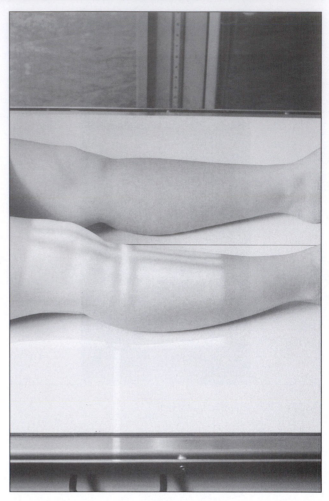

FIGURE 5.111   AP knee.

Tips

1. Non-grid method may be used for a knee that measures less than 11 cm.
2. When the primary interest is the distal femur or the proximal tibia and fibula, the central ray may be directed perpendicular through the knee joint.
3. In cases where the patient is unable to fully extend the knee, a curved cassette is recommended to reduce the part to image receptor distance (Figure 5.114).

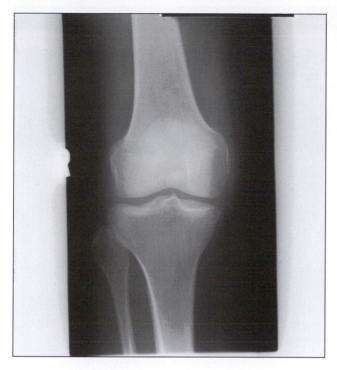

FIGURE 5.112   AP knee.

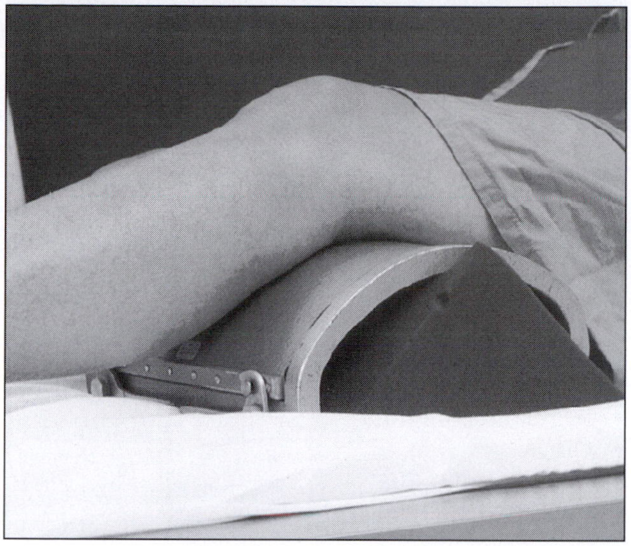

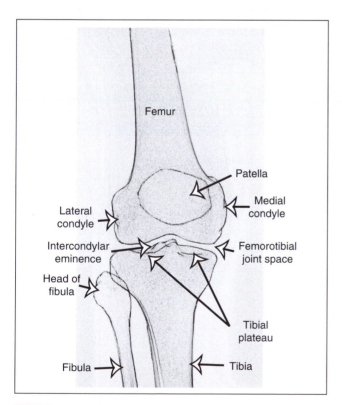

FIGURE 5.113   AP knee.

FIGURE 5.114   AP knee with curved cassette.

KNEE—INTERNAL OBLIQUE POSITION

Exam Rationale The oblique is an alternative position of the knee that is used to provide a different perspective from that of the AP and lateral. Structures demonstrated include the proximal tibia and fibula, the distal femur, and the knee joint. The internal oblique demonstrates particularly well the lateral femoral and tibial condyles, the lateral tibial plateau, and the head of the fibula.

Technical Considerations

- Regular screen/film
- Grid
- kVp range: 60–70
- SID: 40 inch (100 cm)

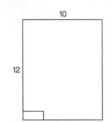

Radiation   AEC
Protection   (Phototiming)

 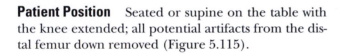

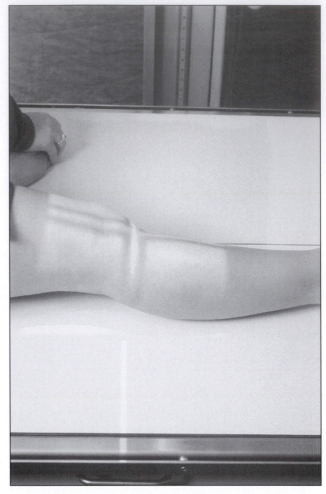

FIGURE 5.115   Internal oblique knee.

Patient Position Seated or supine on the table with the knee extended; all potential artifacts from the distal femur down removed (Figure 5.115).

Part Position With the knee centered to the midline of the table, rotate the affected leg 45° internally; this may require elevation of the hip on the affected side.

Central Ray 5° cephalic to the knee joint (1/2 inch/1 cm distal to patellar apex).

Patient Instructions "Breathe normally but don't move."

Evaluation Criteria (Figures 5.116 and 5.117)

- Tibia and fibula should be separated at their proximal articulation.
- Lateral condyles of the femur and tibia should be visualized.
- Knee joint should be open.

- Both tibial plateaus should be visualized.
- Medial margin of the patella should be projected slightly beyond the medial margin of the femur.

Tip Non-grid method may be used for a knee that measures less than 11 cm.

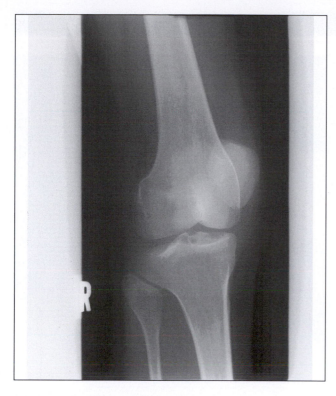

FIGURE 5.116   Internal oblique knee.

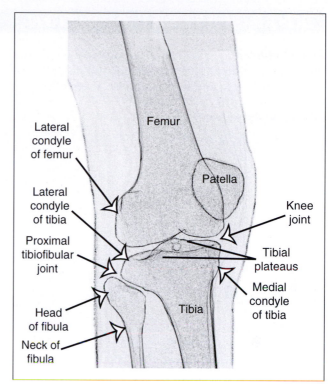

FIGURE 5.117   Internal oblique knee.

KNEE—LATERAL POSITION

Exam Rationale   Structures demonstrated on the lateral projection of the knee include the distal femur, the proximal tibia and fibula, and the knee joint.

Technical Considerations

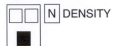

- Regular screen/film
- Grid
- kVp range: 60–70
- SID: 40 inch (100 cm)

Radiation   AEC
Protection   (Phototiming)

 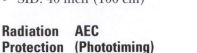 N DENSITY

Patient Position   Lateral recumbent on the affected side with the unaffected leg behind the affected leg; all potential artifacts from the distal femur down removed (Figure 5.118).

Part Position   Rest the knee on its lateral surface and center it to the midline of the table; flex the knee 20° to 30° and adjust it so that the interepicondylar plane is perpendicular to the cassette.

Central Ray   5° cephalic to the knee joint (1/2 inch/1 cm distal to patellar apex).

Patient Instructions   "Breathe normally but don't move."

Evaluation Criteria (Figures 5.119 and 5.120)

- Femoral condyles should be superimposed.
- Patella should be projected in profile.
- Femoropatellar space should be open.
- Fibular head and the tibia should be slightly super-imposed.

Tips

1. A support placed under the heel/ankle of the affected leg helps in maintaining the knee in true lateral position.
2. Non-grid method may be used for a knee that measures less than 11 cm.

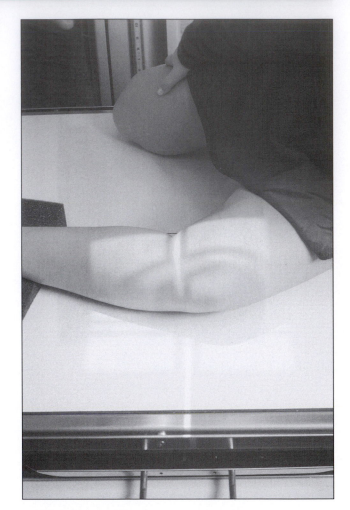

FIGURE 5.118   Lateral knee.

3. In cases of patella fracture, the knee should be flexed no more than 15°.

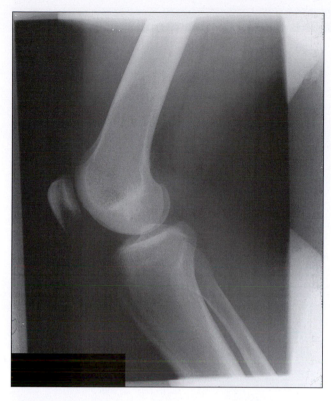

FIGURE 5.119   Lateral knee.

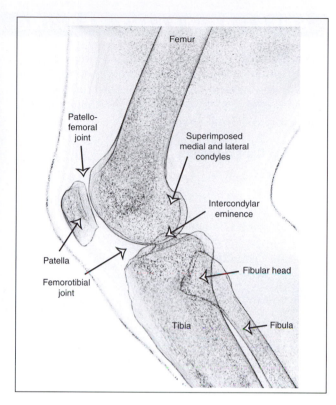

FIGURE 5.120   Lateral knee.

KNEE—AP WEIGHT-BEARING PROJECTION

Exam Rationale Weight-bearing radiographic examination of the knee is commonly indicated in cases of degenerative joint disease. Structures demonstrated include the knee joint, the proximal tibia and fibula, and the distal femur.

Technical Considerations

- Regular screen/film
- Grid
- kVp range: 60–70
- SID: 40 inch (100 cm)

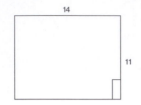

Radiation Protection

Patient Position Erect with the back toward a vertical grid device; the toes should be pointing forward and the feet separated sufficiently to achieve good balance (approximately 6– 8 inches [15–20 cm]); the patient should stand straight with the weight equally distributed on both feet; all potential artifacts from the distal femur down removed (Figure 5.121).

Part Position Center the patellar apices to the midline of the upright grid.

Central Ray Perpendicular to the film midway between the knees at the level of the patellar apices.

Patient Instructions "Breathe normally but don't move."

Evaluation Criteria (Figures 5.122 and 5.123)

- Knees should not be rotated.
- Knee joint space should be centered to the exposed area of the film.

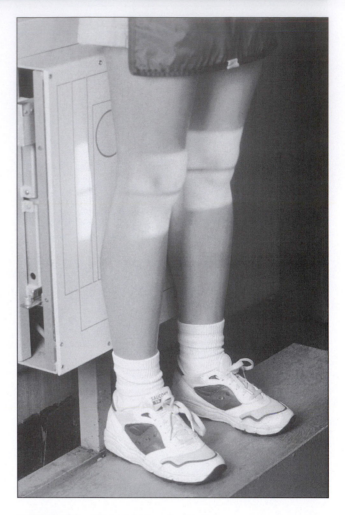

FIGURE 5.121   AP weight-bearing knee.

Tip It is sometimes helpful in evaluating joint space narrowing to do a PA projection with the knees completely extended or with them flexed from 30° to 60° (Figures 5.124 and 5.125).

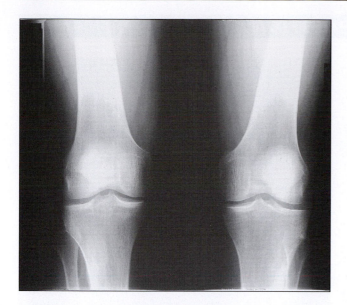

FIGURE 5.122   **AP weight-bearing knee.**

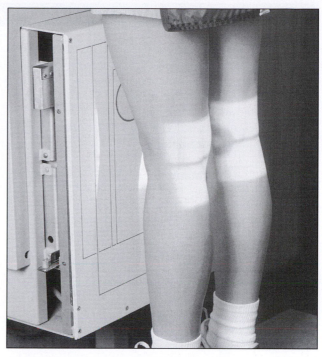

FIGURE 5.124   **PA weight-bearing knee (extended).**

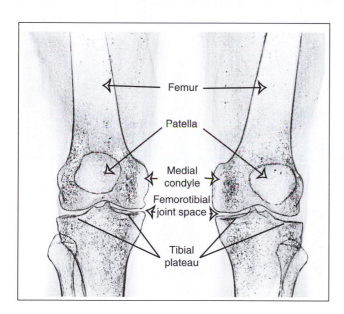

FIGURE 5.123   **AP weight-bearing knee.**

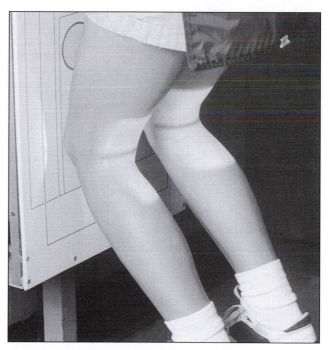

FIGURE 5.125   **PA weight-bearing knee (flexed).**

KNEE—EXTERNAL OBLIQUE POSITION

Exam Rationale   The oblique is an alternative position of the knee that is used to provide a different perspective from that of the AP and lateral. Structures demonstrated include the proximal tibia and fibula, the distal femur, and the knee joint. The external oblique demonstrates the medial femoral and tibial condyles and the lateral tibial plateau.

Technical Considerations

- Regular screen/film
- Grid
- kVp range: 60–70
- SID: 40 inch (100 cm)

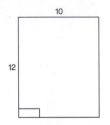

Radiation Protection   AEC (Phototiming)

 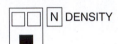 N DENSITY

Patient Position   Seated or supine on the table with the knee extended; all potential artifacts from the distal femur down removed (Figure 5.126).

Part Position   With the knee centered to the midline of the table, rotate the affected leg 45° externally.

Central Ray   5° cephalic to the knee joint (1/2 inch/1 cm distal to patellar apex).

Patient Instructions   "Breathe normally but don't move."

Evaluation Criteria (Figures 5.127 and 5.128)

- Fibula should be nearly completely superimposed by the lateral tibia.
- Medial condyles of the femur and tibia should be visualized.
- Knee joint should be open.
- Both tibial plateaus should be visualized.
- Lateral margin of the patella should be projected slightly beyond the lateral margin of the femur.

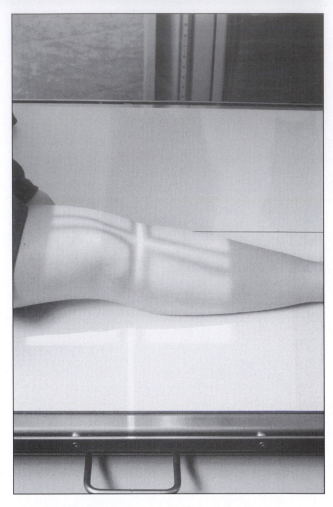

FIGURE 5.126   External oblique knee.

Tip   Non-grid method may be used for a knee that measures less than 11 cm.

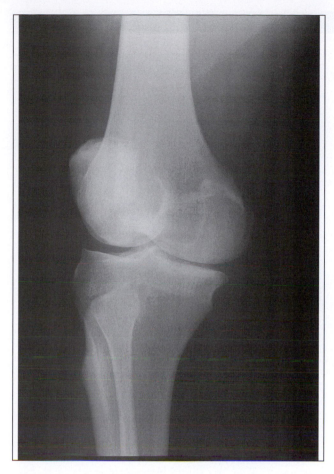

FIGURE 5.127 External oblique knee.

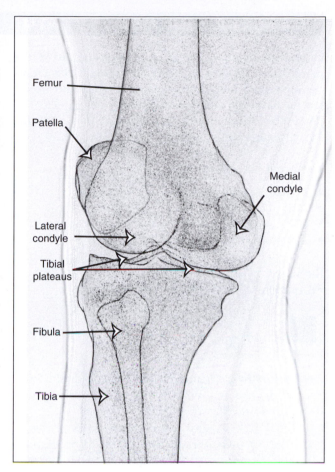

FIGURE 5.128 External oblique knee.

PATELLA—PA PROJECTION

Exam Rationale Radiographic examination of the patella is indicated in cases of trauma. Structures demonstrated include the proximal tibia and fibula, the distal femur, the knee joint, and the patella. The PA projection provides better detail than the routine AP projection of the knee.

Technical Considerations

- Regular screen/film
- Grid
- kVp range: 60–70
- SID: 40 inch (100 cm)

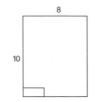

Radiation Protection
AEC (Phototiming)

 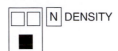 N DENSITY

Patient Position Prone on the table with the knee extended; all potential artifacts from the distal femur down removed (Figure 5.129).

Part Position Center the patella to the midline of the table and adjust it so the patella is parallel with the plane of the film; this usually requires a 5° to 10° lateral rotation of the heel.

Central Ray Perpendicular to the knee joint (1/2 inch/1 cm distal to patellar apex).

Patient Instructions "Breathe normally but don't move."

Evaluation Criteria (Figures 5.130 and 5.131)

- Femorotibial joint space should be open.
- Femur and tibia should not be rotated.
- The head of the fibula should be slightly overlapped by the proximal tibia.
- Patella should be completely superimposed over the femur.

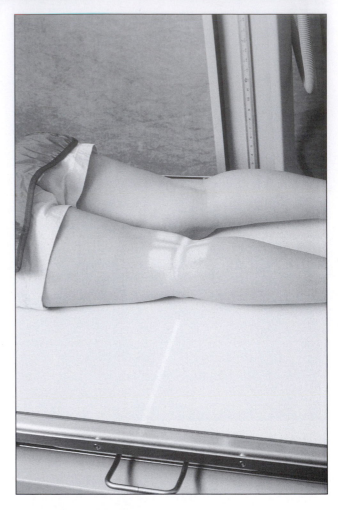

FIGURE 5.129   PA patella.

- In a normal knee, the femorotibial joint space should be equal on both sides.
- Density should be sufficient for the patella to be visualized.

Tip Non-grid method may be used for a knee that measures less than 11 cm.

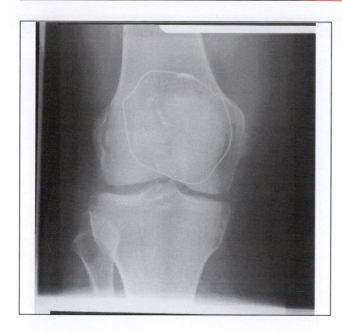

FIGURE 5.130   PA patella.

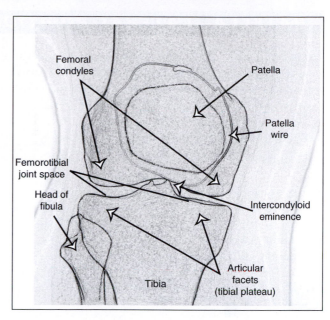

FIGURE 5.131   PA patella.

PATELLA—LATERAL POSITION

Exam Rationale   Structures demonstrated on the lateral projection of the patella include the distal femur, the proximal tibia and fibula, the knee joint, and the patella in profile.

Technical Considerations

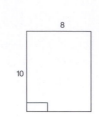

- Regular screen/film
- Grid
- kVp range: 60–70
- SID: 40 inch (100 cm)

Radiation Protection   AEC (Phototiming)

   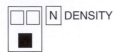

Patient Position   Lateral recumbent on the affected side with the unaffected leg behind the affected leg; all potential artifacts from the distal femur down removed (Figure 5.132).

Part Position   Rest the knee on its lateral surface and center the patella to the midline of the table; flex the knee 5° to 10° and adjust it so the interepicondylar plane is perpendicular to the cassette.

Central Ray   Perpendicular to the femoropatellar joint space.

Patient Instructions   "Breathe normally but don't move."

Evaluation Criteria (Figures 5.133 and 5.134)

- Femoral condyles should be superimposed.
- Patella should be projected in profile.
- Femoropatellar space should be open.
- Fibular head and tibia should be slightly superimposed.

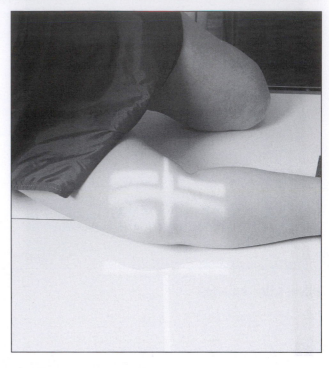

FIGURE 5.132   Lateral patella.

Tips

1. A support placed under the heel/ankle of the affected leg helps in maintaining the knee in true lateral position.
2. Non-grid method may be used for a knee that measures less than 11 cm.

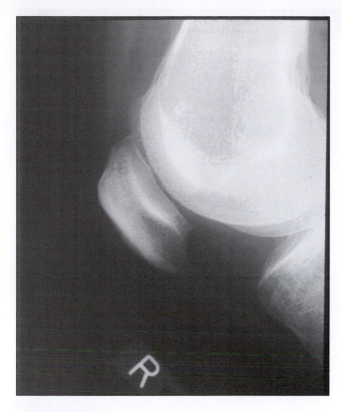

FIGURE 5.133 **Lateral patella.**

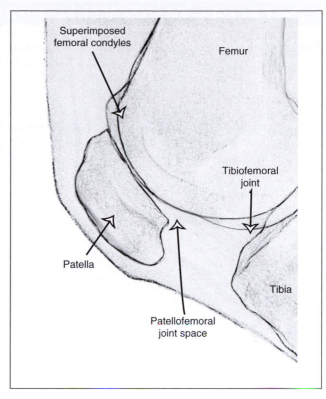

FIGURE 5.134 **Lateral patella.**

PATELLA—TANGENTIAL POSITION (SETTEGAST METHOD)

Exam Rationale   Tangential positions of the patella are used to demonstrate patellar fracture or subluxation. Because of the danger of separation of fractured segments of the patella, this position should not be attempted until a lateral projection has been done to rule out a transverse fracture. This position is used to demonstrate vertical fractures and to evaluate the articulating surfaces of the femur and patella.

Technical Considerations

- Extremity screen/film
- Non-grid
- kVp range: 55–60
- SID: 40 inch (100 cm)

Radiation Protection

Patient Position   Prone on the table with the knee flexed; all potential artifacts from the distal femur down removed (Figure 5.135).

Part Position   Center the patella 2 to 3 inches from the lower edge of the cassette; slowly flex the knee until the patella is perpendicular to the cassette (approximately 100°).

Central Ray   Perpendicular to the space between the patella and the femoral condyles; the degree of angulation will depend on the degree of flexion of the knee.

Patient Instructions   "Breathe normally but don't move."

Evaluation Criteria (Figures 5.136 and 5.137)

- Patellofemoral interspace should be open.
- Patella should be seen in profile.
- Femoral condyles should be visualized.

Tips

1. A gauze strip may be looped around the ankle and used to achieve/maintain the necessary flexion.
2. It is possible to obtain a similar radiograph with the patient in the supine, seated, or lateral position as long as the same part-film and tube-film relationships are maintained (Figures 5.138, 5.139, and 5.140).

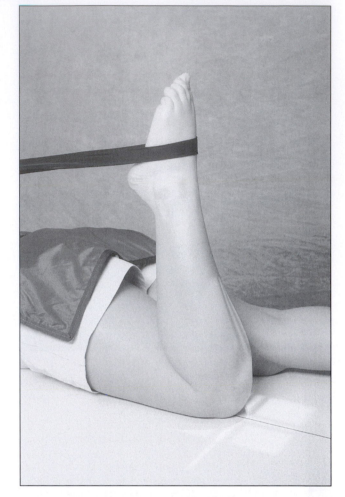

FIGURE 5.135   Tangential patella (Settegast).

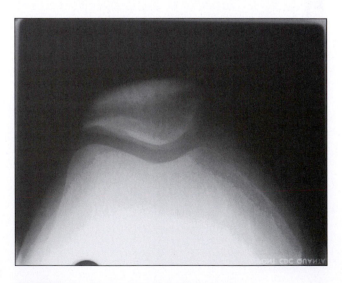

FIGURE 5.136   Tangential patella (Settegast).

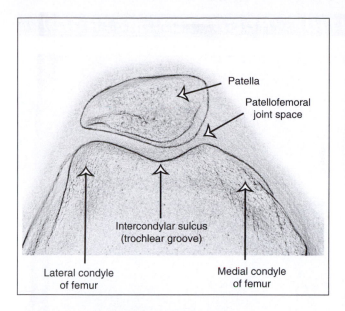

FIGURE 5.137 **Tangential patella (Settegast).**

Patella

Patellofemoral joint space

Intercondylar sulcus (trochlear groove)

Lateral condyle of femur

Medial condyle of femur

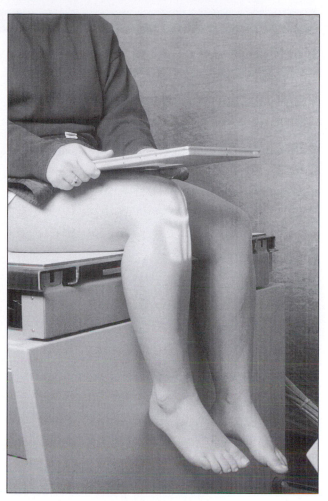

FIGURE 5.139 **Tangential patella (seated).**

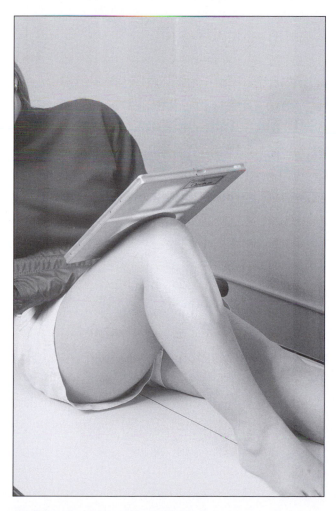

FIGURE 5.138 **Tangential patella (supine).**

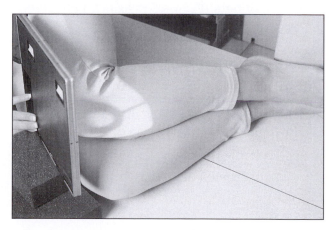

FIGURE 5.140 **Tangential patella (lateral).**

PATELLA—TANGENTIAL POSITION (HUGHSTON METHOD)

Exam Rationale Tangential positions of the patella are used to demonstrate patellar fracture or subluxation. This position demonstrates the patella; Hughston recommends that both knees be examined for comparison.

Technical Considerations

- Extremity screen/film
- Non-grid
- kVp range: 55–60
- SID: 40 inch (100 cm)

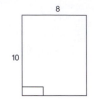

Radiation Protection

Patient Position Prone on the table with the knee extended; all potential artifacts from the distal femur down removed (Figure 5.141).

Part Position Center the patella 2 to 3 inches from the lower edge of the cassette; slowly flex the knee 50° to 60°; adjust the leg so there is no medial or lateral deviation of the leg from the vertical.

Central Ray 45° cephalic to the patellofemoral joint.

Patient Instructions "Breathe normally but don't move."

Evaluation Criteria (Figures 5.142 and 5.143)

- Patellofemoral interspace should be open.
- Patella should be seen in profile.
- Femoral condyles should be visualized.

Tip The foot may be rested on the tube head for support but care must be taken that the surface is not too hot for patient comfort or safety.

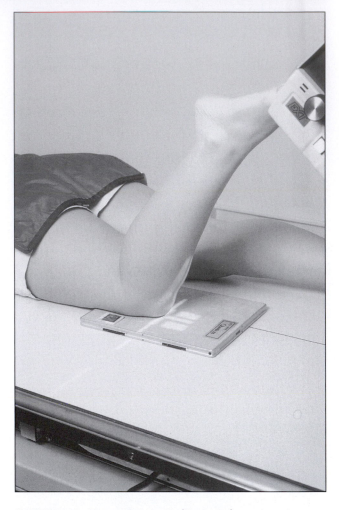

FIGURE 5.141   Tangential patella (Hughston).

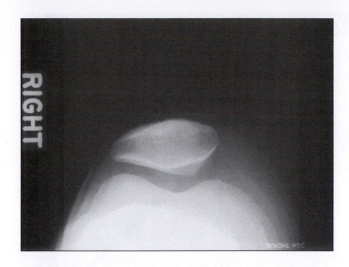

FIGURE 5.142 Tangential patella (Hughston).

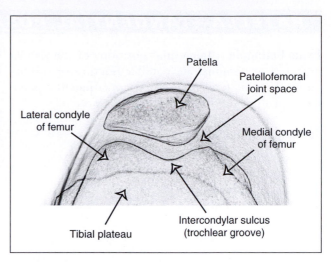

FIGURE 5.143 Tangential patella (Hughston).

PATELLA—TANGENTIAL POSITION (MERCHANT METHOD)

Exam Rationale   Tangential positions of the patella are used to demonstrate patellar fracture or subluxation. This bilateral method demonstrates the patellae in profile and the patellofemoral joints.

Technical Considerations

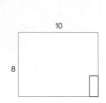

- Extremity screen/film
- Non-grid
- kVp range: 60–65
- SID: 72 inch (180 cm)

Radiation Protection

Patient Position   Supine on the table with the knees flexed and the lower legs hanging off the end of the radiographic table; a special cassette holding device is required; all artifacts from the distal femur down removed (Figure 5.144).

Part Position   Place the femora parallel to the table top by elevating the knees approximately 2 inches and flex the knees 45°; strap the legs together at the calf level to control rotation and help eliminate motion; rest the cassette on the shins perpendicular to them and approximately 1 foot distal to the patellae.

Central Ray   Perpendicular to the cassette midway between the patellae at level of the patellofemoral joint.

Patient Instructions   "Breathe normally but don't move."

Evaluation Criteria (Figures 5.145 and 5.146)

- Patellofemoral interspace should be open.
- Patella should be seen in profile.
- Femoral condyles should be visualized.

Tips

1. Relaxation of the quadriceps femoris is important for accurate diagnosis because tightened muscles may pull the patella into the intercondylar sulcus, giving a false normal appearance.
2. The angle of flexion of the knee should be recorded so it can be reproduced in follow-up films because of the tendency of patellar subluxation to vary with variance in the angle of knee flexion.

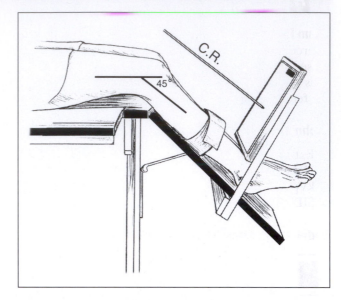

FIGURE 5.144   Tangential patella (Merchant).

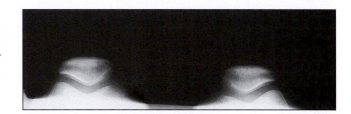

FIGURE 5.145   Tangential patella (Merchant).

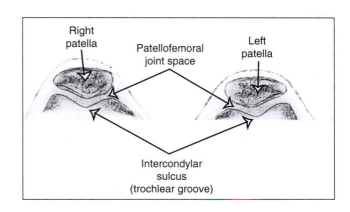

FIGURE 5.146   Tangential patella (Merchant).

INTERCONDYLAR FOSSA—AXIAL PA PROJECTION (HOLMBLAD METHOD)

Exam Rationale Radiographic examination of the intercondylar fossa is indicated in the evaluation of loose bodies in the joint and cartilage abnormalities. This position demonstrates the intercondylar fossa of the femur and the tibial spine.

Technical Considerations

- Extremity screen/film
- Non-grid
- kVp range: 55–65
- SID: 40 inch (100 cm)

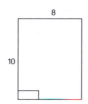

Radiation Protection

Patient Position Kneeling on the table with the knee flexed; all potential artifacts from the distal femur down removed (Figure 5.147).

Part Position Center the patellar apex to the film and flex the knee 70° from full extension (20° from vertical).

Central Ray Perpendicular to the midpoint of the film.

Patient Instructions "Breathe normally but don't move."

Evaluation Criteria (Figures 5.148 and 5.149)

- Fossa should be open and visualized.
- Apex of the patella should not be projected in the fossa.
- Posterior surface of the femoral condyles should be visualized.
- Leg should not be rotated as evidenced by slight overlap of the proximal tibia and fibula.

Tips

1. It is possible to obtain a similar view with the patient standing and resting the flexed knee on the

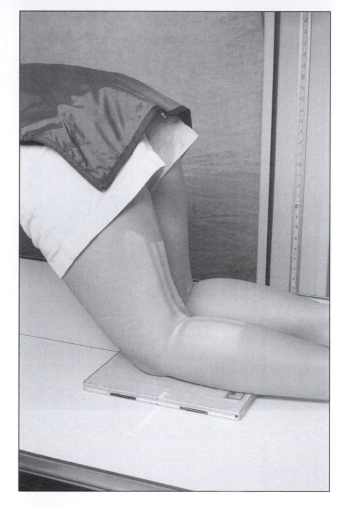

FIGURE 5.147 Intercondylar fossa (Holmblad).

cassette on stool or with patient standing with the flexed knee in contact with the film in front of the knee (Figure 5.150).
2. It is also possible to flex the knee at a 90° angle and use a 20° cephalic angle (Figure 5.151).

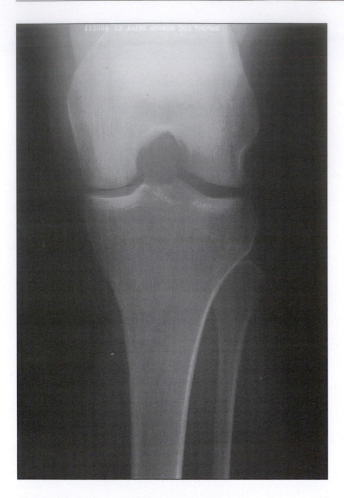

FIGURE 5.148   Intercondylar fossa (Holmblad).

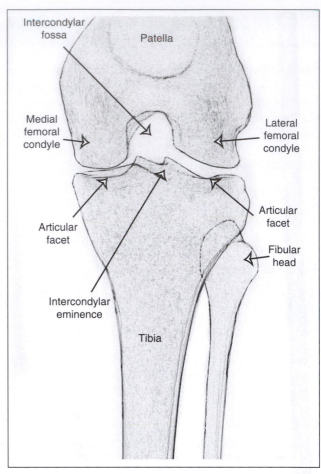

FIGURE 5.149   Intercondylar fossa (Holmblad).

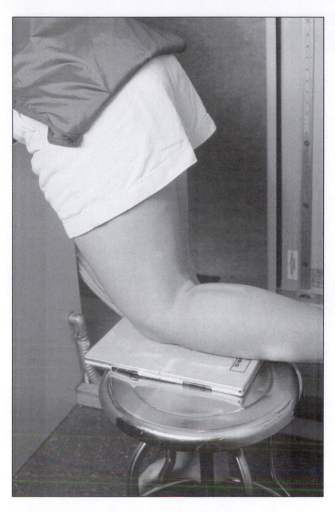

FIGURE 5.150   Intercondylar fossa (standing).

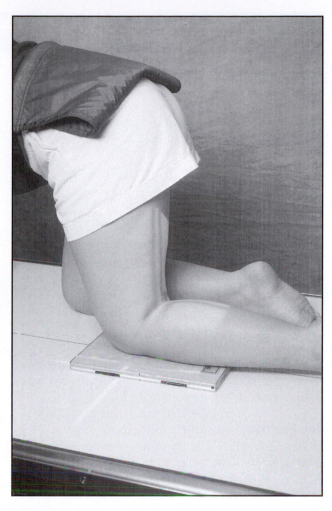

FIGURE 5.151   Intercondylar fossa (with flexion and angulation).

INTERCONDYLAR FOSSA—AXIAL PA PROJECTION (CAMP-COVENTRY METHOD)

Exam Rationale   Radiographic examination of the intercondylar fossa is indicated in the evaluation of loose bodies in the joint and cartilage abnormalities. This position demonstrates the intercondylar fossa of the femur and the tibial spine.

Technical Considerations

- Extremity screen/film
- Non-grid
- kVp range: 55–60
- SID: 40 inch (100 cm)

Radiation Protection

Patient Position   Prone on the table with the knee flexed; all potential artifacts from the distal femur down removed (Figure 5.152).

Part Position   Place the patella approximately 2 to 3 inches (5–8 cm) from the upper border of the cassette; flex the knee approximately 40°, resting the foot on a suitable support; adjust the leg so there is no medial or lateral deviation from the vertical.

Central Ray   Perpendicular to the long axis of the lower leg to the popliteal depression (50° caudad).

Patient Instructions   "Breathe normally but don't move."

Evaluation Criteria (Figures 5.153 and 5.154)

- Fossa should be open and visualized.
- Apex of the patella should not be projected in the fossa.
- Posterior surface of the femoral condyles should be visualized.
- Leg should not be rotated as evidenced by slight overlap of the proximal tibia and fibula.

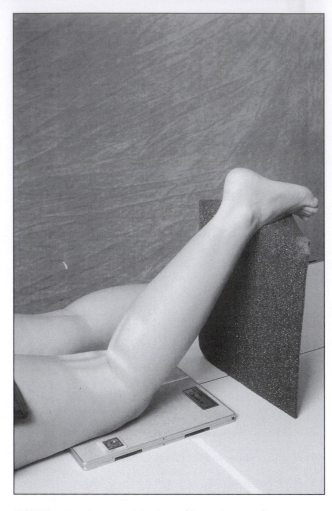

FIGURE 5.152   Intercondylar fossa (Camp-Coventry).

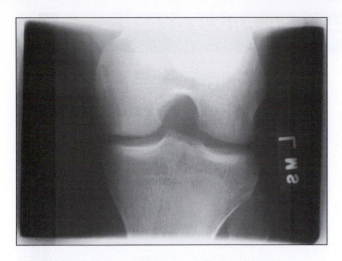

FIGURE 5.153   Intercondylar fossa (Camp-Coventry).

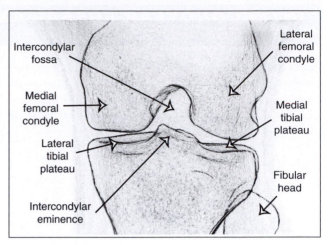

FIGURE 5.154   Intercondylar fossa (Camp-Coventry).

INTERCONDYLAR FOSSA—AXIAL AP PROJECTION (BECLERE METHOD)

Exam Rationale   Radiographic examination of the intercondylar fossa is indicated in the evaluation of loose bodies in the joint and cartilage abnormalities. This position demonstrates the intercondylar fossa of the femur and the tibial spine.

Technical Considerations

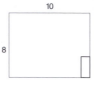

- Extremity screen/film
- A curved cassette is preferred to obtain closer part-film distance than is possible with a regular cassette.
- Non-grid
- kVp range: 55–65
- SID: 40 inch (100 cm)

Radiation Protection

Patient Position   Supine on the table with the knee flexed; all potential artifacts from the distal femur down removed (Figure 5.155).

Part Position   Center the knee joint to the cassette; flex the knee enough to place the long axis of the femur at an angle of 60° to the long axis of the tibia.

Central Ray   Perpendicular to the long axis of the lower leg to the knee joint.

Patient Instructions   "Breathe normally but don't move."

Evaluation Criteria (Figures 5.156 and 5.157)

- Fossa should be open and visualized.
- Apex of the patella should not be projected in the fossa.
- Posterior surface of the femoral condyles should be visualized.
- Leg should not be rotated as evidenced by slight overlap of the proximal tibia and fibula.

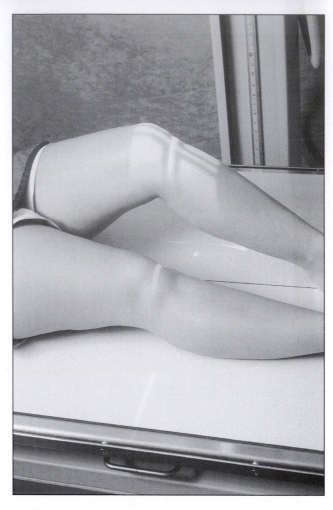

FIGURE 5.155   Intercondylar fossa (Beclere).

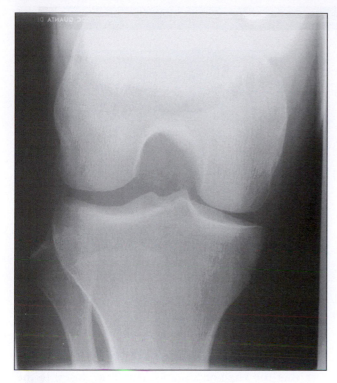

FIGURE 5.156   Intercondylar fossa (Beclere).

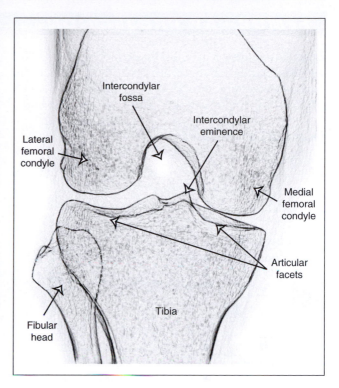

FIGURE 5.157   Intercondylar fossa (Beclere).

FEMUR—AP PROJECTION

Exam Rationale   The most common indication for an examination of the femur is trauma. Structures demonstrated on the AP projection include the entire length of the femur and the knee or hip joint or both.

Technical Considerations

- Regular screen/film
- Grid
- kVp range: 70–80
- SID: 40 inch (100 cm)

Radiation Protection   **AEC (Phototiming)**

 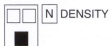 N DENSITY

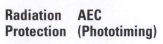

Patient Position   Supine on the table with the knee extended; the patient should be dressed in a patient gown with all clothing from waist down removed (Figure 5.158).

Part Position   Center the thigh to the midline of the table and position it to include both joints when possible or, if not possible, the joint nearest the site of injury or suspected pathology; adjust the femur into the AP position, with the interepicondylar plane parallel to the film, and internally rotate the foot approximately 15°.

Central Ray   Perpendicular to the midpoint of the femur.

Patient Instructions   "Take in a breath; hold your breath. Don't breathe or move."

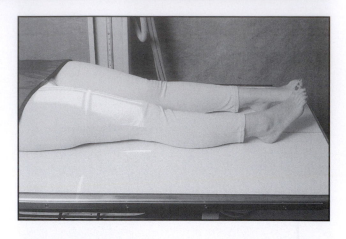

FIGURE 5.158   AP femur.

Evaluation Criteria (Figures 5.159 and 5.160)

- Either the knee or hip joint (the one closest to the injury or suspected pathology) should be included; a separate AP of the other joint may be indicated.
- Little or none of the lesser trochanter should be visible beyond the medial edge of the femur.
- Any orthopedic appliance (e.g., surgical plate) should be seen in its entirety.

Tip   Automatic exposure control should not be used when an orthopedic appliance is in place.

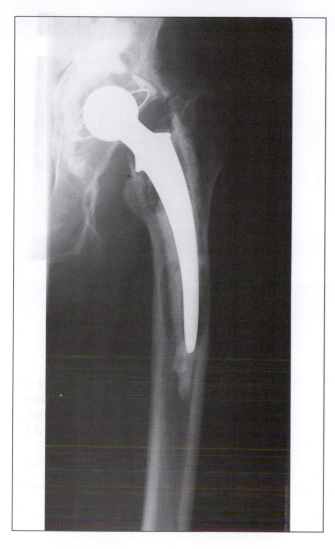

FIGURE 5.159   AP femur.

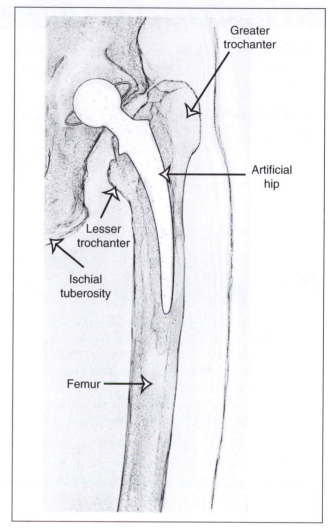

Greater
trochanter

Artificial
hip

Lesser
trochanter

Ischial
tuberosity

Femur

FIGURE 5.160   AP femur.

FEMUR—LATERAL POSITION

Exam Rationale Structures demonstrated on the radiograph include the entire length of the femur and the knee or hip joint or both.

Technical Considerations

- Regular screen/film
- Grid
- kVp range: 70–80
- SID: 40 inch (100 cm)

Radiation Protection

AEC (Phototiming)

 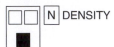 N DENSITY

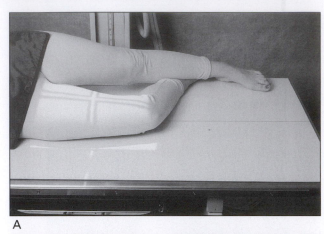

A

Patient Position Lateral recumbent position on the affected side; if the proximal femur is the area of interest, the unaffected leg is placed behind the affected leg (Figure 5.161A); if the distal femur is the area of interest, the unaffected leg is flexed and in front of the affected leg (Figure 5.161B); the patient should be dressed in a patient gown with all clothing from waist down removed.

Part Position Flex the knee and center the thigh to the midline of the table and position it to include both joints when possible or, if not possible, the joint nearest the site of injury or suspected pathology; adjust the femur into the lateral position, with the interepicondylar plane perpendicular to film.

Central Ray Perpendicular to the midpoint of the femur.

Patient Instructions "Take in a breath; hold your breath. Don't breathe or move."

Evaluation Criteria (Figures 5.162 and 5.163)

- Same joint(s) included on the AP should also be included on the lateral; a separate lateral of one joint may be indicated.
- Any orthopedic appliance (e.g., surgical plate) should be seen in its entirety.
- When the knee is included, it should meet the criteria identified in evaluating a lateral knee.
- When the hip is included, the thigh of the unaffected leg should not overlap the area of interest.

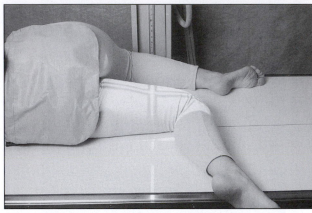

B

FIGURE 5.161   Lateral femur: (A) proximal, (B) distal.

Tips

1. The regular lateral position should not be used when a fracture is suspected because of the possibility of displacing fragments; a translateral should be done instead.
2. Automatic exposure control should not be used when an orthopedic appliance is in place.

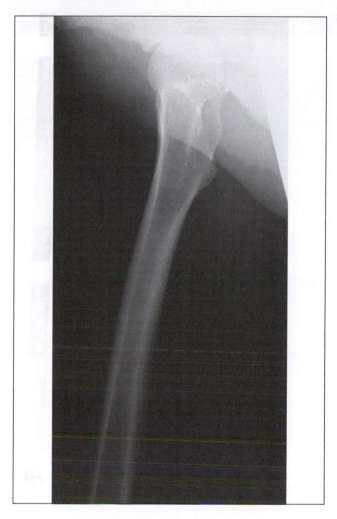

FIGURE 5.162 Lateral femur.

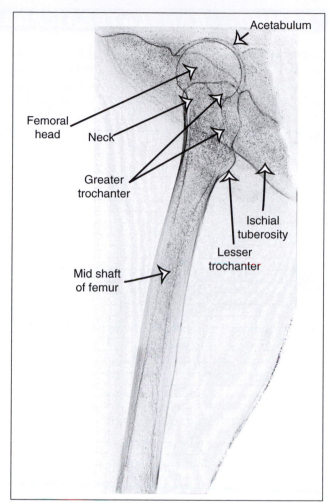

FIGURE 5.163 Lateral femur.

FEMUR—TRANSLATERAL POSITION

Exam Rationale   This lateral position of the femur is indicated when the patient's condition contraindicates turning the patient for a routine lateral. It demonstrates the length of the femur and the knee joint.

Technical Considerations

- Regular screen/film
- Non-grid
- kVp range: 70–80
- SID: 40 inch (100 cm)

Radiation Protection

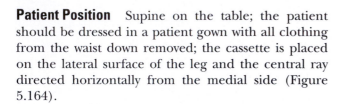

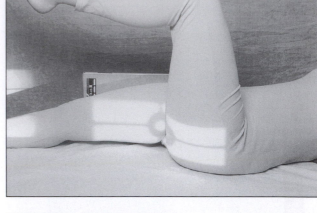

FIGURE 5.164   **Translateral femur.**

Patient Position   Supine on the table; the patient should be dressed in a patient gown with all clothing from the waist down removed; the cassette is placed on the lateral surface of the leg and the central ray directed horizontally from the medial side (Figure 5.164).

Part Position   The knee of the affected leg should be extended.

Central Ray   To the midpoint of the film.

Patient Instructions   "Take in a breath; hold your breath. Don't breathe or move."

Evaluation Criteria (Figures 5.165 and 5.166)

- Knee joint should be included.

Tip   If the proximal femur is the primary area of interest, it is necessary to do a superoinferior view of the hip joint.

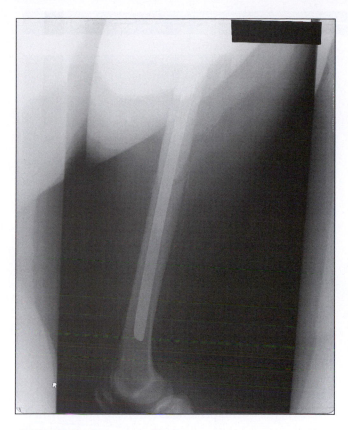

FIGURE 5.165 **Translateral femur.**

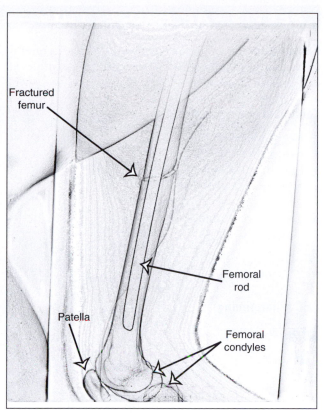

FIGURE 5.166 **Translateral femur.**

Fractured femur

Femoral rod

Patella

Femoral condyles

PELVIS—AP PROJECTION

Exam Rationale   This projection provides a general survey of the bones of the pelvis and the head, neck, and greater trochanter of each of the femora.

Technical Considerations

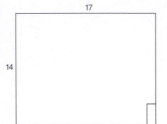

- Regular screen/film
- Grid
- kVp range: 85–90
- SID: 40 inch (100 cm)

Radiation Protection

   Gonadal shielding not possible for female patients.

AEC (Phototiming)

   [N] DENSITY

+ Gas/Distension

Patient Position   Supine on the table; the patient should be dressed in a patient gown with clothing from the waist down removed (Figure 5.167).

Part Position   The midsagittal plane of the body should be centered to the midline of the table; the shoulders should be adjusted to lie in the same transverse plane and the elbows should be flexed with the hands resting on the upper chest; the pelvis should be adjusted to that it is not rotated (distance from anterior superior iliac spine and table top is the same on both sides); the feet should be internally rotated approximately 15°; cassette should be positioned so that its upper border is 1 to 1 1/2 inches (3–4 cm) above the iliac crest.

Central Ray   Perpendicular to the midpoint of the film (approximately 2 inches superior to symphysis pubis).

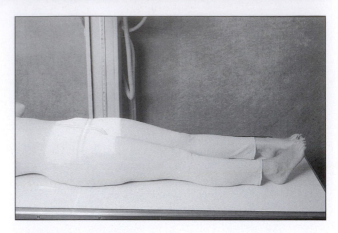

FIGURE 5.167   AP pelvis.

Patient Instructions   "Take in a deep breath and hold it. Don't breathe or move."

Evaluation Criteria (Figures 5.168 and 5.169)

- Entire pelvis and proximal femora should be visualized.
- Pelvis should not be rotated as evidenced by:
  —Symmetrical iliac alae
  —Symmetrical obturator foramina
  —Visualization of ischial spines equally on both sides
  —Sacrum and coccyx aligned with the symphysis pubis
- Little or none of the lesser trochanters should be visible beyond the medial edges of the femora.
- Greater trochanters should be fully visualized.
- Density should be sufficient for femoral heads to be demonstrated through acetabula.

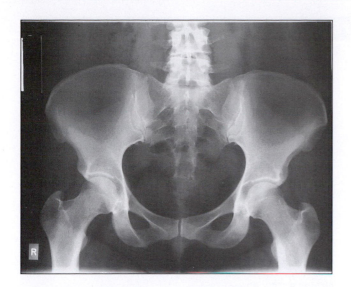

FIGURE 5.168   **AP pelvis.**

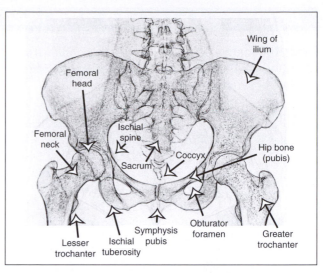

FIGURE 5.169   **AP pelvis.**

PELVIS—AXIAL AP PROJECTION (TAYLOR METHOD)

Exam Rationale This axial projection demonstrates the pubic and ischial rami elongated and magnified but free of superimposition.

Technical Considerations

- Regular screen/film
- Grid
- kVp range: 85–90
- SID: 40 inch (100 cm)

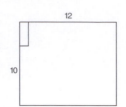

Radiation Protection

AEC (Phototiming)

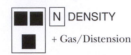

N DENSITY

+ Gas/Distension

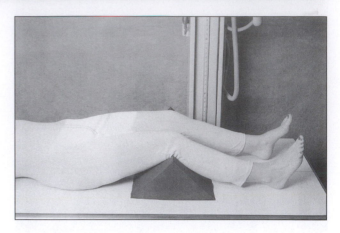

FIGURE 5.170   AP axial pelvis.

Patient Position Supine on the table with the legs extended; the patient should be dressed in a patient gown with all clothing from the waist down removed (Figure 5.170).

Part Position The midsagittal plane of the body should be centered to the midline of the table; the shoulders should be adjusted to lie in the same transverse plane and the elbows should be flexed with the hands resting on the upper chest; the pelvis should be adjusted to that it is not rotated (distance from anterior superior iliac spine and table top is the same on both sides); the cassette should be positioned so that its midpoint will coincide with the central ray.

Central Ray Directed 2 inches (5 cm) distal to the upper border of the symphysis pubis at 25° (for males) and 40° (for females) cephalic angle.

Patient Instructions "Take in a deep breath and hold it. Don't breathe or move."

Evaluation Criteria (Figures 5.171 and 5.172)

- Symmetrical obturator foramina.
- Pubic and ischial bones should be magnified and superimposed over the sacrum and coccyx.
- Hip joints should be included at the edges of the film.

Tip The most prominent lateral portion of the greater trochanter of the femur may be used to determine the level of the central ray.

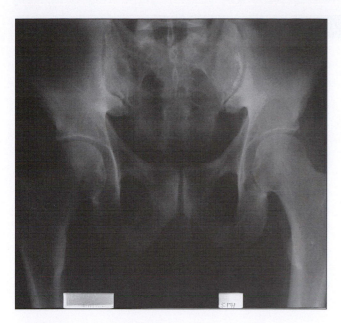

FIGURE 5.171 AP axial pelvis.

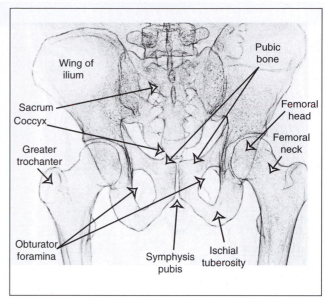

FIGURE 5.172 AP axial pelvis.

HIP—AP PROJECTION

Exam Rationale Structures demonstrated include the head, neck, trochanter, and the proximal third of the femoral shaft.

Technical Considerations

- Regular screen/film
- Grid
- kVp range: 85–90
- SID: 40 inch (100 cm)

10

12

Radiation Protection

AEC (Phototiming)

 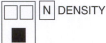 N DENSITY

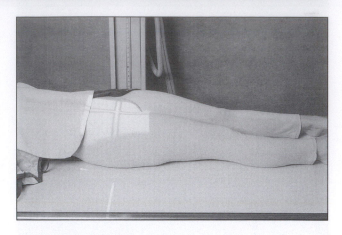

FIGURE 5.173   AP hip.

Patient Position Supine on the table; the patient should be dressed in a patient gown with all clothing from the waist down removed (Figure 5.173).

Part Position The sagittal plane 2 inches medial to the anterior superior iliac spine of the affected side should be centered to the midline of the table; the shoulders should be adjusted to lie in the same transverse plane and the elbows flexed with the hands resting on the upper chest; the pelvis should be adjusted to that it is not rotated (distance from anterior superior iliac spine and table top is the same on both sides); the foot should be internally rotated approximately 15°; the cassette should be centered to the upper limit of the greater trochanter.

Central Ray Perpendicular to the midpoint of the film (approximately 2 inches medial to the ASIS of the affected side at a level just above the greater trochanter).

Patient Instructions "Take in a deep breath and hold it. Don't breathe or move."

Evaluation Criteria (Figures 5.174 and 5.175)

- Little or none of the lesser trochanter should be visible beyond the medial edge of the femur.
- Greater trochanters should be fully visualized.
- Density should be sufficient for the femoral head to be demonstrated through the acetabulum.

Tips

1. In the initial examination of a hip, an AP pelvis is often done to demonstrate the entire pelvic girdle and both upper femora; follow-up studies are confined to the affected side.
2. If an orthopedic appliance is in place, automatic exposure control should not be used; it may also require a larger film to demonstrate the entire prosthesis.

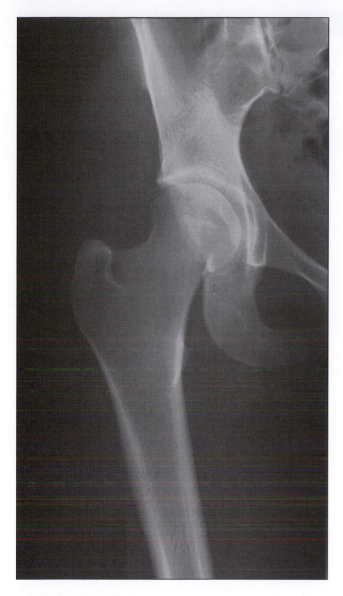

FIGURE 5.174   AP hip.

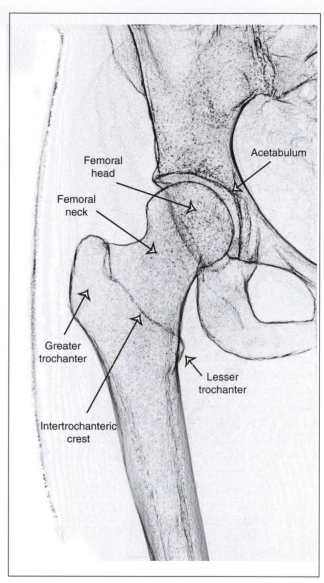

FIGURE 5.175   AP hip.

HIP—LATERAL POSITION

Exam Rationale Structures demonstrated on the radiograph include the proximal femur and the acetabulum. This position is contraindicated in patients with suspected fractures or pathologic hip disease.

Technical Considerations

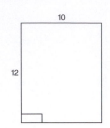

- Regular screen/film
- Grid
- kVp range: 85–90
- SID: 40 inch (100 cm)

Radiation Protection   AEC (Phototiming)

    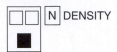

Patient Position Supine on the table; the patient should be dressed in a patient gown with all clothing from the waist down removed (Figure 5.176).

Part Position Patient should flex the knee and turn slightly toward the affected side and abduct the leg to place the femur parallel to the film; center the hip (midway between ASIS and symphysis pubis) to the midline of the table; the unaffected leg should be extended behind the affected leg.

Central Ray Perpendicular to hip.

Patient Instructions "Take in a breath; hold your breath. Don't breathe or move."

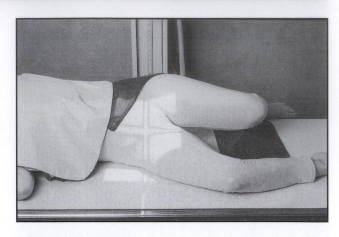

FIGURE 5.176   Lateral hip.

Evaluation Criteria (Figures 5.177 and 5.178)

- Hip joint should be centered to exposed area.
- Any orthopedic appliance (e.g., surgical plate) should be seen in its entirety.

Tips

1. This position should not be used when a fracture is suspected because of the possibility of displacing fragments; a superoinferior projection should be done instead.
2. In the initial examination of a hip, a bilateral frog-leg pelvis is often done to demonstrate the entire pelvic girdle and lateral views of both upper femora; follow-up studies are confined to the affected side.

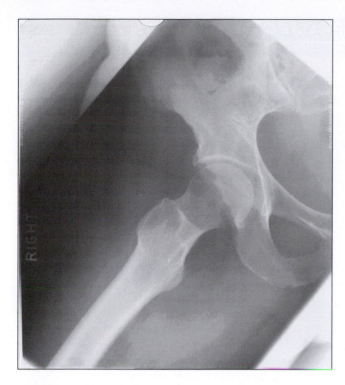

FIGURE 5.177 Lateral hip.

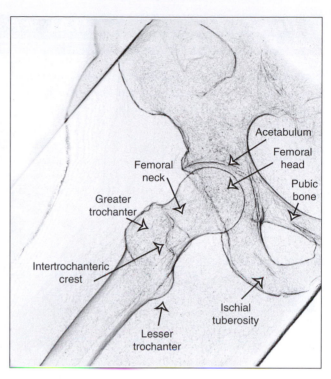

FIGURE 5.178 Lateral hip.

BILATERAL HIPS—AXIAL AP PROJECTION (MODIFIED CLEAVES METHOD)

Exam Rationale This exam is commonly indicated for investigation of congenital hip disease. It is contraindicated in patients with suspected fractures or pathologic hip disease.

Technical Considerations

- Regular screen/film
- Grid
- kVp range: 85–90
- SID: 40 inch (100 cm)

Radiation Protection

  (males)

  (females)

AEC (Phototiming)

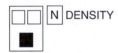 N DENSITY

Patient Position Supine on the table; the patient should be dressed in a patient gown with all clothing from the waist down removed (Figure 5.179).

Part Position The midsagittal plane of the body should be centered to the midline of the table; the shoulders should be adjusted to lie in the same transverse plane and the elbows flexed with the hands resting on the upper chest; the pelvis should be adjusted to that it is not rotated (distance from anterior superior iliac spine and table top is the same on both sides); the knees and hips should be flexed and the feet drawn up as much as possible, allowing the femora to be abducted to approximately a 40° angle from the vertical.

Central Ray Perpendicular to a point 1 inch (2.5 cm) superior to the symphysis pubis.

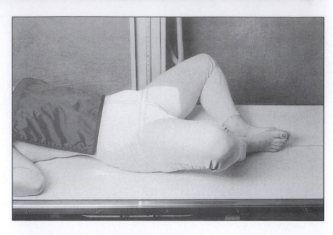

FIGURE 5.179 AP axial bilateral hips.

Patient Instructions "Take a deep breath and hold it. Don't breathe or move."

Evaluation Criteria (Figures 5.180 and 5.181)

- Should include acetabula, femoral heads, and necks.
- Pelvis should not be rotated as evidenced by:
  —Symmetrical iliac alae
  —Visualization of ischial spine equally on both sides
  —Sacrum and coccyx aligned with symphysis pubis
- Lesser trochanter should be projected on the medial side of the femur.

Tip This is a modification of the original Cleaves method, which called for cephalic angulation to parallel the long axis of the femora.

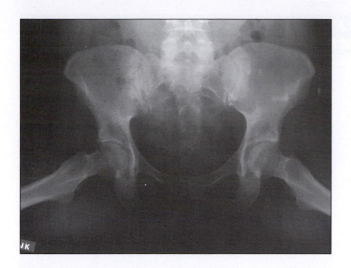

FIGURE 5.180   **AP axial bilateral hips.**

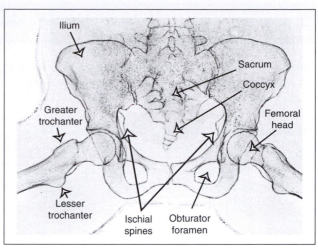

FIGURE 5.181   **AP axial bilateral hips.**

HIP—SUPEROINFERIOR PROJECTION (DANELIUS-MILLER MODIFICATION OF LORENZ METHOD)

Exam Rationale This lateral projection of the hip is indicated when the patient cannot be positioned for a routine lateral.

Technical Considerations

- Regular screen/film
- Grid: stationary
- kVp range: 90–95
- SID: 40 inch (100 cm)

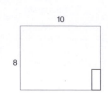

Radiation Protection

(for females)
Gonadal shielding not possible for males.

Patient Position Supine on the table; the patient should be dressed in a patient gown with all clothing from the waist down removed (Figure 5.182).

Part Position The knee of the affected leg should be extended; unless contraindicated, internally rotate the foot of the affected side 15°; flex the knee and hip of the unaffected side and raise the leg, using some suitable support for the leg. The top of the cassette should be at the top of the iliac crest and should be parallel to the femoral neck and perpendicular to the central ray.

Central Ray Horizontal, perpendicular to the hip (about 2 1/2 inches or 7 cm below the intersection of the localization points described below).

Patient Instructions "Take in a breath; hold your breath. Don't breathe or move."

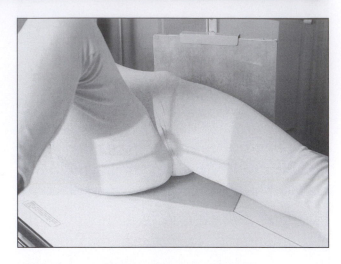

FIGURE 5.182 Axiolateral hip (Danelius-Miller).

Evaluation Criteria (Figures 5.183 and 5.184)

- Proximal femur, hip joint, and acetabulum should be visualized.
- As much as possible of the femoral neck should be visualized.
- Only a small portion of lesser trochanter should be seen on anterior and posterior femur.

Tip To localize the long axis of the femoral neck, draw a line between the ASIS and the superior border of the symphysis pubis and note its center point; palpate the most prominent lateral protrusion of the greater trochanter and note a point 1 inch distal to it; a line drawn between these two points will parallel the long axis of the femoral neck (Figure 5.185).

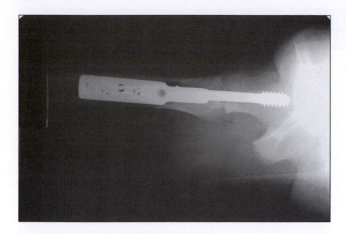

FIGURE 5.183   Axiolateral hip (Danelius-Miller).

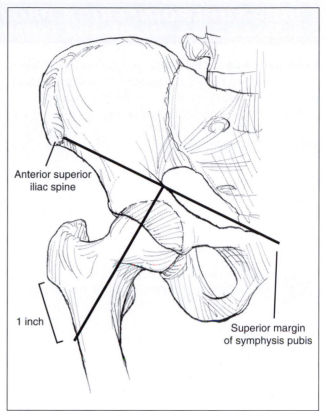

FIGURE 5.185   Localization of the femoral neck.

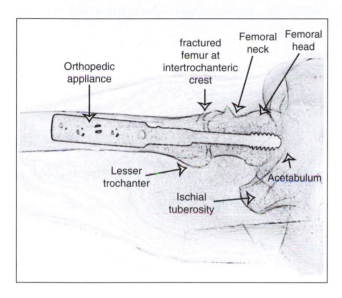

FIGURE 5.184   Axiolateral hip (Danelius-Miller).

HIP—SUPEROINFERIOR PROJECTION (CLEMENTS-NAKAYAMA MODIFICATION)

Exam Rationale This lateral projection of the hip is indicated when both a routine lateral and the axiolateral are contraindicated due to limited movement of both the affected and unaffected leg.

Technical Considerations

- Regular screen/film
- Grid: stationary
- kVp range: 85–95
- SID: 40 inch (100 cm)

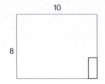

Radiation Protection

  (for females)
Gonadal shielding not possible for males.

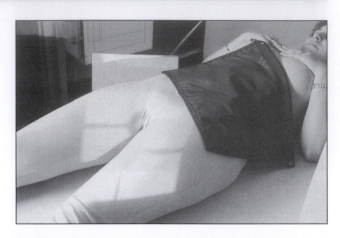

FIGURE 5.186   Axiolateral hip (Clements-Nakayama).

Patient Position Supine, with affected side near the edge of the table, with both legs extended; patient should be dressed in a hospital gown with all clothing from the waist down removed (Figure 5.186).

Part Position Leg remains in neutral position. The cassette should rest on the extended Bucky tray and be placed so top of the cassette is at iliac crest; the cassette should be tilted 15° from the vertical, so it is parallel to the central ray.

Central Ray Aligned perpendicular to femoral neck at 15° posterior angle.

Patient Instructions "Take in a breath; hold your breath. Don't breathe or move."

Evaluation Criteria (Figures 5.187 and 5.188)

- Femoral head, neck, and trochanters should be centered to film area.
- Femoral head and neck should be seen in profile with minimal superimposition by greater trochanter.
- Lesser trochanter should be projected just below femoral shaft.

Tip Care must be taken that the grid is perpendicular to the central ray to prevent grid cutoff.

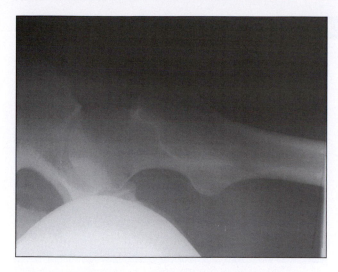

FIGURE 5.187   Axiolateral hip (Clements-Nakayama).

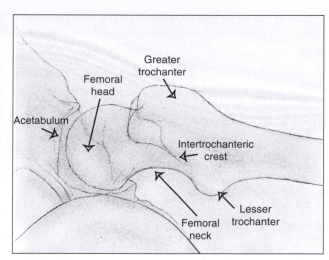

FIGURE 5.188   Axiolateral hip (Clements-Nakayama).

SACROILIAC JOINTS—AXIAL AP PROJECTION

Exam Rationale This projection demonstrates the sacroiliac joints, the L5–S1 junction, and the majority of the sacrum.

Technical Considerations

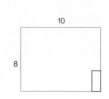

- Regular screen/film
- Grid
- kVp range: 85–95
- SID: 40 inch (100 cm)

Radiation Protection

  (for males)
Gonadal shielding not possible for females.

AEC (Phototiming)

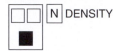 N DENSITY

Patient Position Supine on table with legs extended; patient should be dressed in hospital gown with all clothing from the waist down removed (Figure 5.189).

Part Position The midsagittal plane of the body should be centered to the midline of the table; shoulders should be adjusted to lie in same transverse plane and elbows should be flexed with hands resting on the upper chest; pelvis should be adjusted to that it is not rotated (distance from anterior superior iliac spine and table top is same on both sides).

Central Ray Directed to midline midway between level of ASIS and symphysis pubis at 30° to 35° cephalic angle.

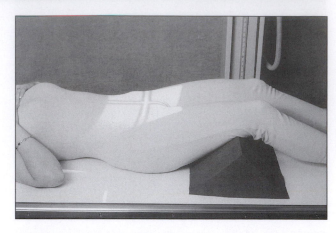

FIGURE 5.189   AP sacroiliac joints.

Patient Instructions "Take in a deep breath and hold it. Don't breathe or move."

Evaluation Criteria (Figures 5.190 and 5.191)

- Sacroiliac joints should be centered to collimation.
- Sacroiliac joint spaces should be open.

Tip This may also be done in the prone position, with the central ray directed to the fourth lumbar segment at a 30° to 35° caudal angle at the level of the iliac crest; in the prone position, the obliquity of the sacroiliac joints more nearly parallels the divergence of the radiation beam (Figure 5.192).

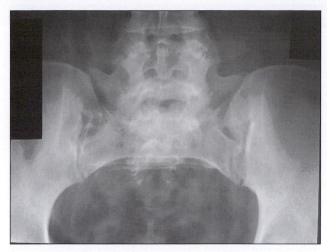

FIGURE 5.190　AP sacroiliac joints.

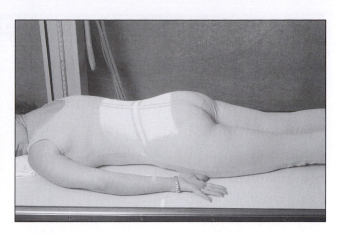

FIGURE 5.192　PA sacroiliac joints.

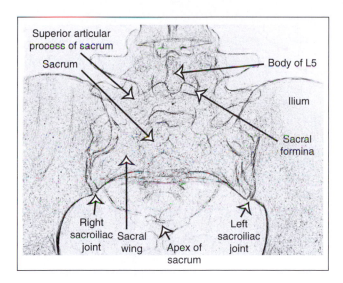

FIGURE 5.191　AP sacroiliac joints.

SACROILIAC JOINTS— OBLIQUE POSITION

Exam Rationale   In the supine position, the sacroiliac joint furthest from the film is demonstrated. Both sides are examined for comparison.

Technical Considerations

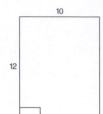

- Regular screen/film
- Grid
- kVp range: 85–95
- SID: 40 inch (100 cm)

Radiation Protection

(for males)
For females, gonadal shielding can be used only on the side not being examined.

AEC (Phototiming)

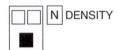 DENSITY

Patient Position   Supine on table; patient should be dressed in hospital gown with all clothing from the waist down removed (Figure 5.193).

Part Position   Raise the side of interest 25° to 30° and center sacroiliac joint to midline of the table; both knees should be slightly flexed.

Central Ray   Perpendicular to point 1 inch (2.5 cm) medial to elevated ASIS.

Patient Instructions   "Take a deep breath and hold it. Don't breathe or move."

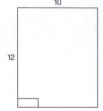

FIGURE 5.193   Oblique sacroiliac joints.

Evaluation Criteria (Figures 5.194 and 5.195)

- There should be no overlap between the ala of the ilium and the sacrum, indicating the proper degree of obliquity.
- Elevated joint space should be open.

Tips

1. To demonstrate the distal portion of the joint more clearly, the central ray may be angled 15° to 20° cephalad.
2. This may also be done in the prone position, with the central ray directed to the vertebral spinous processes at the level of the ASIS; in the prone position, the downside joint will be visualized; to demonstrate the distal portion more clearly in the prone position, the central ray may be angled 15° to 20° caudad (Figure 5.196).

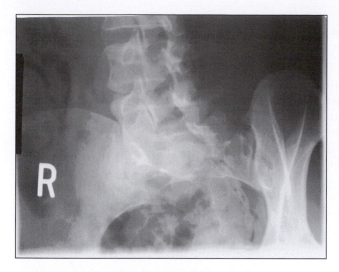

FIGURE 5.194   Oblique sacroiliac joints.

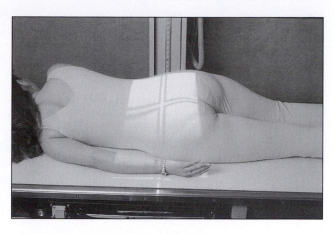

FIGURE 5.196   Prone oblique sacroiliac joints.

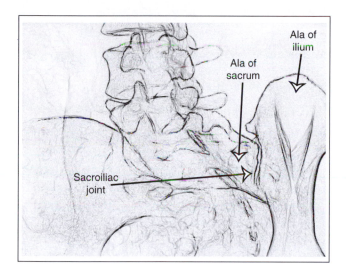

FIGURE 5.195   Oblique sacroiliac joints.

Special Considerations

PEDIATRIC CONSIDERATIONS

When radiographing parts of the lower extremity on pediatric patients, the biggest challenge often comes from flailing arms and legs. Although immobilization may be a time-consuming process and is not always well received by the patient or the parents, immobilization of a patient who is unable or unwilling to cooperate by holding still is highly preferable to the need for repeated radiographs because of motion artifacts.

An effective method of immobilization is to use a mummy wrap on the torso and upper extremities. A heavy sandbag can be used to immobilize the unaffected extremity. The affected extremity can then be held by a parent or other individual (with appropriate radiation protection) (Figure 5.197).

For radiography of the pelvis, the patient's legs can be immobilized with the table's compression band. The parent can hold the patient's humeri as shown in the photograph (Figure 5.198).

GERIATRIC CONSIDERATIONS

The greatest difficulty in radiographing geriatric patients is the potential lack of flexibility. Patients should be assisted in assuming the various positions. Flexing or extending joints should be done slowly and gently and not forced.

COMMON ERRORS

- Failure to dorsiflex the foot on the oblique projection of the ankle results in an image with tibiotalar joint somewhat obscured by overlap (Figure 5.199).
- Failure to internally rotate the femora on AP pelvis when not contraindicated (Figure 5.200).

SELECTED PATHOLOGY

Talipes Equinovarus

This condition, also commonly referred to as congenital clubfoot, is the most common congenital disorder of the lower limb and is twice as prevalent in males as in females. Externally, the foot turns downward (equino) and inward (varus), and the front of the foot has a claw-like appearance. When seen on the radiograph (Figure 5.201), the talus and calcaneus appear shortened, and the front of the foot appears flexed.

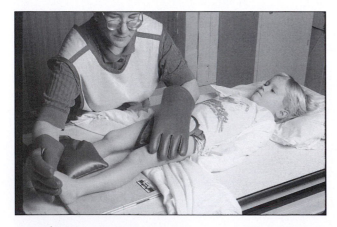

FIGURE 5.197   Immobilization of extremity with sandbag.

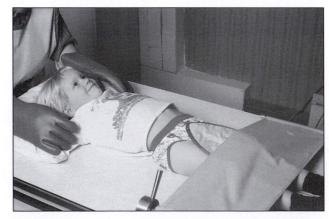

FIGURE 5.198   Immobilization of child for radiograph of pelvis.

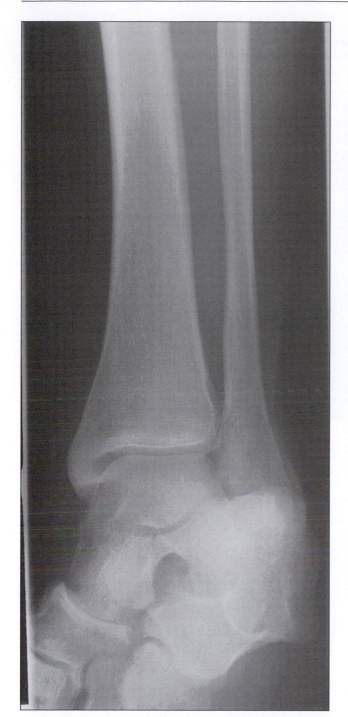

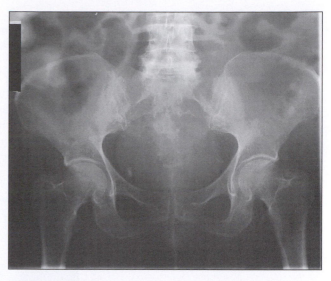

FIGURE 5.200   Femora not internally rotated on AP pelvis.

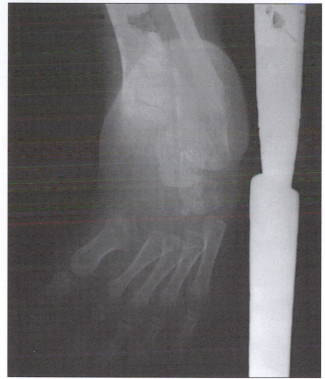

FIGURE 5.199   Lack of dorsiflexion on oblique ankle.

FIGURE 5.201   Talipes equinovarus.

Congenital Hip Dysplasia

This condition is the most common congenital hip disorder and results in a malformation of the acetabulum rather than the femoral head. In some cases, this condition may be diagnosed during a routine physical examination by the presence of extra folds of gluteal tissue. Radiographically, an anteroposterior projection of both hips is routinely used to evaluate whether or not the femoral head is displaced in relation to the acetabulum (Figure 5.202).

Trimalleolar Fracture

This severe fracture of the ankle results from three fractures in the bony structures forming the superior end of the ankle or mortise joint, including the medial malleolus, lateral malleolus, and posterior distal tibia (Figure 5.203).

Intertrochanteric Fracture

In geriatric patients with decreased bone density, fractures in the region of the hip often result from falling accidents. Commonly, this type of fracture is referred to as a broken hip, but it should be noted that the proximal femur is the location of the fracture rather than the hip bone. Although there are several types of hip fractures, one of the most common is a fracture extending between the trochanters (Figure 5.204).

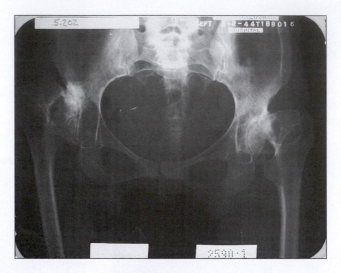

FIGURE 5.202
Congenital hip dysplasia.

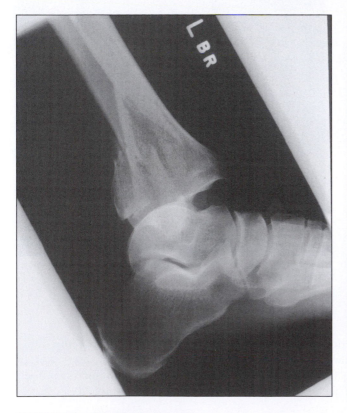

FIGURE 5.203   Trimalleolar fracture.

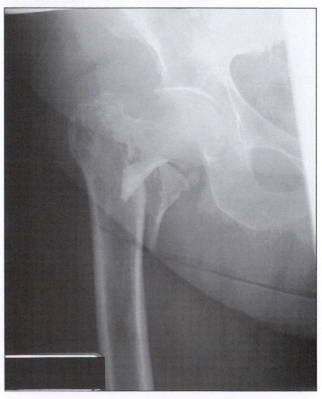

FIGURE 5.204   Intertrochanteric fracture of the hip.

CORRELATIVE IMAGING

Although evaluation of the bony anatomy and joints of the lower limb and pelvis is routinely done with conventional radiography, many conditions require further evaluation with alternative types of diagnostic imaging. In some cases, CT scanning may be necessary to visualize the anatomy in cross section (Figure 5.205). Due to overlapping bone, many regions of the bony lower limb and pelvis are not clearly demonstrated unless seen in cross section.

In contrast, MRI is frequently used to better evaluate the structures associated with the joints. For example, following interpretation of routine x-rays of the knee, many cases necessitate further evaluation with MRI. This procedure, due to its physical characteristics, is better able to demonstrate the soft tissue structures and vascular changes within the region (Figure 5.206).

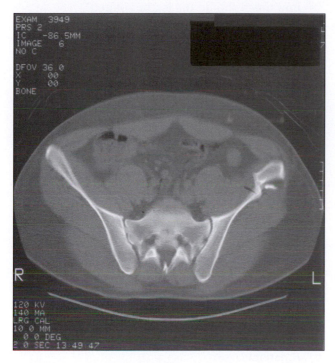

FIGURE 5.205   **CT image of pelvis.**

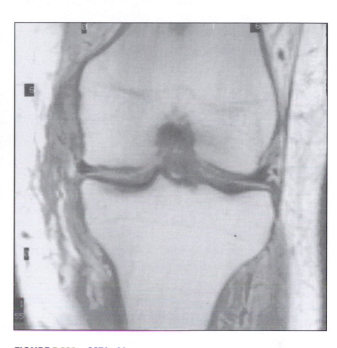

FIGURE 5.206   **MRI of knee.**

Review Questions

1. Which of the following is not a process on the cal-caneus?

   a. tuberosity
   b. sustentaculum tali
   c. shaft
   d. calcaneal sulcus

2. Which of the following is classified as an amphiar-throdial syndesmosis type of joint?

   a. patellar femoral
   b. intertarsal joints
   c. proximal tibiofibular joint
   d. distal tibiofibular joint

3. The ligament in the knee most commonly dam-aged in contact sports is the:

   a. posterior cruciate
   b. anterior cruciate
   c. lateral collateral ligament
   d. medial collateral ligament

4. Which of the following should be included in an examination of the lower limb to reduce the radi-ation exposure of the patient?

   a. contact shielding
   b. limit collimation to area of interest
   c. care when positioning body part to avoid repeating exposure
   d. all of the above

5. For an AP projection of the foot, the central ray is directed to the:

   a. third tarsometatarsal joint
   b. third metatarsophalangeal joint
   c. base of the third metatarsal
   d. head of the third metatarsal

6. Which of the following will display the sesamoid bones of the foot free of superimposition?

   a. AP
   b. oblique
   c. lateral
   d. tangential

7. On an axial (plantodorsal) calcaneus, the central ray is angled:

   a. 20° cephalad
   b. 20° caudad
   c. 40° cephalad
   d. 40° caudad

8. Which view is used to demonstrate the longitudi-nal arch of the foot?

   a. oblique
   b. anteroposterior
   c. posteroanterior weight-bearing
   d. lateral weight-bearing

9. For an internal oblique projection of the ankle, how much should the leg be rotated?

   a. 15°
   b. 30°
   c. 45°
   d. 60°

10. On a routine lateral of the ankle, the central ray should be directed to:

    a. the medial malleolus
    b. a point two inches superior to the medial mal-leolus
    c. a point one inch inferior to the medial malleo-lus
    d. a point one inch anterior to the medial malleo-lus

11. Which position/projection of the lower leg best demonstrates the tibiofibular articulation?

    a. AP
    b. PA
    c. oblique
    d. lateral

12. When performing the weight-bearing AP projec-tion of the knees, the feet should be:

    a. close together
    b. 6–8 inches apart
    c. at least 12 inches apart

13. For oblique positions of the knee, the leg should be rotated

    a. 30°
    b. 45°
    c. 60°
    d. 90°

14. Which of the tangential methods of radiograph-ing the patella requires use of a special cassette holding device?

    a. Hughston
    b. Merchant
    c. Settegast

15. Which position/projection of the knee demonstrates the head of the fibula largely free of superimposition?

    a. AP
    b. internal oblique
    c. external oblique
    d. lateral

16. On the lateral knee, the knee should be flexed:

    a. 20–30°
    b. 35°
    c. 45°
    d. 90°

17. In the Camp-Coventry method of radiographing the intercondyloid fossa, the patient is _____, and the knee is flexed _____ degrees.

    a. kneeling   a. 20
    b. prone   b. 40
    c. supine   c. 60

18. Which of the following positions/projections of the knee should not be attempted until a lateral has been done to rule out a transverse fracture of the patella?

    a. external oblique
    b. internal oblique
    c. PA
    d. tangential (Settegast)

19. Which of the following technical factors would not be generally considered for the average patient in radiographic examinations of the femur?

    a. kVp in the range of 40–45
    b. 7 × 17 (20 × 45 cm) film size
    c. SID: 40 inch
    d. grid

20. When radiographing the femur, which should be included?

    a. knee
    b. hip
    c. either knee or hip
    d. both knee and hip

21. Which of the following is contraindicated in patients suspected of having a fracture?

    a. axiolateral hip
    b. AP hip
    c. axial AP hip (modified Cleaves)
    d. none of the above

22. Which of the following is true when positioning the patient for an AP hip?

    a. foot of the affected side should be rotated medially 15°
    b. foot of the affected side should be rotated laterally 15°
    c. plantar surfaces of foot should be perpendicular to the film
    d. none of the above

23. When viewing an AP pelvis radiograph, most of the lesser trochanters are visible. Which of the following is true?

    a. patient was positioned correctly
    b. patient/pelvis was rotated
    c. hips are fractured
    d. feet were not properly rotated

24. On an AP pelvis, the central ray should be directed to:

    a. the symphysis pubis
    b. a point 2 inches inferior to the symphysis pubis
    c. a point 2 inches superior to the symphysis pubis
    d. to the iliac crest

25. The patella articulates with both the femur and the tibia.

    a. true
    b. false

26. The female pelvis is generally narrower than that of the male.

    a. true
    b. false

27. The position of the foot is the same for both a lateral of the foot and a lateral of the calcaneus.

    a. true
    b. false

28. The weight-bearing AP projection of the foot involves a double-exposed image with two different central ray angulations.

    a. true
    b. false

29. On an AP projection of the ankle, the foot should be dorsiflexed until the plantar surface is perpendicular to the cassette.

    a. true
    b. false

30. When radiographing the lower leg, both the knee and ankle joints should be in true AP position.

    a. true
    b. false

31. On a lateral knee, the femoropatellar space should be open.

    a. true
    b. false

32. When radiographing a femur or hip that contains an orthopedic appliance, it is important to visualize the entire appliance.

    a. true
    b. false

33. Sacroiliac joints can be radiographed with the patient in either the supine or prone position.

    a. true
    b. false

34. Toes 2 to 5 each consists of _____ (#) of phalanges.

35. The arches of the foot are found in two directions: _____ and _____ .

36. The _____ is the largest joint in the body.

37. The longest, strongest, and heaviest bone in the body is the _____ .

38. For the oblique position, the foot should be rotated _____ degrees medially.

39. An AP stress study of the ankle involves two exposures, one with the foot _____ and the other with the foot _____ .

40. When radiographing the ankle in the AP mortise projection, the entire leg and foot should be rotated _____ degrees _____ to place the intermalleolar plane parallel to the film.

41. For radiography of the knee, a grid should be used for knees that measure _____ cm or more.

42. In the tangential position for the patella (Hughston method), the knee is slowly flexed _____ degrees to best demonstrate the patella.

43. In the AP projection of the knee the central ray should be directed _____ at a _____ degree angle.

44. Radiographic examination of the femur is most commonly done to evaluate _____ .

45. For an axiolateral of the hip, the cassette should be _____ to the femoral neck and _____ to the central ray.

46. On the axial AP sacroiliac joints, the central ray is angled _____ degrees in the _____ direction.

47. When performing oblique sacroiliac joints with the patient in the supine position, the side of interest is elevated _____ degrees.

48. What group of bones comprise the instep of the foot?

49. What three bones comprise the ankle joint?

50. The medial malleolus is a process located on which bone of the lower leg?

51. On an AP hip, the central ray should be directed to what point?

52. For each of the following body parts, list the routine positions/projections required at your clinical facility.

a. foot

b. ankle

c. lower leg

d. knee

e. femur

f. hip

g. pelvis

h. sacroiliac joints

References and Recommended Reading

Anderson, J. E. (1983). *Grant's atlas of anatomy* (8th ed.). Baltimore: Williams & Wilkins.

Ballinger, P. W. (1995). *Merill's atlas of radiographic positions and radiologic procedures* 8th ed., (Vols. 1–3). St. Louis: Mosby-Year Book.

Basmajian, J. V. (1980). (Ed.). *Grant's method of anatomy* (10th ed.). Baltimore: Williams & Wilkins.

Bates, B. (1983). *A guide to physical examination* (3rd ed.). Philadelphia: Lippincott.

Bo, W., Wolfman, N., Krueger, W., & Meschan, I. (1990). *Basic atlas of sectional anatomy with correlated imaging* (2nd ed.). Philadelphia: Saunders.

Bontrager, K. L. (1993). *Textbook of radiographic positioning and related anatomy* (3rd ed.). St. Louis: Mosby-Year Book.

Cahill, D. R., & Orland, M. J. (1984). *Atlas of human cross-sectional anatomy*. Philadelphia: Lea & Febiger.

Dorland's illustrated medical dictionary. (28th ed.). Philadelphia: Saunders.

Eisenberg, R. L. (1992). *Clinical imaging: An atlas of differential diagnosis* (2nd ed.).Gaithersburg, MD: Aspen.

Gardner, E., Gray, D. J., & O'Rahilly, R. (1975). *Anatomy: A regional study of human structure* (4th ed.). Philadelphia: Saunders.

Gerhart, P., & VanKaich, G. (1979). *Total body computed tomography* (2nd ed.). Stuttgart: Georg Thieme.

Gray, H. (1985). In C. D. Clemente (Ed.), *Anatomy of the human body* (30th ed.).Philadelphia: Lea & Febiger.

International Anatomical Nomenclature Committee. (1989). *Nomina anatomica* (6th ed.). Baltimore: Waverly Press.

Laudicina, P. F. (1989). *Applied pathology for radiographers*. Philadelphia: Saunders.

Meschan, I. (1975). *An atlas of anatomy basic to radiology*. Philadelphia: Lea & Febiger.

O'Rahilly, R. (1983). *Basic human anatomy*. Philadelphia: Saunders.

Pansky, B. (1984). *Review of gross anatomy* (5th ed.). New York: Macmillan.

Robbins, S. L., & Kumar, V. (1987). *Basic Pathology* (4th ed.). Philadelphia: Saunders.

Snell, R. S. (1981). *Clinical anatomy for medical students* (2nd ed.). Boston: Little, Brown.

Tortora, G. R., & Anagnostakos, N. P. (1984). *Principles of anatomy and physiology* (4th ed.). New York: Harper & Row.

Williams, P. L., & Warwick, R. (1980) (Eds.). *Gray's anatomy* (36th ed.). Philadelphia: Saunders.

Woodburne, R. T. (1983). *Essentials of human anatomy* (7th ed.). New York: Oxford University Press.

Woodburne, R. T., & Burkel, W. E. (1988) *Essentials of human anatomy* (8th ed.). New York: Oxford University Press.

Ribs and Sternum

DENNIS F. SPRAGG, MSEd, RT(R)(ARRT)

JOANNE S. GREATHOUSE, EdS, RT(R)(ARRT), FASRT

ANATOMY

The Bony Thorax

RIBS—ROUTINE POSITIONS/PROJECTIONS

AP Above Diaphragm

AP Below Diaphragm

PA Above Diaphragm

Oblique

STERNUM—ROUTINE POSITIONS/PROJECTIONS

Right Anterior Oblique

Lateral

STERNOCLAVICULAR ARTICULATIONS—ROUTINE PROJECTIONS

PA

Oblique

SPECIAL CONSIDERATIONS

Trauma Considerations

Pediatric Considerations

Geriatric Considerations

Common Errors

Correlative Imaging

OBJECTIVES

At the completion of this chapter, the student should be able to:

1. List and describe anatomic structures of the ribs and sternum.

2. Given drawings and radiographs, locate anatomic structures and landmarks.

3. Explain the rationale for each projection.

4. Explain the patient preparation required for each examination.

5. Describe the positioning used to visualize anatomic structures of the bony thorax.

6. List or identify the central location and identify the extent of field necessary for each projection.

7. Explain the protective measures that should be taken for each examination.

8. Recommend the technical factors for producing an acceptable radiograph for each projection.

9. State the patient instructions for each projection.

10. Given radiographs, evaluate positioning and technical factors.

11. Describe modifications of procedures for atypical or impaired patients to better demonstrate the anatomic area of interest.

Anatomy

THE BONY THORAX

The bony thorax is comprised of twelve pairs of ribs, the sternum anteriorly and the thoracic vertebrae posteriorly. These structures protect the thoracic **viscera** (vĭs´ĕr-ă) and upper abdominal viscera (organs) from injury (Figure 6.1).

The Ribs

Posteriorly, the twelve pairs of ribs articulate directly with the thoracic vertebrae. The heads of the ribs articulate with the bodies of the thoracic vertebrae, forming the costovertebral articulations (Figure 6.2). The tubercles articulate with the transverse processes, forming the costotransverse articulations. At their posterior aspect, the ribs assume a somewhat horizontal orientation as they come off the thoracic vertebrae and continue laterally and then anteriorly to form the lateral axillary margin of the rib cage. As the ribs continue anteriorly to articulate with the sternum, they

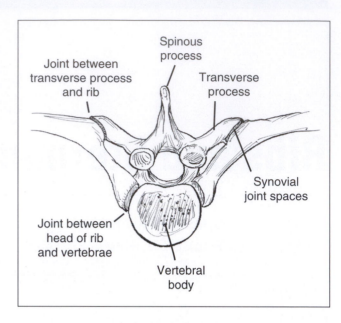

FIGURE 6.2   Costovertebral articulation.

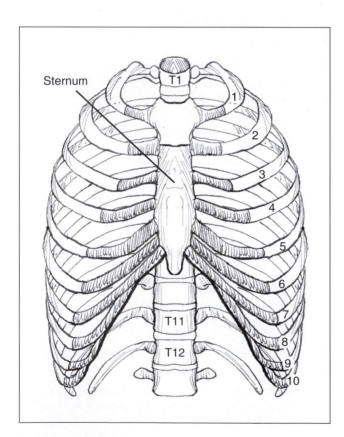

FIGURE 6.1   Bony thorax.

assume an oblique downward direction as they approach the midline. The thorax is widest at the level of the eighth and ninth pairs of ribs.

Anteriorly, the first seven pairs of ribs attach directly to the sternum (Figure 6.3). The first pair of ribs, which are the shortest and broadest, articulate directly with the manubrium (mă-nū´brē-ŭm). The second through seventh pairs of ribs articulate with the sternum via costochondral cartilage. Because the first seven pairs of ribs articulate directly with the sternum, they are referred to as "true" ribs. The eighth, ninth, and tenth ribs articulate indirectly with the sternum via cartilage that attaches to the cartilage of the seventh rib and are considered "false" ribs. The eleventh and twelfth ribs have no cartilage at the anterior ends and have no anterior sternal attachment. These last two rib pairs are considered not only "false" ribs but also "floating" ribs.

The Sternum

The sternum is a thin flat bone that lies longitudinally in the midsagittal plane. Superiorly the sternum is tilted backward or posteriorly and then assumes an anterior direction as it descends (Figure 6.4).

Approximately 6 inches in length, the sternum is comprised of three distinct parts (Figure 6.5). The most superior portion is the manubrium. Quadrilat-

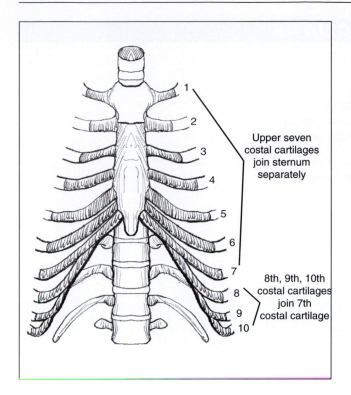

FIGURE 6.3   **Sternum and costal cartilages.**

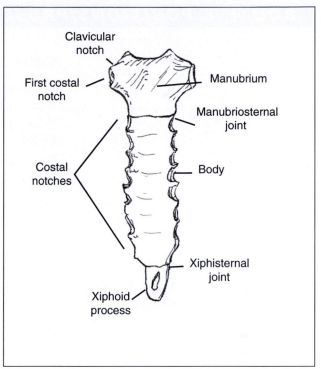

FIGURE 6.5   **Sternum (anterior view).**

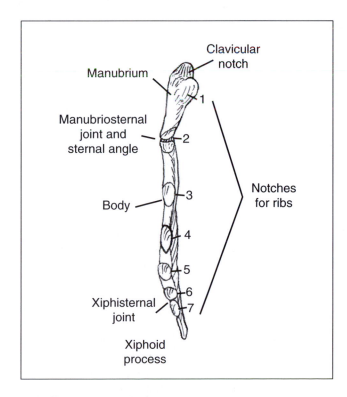

FIGURE 6.4   **Sternum (lateral view).**

eral in shape, the manubrium has a distinct concavity on its superior border called the manubrial notch, suprasternal notch, or jugular notch. Corresponding to the intervertebral disk space between the second and third thoracic vertebrae, this notch is an important positioning landmark for many radiographic examinations. The clavicles articulate with the manubrium to form the sternoclavicular articulations.

The middle portion of the sternum is called the body, corpus, or gladiolus. This is the longest of the three sternal sections and attaches superiorly to the manubrium to form the positioning landmark known as the sternal angle. This landmark corresponds to the vertebral disk space between the fourth and fifth thoracic vertebrae. The lateral margins of the corpus appear to be serrated due to the presence of sternal notches, which provide articulation with the costochondral cartilage of the anterior ends of the ribs.

The smallest and most inferior portion of the sternum is the xiphoid (zĭf´oyd) or ensiform (ĕn´sĭ-form) process. It is comprised of cartilage and represents another important radiographic positioning landmark corresponding to the level of the tenth thoracic vertebra.

ROUTINE POSITIONS/PROJECTIONS

RIBS—AP PROJECTION (ABOVE DIAPHRAGM)

Exam Rationale   Although the most common indication for radiographic examination of the ribs is trauma, rib projections may also be ordered for pathologic investigations. This position best demonstrates the upper, posterior ribs.

Technical Considerations

- Regular screen/film
- Grid
- kVp range: 65–70
- SID: 40 inch (100 cm)

Radiation Protection

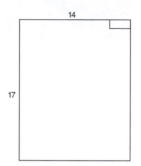

Patient Position   Erect with back against Bucky with all potential artifacts removed from area of interest (Figure 6.6).

Part Position   Arms slightly abducted and weight equally distributed on both feet with no rotation; midsagittal plane aligned to midline of Bucky and perpendicular to the plane of the film; shoulders rotated anteriorly to reduce superimposition on the upper ribs.

Central Ray   Upper border of cassette 2 inches (5 cm) above the upper border of the shoulders; central ray directed perpendicularly to the plane of the film at the level of the seventh thoracic vertebra.

Patient Instructions   "Take in a breath. Let it out. Take in another breath and hold it. Don't breathe or move."

Evaluation Criteria   (Figures 6.7 and 6.8)

- First nine or ten pairs of posterior ribs inclusive of the axillary margin should be visualized with no evidence of motion or rotation.

Tip   The same procedure may be done with the patient in a recumbent position.

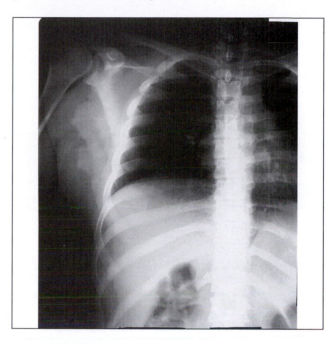

FIGURE 6.7   AP (above diaphragm) ribs.

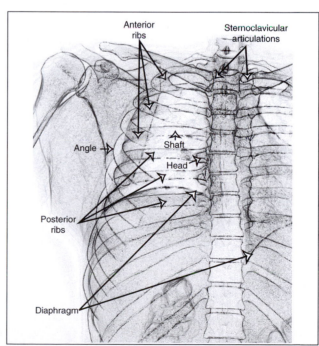

FIGURE 6.8   AP (above diaphragm) ribs.

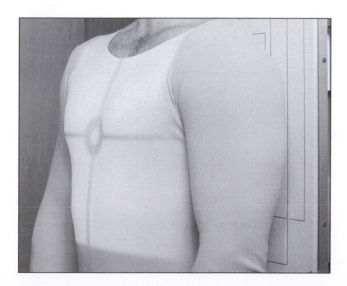

FIGURE 6.6   AP (above diaphragm) ribs.

RIBS—AP PROJECTION (BELOW DIAPHRAGM)

Exam Rationale   Because the lower ribs are superimposed by the diaphragm, it is necessary to expose the lower ribs using a darker density setting. The exposure is made on patient exhalation to allow the diaphragm excursion to be at its most superior extreme to demonstrate as many pairs of ribs as possible on the more dense setting.

Technical Considerations

- Regular screen/film
- Grid
- kVp range: 75–80
- SID: 40 inch (100 cm)

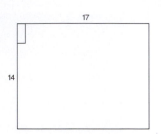

(may be lengthwise for smaller patients)

Radiation Protection

Patient Position   Erect with back against Bucky with all potential artifacts removed from area of interest (Figure 6.9).

Part Position   Arms slightly abducted and weight equally distributed on both feet with no rotation; midsagittal plane aligned to midline of Bucky and perpendicular to the plane of the film.

Central Ray   Lower border of cassette 2 inches (5 cm) below the inferior rib margin; central ray directed perpendicularly to the plane of the film at the level of the twelfth thoracic vertebra for crosswise film placement or the tenth thoracic vertebra for lengthwise film placement.

Patient Instructions   "Take in a breath. Let it out. Hold it out. Don't breathe or move."

Evaluation Criteria (Figures 6.10 and 6.11)

- Eighth through twelfth pairs of posterior ribs inclusive of the axillary margins should be visualized with no evidence of motion or rotation.

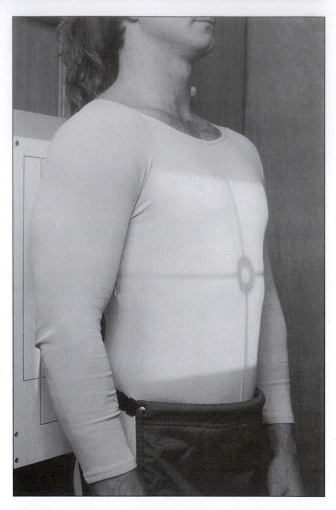

FIGURE 6.9   AP (below diaphragm) ribs.

Tips

1. Be sure lead shielding does not superimpose lower ribs.
2. The same procedure may be done with the patient in a recumbent position.

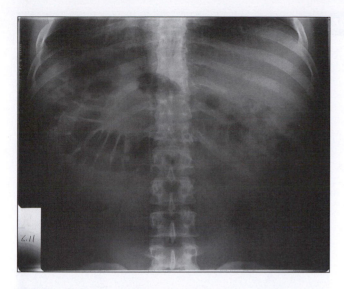

FIGURE 6.10   AP (below diaphragm) ribs.

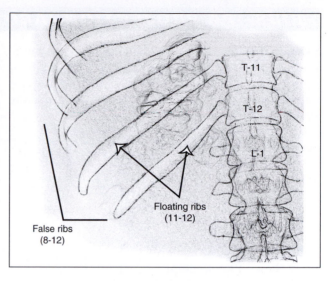

FIGURE 6.11   AP (below diaphragm) ribs.

RIBS—PA PROJECTION (ABOVE DIAPHRAGM)

Exam Rationale   Although the most common indication for radiographic examination of the ribs is trauma, rib projections may also be ordered for pathologic investigations. This position best demonstrates the upper, anterior ribs.

Technical Considerations

- Regular screen/film
- Grid
- kVp range: 65–70
- SID: 40 inch (100 cm)

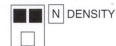

Radiation Protection   AEC (Phototiming)

 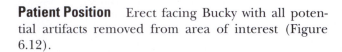 N DENSITY

Patient Position   Erect facing Bucky with all potential artifacts removed from area of interest (Figure 6.12).

Part Position   Arms slightly abducted and weight equally distributed on both feet with no rotation; midsagittal plane aligned to midline of Bucky and perpendicular to the plane of the film; shoulders rotated anteriorly to reduce superimposition on the upper ribs.

Central Ray   Upper border of cassette 2 inches (5 cm) above the upper border of the shoulders; central ray directed perpendicularly to the plane of the film at the level of the seventh thoracic vertebra.

Patient Instructions   "Take in a breath. Let it out. Take in another breath and hold it. Don't breathe or move."

Evaluation Criteria (Figures 6.13 and 6.14)

- First nine or ten pairs of anterior ribs inclusive of the axillary margins should be visualized with no evidence of motion or rotation.
- Should be no rotation as evidenced by the sternoclavicular articulations on each side being equidistant from the midsagittal plane.

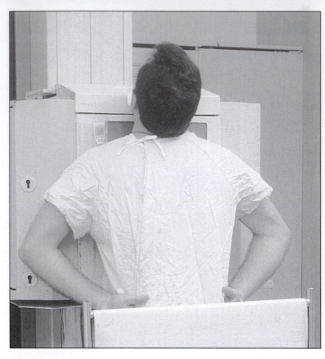

FIGURE 6.12   PA ribs.

Tips

1. The neck can be extended to lift the chin off the upper ribs.
2. The same procedure may be adapted for the patient in a recumbent position.

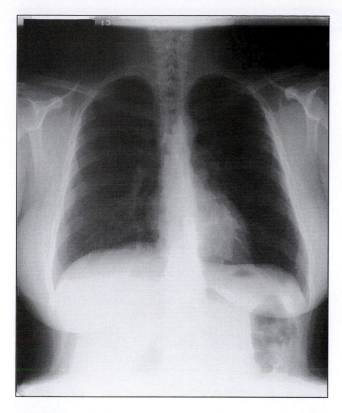

FIGURE 6.13 PA ribs.

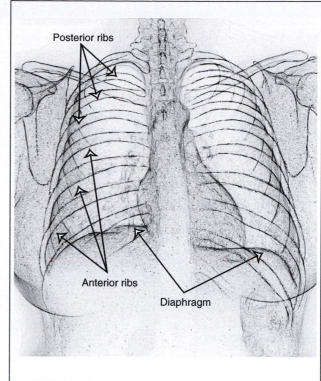

FIGURE 6.14 PA ribs.

RIBS—OBLIQUE (RPO/LPO POSITIONS)

Exam Rationale Because the rib cage completely encircles the thoracic cavity, superimposition of the anterior and posterior ribs is always evident in AP or PA projections. It is necessary to oblique the thorax relative to the plane of the film to project the ribs free of superimposition and to demonstrate the axillary portion of the ribs. These projections/positions are selected in cases of trauma to the posterior or axillary aspects of the ribs.

Technical Considerations

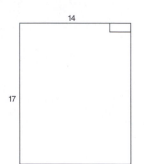

- Regular screen/film
- Grid
- kVp range: 65–70 (for ribs above diaphragm), 75–80 (for ribs below diaphragm)
- SID: 40 inch (100 cm)

Radiation Protection

Patient Position Erect with posterior of side of interest against Bucky with all potential artifacts removed from area of interest.

Part Position Arms slightly abducted and hand of affected side behind head to move scapula off upper ribs; midsagittal plane at a 45° angle with the plane of the film; sagittal plane that lies halfway between the midsagittal plane and the lateral margin of the affected ribs aligned with the longitudinal midline of cassette.

Central Ray

- Upper ribs: upper border of cassette 2 inches (5 cm) above the upper border of the shoulders; central ray directed perpendicularly to a sagittal plane halfway between the midsagittal plane and the lateral margin of the affected ribs at the level of the seventh thoracic vertebra (Figure 6.15).
- Lower ribs: lower border of cassette 2 inches (5 cm) below inferior margin of the ribs; central ray directed perpendicularly to a sagittal plane halfway between the midsagittal plane and the lateral margin of the affected ribs at the level of the tenth thoracic vertebra.

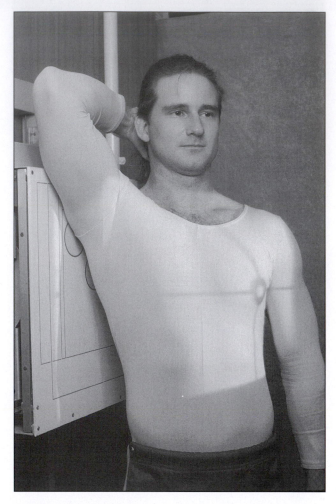

FIGURE 6.15   RPO upper ribs.

Evaluation Criteria

- Upper ribs: first nine or ten pairs of ribs inclusive of the axillary margins should be visualized above the diaphragm with no evidence of motion; distance between the spine and the axillary margin of the affected side will appear to be double that of the distance between the same structures on the unaffected side (Figures 6.16 and 6.17).
- Lower ribs: eighth through the twelfth ribs inclusive of the axillary margins should be visualized below the diaphragm with no evidence of motion; distance between the spine and the axillary margin of the affected side wall will appear to be double that of the distance between the same structures on the unaffected side.

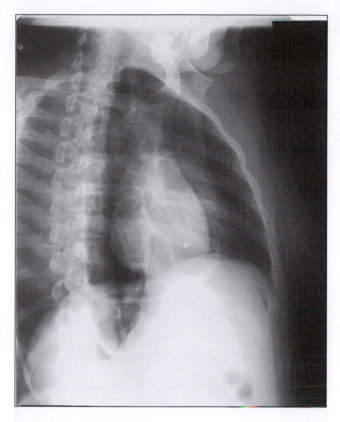

FIGURE 6.16   **LPO upper ribs.**

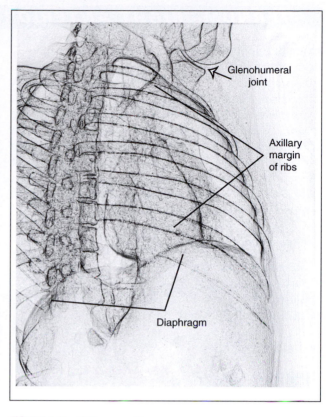

FIGURE 6.17   **LPO upper ribs.**

Tips

1. Always rotate the spine *away* from side of interest.
2. Make sure the lead shield does not superimpose the lower ribs.
3. For a patient unable to stand, the same procedures may be adapted for the recumbent position.
4. The oblique may also be done in the PA projection. The patient begins in the erect position facing the Bucky and is rotated 45° away from the injured side.

STERNUM—RIGHT ANTERIOR OBLIQUE POSITION

Exam Rationale   Because the sternum is a relatively thin, flat bone, it is completely obliterated by the superimposition of the thoracic vertebrae in a true PA projection. To obtain a PA projection of the sternum, it is necessary to slightly rotate the patient to move the thoracic vertebrae off the sternum. The RAO position is routinely selected because it projects the sternum through the heart shadow, which takes advantage of the more homogeneous anatomic density of the heart muscle to allow improved demonstration of the sternum relative to radiographic density.

Technical Considerations

- Regular screen/film
- Grid
- kVp range: 65–70
- SID: 40 inch (100 cm)

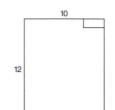

Radiation Protection

Patient Position   Erect facing Bucky with all potential artifacts removed from area of interest (Figure 6.18).

Part Position   With the right anterior aspect of the patient's chest against the Bucky, rotate patient 15° to 20°; align long axis of sternum to long axis of cassette.

Central Ray   Upper border of cassette 1 1/2 inches (4 cm) above manubrial notch; align central ray perpendicularly to the plane of the film at the level of the seventh thoracic vertebra (approximately 1 1/2 to 2 inches (4–5 cm) to the left of the midsagittal plane).

Patient Instructions   "Continue to breathe gently during the exposure. Don't move."

Evaluation Criteria (Figures 6.19 and 6.20)

- Entire sternum should be projected through the blurred heart shadow free of superimposition with the thoracic vertebrae.
- Lung markings and ribs should appear blurred.

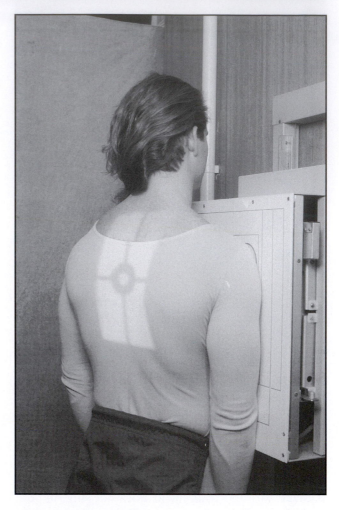

FIGURE 6.18   RAO sternum.

Tips

1. Palpate the thoracic vertebral spinous processes with one hand and the manubrial notch with the other when rotating patient. This will serve as a guide to ensure appropriate rotation of the thoracic spine away from the sternum.
2. A long exposure time (2–3 seconds) will ensure adequate blurring of ribs, pulmonary markings, and the heart shadow.
3. For a patient who is unable to stand, the patient may be examined in the recumbent position.

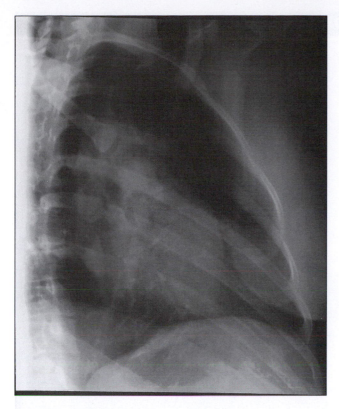

FIGURE 6.19 RAO sternum.

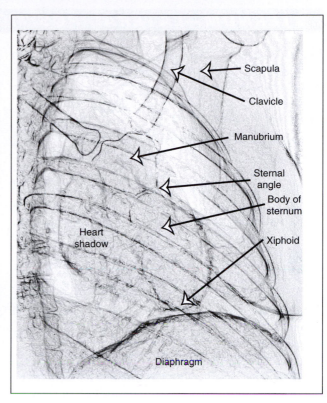

FIGURE 6.20 RAO sternum.

STERNUM—LATERAL POSITION

Exam Rationale This position allows the sternum to be visualized in a lateral orientation that complements the RAO.

Technical Considerations

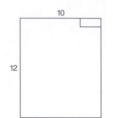

- Regular screen/film
- Grid
- kVp range: 70–75
- SID: 40 inch (100 cm)

Radiation Protection

Patient Position Erect right or left lateral with all potential artifacts removed from area of interest (Figure 6.21).

Part Position With midsagittal plane parallel to the plane of the film, align sternum to midline of cassette; have patient clasp hands behind back to move shoulders posteriorly and to project the sternum anteriorly.

Central Ray With upper border of cassette 1 1/2 inches above manubrial notch, align central ray perpendicularly to the lateral border of the sternum midway between the manubrial notch and the xiphoid process.

Patient Instructions "Take in a breath and hold it in. Don't breathe or move."

Evaluation Criteria (Figures 6.22 and 6.23)

- Entire sternum should be visualized with no evidence of rotation or motion.

Tips

1. Be sure patient is in contact with Bucky but not leaning against it to ensure there is no forward or backward swaying during the exposure.
2. For female patients, it may be necessary to move the breasts to the side and secure them with a wide

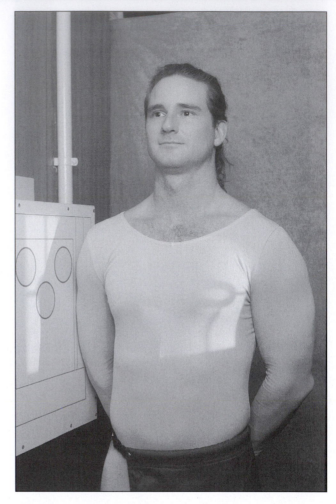

FIGURE 6.21 Lateral sternum.

bandage to prevent superimposition of breast shadows over sternum.
3. For the patient who is unable to stand, this procedure may be done in the recumbent position.

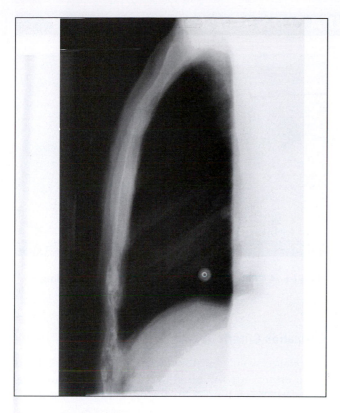

FIGURE 6.22   Lateral sternum.

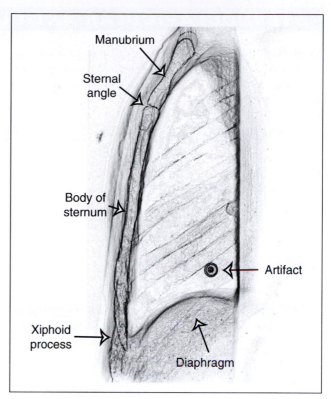

FIGURE 6.23   Lateral sternum.

STERNOCLAVICULAR ARTICULATIONS—PA PROJECTION

Exam Rationale   Occasionally, radiographic visualization of the sternoclavicular articulations may be desirable to demonstrate possible traumatic or pathologic (arthritic) changes.

Technical Considerations

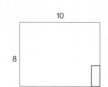

* Regular screen/film
* kVp range: 65–70
* SID: 40 inch (100 cm)

Radiation Protection

Patient Position   Recumbent with MSP centered to midline of table and with all potential artifacts removed from area of interest (Figure 6.24).

Part Position   Chin should be extended; adjust midsagittal plane perpendicular to plane of film.

Central Ray   Perpendicular to the third thoracic vertebra.

Patient Instructions   "Take in a breath. Blow it out and hold it out. Don't breathe or move."

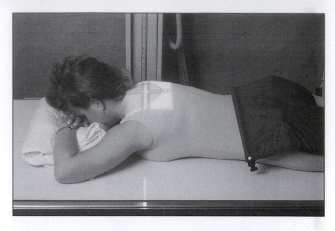

FIGURE 6.24   Recumbent PA sternoclavicular articulations.

Evaluation Criteria (Figures 6.25 and 6.26)

* Sternoclavicular articulations should be visualized on either side of and equidistant from the midsagittal plane with no evidence of rotation or motion.

Tips   The same procedure may be adapted for the erect position.

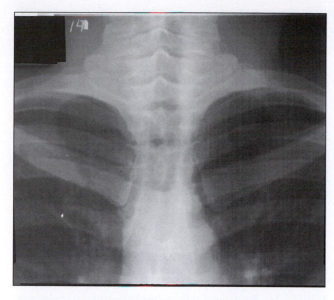

FIGURE 6.25   **PA sternoclavicular articulations.**

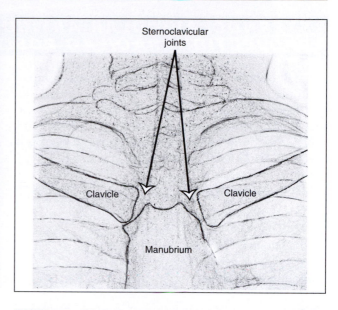

FIGURE 6.26   **PA sternoclavicular articulations.**

STERNOCLAVICULAR ARTICULATIONS—OBLIQUE PA PROJECTION (RAO/LAO POSITIONS)

Exam Rationale The oblique projections complement the PA projection by projecting the sternoclavicular articulations to one side of the thoracic vertebrae, which reduces superimposition and "opens" the joint space for better visualization. Both sides are examined for comparison.

Technical Considerations

- Regular screen/film
- kVp range: 65–70
- SID: 40 inch (100 cm)

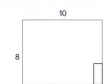

Radiation Protection

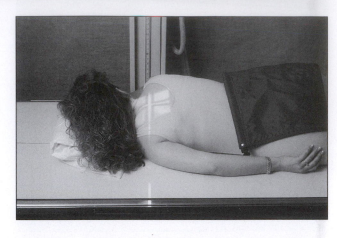

FIGURE 6.27 Recumbent oblique sternoclavicular articulations.

Patient Position Recumbent with all potential artifacts removed from area of interest (Figure 6.27).

Part Position Rotate patient 15° to place side of interest closest to Bucky; midsagittal plane forms 15° angle with plane of film.

Central Ray Perpendicular to the third thoracic vertebra.

Patient Instructions "Take in a breath. Blow it out and hold it out. Don't breathe or move."

Evaluation Criteria (Figures 6.28 and 6.29)

- Sternoclavicular articulation, manubrium, and proximal clavicle should be demonstrated with the joint space "open" and free of superimposition with thoracic vertebrae.
- No evidence of rotation or motion.

Tips

1. Rotate the patient's head more than the patient's body to allow for patient comfort and to reduce magnification.
2. The same procedure may be adapted for the erect position.

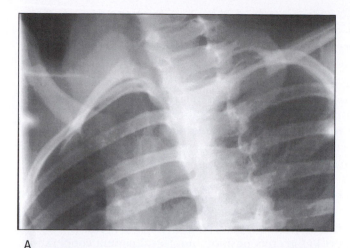

A

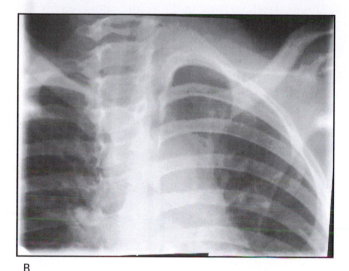

B

FIGURE 6.28A and B Oblique sternoclavicular articulations.

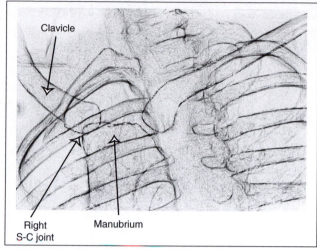

A

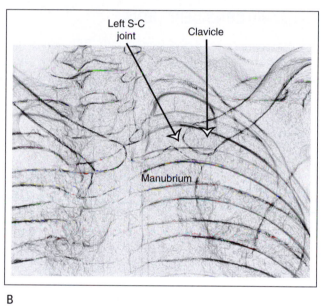

B

FIGURE 6.29A and B Oblique sternoclavicular articulations.

Special Considerations

TRAUMA CONSIDERATIONS

Injury to the ribs can be very painful due to the constant movement of respiration and, if severe enough, can be life-threatening. For this reason, perhaps the single most important radiograph in a rib examination series may be a routine, erect chest projection. If at all possible, it is important to radiograph the patient upright (or at least with some type of horizontal central projection) to rule out the possibility of **pneumothorax** (presence of air in the pleural cavity) or **hemothorax** (presence of blood in the pleural cavity) resulting from possible laceration of the lung tissue. It is more important to obtain this diagnostic information than to check for rib fractures. Once the patient is stabilized, a complete series of radiographs can be obtained.

Because rib and sternal injuries may be painful, it is generally more comfortable for the patient to stand in front of a Bucky than to lie on the painful injured side on the radiographic table. The area of interest is always placed closest to the recording medium (film). If the study is performed erect, the patient is not forced into uncomfortable positions. Because of the increased comfort in the erect position, improved patient cooperation helps realize improved radiographs studies (i.e., reduction of repeat radiographs, faster examinations, etc.).

PEDIATRIC CONSIDERATIONS

Because the bones of children are not fully **ossified** (changed to bone), children are not as susceptible to fractures resulting from trauma as are adults. This is particularly true in the thorax, which is designed for flexibility to facilitate the respiration process. Radiographic examinations of the ribs are rarely ordered for pediatric patients.

GERIATRIC CONSIDERATIONS

Considerations when examining a geriatric patient are lack of mobility and flexibility. Patience and respect are the most important skills a radiographer can use to facilitate the examination. It is much more comfortable for the patient and quicker for the radiographer to radiograph the geriatric patient standing at the upright Bucky as opposed to examining the patient on a radiographic table.

COMMON ERRORS

Ribs

- Failure to examine anterior ribs with anterior aspect closest to recording medium.
- Failure to rotate the spine away from the side of interest on oblique projections.

Sternum

- Failure to select appropriate density/contrast settings for diagnostic exposure.

CORRELATIVE IMAGING

Typically, diagnostic information of the ribs and sternum is obtained via radiographic studies. Due to the curving shape of the rib cage, the bony thorax does not lend itself well to sectional imaging modalities. The one exception may be CT examinations for visualizing **retrosternal** (behind the sternum) and sternoclavicular articulation trauma. Excellent images of this anatomy can be obtained with small section CT using bone **algorithms** (a mathematical progression that is programmed for a computer).

Review Questions

1. How many pairs of ribs connect directly to the sternum by way of their own costochondral cartilage?

   a. 5
   b. 6
   c. 7
   d. 8

2. Which pairs of ribs are identified as "floating" ribs?

   a. 1, 2, 3, 4, 5, 6, and 7
   b. 8, 9, and 10
   c. 10, 11, and 12
   d. 11 and 12

3. The thorax is widest at the level of which ribs?

   a. 4th and 5th
   b. 6th and 7th
   c. 8th and 9th
   d. 10th and 11th

4. The articulation between the tubercle of a rib and a transverse process of a thoracic vertebra is called:

   a. costovertebral articulation
   b. costotransverse articulation
   c. costosternal articulation
   d. zygapophyseal articulation

5. Which thoracic vertebra(e) is at the same level as the ensiform process?

   a. 4th and 5th intervertebral disk space
   b. 7th
   c. 10th
   d. 12th

6. The concavity which serves as positioning landmark at the margin of the manubrium is called:

   a. suprasternal notch
   b. xiphoid notch
   c. xiphoid tip
   d. ensiform process

7. The articulation between the head of a rib and the body of a thoracic vertebra is called:

   a. costovertebral articulation
   b. costotransverse articulation
   c. costosternal articulation
   d. zygapophyseal articulation

8. To demonstrate the upper ribs on an AP projection, the central ray is centered at:

   a. 4th thoracic vertebra
   b. 7th thoracic vertebra
   c. 10th thoracic vertebra
   d. 12th thoracic vertebra

9. Which oblique position should be used for an injury to the left anterior ribs?

   a. RAO
   b. LAO
   c. RPO
   d. LPO

10. How many degrees is the patient rotated for an oblique position of the ribs?

    a. 15–20
    b. 25–30
    c. 45
    d. 70

11. Which of the following positions/projections is taken when a fracture to the posterior portion of the right 5th and 6th ribs is suspected?

    1. erect PA chest
    2. AP ribs (above diaphragm)
    3. oblique (RPO) ribs (above diaphragm)

    a. 1 and 2
    b. 1 and 3
    c. 2 and 3
    d. 1, 2, and 3

12. What are the basic positions/projections for a sternum examination?

    a. AP and RAO
    b. AP and LAO
    c. AP and lateral
    d. RAO and lateral

13. How much is the patient rotated on the oblique position for the sternoclavicular joints?

    a. 15°
    b. 25°
    c. 30°
    d. 45°

14. AP, PA, and oblique ribs may be taken in either the erect or recumbent position.

    a. true
    b. false

15. The AP projection of the ribs below the diaphragm should be taken on suspended expiration.

    a. true
    b. false

16. The clavicle articulates with what section of the sternum to form the sternoclavicular joint?

17. An AP projection of the ribs above the diaphragm should demonstrate how many pairs of posterior ribs?

18. How many degrees is the patient rotated for an oblique sternum?

19. What is the central ray location for a lateral sternum?

20. What are the basic projections for an exam of the sternoclavicular joints?

21. Why is it necessary to rotate the body from a true PA position for a frontal projection of the sternum?

22. When radiographing the sternum, why is an RAO position preferable to an LAO position?

References and Recommended Reading

Ballinger, P. W. (1995). *Merrill's atlas of radiographic positions and radiologic procedures* (8th ed.). St. Louis: Mosby-Year Book.

Bontrager, K. L. (1993). *Textbook of radiographic positioning and related anatomy* (3rd ed.). St. Louis: Mosby-Year Book.

Dowd, S. B., & Wilson, B. G. (1995). *Encyclopedia of radiographic positioning* (2nd ed.). Boston: Little, Brown.

Eisenberg, R. L., Dennis, C. A., & May, C. R. (1995). *Radiographic positioning* (2nd ed.). Boston: Little, Brown.

McDonough, J. T., Jr. (Ed.). (1995). *Stedman's concise medical dictionary.* Baltimore: Williams & Wilkins.

SECTION IV

VERTEBRAL COLUMN

Cervical Spine

JOANNE S. GREATHOUSE, EdS, RT(R)(ARRT), FASRT
MICHAEL MADDEN, PhD, RT(R)(ARRT)

ANATOMY
Typical Cervical Vertebrae
Atypical Cervical Vertebrae
Routine Positions/Projections
AP
AP Open Mouth
Oblique
Lateral

ALTERNATE POSITIONS/PROJECTIONS
Flexion/Extension Laterals
AP wagging jaw (Otonello)

AP Odontoid Process (Fuchs)
PA Odontoid Process (Judd)
AP Vertebral Arch

SPECIAL CONSIDERATIONS
Pediatric Considerations
Common Errors
Selected Pathology
Correlative Imaging

OBJECTIVES

At the completion of this chapter, the student should be able to:

1. List and describe the bony anatomy of the cervical spine.

2. Given drawings and radiographs, locate anatomic structures and landmarks.

3. Explain the rationale for each projection.

4. Explain the patient preparation required for each examination.

5. Describe the positioning used to visualize anatomic structures of the cervical spine.

6. List or identify the central ray location and identify the extent of field necessary for each projection.

7. Explain the protective measures that should be taken for each projection.

8. Recommend the technical factors for producing an acceptable radiograph for each projection.

9. State the patient instructions for each projection.

10. Given radiographs, evaluate positioning and technical factors for radiographs of the cervical spine.

11. Describe modifications for procedures for atypical or impaired patients to better demonstrate the anatomic area of interest.

Anatomy

The vertebral column is comprised of approximately thirty-three separate bones, called vertebrae (věr´tē-brā). The vertebrae are generally considered in four primary divisions, with the bones in each division having distinguishing features: cervical, thoracic, lumbar, and sacrum and coccyx.

When viewed from the lateral perspective, the vertebral column forms a series of alternating curves. The cervical spine is concave, the thoracic spine convex, the lumbar spine concave, and the sacrum and coccyx convex. These normal curvatures of the spine increase its strength and stability (Figure 7.1).

The uppermost seven vertebrae, the cervical vertebrae, have little resemblance to the other vertebrae. The most easily identified distinctive feature of the cervical vertebrae is the foramen in the transverse

process, called the transverse foramen. Also, the cervical vertebrae are the smallest of the moving vertebrae, which is all the vertebrae except the coccygeal. This discussion begins with the typical cervical vertebrae, the third through the sixth, and is followed by individual descriptions of the atypical vertebrae: the first, the second, and the seventh.

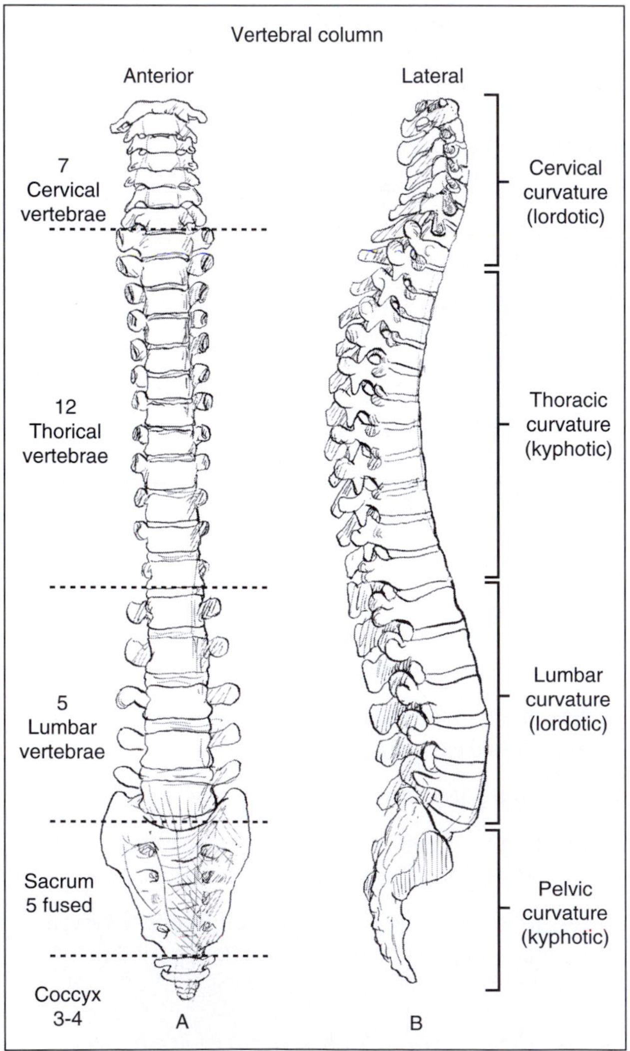

TYPICAL CERVICAL VERTEBRAE

The typical cervical vertebra has two main parts, a body and a vertebral arch. The vertebral arch surrounds the vertebral foramen, which is comparatively large and triangular rather than round. The vertebral foramina protect and house the spinal cord and its surrounding structures (Figures 7.2 and 7.3).

Body
The body is the largest and heaviest part of the bone and is roughly cylindrical in shape. The flattened ends of the body are adjacent to the cartilaginous intervertebral disks.

Vertebral Arch
Also known as the neural arch, the vertebral arch is the bony process posterior to the vertebral body. It includes two pedicles, two laminae, and seven processes: one spinous, two transverse, and four articular.

Vertebral column

Anterior | Lateral

7
Cervical
vertebrae

Cervical
curvature
(lordotic)

12
Thorical
vertebrae

Thoracic
curvature
(kyphotic)

5
Lumbar
vertebrae

Lumbar
curvature
(lordotic)

Sacrum
5 fused

Pelvic
curvature
(kyphotic)

Coccyx
3-4

A   B

FIGURE 7.1   (A) Anterior spine (B) Lateral spine.

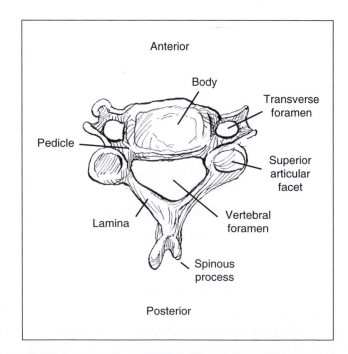

FIGURE 7.2   Superior view of typical cervical vertebra.

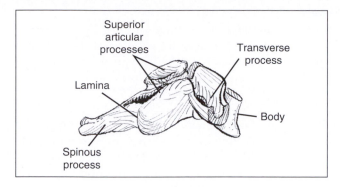

FIGURE 7.3 **Lateral view of typical cervical vertebra.**

Pedicle (pĕd´ĭ-k´l) This bony structure attaches to the posterolateral margin of the body and extends to the lamina. The concave superior and inferior surfaces of the bone form the vertebral notches between adjacent vertebrae, creating the intervertebral foramina, which are equal in depth and project at a 45° angle from the median plane.

Lamina (lăm´ĭ-nă) These are the relatively long narrow bony structures with a thin upper margin that extends posteriorly and medially from the pedicles, forming much of the posterior border of the vertebral foramen.

Spinous Process This bony process is directly posterior to the union of the laminae and extends caudally. The spinous processes of the cervical vertebrae, other than those of C6 and C7, are shorter than those of other vertebrae. The spinous processes of C6 and C7 are longer. In white persons, the terminal process is usually bifid, and the resulting tubercles are often unequal in size. In black persons, the spinous process is usually not bifid but has a single tubercle at its terminus.

Transverse Process The most distinctive feature of cervical vertebrae, the transverse foramen, is located centrally and encases the vertebral artery and veins.

Articular Processes These processes are directly lateral to the vertebral foramen and extend both upward and downward from the points where the pedicles and laminae join. The upward projection, the superior articular process, has the articular surface facing posteriorly; the articular surface of the inferior articular process faces anteriorly. Together, the processes form the **zygapophyseal joints** between adjacent vertebrae.

Zygapophyseal Joints 2–7 (zī´´gă-pō-fĭz´ē-ăl) These amphiarthrodial joints between the articular processes of the vertebrae are lateral to the vertebral foramina. The articular processes align and form the articular pillars, which are the site of the joints on the lateral side (Figure 7.4).

Intervertebral Foramina In contrast to the other vertebrae, the pedicles and intervertebral foramina of the cervical vertebrae are not well visualized in a lateral view but are better seen from the anterolateral aspect. The foramina are directed anteriorly at a 45° angle and also slope approximately 15° inferiorly as they project from the vertebral foramen.

ATYPICAL CERVICAL VERTEBRAE

Atlas
The first cervical vertebra, which supports the head, is named for Atlas, a mythical Greek titan who was thought to have supported the world. The **atlas** is the

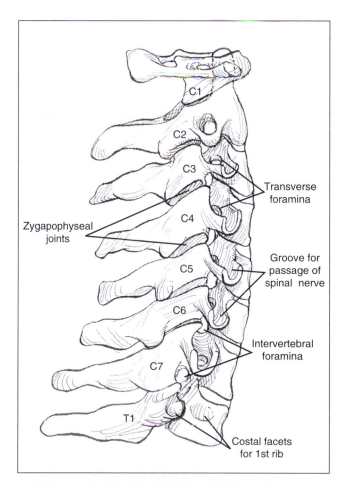

FIGURE 7.4 **Anterolateral view of zygapophyseal joints.**

most atypical vertebrae in the body because it lacks a body and a true spinous process. It is roughly circular in shape. The front and back of the vertebra are formed by the anterior and posterior arches, with the sides consisting of the lateral masses (Figure 7.5).

Anterior Arch This marked feature of the atlas is an arch of bone with a central expanded area, the anterior tubercle. In the adult vertebral column, the centrum, which would have given rise to the body of the atlas, is fused to the second cervical vertebral body and is located directly posterior to the end of the anterior arch.

Posterior Arch This arch does not have a true spinous process but instead has a much smaller posterior tubercle.

Lateral Masses These bulky bony structures are lateral to the vertebral foramen and contain the articular facets. The superior articular facets, which correspond with the occipital condyles, are very large concave oval structures facing medially and superiorly. They are usually constricted in the middle and may be divided. The inferior articular facets are large and roughly round in shape.

Atlanto-occipital Joints These are the paired synovial joints between the superior articular surfaces of the atlas and the occipital condyles. The large articular surfaces partially enable nodding and lateral movements of the head.

Axis

The second cervical vertebrae or epistropheus (ĕp´´i-strō´fē-ŭs) forms the pivot for rotation of the atlas and the head. The **axis** is easily distinguished by its long body that extends superiorly, forming the dens or odontoid process (Figures 7.6 and 7.7).

Dens This bony structure, which is roughly 1 1/2 inches (4 cm) long, projects from the vertebral body of the axis and acts as the body for the atlas. The dens is highly involved in the rotational and nodding movements of the head and is often the sight of trauma. In instances where the head is forced into hyperflexion or hyperextension, as in "**whiplash**" injuries, the dens may become fractured. Because the dens form the anterior wall of the spinal foramen, this injury may

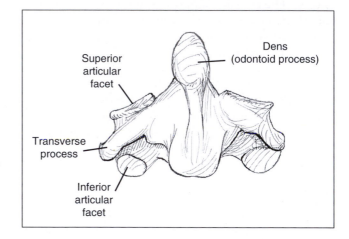

FIGURE 7.6   Anterior view of second cervical vertebra.

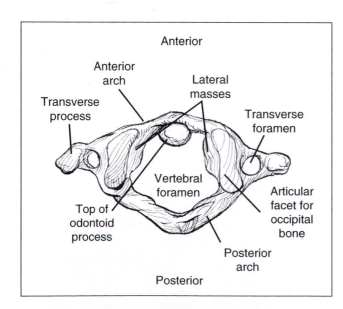

FIGURE 7.5   Superior view of first cervical vertebra.

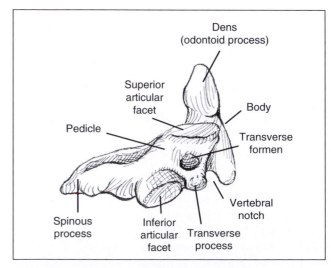

FIGURE 7.7   Lateral view of second cervical vertebra.

becoming life-threatening if the spinal cord is involved. This is the reason immobilization is critical in cases where neck injury is suspected.

Pedicles   These very thick, strong bony structures are fused to the sides of the body and the dens. Their upper surface forms the large superior articular facets, large oval structures that match with the inferior facets projecting from the lateral masses of the atlas. The articular facets of the atlas and axis are not aligned in the articular pillars formed by the other vertebrae.

Spinous Process   This bony projection is horizontal and is a short, blunt process with a single tubercle terminus.

Atlantoaxial Joint   Also referred to as the first zygapophyseal joint, this is actually three synovial joints: one on each side between the inferior articular facet of the lateral mass of the atlas and the superior articular facet of the axis and one between the dens and the anterior arch. Due to the unique structure, the lateral joints are best demonstrated in a true frontal view, immediately lateral to the anterior tubercle and dens.

Vertebra Prominens

The seventh cervical vertebra is the most distinctive of the lower cervical vertebrae due primarily to its spinous process. In comparison, the process is a very thick bony projection extending in a horizontal fashion posteriorly and can be easily palpated on the posterior base of the neck. In contrast to the typical vertebrae, the spinous process is not bifid but ends in a single tubercle.

ROUTINE AND ALTERNATIVE POSITIONS/PROJECTIONS

Part	Routine	Page	Alternative	Page
Cervical spine	AP	347		
	AP open mouth	349	AP wagging jaw (Otonello)	356
			AP odontoid process (Fuchs)	358
			PA odontoid process (Judd)	359
	Oblique	350		
	Lateral	352	Flexion/extension laterals	354
			AP vertebral arch	360

CERVICAL SPINE—AP PROJECTION

Exam Rationale   Examination of the cervical spine may be indicated in the investigation of degenerative disease or in cases of trauma.

Technical Considerations

- Regular screen/film
- Grid
- kVp range: 75–80
- SID: 40 inch (100 cm)

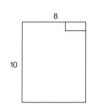

Radiation Protection   AEC (Phototiming)

    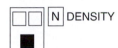   N DENSITY

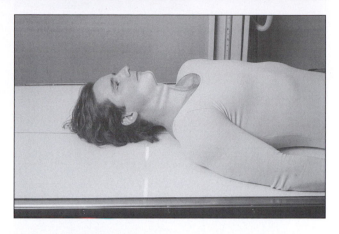

FIGURE 7.8   AP cervical spine.

Patient Position   Supine with midsagittal plane (MSP) centered to the midline of the table (Figure 7.8).

Part Position   Adjust so there is no rotation of the head or body; extend the neck so that a line from the lower edge of the upper incisors to the mastoid tips is perpendicular to the table.

Central Ray   Directed to C5 (thyroid cartilage) at a 15° to 20° cephalic angle.

Patient Instructions   "Breathe normally but don't move."

Evaluation Criteria (Figures 7.9 and 7.10)

- Should include C3–T2.
- There should be no rotation as evidenced by equal distance from spinous processes to spinous border on each side.
- Intervertebral disk spaces should be open.
- Base of skull and mandible will overlap C1 and C2.

Tip   This projection may also be done with the patient in an erect position.

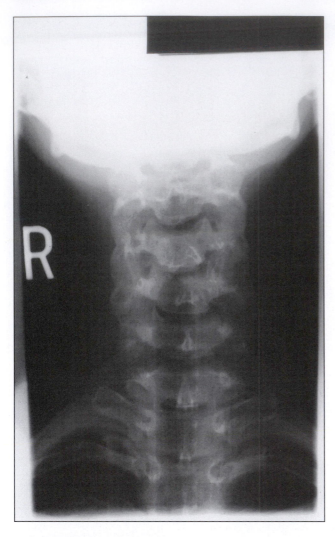

FIGURE 7.9   AP cervical spine.

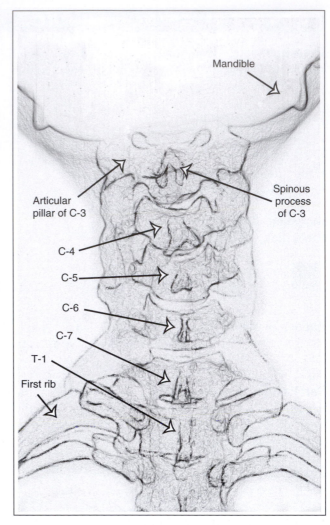

FIGURE 7.10   AP cervical spine.

CERVICAL SPINE—AP OPEN MOUTH (ATLAS AND AXIS) PROJECTION

Exam Rationale   This projection demonstrates the first two cervical vertebrae free of superimposition.

Technical Considerations

- Regular screen/film
- Grid
- kVp range: 70–75
- SID: 40 inch (100 cm)

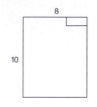

Radiation Protection   **AEC (Phototiming)**

 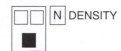 N DENSITY

Patient Position   Supine with MSP centered to the midline of the table (Figure 7.11).

Part Position   Adjust so there is no rotation of the head or body; extend the neck so that a line from the lower edge of the upper incisors to the mastoid tips is perpendicular to the table; have the patient open mouth by lowering the lower mandible.

Central Ray   Directed through the center of the open mouth.

Patient Instructions   "Stop breathing; don't breathe or move."

Evaluation Criteria (Figures 7.12 and 7.13)

- C1 and C2 should be clearly demonstrated through the open mouth.
- C1–2 zygapophyseal joint should be clearly visible.
- If the lower edge of the upper incisors and the base of the skull are superimposed, the position cannot be improved.

Tips

1. The patient should not open his mouth until just before the exposure is made because this position is somewhat uncomfortable and difficult to maintain.
2. Care must be taken that only the lower jaw is moved when the mouth is opened, maintaining the position of the spine.
3. If the upper incisors obscure the vertebrae, the chin needs to be elevated. If the base of the skull obscures the vertebrae, the chin must be depressed more.
4. Take care that center AEC has full primary beam collimation.

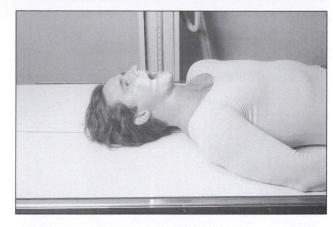

FIGURE 7.11   AP open mouth cervical spine.

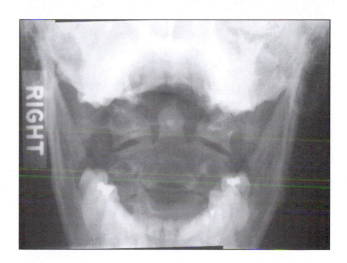

FIGURE 7.12   AP open mouth cervical spine.

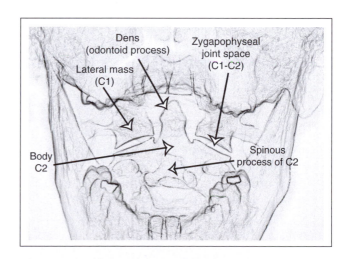

FIGURE 7.13   AP open mouth cervical spine.

CERVICAL SPINE—OBLIQUE POSITION (PA)

Exam Rationale This position demonstrates the open intervertebral foramina and pedicles closest to the film (the down side). Both sides are examined for comparison.

Technical Considerations

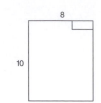

- Regular screen/film
- Grid
- kVp range: 75–80
- SID: 40 inch (100 cm)

Radiation Protection

AEC (Phototiming)

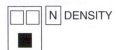 N DENSITY

Patient Position Erect or seated with the body at a 45° angle from the PA position (Figure 7.14).

Part Position Adjust so the whole body forms an angle of 45° with the plane of the film; the head should look straight ahead; chin should be extended slightly.

Central Ray Directed to C4 (upper margin of the thyroid cartilage) at 15° to 20° caudal angle.

Patient Instructions "Breathe normally but don't move."

Evaluation Criteria (Figures 7.15 and 7.16)

- Intervertebral foramina and disk spaces should be open.
- All seven cervical vertebrae should be seen.
- Chin should be sufficiently elevated so the mandibular rami do not overlap C1.
- Cervical pedicles should be well demonstrated.

Tips

1. These projections may also be done with the patient in a recumbent position, although the erect or seated position is preferred.
2. These projections may also be done with the patient rotated 45° from the AP position (Figure

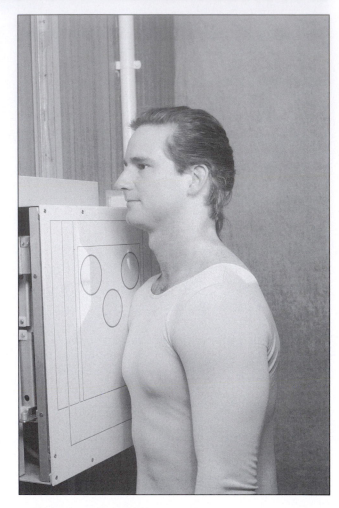

FIGURE 7.14   PA oblique cervical spine.

7.17); the central ray is then directed to C4 at a 15° to 20° cephalic angle.
3. Some department protocols call for these projections to be done at a 72-inch (180 cm) focus film distance (as with the lateral).
4. Take care that patient remains centered to AEC.

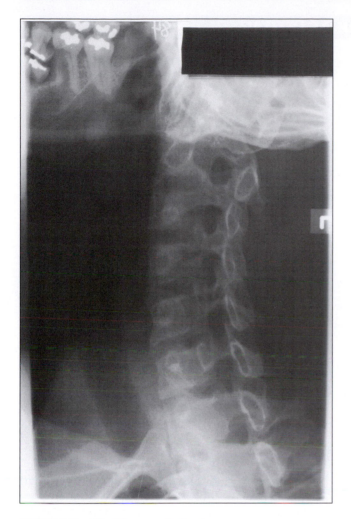

FIGURE 7.15   PA oblique cervical spine.

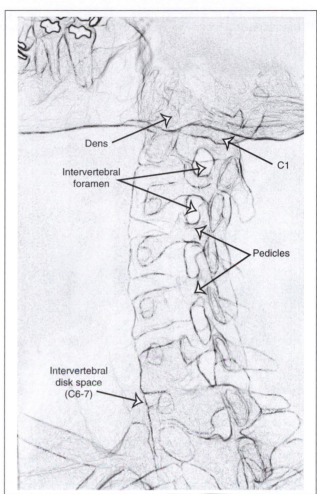

Dens

Intervertebral foramen

C1

Pedicles

Intervertebral disk space (C6-7)

FIGURE 7.16   PA oblique cervical spine.

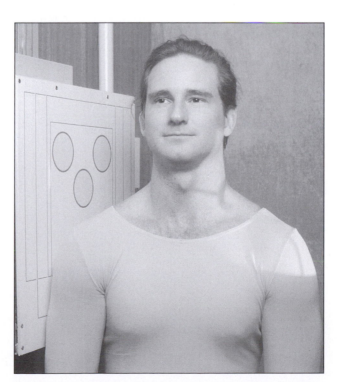

FIGURE 7.17
AP oblique cervical spine.

CERVICAL SPINE—LATERAL POSITION

Exam Rationale This position shows the vertebral bodies in a lateral position, the intervertebral joint spaces, the articular pillars, the spinous processes, and the articular facets of the lower five vertebrae.

Technical Considerations

- Regular screen/film
- Grid
- kVp range: 75–80
- SID: 72 inch (180 cm)

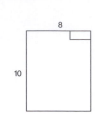

Radiation Protection   AEC (Phototiming)

 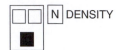 N DENSITY

Patient Position Erect or seated with left side against film (Figure 7.18).

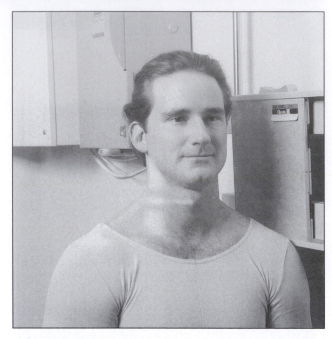

FIGURE 7.18   Lateral cervical spine.

Part Position Center the midcoronal plane to the midline of the film; adjust the body so its MSP is parallel to the film; depress the shoulders; raise the chin slightly to prevent overlap of the mandibular rami on the upper vertebrae.

Central Ray Top of cassette should be placed about 2 inches (5 cm) above EAM; central ray is directed to center of film at the level of the upper margin of the thyroid cartilage.

Patient Instructions "Take in a deep breath; let it all out. Don't breathe or move."

Evaluation Criteria (Figures 7.19 and 7.20)

- Should include all seven cervical vertebrae.
- There should be no rotation as evidenced by superimposition or close approximation of the two mandibular rami.
- Mandibular rami should not be superimposed over upper cervical vertebrae.

Tips

1. To help depress the shoulders, the patient can hold equal weights (sandbags) in each hand or pull up with both hands on a long strip of gauze under the feet.
2. If it is not possible to depress the shoulders sufficiently to visualize the lower cervical vertebrae, a separate swimmer's lateral should be done (see page 378).

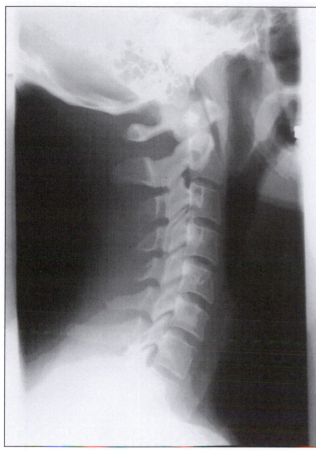

FIGURE 7.19   Lateral cervical spine.

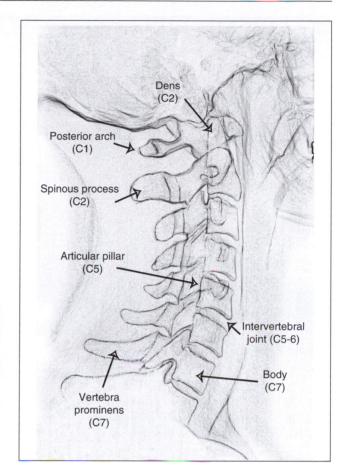

Dens
(C2)

Posterior arch
(C1)

Spinous process
(C2)

Articular pillar
(C5)

Intervertebral
joint (C5-6)

Body
(C7)

Vertebra
prominens
(C7)

FIGURE 7.20   Lateral cervical spine.

CERVICAL SPINE—LATERAL POSITION WITH HYPER-FLEXION AND HYPEREXTENSION

Exam Rationale These positions are functional studies to demonstrate the range of motion of the cervical vertebrae.

Technical Considerations

- Regular screen/film
- Grid
- kVp range: 75–80
- SID: 72 inch (180 cm)

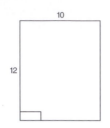

Radiation Protection

AEC (Phototiming)

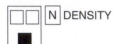 N DENSITY

Patient Position Erect or seated with left side against film.

Part Position Center the midcoronal plane to the midline of the film; adjust the body so the MSP is parallel with the film; depress the shoulders.

- Exposure 1: the patient's head is dropped forward as close to the chest as possible (Figure 7.21).
- Exposure 2: the patient's head is leaned backward as much as possible (Figure 7.22).

Central Ray Top of cassette should be placed about 2 inches (5 cm) above EAM; central ray is directed to center of film at the level of the upper margin of the thyroid cartilage.

Patient Instructions "Take in a deep breath; let it all out. Don't breathe or move."

Evaluation Criteria (Figures 7.23 through 7.26)

- Should include all seven cervical vertebrae.
- There should be no rotation as evidenced by superimposition or close approximation of the two mandibular rami.

Tips

1. Care should be taken that only the head and neck are moved, not the shoulders or whole body.
2. These manipulations should not be done on any patient without first ruling out fracture.

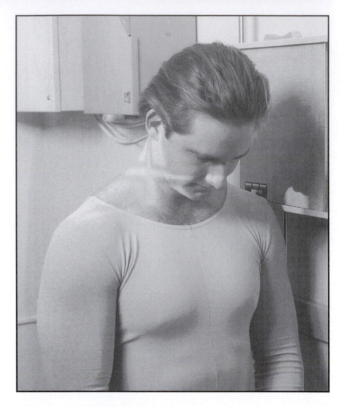

FIGURE 7.21   Flexion lateral cervical spine.

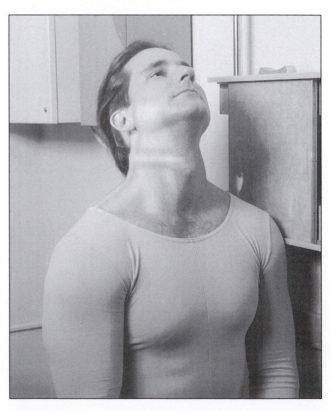

FIGURE 7.22   Extension lateral cervical spine.

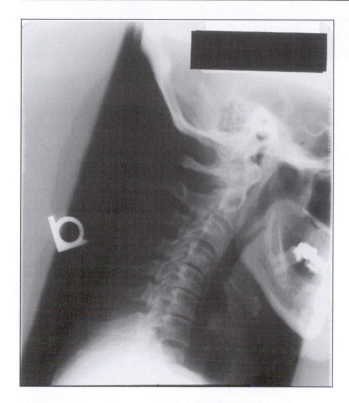

FIGURE 7.23   Flexion lateral cervical spine.

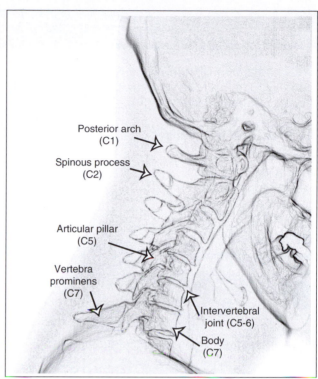

FIGURE 7.25   Flexion lateral cervical spine.

Posterior arch
(C1)

Spinous process
(C2)

Articular pillar
(C5)

Vertebra
prominens
(C7)

Intervertebral
joint (C5-6)

Body
(C7)

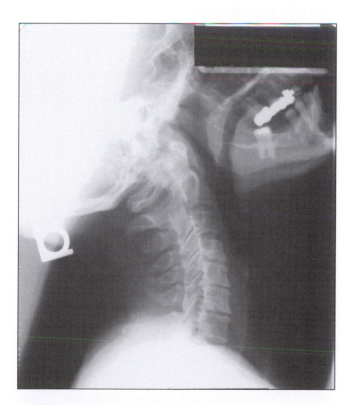

FIGURE 7.24   Extension lateral cervical spine.

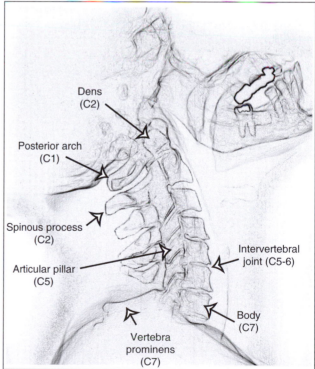

FIGURE 7.26   Extension lateral cervical spine.

Dens
(C2)

Posterior arch
(C1)

Spinous process
(C2)

Articular pillar
(C5)

Intervertebral
joint (C5-6)

Body
(C7)

Vertebra
prominens
(C7)

CERVICAL SPINE—AP "WAGGING JAW" PROJECTION (OTONELLO METHOD)

Exam Rationale This projection demonstrates the entire cervical spine with the shadow of the mandible blurred or obliterated by motion.

Technical Considerations

- Regular screen/film
- Grid
- kVp range: 80–85
- SID: 40 inch (100 cm)

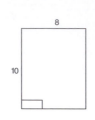

Radiation Protection

AEC (Phototiming)

 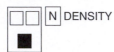 N DENSITY

Patient Position Supine with MSP centered to the midline of the table (Figure 7.27).

Part Position Adjust so there is no rotation of the head or body; extend the neck so that a line from the lower edge of the upper incisors to the mastoid tips is perpendicular to the table.

Central Ray Directed to C4 (lower margin of the thyroid cartilage).

Patient Instructions "Hold your breath and keep your lower jaw moving."

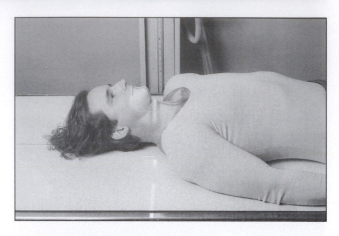

FIGURE 7.27 AP Otonello cervical spine.

Evaluation Criteria (Figures 7.28 and 7.29)

- Should visualize all seven vertebrae, although primary area of interest is C1-C2.
- Mandible should be blurred and first two cervical vertebrae should be visualized through it.
- There should be no motion of head or cervical spine.

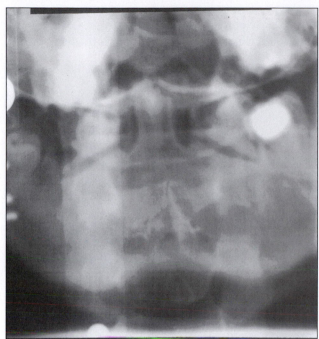

FIGURE 7.28   AP Otonello cervical spine.

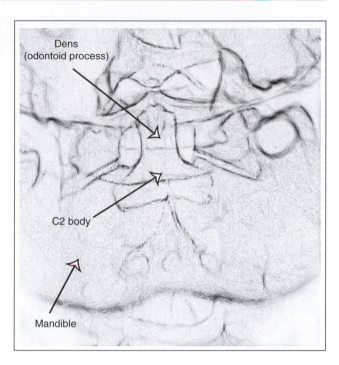

FIGURE 7.29   AP Otonello cervical spine.

CERVICAL SPINE—AP ODONTOID PROCESS PROJECTION (FUCHS METHOD)

Exam Rationale This method demonstrates the odontoid process projected within the foramen magnum.

Technical Considerations

- Regular screen/film
- Grid
- kVp range: 75–80
- SID: 40 inch (100 cm)

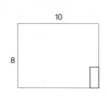

Radiation Protection

AEC (Phototiming)

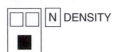 N DENSITY

Patient Position Supine with MSP centered to the midline of the table (Figure 7.30).

Part Position Adjust so there is no rotation of the head or body; extend the neck so that a line from the chin to the mastoid tips is perpendicular to the table.

Central Ray Center the cassette to the mastoid tips; the central ray is directed to the center of the film, entering the neck just distal to the chin.

Patient Instructions "Breathe normally but don't move."

Evaluation Criteria (Figures 7.31 and 7.32)

- Odontoid process should be seen in the foramen magnum.
- There should be no rotation of head or neck.

Tip This position should not be attempted with a patient who has a suspected fracture or degenerative disease.

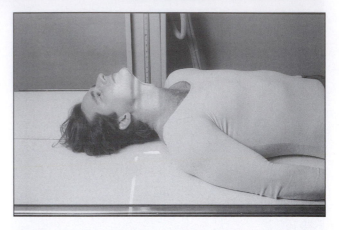

FIGURE 7.30 Odontoid process (Fuchs method).

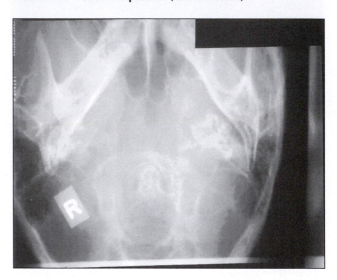

FIGURE 7.31 Odontoid process (Fuchs method).

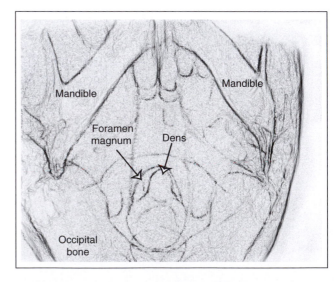

FIGURE 7.32 Odontoid process (Fuchs method).

CERVICAL SPINE—PA ODONTOID PROJECTION (JUDD METHOD)

Exam Rationale This method demonstrates the odontoid process projected within the foramen magnum.

Technical Considerations

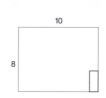

- Regular screen/film
- Grid
- kVp range: 75–80
- SID: 40 inch (100 cm)

Radiation Protection   AEC (Phototiming)

 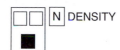 N DENSITY

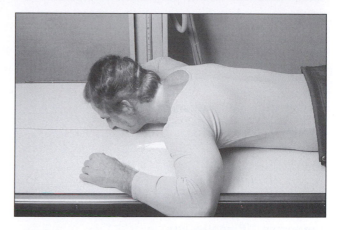

FIGURE 7.33   Odontoid process (Judd method).

Patient Position Prone with MSP centered to the midline of the table (Figure 7.33).

Part Position Adjust so there is no rotation of the head or body; with the chin resting on the table, extend the neck so that a line from the chin to the mastoid tips is perpendicular to the table (the orbitomeatal line will be approximately 37° to the plane of the film).

Central Ray Center the cassette to the mastoid tips; the central is directed to the center of the film, entering just posterior to the mastoid tips.

Patient Instructions "Breathe normally but don't move."

Evaluation Criteria (Figures 7.34 and 7.35)

- Odontoid process should be seen in the foramen magnum.
- There should be no rotation of head or neck.

Tip This position should not be attempted with a patient who has a suspected fracture or degenerative disease.

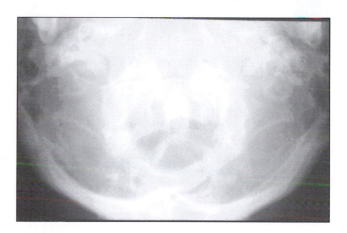

FIGURE 7.34   Odontoid process (Judd method).

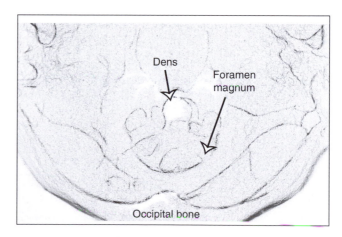

FIGURE 7.35   Odontoid process (Judd method).

CERVICAL SPINE—AP VERTEBRAL ARCH PROJECTION

Exam Rationale   This projection, sometimes also referred to as the pillar projection, demonstrates the posterior elements of the cervical and upper thoracic spine, including the lateral masses, the zygapophyseal joints, the articular pillars and facets, and the spinous processes.

Technical Considerations

- Regular screen/film
- Grid
- kVp range: 75–80
- SID: 40 inch (100 cm)

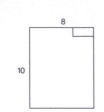

Radiation   AEC
Protection   (Phototiming)

 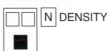 N DENSITY

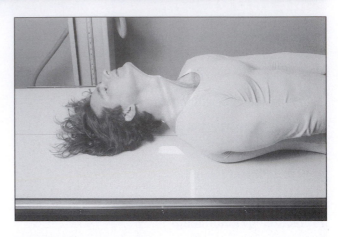

FIGURE 7.36   Vertebral arch.

Patient Position   Supine with MSP centered to the midline of the table (Figure 7.36).

Part Position   Adjust so there is no rotation of the head or body; hyperextend the neck; a long strip of bandage should be looped around the patient's feet with the knees flexed; the patient should grasp both ends of the bandage and extend the knees, depressing the shoulders.

Central Ray   Directed to C5 (thyroid cartilage) at a 25° caudal angle.

Patient Instructions   "Breathe normally but don't move."

Evaluation Criteria (Figures 7.37 and 7.38)

- Vertebral arches should be seen without superimposition from the vertebral bodies or transverse processes.
- The zygapophyseal joints should be open.

Tip   A patient with greater or lesser cervical lordosis may require more or less angulation of the central ray to achieve the goal of making it parallel with the plane of the articular facets.

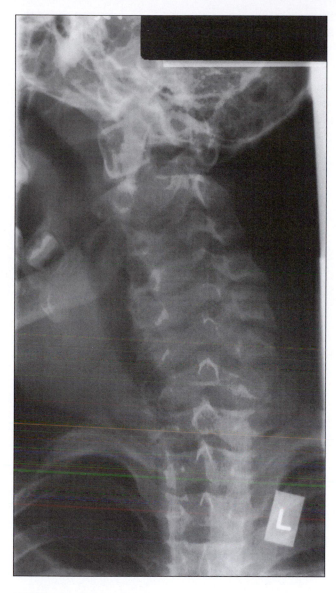

FIGURE 7.37   Vertebral arch.

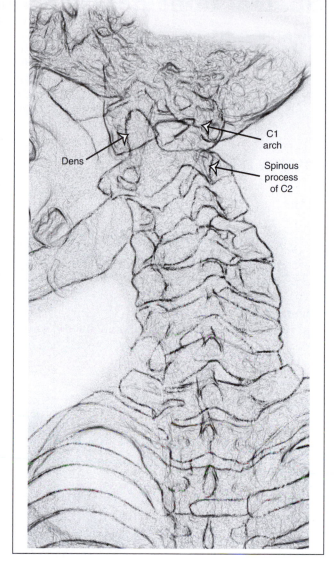

FIGURE 7.38   Vertebral arch.

Dens

C1 arch

Spinous process of C2

Special Considerations

PEDIATRIC CONSIDERATIONS

Although cervical spine films are seldom done on young children, they are occasionally required. With children too young to hold very still, it is easier to do all of them, including the lateral, with the patient in the recumbent position. The lateral, difficult to obtain on adults in the recumbent position, is easier with children due to their greater flexibility. With the patient's torso and extremities in a mummy wrap, it is then necessary to only immobilize the child's head and neck.

COMMON ERRORS

- Failure to angle on the AP cervical projection will cause the mandible to obstruct the view of the upper cervical vertebrae (Figure 7.39).
- Instead of maintaining the position of the head in alignment with the rest of the body, it is turned, giving a rotated image of the upper cervical vertebrae (Figure 7.40).

SELECTED PATHOLOGY

Whiplash Injury

This is a common term used to describe injury of the spine and spinal cord at the junction of the fourth and fifth cervical vertebrae, resulting from rapid acceleration and deceleration of the body (Figure 7.41). The term origi-

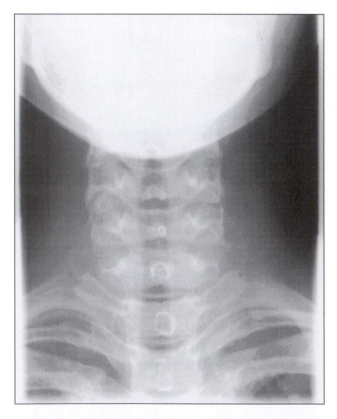

FIGURE 7.39   **Mandible superimposes upper cervical vertebrae on AP projection due to failure to angle central ray.**

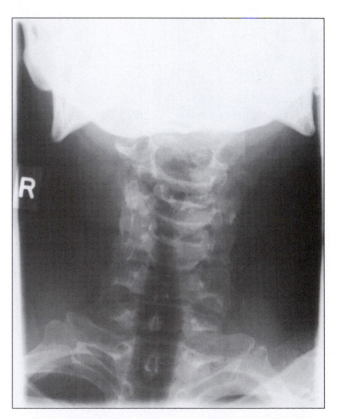

FIGURE 7.40   **Head is not maintained in alignment with rest of body, giving rotated image to upper cervical vertebrae.**

nated from the actions of the cervical vertebrae: the rigidity of the three lower vertebrae act as a handle to the whip, and the flexibility of the upper four vertebrae allow them to act as a lash.

In cases of suspected trauma to the neck, the integral relationship between the spine and the spinal cord necessitate complete immobilization of the cervical spine until possible fractures can be ruled out. Routinely, this preliminary evaluation is done with a lateral view, which is interpreted before moving the patient for any subsequent views (see Chapter 10).

CORRELATIVE IMAGING

Conventional radiography is routinely done in preliminary evaluation of the cervical spine and spinal cord. However, in some cases, additional diagnostic information may be necessary and will most often be obtained with either CT or MRI. In the cervical spine, CT images often provide useful information and can demonstrate fractures of the spine or the location of the resulting bony fragments (Figure 7.42). By comparison, MRI is routinely used to evaluate the cervical spine and provides much better visualization of the spinal cord and its position within the spinal canal (Figure 7.43).

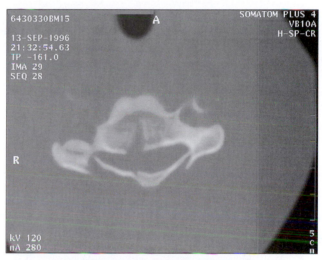

FIGURE 7.42   **CT axial image demonstrating comminuted fracture of cervical body.**

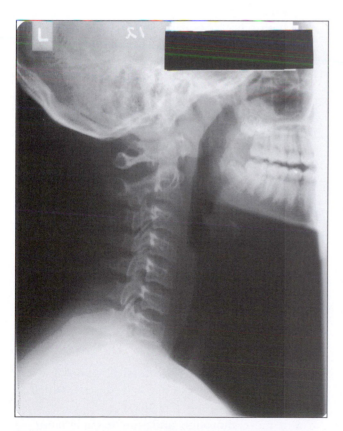

FIGURE 7.41   **Lateral cervical spine showing whiplash injury between C4 and C5.**

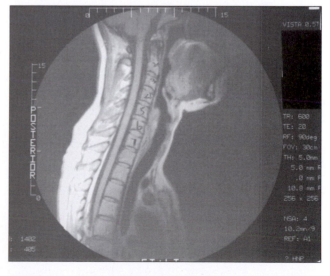

FIGURE 7.43   **MRI sagittal image in medial plane demonstrating a herniated cervical disk (C5-C6).**

Review Questions

1. Which of the following is not a part of the bony vertebral arch?

   a. body
   b. pedicle
   c. lamina
   d. spinous process

2. What part of the typical cervical vertebra extends from the posterolateral margin of the body to the lamina?

   a. pedicle
   b. spinous process
   c. transverse process

3. What is the most distinctive feature of the cervical vertebrae?

   a. lamina
   b. pedicle
   c. transverse foramen
   d. vertebral foramen

4. Which of the following is not found on the atlas?

   a. body
   b. anterior arch
   c. posterior arch
   d. lateral mass

5. Which cervical vertebra acts as the major pivot point for the rotation of the head?

   a. atlas
   b. axis
   c. third cervical vertebra
   d. vertebral prominens

6. Which of the following is true about an AP open mouth projection of the cervical spine?

   a. demonstrates the first two cervical vertebrae
   b. demonstrates all of the cervical vertebrae
   c. central ray should be directed at C4
   d. More than one of the above answers is correct.

7. Which of the following technical factors would not generally be considered for the average patient for a lateral cervical spine?

   a. kVp in the range of 75–80
   b. SID: 40 inch
   c. 8 × 10 (20 × 25 cm) film lengthwise
   d. grid

8. How much is the patient rotated for an oblique cervical spine?

   a. 10°
   b. 20°
   c. 30°
   d. 45°

9. To best visualize the intervertebral foramen, which of the following positions/projections should be done?

   a. oblique (RPO, LPO) with 30 degree cephalic angle
   b. oblique (RAO, LAO) with 30 degree caudal angle
   c. oblique (RAO, LAO) with 15 degree cephalic angle
   d. lateral

10. In an oblique (RPO, LPO) of the cervical spine, which intervertebral foramina and intervening pedicles are best demonstrated?

    a. side up or farthest from the film
    b. side down or closest to the film
    c. both sides are equally well seen
    d. neither side is particularly well seen

11. When evaluating an AP odontoid process projection (Fuch's method), which of the following evaluation criteria would be used?

    a. should be no rotation of head or neck
    b. odontoid process should be seen in foramen magnum
    c. the mandible should be seen below the odontoid process
    d. both a and b
    e. all of the above

12. Which of the following would demonstrate open zygapophyseal joints of the cervical spine?

    a. AP
    b. oblique
    c. lateral
    d. vertebral arch position

13. When radiographing the cervical spine of a very young child (between the ages of 2-4), which of the following should be considered?

    a. a more thorough and simple explanation of the procedure
    b. additional positioning aids

c. may require restraint

d. all of the above

14. In a properly positioned anteroposterior projection of the cervical spine, C1 and C2 will often overlap with other bony structures and will not be clearly demonstrated.

    a. true

    b. false

15. The intervertebral foramina are well visualized on the lateral cervical spine.

    a. true

    b. false

16. The joints between the superior and inferior articular processes of the vertebrae are called the

    _____ .

17. In an oblique (RPO, LPO) cervical spine, the central ray should be directed at _____ and angled _____ .

18. When positioning the patient for an AP projection of the cervical spine, the central ray should be directed at _____ and angled _____ degrees _____ (cephalad/caudad).

19. Hyperflexion and hyperextension laterals of the cervical spine are done to demonstrate what?

20. After positioning the patient for an anteroposterior "wagging jaw" (Otonello) projection, what verbal instructions would you give the patient before making the exposure?

21. What simple error might cause the mandible to overlap C1 through C4 on an AP projection of the cervical spine?

22. If the patient has suffered trauma and is unable to remain erect for an oblique cervical spine, what alternative patient position might be used?

23. In cases of suspected trauma to the cervical spine, why should a lateral cervical spine be taken and interpreted prior to moving the patient for other positions/projections?

24. List the routine positions/projections for a cervical spine examination at your clinical facility.

References and Recommended Reading

Anderson, J. E. (1983). *Grant's atlas of anatomy* (8th ed.). Baltimore: Williams & Wilkins.

Ballinger, P. W. (1995). *Merrill's atlas of radiographic positions and radiologic procedures* (8th ed.). St. Louis: Mosby-Year Book.

Bates, B. (1983). *A guide to physical examination* (3rd ed.). Philadelphia: Lippincott.

Bo, W., Wolfman, N., Krueger, W., & Meschan, I. (1990). *Basic atlas of sectional anatomy with correlated imaging* (2nd ed.). Philadelphia: Saunders.

Bontrager, K. L. (1997). *Textbook of radiographic positioning and related anatomy* (4th ed.). St. Louis: Mosby-Year Book.

Cahil, D. R., and Orland, M. J. (1984). *Atlas of human cross-sectional anatomy.* Philadelphia: Lea & Febiger.

Dorland's illustrated medical dictionary (28th ed.). (1995). Philadelphia: Saunders.

Eisenberg, R. L. (1992). *Clinical imaging: an atlas of differential diagnosis* (2nd ed.). Gaithersburg, MD: Aspen.

Eisenberg, R., & Dennis, C. (1990). *Comprehensive radiographic pathology.* St. Louis: Mosby.

Gardner, E., Gray, D. J., & O'Rahilly, R. (1975). *Anatomy: A regional study of human structure* (4th ed.). Philadelphia: Saunders.

Gray, H. (1985). In C. D. Clements (Ed.), *Anatomy of the human body* (30th ed.). Philadelphia: Lea & Febiger.

Hollinshead, W. H., & Rosse, C. (1985). *Textbook of anatomy* (4th ed.). New York: Harper & Row.

International Anatomical Nomenclature Committee. (1989). *Nomina anatomica* (6th ed.). Baltimore: Waverly Press.

Juhl, J. H. (1981). *Paul and Juhl's essentials of roentgen interpretation* (4th ed.). Philadelphia: Harper & Row.

Laudicina, P. F. (1989). *Applied pathology for radiographers.* Philadelphia: Saunders.

Long, B. W., & Rafert, J. A. (1995). *Orthopaedic radiography.* Philadelphia: Saunders.

Mace, D. M., & Kowalczyk, N. (1995). *Radiographic pathology for technologists* (2nd ed.). St. Louis: Mosby-Year Book.

Meschan, I. (1975). *An atlas of anatomy basic to radiology.* Philadelphia: Lea & Febiger.

Norkin, C., & LeVange, P. (1983). *Joint structure & function: A comprehensive analysis.* Philadelphia: Davis.

Pansky, B. (1996). *Review of gross anatomy* (6th ed.). New York: Macmillan Publishing.

Robins, S. L., & Vinay, K. (1987). *Basic pathology* (4th ed.). Philadelphia: Saunders.

Snell, R. S. (1992). *Clinical anatomy for medical students* (4th ed.). Boston: Little, Brown.

Tortora, G. R., & Anagnostakos, N. P. (1984). *Principles of anatomy and physiology* (4th ed.). New York: Harper & Row.

Williams, P. L., & Warwick, R. (Eds.). (1980). *Gray's anatomy* (36th ed.). Philadelphia: Saunders.

Woodburne, R. T. (1983). *Essentials of human anatomy* (7th ed.). New York: Oxford University Press.

Woodburne, R. T., & Burkel, W. E. (1988). *Essentials of human anatomy* (8th ed.). New York: Oxford University Press.

Thoracic Spine

MICHAEL PATRICK ADAMS, PhD, RT(R)(ARRT)

ANATOMY

Typical thoracic Vertebrae

Topographic Landmarks

ROUTINE POSITIONS/PROJECTIONS

AP

Lateral

ALTERNATE PROJECTIONS

Oblique

Swimmer's Lateral

SPECIAL CONSIDERATIONS

Geriatric Considerations

Common Errors

Correlative Imaging

OBJECTIVES

At the completion of this chapter, the student should be able to:

1. List and describe the bony anatomy of the thoracic spine.

2. Given drawings and radiographs, locate anatomic structures and landmarks.

3. Explain the rationale for each projection.

4. Explain the patient preparation required for each examination.

5. Describe the positioning used to visualize anatomic structures in the thoracic spine.

6. List or identify the central ray location and identify the extent of the field necessary for each projection.

7. Explain the protective measures that should be taken for each examination.

8. Recommend the technical factors for producing an acceptable radiograph for each projection.

9. State the patient instructions for each projection.

10. Given radiographs, evaluate positioning and technical factors.

11. Describe modifications of procedures for atypical or impaired patients to better demonstrate the anatomic area of interest.

Anatomy

The thoracic (thō-răs´ik) spine consists of twelve vertebrae. At the superior end the vertebrae are small and resemble cervical vertebrae. As the vertebrae become larger toward the inferior end they tend to resemble a typical lumbar vertebra. Other than size, each of the thoracic vertebrae have similar bony processes. Unlike the cervical vertebrae they possess no transverse foramina (Figure 8.1).

The thoracic spine normally has a convex curvature. Abnormal accentuation of this curvature is called **kyphosis** (kī-fō´sĭs) and may result in a hunchback deformity. Abnormal lateral curvature of the thoracic spine is called **scoliosis** (skō´´lē-ō´sĭs). Kyphosis may occur in isolation or may occur with scoliosis (**kyphoscoliosis**), increasing the thoracic deformity (Figure 8.2).

The remainder of this section describes the anatomy of the thoracic vertebrae, emphasizing structural differences between them and the cervical and lumbar vertebrae. The student should refer to the chapters on the cervical and lumbar spines for more detailed information on the anatomy of a typical vertebrae.

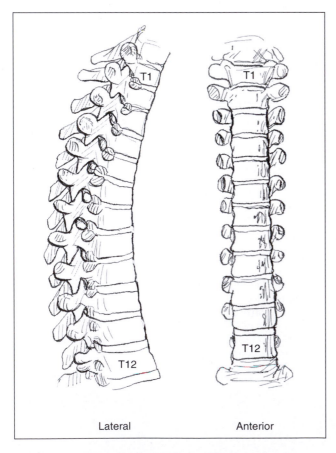

FIGURE 8.1 Lateral and frontal views of the thoracic spine.

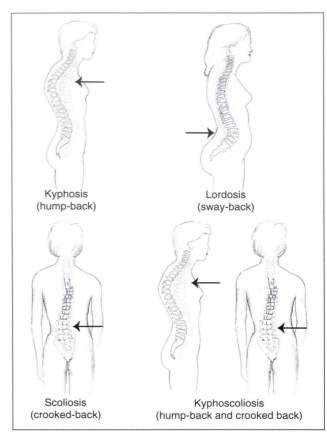

FIGURE 8.2 Curvatures of the thoracic spine.

TYPICAL THORACIC VERTEBRA

Body

The large anterior portion of a thoracic vertebra is called the body, which provides a relatively flat surface for the intervertebral disk. The vertebral arch extends posteriorly from the body to form the vertebral foramen, which serves as a conduit for the spinal cord. The lamina and pedicles of the thoracic vertebra are the same as those described for cervical and lumbar vertebra. On frontal projections of the thoracic spine, the pedicles appear as bilateral, oval-shaped structures. The distance between the pedicles, called the interpedicular distance, is used to check for symmetry and rotation on the radiograph.

Transverse Processes

Like cervical and lumbar vertebra, each thoracic vertebra has a pair of transverse processes that arise from the lateral portion of the vertebral arch near the junction of the lamina and pedicle. Unlike the cervical and lumbar spines, however, the transverse processes of the first ten thoracic vertebrae articulate with ribs (Figure 8.3).

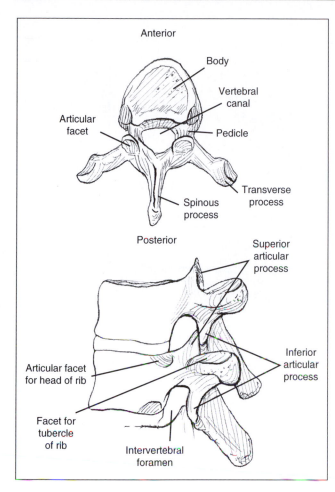

FIGURE 8.3   Superior and lateral views of a typical thoracic vertebra.

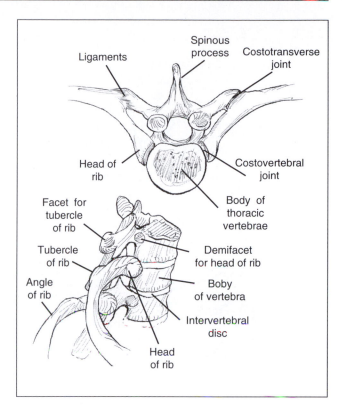

FIGURE 8.4   Rib articulations with the thoracic vertebrae.

Spinous Process

Each thoracic vertebra has a single spinous process, which originates at the junction of the laminae and continues posteriorly. Compared to lumbar vertebrae, thoracic spinous processes are generally longer and point sharply downward. Radiographically, the spinous processes are generally obscured by the ribs, which curve posteriorly and overlie them.

Rib Articulations

The one feature that truly distinguishes thoracic vertebrae from cervical or lumbar vertebrae is the presence of rib articulations (Figure 8.4). The two types of rib articulations are called costovertebral (kŏs´´tō-vĕr´tĕ-brăl) and costotransverse (kŏs´´tō-trăns-vĕrs´) joints. They are both classified as gliding diarthrodial joints.

Costovertebral Joints   A typical thoracic vertebra has two facets (făs´ĕt), commonly called demifacets, on each side of the vertebral body, one on the superior edge and the other on the inferior edge. The costovertebral joint is formed by the head of a rib articulating with the inferior demifacet of one vertebra and the superior demifacet of the vertebra immediately below. The bodies of the last three thoracic vertebrae have only one facet on each side. The first thoracic vertebra has a whole facet for rib one and an inferior demifacet for rib two.

Costotransverse Joints   A costotransverse joint is formed by the articulation of a transverse process with the tubercle of an adjacent rib. Thoracic vertebrae eleven and twelve do not have costotransverse joints.

Zygapophyseal Joints

The zygapophyseal (zī´´gă-pō-fĭz´ē-ăl) joints of the thoracic spine are formed by the superior articulating process of one vertebra and the inferior articulating process of the vertebra immediately below (Figure 8.5). In the thoracic region, the planes of the zygapophyseal joints generally form a 70° to 75° angle to the MSP. Radiographic demonstration of these joints requires a different oblique patient angle than the same joints in the cervical or lumbar spine. The inferior zygapophyseal joint of the twelfth thoracic vertebra is an exception, forming an angle of about 45°.

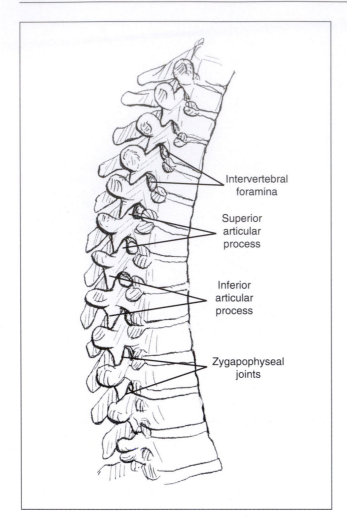

FIGURE 8.5 Zygapophyseal joints of the thoracic spine.

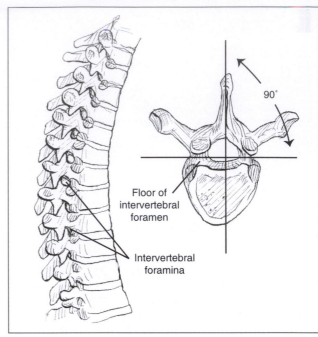

FIGURE 8.6 Intervertebral foramina of the thoracic spine.

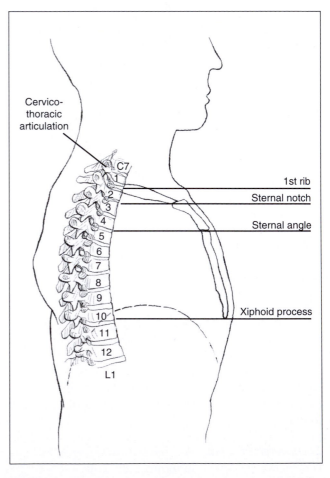

FIGURE 8.7 Topographic landmarks for positioning the thoracic spine.

Intervertebral Foramina

The intervertebral foramina in the thoracic region are formed by the inferior vertebral notch of one vertebra and the superior vertebral notch of the vertebra below (Figure 8.6). The thoracic intervertebral foramina are best visualized when the spine is placed in a lateral position, 90° to the MSP.

TOPOGRAPHIC LANDMARKS

Several bony landmarks on the sternum aid the radiographer in positioning the thoracic spine. The easily palpable manubrial (mă-nū′brē-ăl) or jugular notch lies at the level of T2–T3. The less obvious sternal angle lies about 2 inches (5 cm) below the jugular notch and corresponds to the level of T4–T5. The xiphoid (zĭf′oyd) tip lies at the level of T10 (Figure 8.7).

ROUTINE AND ALTERNATIVE POSITIONS/PROJECTIONS

THORACIC SPINE—AP PROJECTION

Exam Rationale   The most common indications for thoracic spine examinations are trauma and degenerative disease. Structures best demonstrated on the AP include the vertebral bodies, transverse processes, pedicles, and intervertebral disk spaces.

Technical Considerations

- Regular screen/film
- Grid
- kVp range: 75–80
- SID: 40 inch (100 cm)

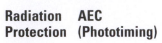

Radiation Protection   **AEC (Phototiming)**

    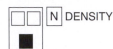 N DENSITY

Patient Position   Supine with the MSP centered to the midline of the table; arms are placed at the patient's sides (Figure 8.8).

Part Position   Scapulae and upper spine are flat on table with no rotation; knees may be flexed to bring the spine in closer contact with the table.

Central Ray   Perpendicular and directed 3 to 4 inches (8–10 cm) below the jugular notch to the sixth thoracic vertebra. The top of the film should be 1 to 2 inches (3–5 cm) above the top of the shoulder.

Patient Instructions   "Take in a breath and let it out. Don't breathe or move."

Evaluation Criteria (Figures 8.9 and 8.10)

- Must include all thoracic vertebrae.
- Transverse processes, pedicles, vertebral bodies, and intervertebral disk spaces should be demonstrated.
- Although visible, the transverse processes are normally superimposed on the heads of the ribs.

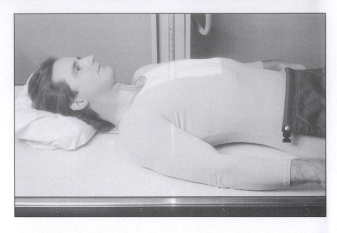

FIGURE 8.8   Thoracic spine, AP projection.

- Rotation, as evidenced by the asymmetrical appearance of the transverse processes or pedicles, should not be observed.
- Spinous processes should be in the midline.

Tips

1. Patients with severe kyphosis may be examined prone, with a PA projection.
2. Some department protocols require collimation to the edge of the transverse processes; others prefer the collimator to be left open to view the entire thorax, on a 14 × 17 inch film.
3. Radiographic densities in the thoracic region vary considerably. The air-filled trachea overlies the upper vertebrae; the fluid-filled heart overlies the mid and lower vertebrae. A wedge filter or the anode-heel effect may be used to help maintain even levels of density from T1–T12.
4. Care should be taken not to elevate the head too much because the chin may overlie vertebral bodies.
5. If a pillow is used, care must be taken not to place it under the thoracic vertebra.

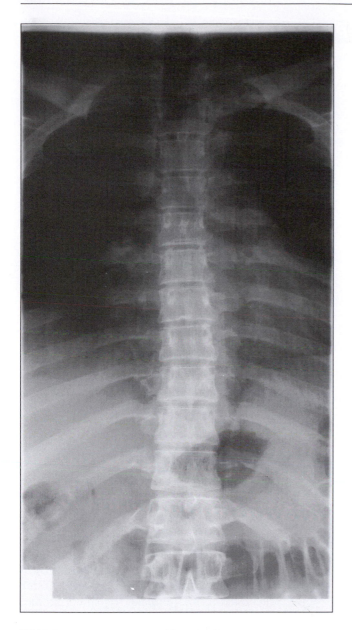

FIGURE 8.9 Thoracic spine, AP projection.

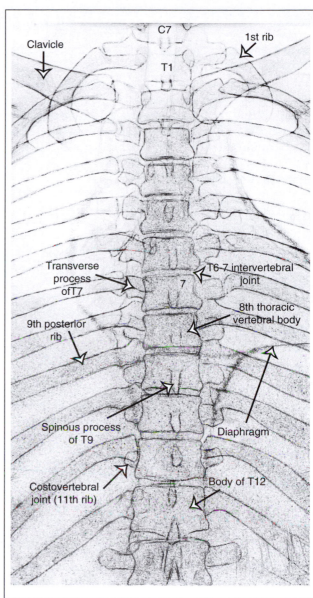

FIGURE 8.10 Thoracic spine, AP projection.

THORACIC SPINE—LATERAL POSITION

Exam Rationale   The lateral is taken at 90° to the AP. Structures best demonstrated include the vertebral bodies, intervertebral disk spaces, and intervertebral foramina. The spinous processes are not well visualized due to their superimposition on ribs. The upper three to four vertebrae are not visualized due to superimposition from shoulder structures.

Technical Considerations

- Regular screen/film
- Grid
- kVp range: 75–80
- SID: 40 inch (100 cm)

Radiation Protection   **AEC (Phototiming)**

  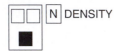 N DENSITY

Patient Position   Recumbent left lateral with knees and hips flexed for comfort; arms are drawn forward at right angles to the body to prevent the scapulae from superimposing on the thoracic spine (Figure 8.11).

Part Position   Place the long axis of the spine parallel to the table; the sagittal plane should be parallel and the coronal plane perpendicular to the table. The midaxillary line should be centered to the table.

Central Ray   Perpendicular and directed 4 inches (10 cm) below the jugular notch to the seventh thoracic vertebra. The top of the film should be 1/2 to 1 inch (1–3 cm) above the top of the shoulder.

Patient Instructions   "Breathe normally but don't move." The patient is allowed to continue normal breathing during the exposure, as this will blur thorax shadows, which frequently obscure bony detail. At

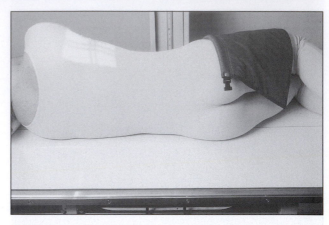

FIGURE 8.11   Thoracic spine, lateral projection.

least 2 seconds of exposure time is needed to accommodate the breathing technique.

Evaluation Criteria (Figures 8.12 and 8.13)

- Must include at least T4–T12.
- The posterior ribs should be mostly superimposed, indicating minimal rotation.
- Intervertebral disk spaces and intervertebral foramina should be clearly demonstrated.

Tips

1. If a visible downward sag is present in the spine after placing the patient into a lateral position, a small radiolucent sponge should be placed under the thoracolumbar area to make the spine parallel to the table.
2. To visualize the upper three to four vertebrae, a swimmer's lateral must be taken.
3. If a pillow is used, care must be taken not to place it under the thoracic vertebra.
4. If the patient is unable to lie on the left side, a right lateral may be substituted.

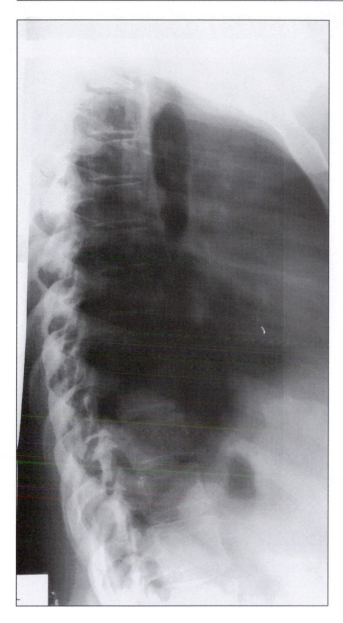

FIGURE 8.12   Thoracic spine, lateral projection.

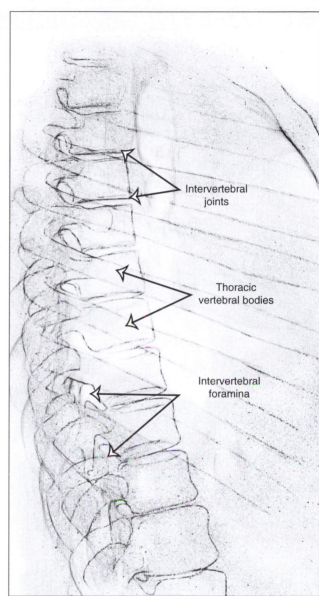

Intervertebral joints

Thoracic vertebral bodies

Intervertebral foramina

FIGURE 8.13   Thoracic spine, lateral projection.

THORACIC SPINE—OBLIQUE AP PROJECTION

Exam Rationale   Oblique projections of the thoracic spine are usually done to demonstrate the zygapophyseal joints. They are occasionally done to demonstrate mediastinal structures or to remove mediastinal shadows from obscuring thoracic spine anatomy. Both right and left obliques are done.

Technical Considerations

- Regular screen/film
- Grid
- kVp range: 75–80
- SID: 40 inch (100 cm)

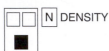

Radiation Protection

AEC (Phototiming)

N DENSITY

Patient Position   Semi-supine, RPO/LPO (Figures 8.14 and 8.15).

Part Position   Place the spine at a 70° to 75° angle to the film (15–20° from the true lateral); center the spine to the midline of the table.

Central Ray   Perpendicular and directed 3 inches (8 cm) below the jugular notch to the sixth thoracic vertebra. The top of the film should be 1 to 2 inches (3–5 cm) above the top of the shoulder.

Patient Instructions   "Take in a breath and let it out. Don't breathe or move."

Evaluation Criteria (Figures 8.16 and 8.17)

- Must include all thoracic vertebrae.
- In the RPO and LPO positions, the zygapophyseal joints on the side farthest from the table should be clearly opened (this is the same as cervical spine obliques, but differs from lumbar spine obliques).
- Superior and inferior articulating processes, pedicles, laminae, pars interarticularis, vertebral bodies, and disk spaces should be demonstrated.

Tips

1. If the patient cannot be placed supine, oblique PA projections may be performed with the patient semiprone (RAO/LAO); in the RAO/LAO posi-

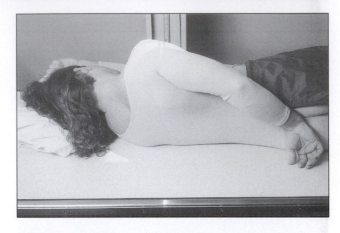

FIGURE 8.14   Thoracic spine, oblique projection: LPO.

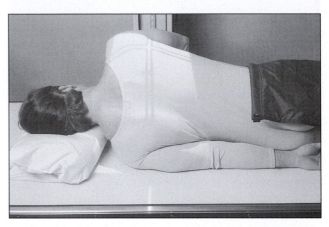

FIGURE 8.15   Thoracic spine, oblique projection: LAO.

tions, the zygapophyseal joint visualized is the one nearest the table.
2. To demonstrate the inferior zygapophyseal joints of T12, a 45° patient rotation is required.
3. Kyphosis or scoliosis of the thoracic spine requires varying patient rotation to demonstrate the zygapophyseal joints.

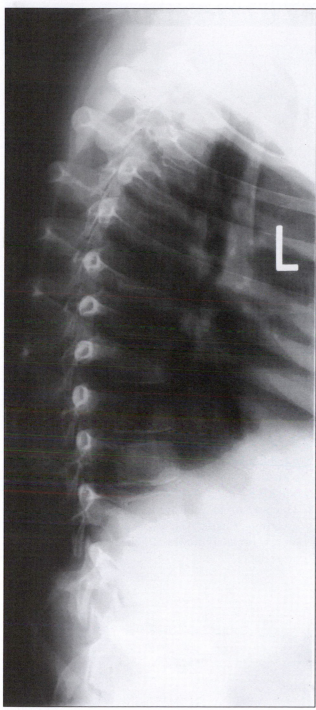

FIGURE 8.16   Thoracic spine, oblique projection.

Zygapophyseal joints

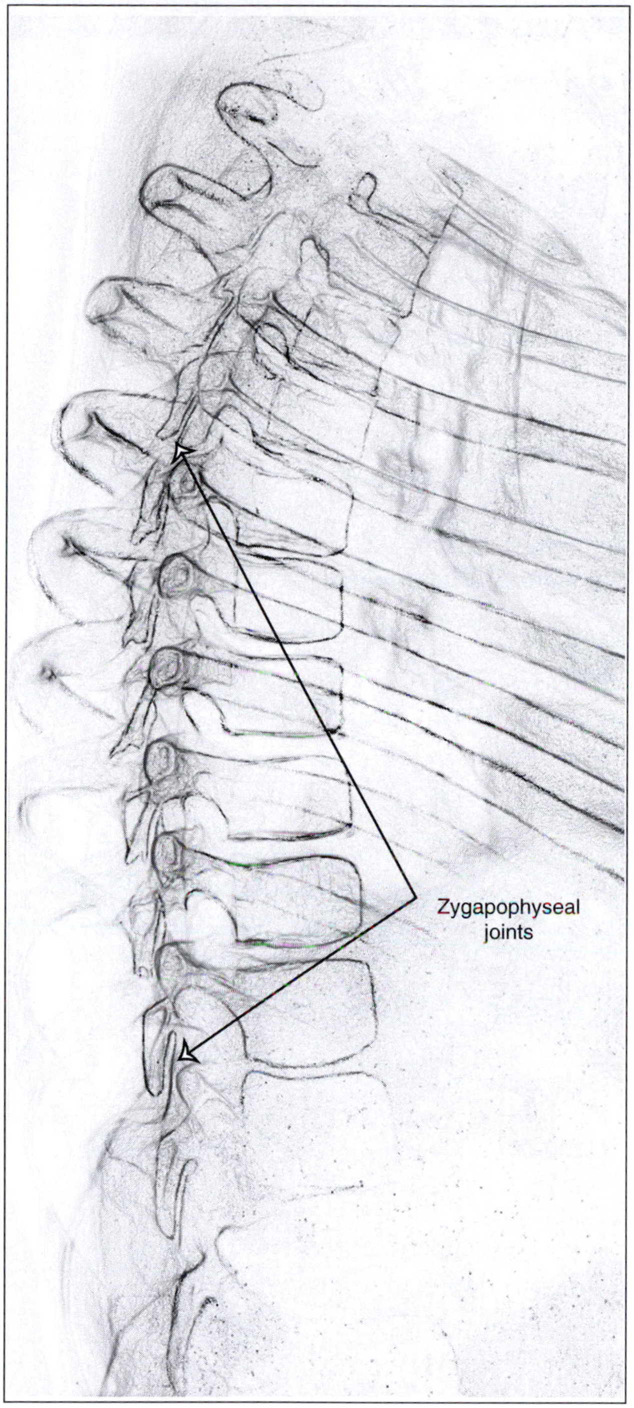

FIGURE 8.17   Thoracic spine, oblique projection.

THORACIC SPINE—SWIMMER'S LATERAL POSITION

Exam Rationale The most common indication for the swimmer's lateral is trauma to the upper thoracic or lower cervical vertebra. The swimmer's lateral will demonstrate the junction between C7 and T1 and the first three to four thoracic vertebrae, which are not visualized on routine lateral thoracic spine radiographs.

Technical Considerations

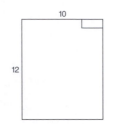

- Regular screen/film
- Grid
- kVp range: 80–90
- SID: 40 inch (100 cm)

Radiation Protection   AEC (Phototiming)

  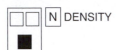 N DENSITY

Patient Position Left lateral recumbent (Figure 8.18).

Part Position True lateral position with the MSP parallel to the table; the arm closest to the table is abducted far above the head while the shoulder farthest from the film should be depressed as much as possible; rotate the depressed shoulder forward slightly and the raised shoulder backward slightly to prevent superimposition of the humeral heads on the vertebral bodies.

Central Ray Directed at a 5° to 10° caudal angle to the level of T1–T2.

Patient Instructions "Take in a breath and let it out. Don't breathe or move."

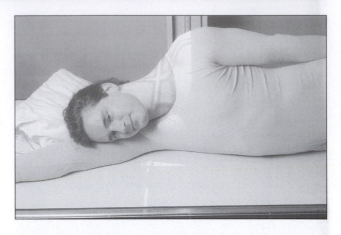

FIGURE 8.18 Swimmer's projection, thoracic spine.

Evaluation Criteria (Figures 8.19 and 8.20)

- The disk space between C7 and T1 and the first three to four thoracic vertebrae must be visualized.
- The humeral heads should not be superimposed on the vertebral bodies.

Tips

1. A pillow or sponge should be placed under the patient's head to prevent it from tilting toward the table.
2. The patient may be allowed to continue normal breathing during the exposure because this will blur thorax shadows, which frequently obscure bony detail.

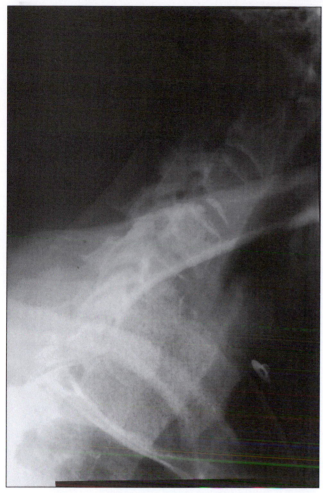

FIGURE 8.19   Swimmer's projection, thoracic spine.

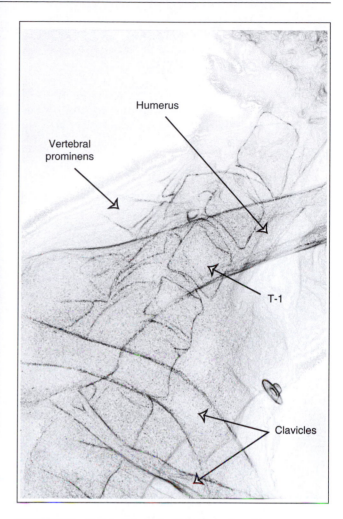

FIGURE 8.20   Swimmer's projection, thoracic spine.

Special Considerations

GERIATRIC CONSIDERATIONS

Several major degenerative diseases affect the spine of geriatric patients. These diseases reduce the patient's flexibility and mobility. To obtain optimum films, the radiographer needs to adapt routines to compensate for this loss of vertebral motion. Several common geriatric diseases are illustrated in Figures 8.21, 8.22, and 8.23.

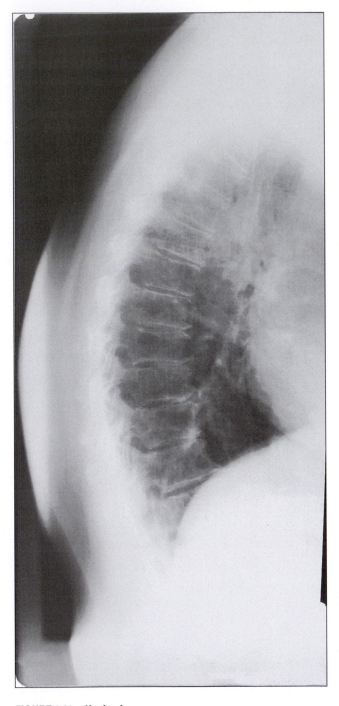

FIGURE 8.21   Kyphosis.

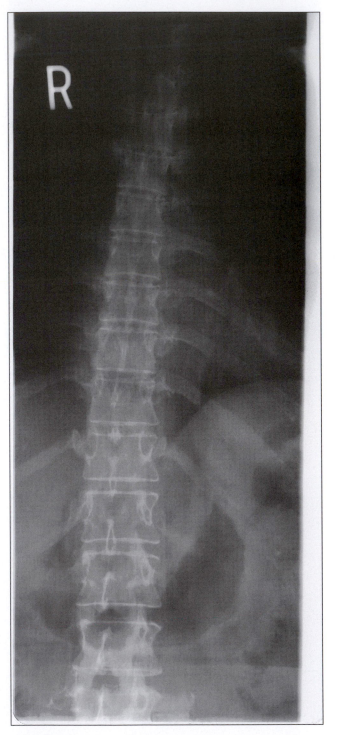

FIGURE 8.22   Osteoporosis of thoracic spine.

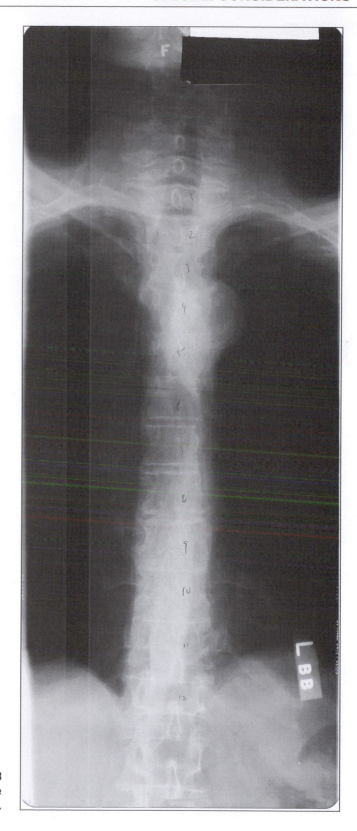

FIGURE 8.23
Pathologic fracture of thoracic spine
due to osteoporosis.

COMMON ERRORS

Rotation on lateral radiographs is one of the most common errors in spine radiography (Figure 8.24). Another commonly repeated thoracic spine position is the swimmer's position, which takes considerable skill and experience on the part of the radiographer to position correctly (Figure 8.25).

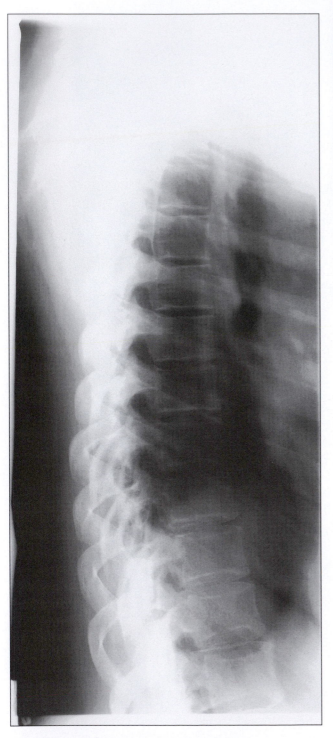

FIGURE 8.24   Rotation on a lateral thoracic spine.

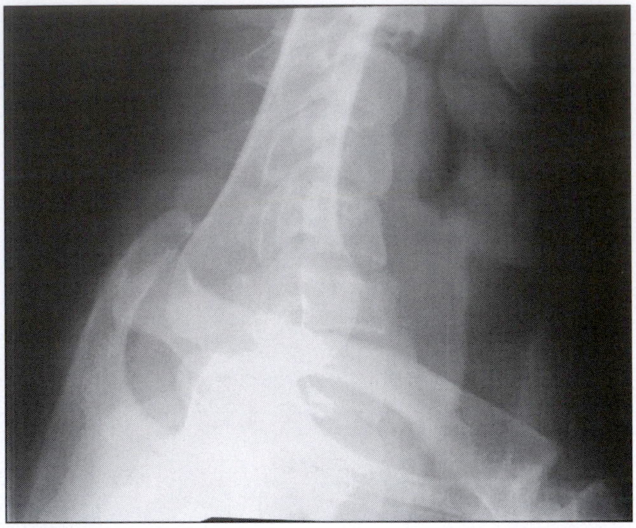

FIGURE 8.25   Humeral head superimposed on spine on swimmer's projection.

CORRELATIVE IMAGING

Bone can be imaged by a number of modalities. MRI of the thoracic spine is able to demonstrate the spinal cord and other soft tissues surrounding the vertebrae (Figure 8.26). Nuclear medicine is able to visualize the physiology of bone and identify areas of increased or decreased bone cell activity (Figure 8.27).

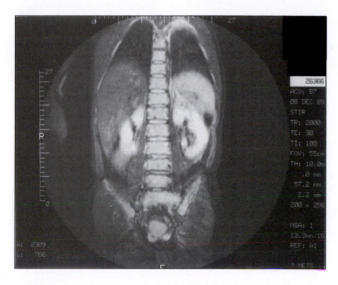

FIGURE 8.26   MRI of the thoracic spine.

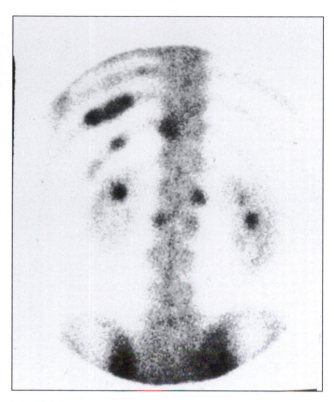

FIGURE 8.26   Nuclear medicine scan illustrating tumor of thoracic spine.

Review Questions

1. Which of the following is an abnormal "hunch-back" curve of the thoracic spine?

   a. kyphosis
   b. lordosis
   c. scoliosis

2. What is the name of the joint formed between the tubercle of the rib and the transverse process of the thoracic spine?

   a. costotransverse
   b. costovertebral
   c. intervertebral
   d. zygapophyseal

3. The structures on a thoracic vertebra that articulate with ribs at costovertebral joints are called:

   a. demifacets
   b. pedicles
   c. transverse processes
   d. vertebral notches

4. The xiphoid tip is at the level of:

   a. T2
   b. T7
   c. T10
   d. T12

5. The large space through which the spinal cord passes is called the:

   a. intervertebral foramen
   b. vertebral arch
   c. vertebral foramen
   d. vertebral notch

6. For the AP projection of the thoracic spine, the central ray passes through:

   a. one inch inferior to the jugular notch
   b. T4
   c. T6
   d. T10

7. For the lateral thoracic spine, the central ray should be directed to:

   a. one inch inferior to the vertebral notch
   b. T4
   c. T7
   d. T10

8. For the swimmer's lateral thoracic spine, the central ray is angled:

   a. 5–10° cephalad
   b. 5–10° caudad
   c. 15–20° cephalad
   d. 15–20° caudad

9. For the oblique (LAO, RAO) thoracic spine, the spine should be at a _____ degree angle with the plane of the film.

   a. 15
   b. 30
   c. 45
   d. 70

10. A breathing technique is sometimes used for a lateral thoracic spine to:

    a. blur lung markings
    b. blur the thoracic spine
    c. magnify the image
    d. all of the above

11. Which position/projection best demonstrates the left intervertebral foramina of the thoracic spine?

    a. AP
    b. RAO
    c. RPO
    d. lateral

12. Thoracic vertebrae do not possess transverse foramen.

    a. true
    b. false

13. For the lateral thoracic spine, the sagittal plane should be perpendicular to the table.

    a. true
    b. false

14. Why might it be necessary to perform a swimmer's lateral of the thoracic spine?

15. List the routine positions/projections required for a thoracic spine examination at your clinical facility.

References and Recommended Reading

Ballinger, P. W. (1991). *Merrill's atlas of radiographic positions and radiologic procedures* (8th ed.). (Vol. 2). St. Louis: Mosby-Year Book.

Bontrager, K. L. (1993). *Textbook of radiographic positioning and related anatomy* (4th ed.). St. Louis: Mosby-Year Book.

Marieb, E. N. (1995). *Human anatomy and physiology* (3rd ed.). Redwood City: Benjamin/Cummings Publishing Company.

McInnes, J. (1973). *Clark's positioning in radiography* (9th ed.). (Vol. 1). Chicago: Year Book Medical Publishers.

Meschan, I. (1975). *An atlas of anatomy basic to radiology.* Philadelphia: Lea and Febiger.

Lumbar Spine, Sacrum, and Coccyx

MICHAEL PATRICK ADAMS, PhD, RT(R)(ARRT)

OBJECTIVES

At the completion of this chapter, the student should be able to:

1. List and describe the anatomy of the lumbar spine, sacrum, and coccyx.

2. Given drawings and radiographs, locate anatomic structures and landmarks.

3. Explain the rationale for each projection.

4. Explain the patient preparation required for each examination.

5. Describe the positioning used to visualize anatomic structures in the lumbar spine, sacrum, and coccyx.

6. List or identify the central ray location and the extent of the field necessary for each projection.

7. Explain the protective measures that should be taken for each examination.

8. Recommend the technical factors for producing an acceptable radiograph for each projection.

9. State the patient instructions for each projection.

10. Given radiographs, evaluate positioning and technical factors.

11. Describe modifications of procedures for atypical or impaired patients to better demonstrate the anatomic area of interest.

Anatomy

The lower spine consists of five lumbar vertebrae, five fused sacral vertebrae, and three to five fused coccygeal vertebrae. The normal curvature of the lower spine changes from concave in the lumbar area to convex in the sacral region (Figure 9.1).

The lumbar spine normally has a concave curvature. Abnormal accentuation of this curvature is called **lordosis** (lor´dō-sĭs) or swayback (Figure 9.2).

TYPICAL LUMBAR VERTEBRA

Each of the five lumbar vertebrae have identical processes. They possess no transverse foramen, as do the cervical vertebrae, or rib facets, as do the thoracic vertebrae.

Body

As with cervical and thoracic vertebrae, the most massive portion is called the body. The large size of the lumbar bodies reflects their weight-bearing function. The vertebral body serves as a relatively flat surface for the intervertebral disk, which cushions the spine during body movements (Figure 9.3).

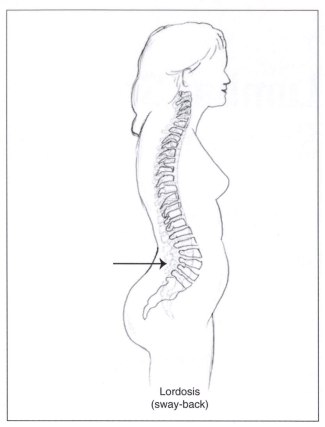

Lordosis
(sway-back)

FIGURE 9.2　Lordosis.

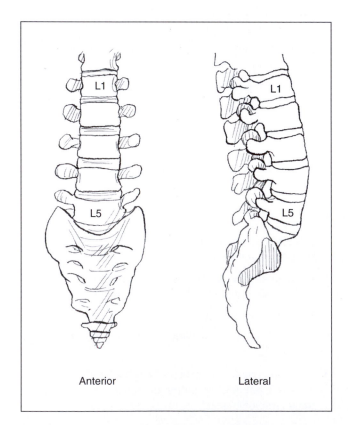

FIGURE 9.1　Anterior and lateral views of the lumbar spine.

Vertebral (Neural) Arch

The vertebral arch extends posteriorly from the body. Together with the posterior portion of the body, the arch forms a somewhat circular opening called the **vertebral foramen** (věr´tē-brăl for-ā´měn). These structures give excellent bony protection for the spinal cord, which travels through the vertebral foramen.

Pedicle　The pedicles (pěd´ĭ-k´l) arise posteriorly from the vertebral body to form the anterior, lateral sides of the vertebral arch. The pedicles have two notches, the inferior and superior vertebral notches. The inferior vertebral notch is much larger than the superior.

Lamina　The laminae (lăm´ĭ-nē) project from the pedicles to form the posterior portion of the vertebral arch. They are longer than the pedicles. Posteriorly, the two laminae fuse to form the spinous process. Failure of the laminae to unite results in a congenital disease known as **spina bifida** (spī´nă bĭ´fĭ-dă).

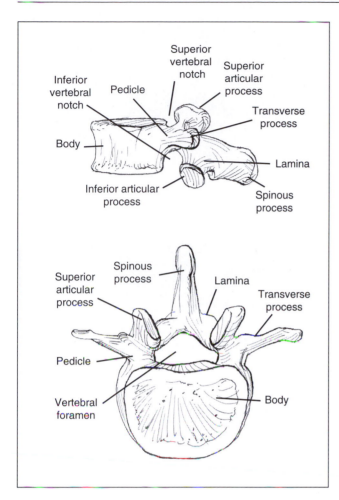

FIGURE 9.3　Lateral and superior views of a typical lumbar vertebra.

foramina serve as important openings through which spinal nerves pass. In the lumbar area, the intervertebral foramina are best visualized when the spine is placed 90° to the MSP or in a lateral position. The intervertebral foramen of L5 is atypical and generally requires the patient to be slightly obliqued for optimum radiographic visualization (Figure 9.4).

LUMBAR SPINE ARTICULATIONS

Superior Articulating Process
Each vertebra articulates with the vertebra above and the vertebra below. The two superior articulating processes project superiorly near the junction of the lamina and pedicle. Their flat articulating surfaces, called facets, face posteriorly where they articulate with the inferior articulating processes of the vertebra above (Figure 9.5).

Inferior Articulating Process
The two inferior articulating processes project inferiorly near the junction of the lamina and pedicle. Their facets face anteriorly, where they articulate with the superior articulating processes of the vertebra below.

Pars Interarticularis
The pars interarticularis (părz ĭn´´tĕr-ăr-tĭk´ū-lăr´ĭs) is a small region of bone lying between the superior and inferior articulating processes.

Spinous Process　Each lumbar vertebra has a single, large spinous process that originates at the junction of the laminae and continues posteriorly. The spinous process lies in the approximate midline of the vertebra, which is useful in evaluating positioning accuracy on frontal projections.

Transverse Process　The two transverse processes project from the lateral portion of the vertebral arch near the junction of the lamina and pedicle. Like the spinous process, the transverse processes serve as important sites for muscle attachment.

Intervertebral Foramina
The inferior vertebral notch of one vertebra and the superior vertebral notch of the vertebra below form an opening called the intervertebral foramen. These

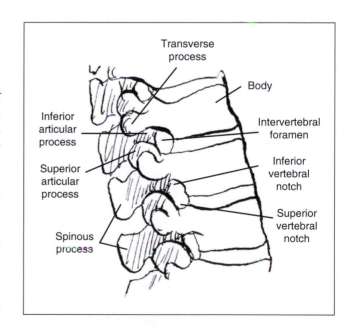

FIGURE 9.4　Intervertebral foramina.

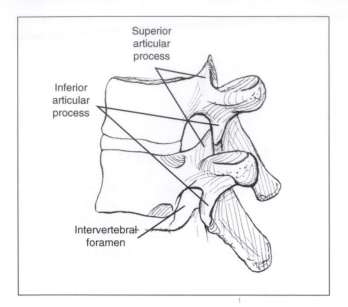

FIGURE 9.5   Detailed structure of articulating processes.

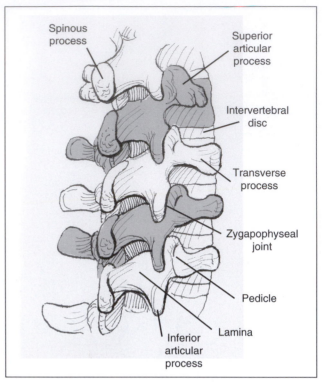

FIGURE 9.6   Zygapophyseal joints.

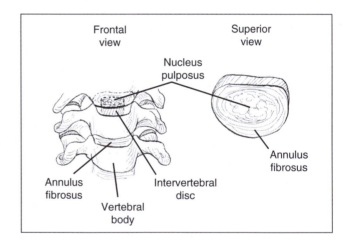

FIGURE 9.7   Intervertebral disks.

Zygapophyseal Joints

The zygapophyseal (zĭ˝gă-pō-fĭz´ē-ăl) joints are diarthrodial joints formed by the superior articulating process of one vertebra and the inferior articulating process of the vertebra below. In the lumbar area the planes of the zygapophyseal joints form a 30° to 50° angle to the midsagittal plane, with the joint between L5 and S1 tending to be more variable than the others. The zygapophyseal joints are essential for proper spine mobility, and their integrity is often examined radiographically (Figure 9.6).

Intervertebral Disks

The intervertebral disks are located between each of the vertebrae and serve as very effective shock absorbers. They consist of an outer tough fibrocartilaginous ring called the annulus fibrosis (ăn´ū-lŭs fī-brō´sĭs) and an inner gel-like portion called the nucleus pulposus (nū´klē-ŭs pŭl-pō´sŭs). The annulus fibrosis connects the two vertebrae and helps form an amphiarthrodial joint. About 25% of the total length of the vertebral column is comprised by the disks. This explains why body height can decrease with age, as the disks begin to degenerate. Unless calcified, the intervertebral disks are radiolucent and only the intervertebral space is visualized (Figure 9.7).

Scotty Dog

When viewed at a 45° oblique angle, the structures of the lumbar spine take on a "Scotty dog" appearance (Figure 9.8). Because its clear presence signifies correct positioning on oblique projections, the radiographer should become familiar with the radiographic appearance of all the parts of the "Scotty dog."

SACRUM

The sacrum is a triangular-shaped bone consisting of five fused segments. The sacrum forms the posterior wall of the pelvis and its somewhat massive structure supports the pelvis and spine (Figure 9.9).

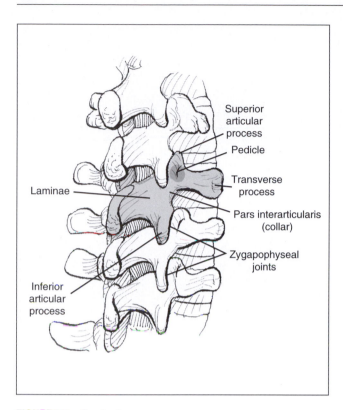

FIGURE 9.8　Scotty dog.

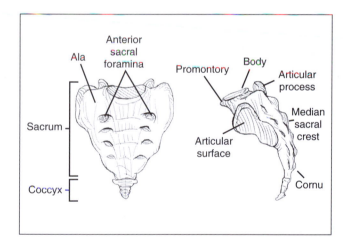

FIGURE 9.9　Anterior and lateral views of the sacrum.

Body

The large center portion is called the body. This single region represents the fused bodies of the five sacral vertebrae.

Alae

The large, lateral portions of the sacrum are called ala (ā´lă) or wings.

Promontory

The flat promontory (prŏm´ŏn-tor´´ē) is located at the superior portion of the sacrum, anteriorly.

Sacral Foramina

The anterior sacrum contains a series of openings called the anterior sacral foramina, which convey blood vessels and nerves. These foramina, when viewed from the back, are called the posterior sacral foramina.

Sacral Crest

Posteriorly, the sacrum has a prominent bony ridge called the median sacral crest. This crest, which consists of the fused sacral spinous processes, can be easily palpated on many patients.

Sacral Canal

The sacral canal is a continuation of the vertebral canal that contains nerves.

Articulations

The two superior articulating processes of the sacrum articulate with the inferior articulating processes of L5 to form the final zygapophyseal joint. Laterally, the sacrum has two articulating surfaces that join with the ilium to form the sacroiliac joints. The sacroiliac joints slant obliquely at a highly variable angle, usually between 15° and 30°. Inferiorly, the sacrum articulates with the coccyx.

Coccyx

The tiny coccyx (kŏk´sĭks) is a triangular-shaped bone that consists of approximately four fused vertebrae (Figure 9.10). Like the sacrum, the portion of the triangle pointing inferiorly is called the apex. It has two

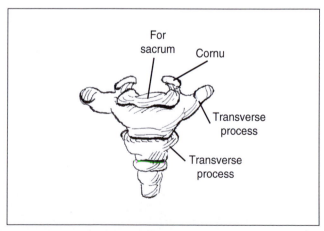

FIGURE 9.10　Anterior view of the coccyx.

small transverse processes that project laterally from the superior base of the coccyx.

TOPOGRAPHIC LANDMARKS

Several bony landmarks are available to assist the radiographer in positioning the lower spine (Figure 9.11). The most superior of the landmarks is the lower costal margin, which lies at the level of L2–L3. The iliac crest, probably the most widely used of the landmarks, lies at the level of L4–L5. The ASIS is normally easily palpable and lies at the midsacrum. Less easily palpated but nevertheless important in positioning is the symphysis pubis, lying at the level of the coccyx.

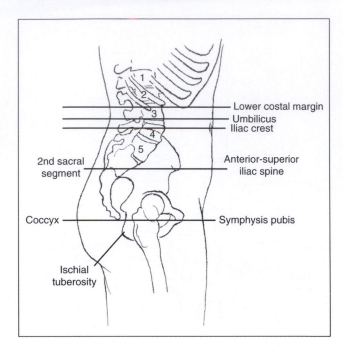

FIGURE 9.11   Topographic landmarks.

ROUTINE AND ALTERNATIVE POSITIONS/PROJECTIONS

LUMBAR SPINE—AP PROJECTION

Exam Rationale   The most common indications for lumbar spine examinations are trauma and degenerative disease. Structures best demonstrated on the AP include the vertebral bodies, transverse processes, pedicles, and intervertebral disk spaces.

Technical Considerations

- Regular screen/film
- Grid
- kVp range: 75–80
- SID: 40 inch (100 cm)

Radiation Protection

AEC (Phototiming)

  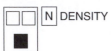

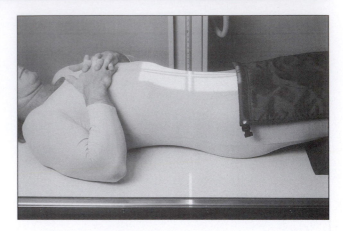

FIGURE 9.12   Lumbar spine; AP projection.

Patient Position   Supine with the MSP centered to the midline of the table; arms are placed at the patient's sides or high on the chest (Figure 9.12).

Part Position   Flex the knees to place the small of the back in contact with the surface of the table and to help reduce rotation.

Central Ray   Perpendicular and centered at the level of the iliac crest.

Patient Instructions   "Take in a breath and let it out. Don't breathe or move."

Evaluation Criteria (Figures 9.13 and 9.14)

- Must include all lumbar vertebrae and part of the sacrum.
- Rotation, as evidenced by the asymmetrical appearance of the sacroiliac joints, pedicles, or transverse processes, should not be observed.

- Transverse processes, pedicles, vertebral bodies, and intervertebral disk spaces should be demonstrated.
- Spinous processes should be in the midline.

Tips

1. If the patient cannot be placed supine, the PA projection may be performed with the patient prone. The PA will result in more magnification but may more clearly demonstrate the intervertebral disk spaces.
2. Some department protocols require collimation to the edge of the transverse processes, whereas others prefer the collimator to be left open to view the entire abdomen.

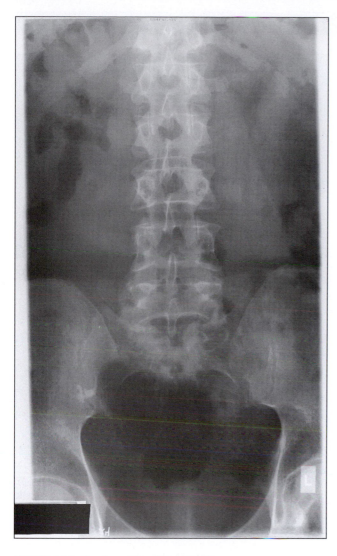

FIGURE 9.13 Lumbar spine; AP projection.

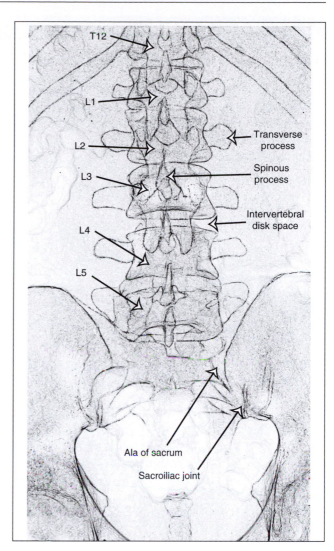

FIGURE 9.14 Lumbar spine; AP projection.

LUMBAR SPINE—OBLIQUE POSITION

Exam Rationale   The oblique is a routine position of the lumbar spine that gives a different perspective from the AP, that of a 45° oblique. Both right and left obliques are performed because each demonstrates structures in a slightly different perspective.

Technical Considerations

- Regular screen/film
- Grid
- kVp range: 75–80
- SID: 40 inch (100 cm)

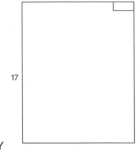

Radiation Protection   AEC (Phototiming)

 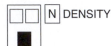 N DENSITY

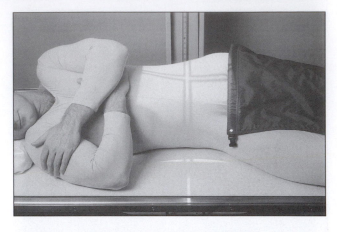

FIGURE 9.15   Lumbar spine; AP oblique projection.

Patient Position   Semi-supine. Arms are placed at the patient's sides or high on the chest (Figures 9.15 and 9.16).

Part Position   Place the spine at a 45° angle to the film; the sagittal plane 1 to 2 inches (3–5 cm) medial to the elevated anterior superior iliac spine is centered to the table.

Central Ray   Perpendicular and centered at the level of the iliac crest.

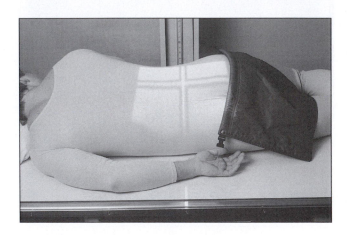

FIGURE 9.16   Lumbar spine; PA oblique projection.

Patient Instructions   "Take in a breath and let it out. Don't breathe or move."

Evaluation Criteria (Figures 9.17 and 9.18)

- Must include all lumbar vertebrae and part of the sacrum.
- In the RPO and LPO positions, the zygapophyseal joints on the side nearer the table should be clearly opened.
- "Scotty dog" sign should be evident for all five lumbar vertebrae.
- Superior and inferior articulating processes, pedicles, laminae, pars interarticularis, vertebral bodies, and disk spaces should be demonstrated.

Tips

1. A radiolucent 45° angle sponge may be placed behind the spine to assist the patient in maintaining this position.
2. If the patient cannot be placed supine, oblique PA projections may be performed with the patient semiprone (RAO/LAO). The spine is centered to the midline of the table by placing the central ray 1 inch (3 cm) to the left (for the RAO position) or right (for the LAO position) of the spinous processes (Figure 9.16). The open zygapophyseal joint is the one farthest from the table (this differs from cervical and thoracic spine obliques).
3. Optimum visualization of the zygapophyseal joint between L5 and S1 may require a 30° patient angle.

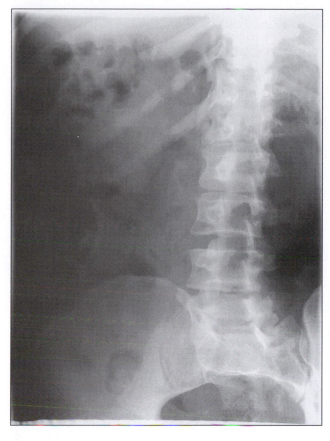

FIGURE 9.17 Lumbar spine; oblique AP projection.

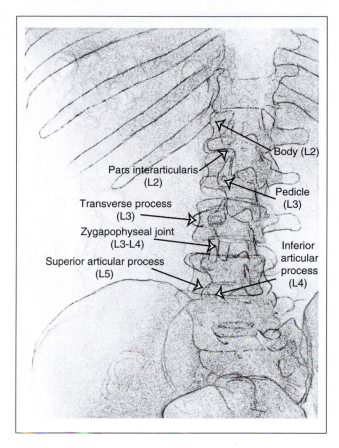

Body (L2)

Pars interarticularis
(L2)

Pedicle
(L3)

Transverse process
(L3)

Zygapophyseal joint
(L3-L4)

Superior articular process
(L5)

Inferior
articular
process
(L4)

FIGURE 9.18 Lumbar spine; oblique AP projection.

LUMBAR SPINE—LATERAL POSITION

Exam Rationale   The lateral is taken at 90° to the AP. Structures best demonstrated include the vertebral bodies, intervertebral disk spaces, spinous processes, and intervertebral foramina.

Technical Considerations

- Regular screen/film
- Grid
- kVp range: 75–80
- SID: 40 inch (100 cm)

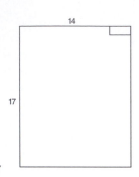

Radiation Protection

AEC (Phototiming)

 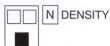 N DENSITY

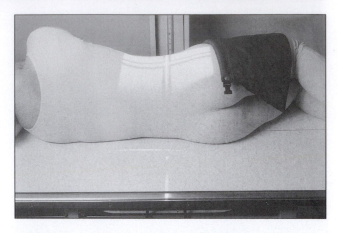

FIGURE 9.19   Lumbar spine; lateral projection.

Patient Position   Recumbent left lateral with knees and hips flexed for comfort; arms are placed at right angles to the body with elbows flexed (Figure 9.19).

Part Position   Place the long axis of the spine parallel to the table; the sagittal plane should be parallel and the coronal plane perpendicular to the table; the plane approximately 3 inches (8 cm) anterior to the spinous processes should be centered to the table.

Central Ray   Perpendicular and centered at the level of the iliac crest.

Patient Instructions   "Take in a breath and let it out. Don't breathe or move."

Evaluation Criteria (Figures 9.20 and 9.21)

- Must include all lumbar vertebrae and part of the sacrum.
- Vertebral bodies, intervertebral disk spaces, spinous processes, and intervertebral foramina should be clearly demonstrated.
- The iliac crests and acetabula should be mostly superimposed, indicating minimal rotation.

Tips

1. If a visible downward sag in the spine is present after placing the patient into a lateral position, a radiolucent sponge should be placed under the thoracolumbar area to make the spine parallel to the table.
2. To better open the intervertebral disk spaces, a 5° caudal angle may be used.
3. If the patient is unable to lie on the left side, a right lateral may be substituted.

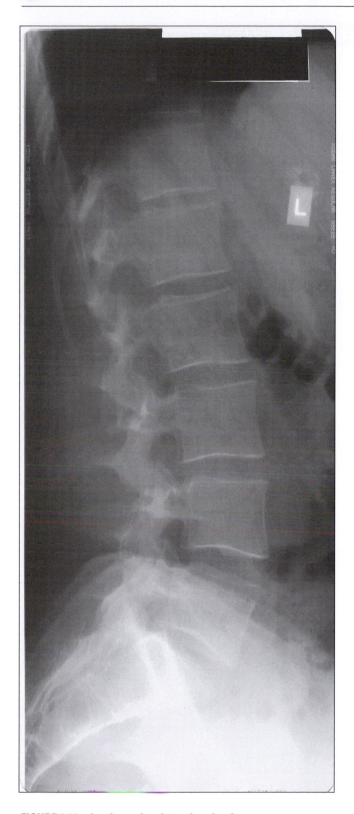

FIGURE 9.20   Lumbar spine; lateral projection.

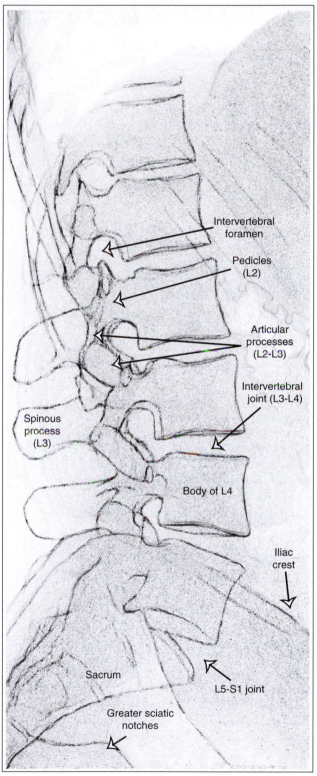

Intervertebral
foramen

Pedicles
(L2)

Articular
processes
(L2–L3)

Intervertebral
joint (L3–L4)

Spinous
process
(L3)

Body of L4

Iliac
crest

Sacrum

L5–S1 joint

Greater sciatic
notches

FIGURE 9.21   Lumbar spine; lateral projection.

LUMBAR SPINE—LATERAL POSITION OF L5–S1 JUNCTION

Exam Rationale The fifth lumbar vertebra and the intervertebral disk between L5 and the sacrum is a common site of pathology. The region is often not well visualized on the lateral lumbar spine because it is much denser than the rest of the lumbar spine and lies at the end of the film, causing the disk space to be closed by the diverging x-ray beam.

Technical Considerations

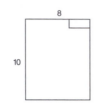

- Regular screen/film
- Grid
- kVp range: 90–100
- SID: 40 inch (100 cm)

Radiation   AEC
Protection   (Phototiming)

 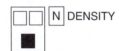 N DENSITY

Patient Position Recumbent left lateral with knees and hips flexed for comfort; arms are placed at right angles to the body with elbows flexed (Figure 9.22).

Part Position Place the long axis of the spine parallel to the table; the sagittal plane should be parallel and the coronal plane perpendicular to the table; a plane 1 1/2 inches (4 cm) posterior to the midaxillary line should be centered to the table.

Central Ray Directed at a 5° to 10° caudal angle to enter at the L5–S1 joint space; this space is located halfway between the anterior superior iliac spine and the iliac crest and 2 inches (5 cm) anterior to the palpated spinous processes.

Patient Instructions "Take in a breath and hold it. Don't breathe or move."

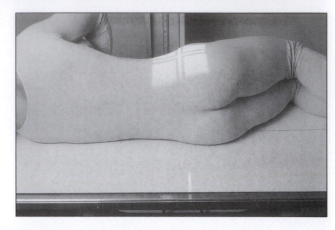

FIGURE 9.22   Lumbar spine; lateral L5–S1 junction.

Evaluation Criteria (Figures 9.23 and 9.24)

- L5–S1 joint space should be open.
- The acetabula should be mostly superimposed, indicating minimal rotation.

Tips

1. Angulation is not always necessary if the spine is placed parallel to the table.
2. Females may require an increased caudal angle to better open the joint space.
3. To obtain a more uniform density, a lead strip may be placed on the table top behind the patient to limit scatter radiation.

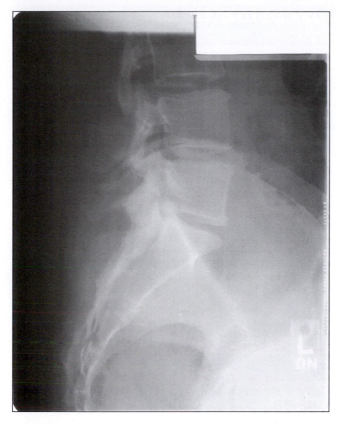

FIGURE 9.23   Lumbar spine; lateral L5–S1 junction.

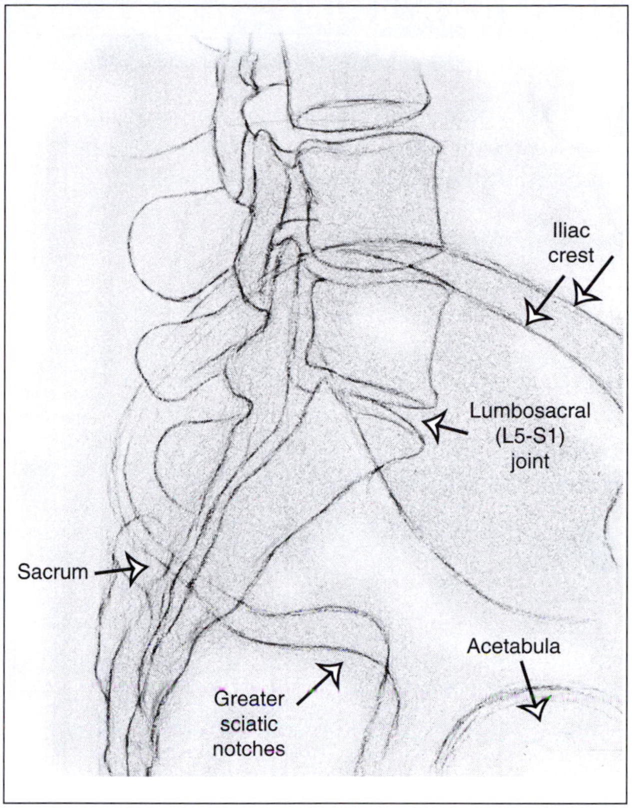

FIGURE 9.24   Lumbar spine; lateral L5–S1 junction.

Iliac
crest

Lumbosacral
(L5-S1)
joint

Sacrum

Greater
sciatic
notches

Acetabula

LUMBAR SPINE—AXIAL AP PROJECTION OF L5–S1 JUNCTION

Exam Rationale Because the sacrum curves posteriorly, this projection is often necessary to open the intervertebral disk space between L5 and S1.

Technical Considerations

- Regular screen/film
- Grid
- kVp range: 80–85
- SID: 40 inch (100 cm)

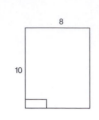

Radiation Protection

AEC (Phototiming)

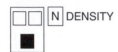

N DENSITY

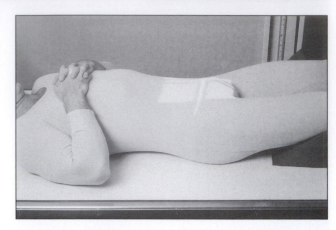

FIGURE 9.25 Lumbar spine; axial AP projection of L5–S1 junction.

Patient Position Supine with the MSP centered to the midline of the table; arms are placed at the patient's sides or high on the chest (Figure 9.25).

Part Position Flex the knees to place the small of the back in contact with the surface of the table and to help reduce rotation.

Central Ray Directed at a 30° to 35° cephalad angle to enter at the level of the L5–S1 joint space.

Patient Instructions "Take in a breath and hold it. Don't breathe or move."

Evaluation Criteria (Figures 9.26 and 9.27)

- L5–S1 joint space should be open.
- Rotation, as evidenced by the asymmetrical appearance of the sacroiliac joints, pedicles, or transverse processes, should not be observed.

Tips

1. Females may require an increased cephalad angle to better open the joint space.
2. If the patient cannot be placed supine, a frontal view may be obtained with the patient prone using a 30° to 35° caudal angle. This results in a more magnified view of the L5–S1 disk space.

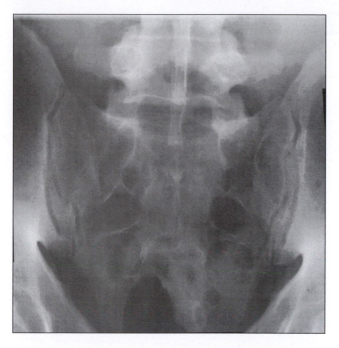

FIGURE 9.26   Lumbar spine; axial AP projection of L5–S1 junction.

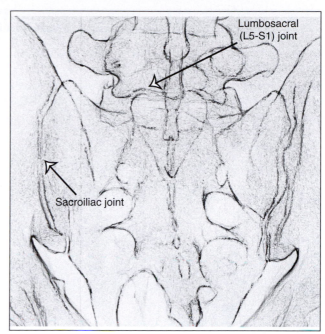

FIGURE 9.27   Lumbar spine; axial AP projection of L5–S1 junction.

LUMBAR SPINE—BENDING EXAMINATIONS

Exam Rationale   Bending films are taken to demonstrate the degree of mobility of the vertebrae. Indications for this examination may include scoliosis or postspinal fusion. Both right and left bending films are taken for comparison.

Technical Considerations

- Regular screen/film
- Grid
- kVp range: 80–90
- SID: 40 inch (100 cm)

Radiation Protection   **AEC (Phototiming)**

 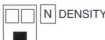 N DENSITY

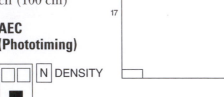

Patient Position   Supine with arms at the patient's sides (Figure 9.28).

Part Position   Begin with the MSP centered to the film; have the patient bend to the right as much as possible while keeping the pelvis straight to avoid rotation; a second film is taken with the patient bending to the left to the maximum extent possible.

Central Ray   Perpendicular and centered at the level 1 to 2 inches (3–5 cm) above the iliac crest.

Patient Instructions   "Take in a breath and let it out. Don't breathe or move."

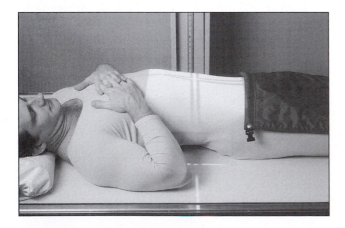

FIGURE 9.28   Lumbar spine; bending exam.

Evaluation Criteria (Figures 9.29 and 9.30)

- All vertebrae affected by the scoliosis or spinal fusion must be visualized.
- Rotation, as evidenced by the asymmetrical appearance of the ilia and sacroiliac joints, should not be observed.

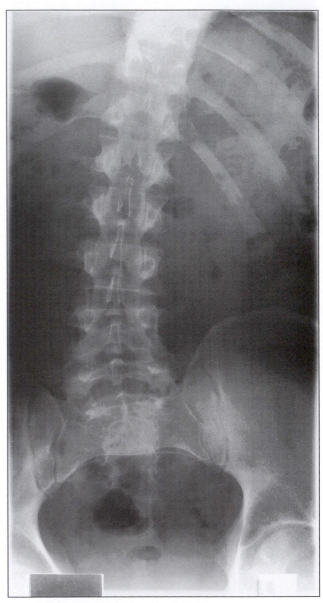

FIGURE 9.29A   Lumbar spine; bending exam; bending to left.

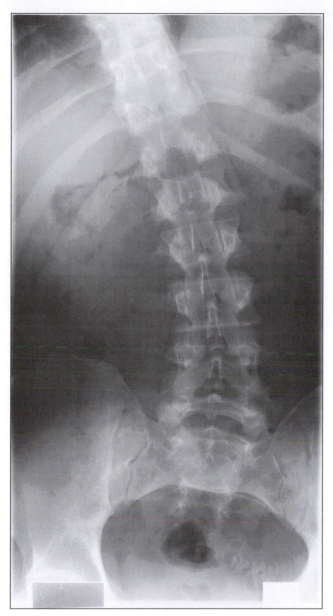

FIGURE 9.29B   Lumbar spine; bending exam; bending to right.

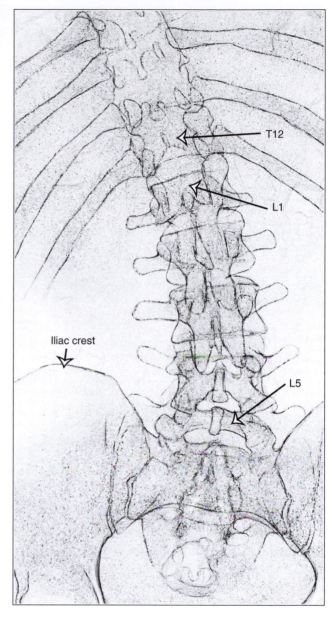

FIGURE 9.30   Lumbar spine; bending exam.

Tips

1. The PA projection gives the patient less radiation than the AP and is therefore called for by some department protocols.
2. Weight-bearing bending films are taken with the patient standing with the weight equally distributed on both legs.

LUMBAR SPINE—HYPEREXTENSION AND HYPERFLEXION EXAMINATIONS

Exam Rationale   Hyperextension and hyperflexion films are taken to demonstrate the degree of mobility of the vertebrae after spinal fusion.

Technical Considerations

- Regular screen/film
- Grid
- kVp range: 80–90
- SID: 40 inch (100 cm)

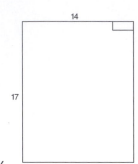

14

17

Radiation Protection   AEC (Phototiming)

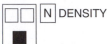 N DENSITY

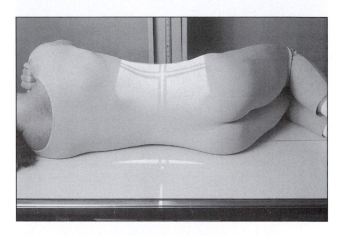

FIGURE 9.31   Lumbar spine; hyperflexion.

Patient Position   Recumbent left lateral; arms placed at right angles to the body with elbows flexed.

Part Position   Place the long axis of the spine parallel to the table; the sagittal plane should be parallel and the coronal plane perpendicular to the table; the plane 3 inches (8 cm) anterior to the spinous processes is centered to the table; have the patient hyperflex the spine by bending forward as much as possible (Figure 9.31); a second film is taken in hyperextension, with the patient bending backward to the maximum extent possible (Figure 9.32).

Central Ray   Perpendicular and centered at the level 1 to 2 inches (3–5 cm) above the iliac crest.

Patient Instructions   "Take in a breath and let it out. Don't breathe or move."

FIGURE 9.32   Lumbar spine; hyperextension.

Evaluation Criteria (Figures 9.33 through 9.36)

- All vertebrae affected by the spinal fusion must be visualized.
- The iliac crests and acetabula should be mostly superimposed, indicating minimal rotation.
- Vertebral bodies, intervertebral disk spaces, spinous processes, and intervertebral foramina should be clearly visible.

Tips

1. If the patient is unable to lie on the left side, a right lateral may be substituted without any degradation in image quality.
2. To better open the intervertebral disk spaces, a 5° caudal angle may be used.
3. Some department protocols prefer that the films be taken with the patient standing.

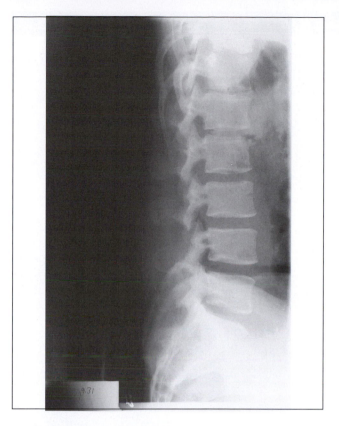

FIGURE 9.33   Lumbar spine; hyperflexion.

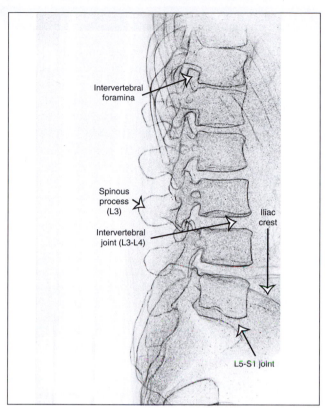

FIGURE 9.35   Lumbar spine; hyperflexion.

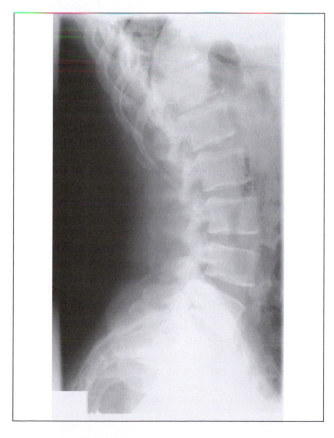

FIGURE 9.34   Lumbar spine; hyperextension.

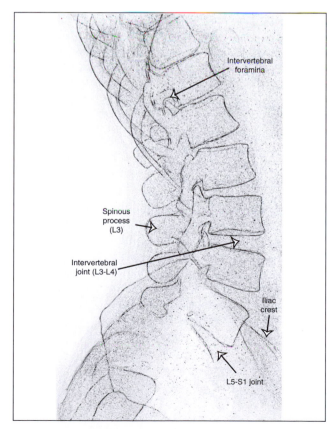

FIGURE 9.36   Lumbar spine; hyperextension.

LUMBAR SPINE—SCOLIOSIS SERIES

Exam Rationale   Scoliosis, a lateral curvature of the spine, is common. Scoliosis films are taken to periodically monitor the progress of the disease or its treatment. Often a single AP or PA projection is taken to include both the lumbar and thoracic spines because the abnormal curvature usually affects both regions. A lateral film may also be requested.

Technical Considerations

- Regular screen/film
- Grid
- kVp range: 80–90
- SID: 40 inch (100 cm)

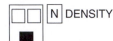

Radiation Protection   **AEC (Phototiming)**

 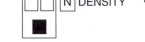

Patient Position   Standing facing the cassette with arms at the patient's sides; shoes should be removed (Figure 9.37).

Part Position   The MSP is centered to the midline of the film.

Central Ray   Perpendicular and centered at a level approximately 4 to 5 inches (10–13 cm) above the iliac crest; the bottom of the film should be placed 2 inches (5 cm) below the level of the iliac crest.

Patient Instructions   "Take in a breath and let it out. Don't breathe or move."

Evaluation Criteria (Figures 9.38 and 9.39)

- All vertebrae affected by the abnormal curvature must be visualized; this normally includes the entire thoracic and lumbar spine.
- Excessive rotation, as evidenced by the asymmetrical appearance of the sacroiliac joints, pedicles, or transverse processes, should not be observed; some degree of rotation will likely be present due to the abnormal curvature of the spine.

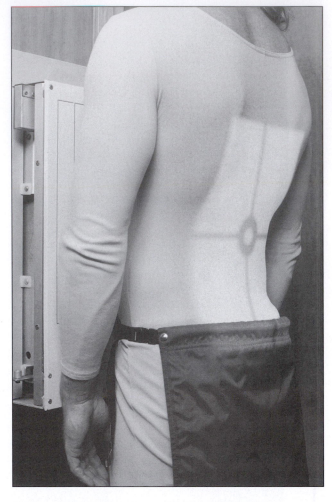

FIGURE 9.37   Lumbar spine; scoliosis series.

Tips

1. A lateral film may also be requested.
2. Because most patients receive this series over an extended period of time, radiation protection is especially critical. Departments that perform many scoliosis series usually have special shields to cover both the breast and gonadal areas.
3. The PA projection is preferred by most departments because the patient receives less radiation than with an AP.

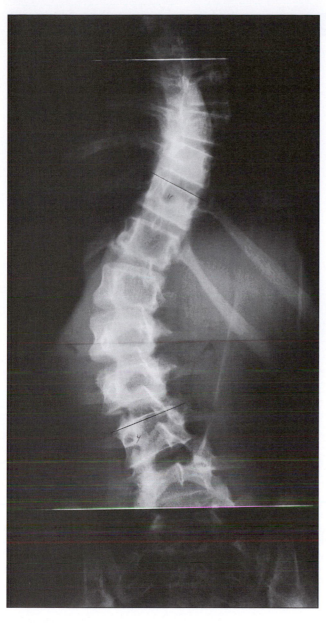

FIGURE 9.38　Lumbar spine; scoliosis series.

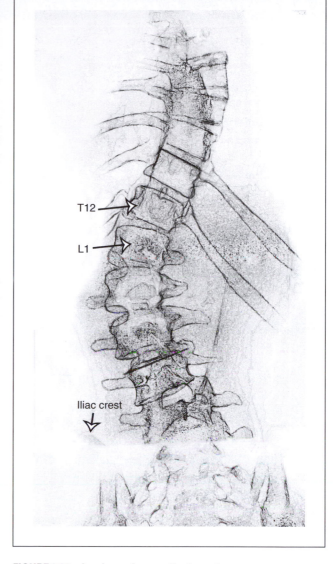

T12

L1

Iliac crest

FIGURE 9.39　Lumbar spine; scoliosis series.

SACRUM—AP PROJECTION

Exam Rationale The most common indication for sacrum examinations is trauma. Structures best demonstrated include the ala, promontory, anterior sacral foramina, and the L5–S1 joint space.

Technical Considerations

- Regular screen/film
- Grid
- kVp range: 80–90
- SID: 40 inch (100 cm)

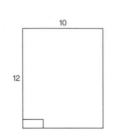

Radiation Protection

AEC (Phototiming)

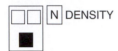

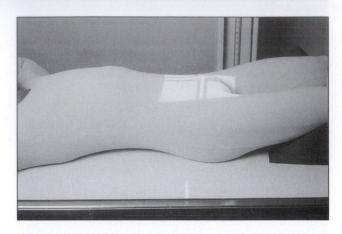

FIGURE 9.40 Sacrum; AP projection.

Patient Position Supine with arms placed at the patient's sides or high on the chest (Figure 9.40).

Part Position The MSP is centered to the midline of the table; the knees may be flexed to place the small of the back in contact with the surface of the table and to help reduce rotation.

Central Ray Directed at a 15° cephalad angle, entering at a level midway between the symphysis pubis and the anterior superior iliac spine.

Patient Instructions "Take in a breath and hold it. Don't breathe or move."

Evaluation Criteria (Figures 9.41 and 9.42)

- Entire sacrum must be included.
- Sacrum should appear more elongated than on an AP lumbar spine projection.
- Rotation, as evidenced by the asymmetrical appearance of the sacroiliac joints and ilia, should not be observed.

Tips

1. Injury to the sacrum may prevent a patient from lying supine. An alternative PA projection can be obtained with the patient lying prone and using a 15° caudal angle, although more radiographic magnification will be evident.
2. Because fecal shadows often overlie the sacrum, the bowel may require cleansing before the radiographic examination to obtain a film of optimum radiographic quality.

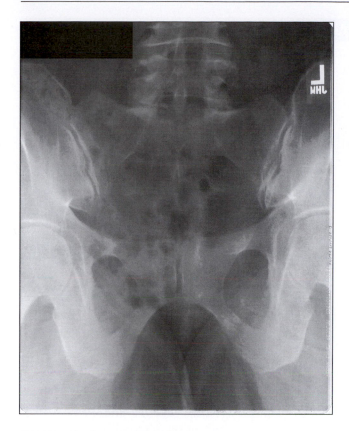

FIGURE 9.41   Sacrum; AP projection.

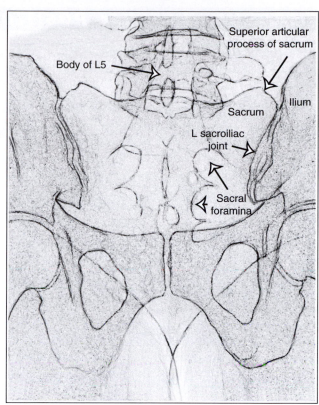

FIGURE 9.42   Sacrum; AP projection.

SACRUM—LATERAL POSITION

Exam Rationale   The lateral sacrum is taken at 90° to the AP. Structures best demonstrated include the body and median sacral crest.

Technical Considerations

- Regular screen/film
- Grid
- kVp range: 80–90
- SID: 40 inch (100 cm)

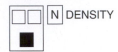

Radiation   AEC
Protection   (Phototiming)

    □ □ □ N DENSITY
                         □ ■ □

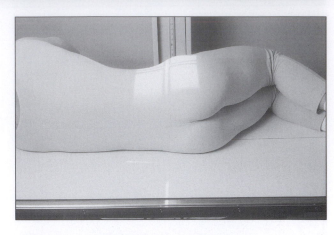

FIGURE 9.43   Sacrum; lateral projection.

Patient Position   Recumbent left lateral with knees and hips flexed for comfort; arms are placed at right angles to the body with elbows flexed (Figure 9.43).

Part Position   Place the long axis of the spine parallel to the table; the sagittal plane should be parallel and the coronal plane perpendicular to the table; a plane approximately 3 inches (8 cm) posterior to the midaxillary line should be centered to the table.

Central Ray   Perpendicular to the midsacrum, 2 inches (5 cm) anterior to the palpated sacral crest and 1 inch (3 cm) below the ASIS.

Patient Instructions   "Take in a breath and hold it. Don't breathe or move."

Evaluation Criteria (Figures 9.44 and 9.45)

- The entire sacrum must be included.
- All or part of the L5–S1 joint space must be included.
- The iliac crests and acetabula should be mostly superimposed, indicating minimal rotation.

Tips

1. To obtain a more uniform density, lead blockers may be placed on the table top behind the patient to limit scatter radiation.
2. Close collimation is essential to limit scatter radiation.

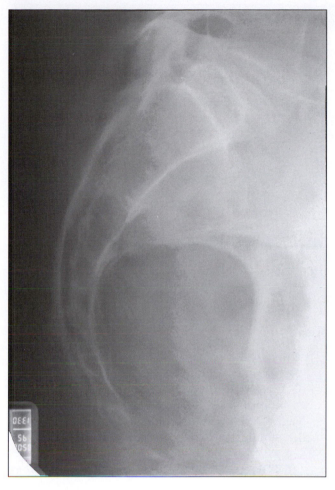

FIGURE 9.44   Sacrum; lateral projection.

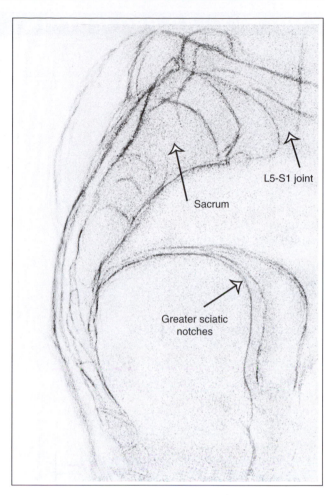

FIGURE 9.45   Sacrum; lateral projection.

COCCYX—AP PROJECTION

Exam Rationale The most common indication for radiographic examination of the coccyx is trauma. The AP is one of two routine positions.

Technical Considerations

- Regular screen/film
- Grid
- kVp range: 75–80
- SID: 40 inch (100 cm)

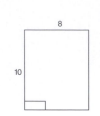

Radiation Protection   AEC (Phototiming)

 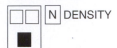 N DENSITY

Patient Position Supine with the MSP centered to the midline of the table; arms are placed at the patient's sides or high on the chest (Figure 9.46).

Part Position The MSP is centered to the midline of the table.

Central Ray Directed at a 10° caudal angle, entering at a level midway between the symphysis pubis and the anterior superior iliac spine.

Patient Instruction "Take in a breath and hold it. Don't breathe or move."

Evaluation Criteria (Figures 9.47 and 9.48)

- Entire coccyx must be included.
- Coccyx should appear more elongated than on an AP lumbar spine examination.
- Rotation, as evidenced by the asymmetrical appearance of the ischial or pubic rami and the obturator foramina, should not be observed.

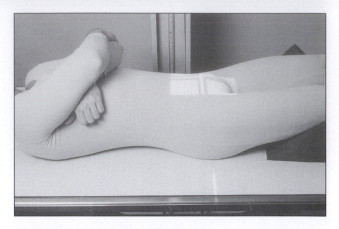

FIGURE 9.46   Coccyx; AP projection.

Tips

1. Injury to the coccyx may prevent a patient from lying supine. An alternative PA projection can be obtained with the patient lying prone and using a 10° cephalad angle, although more radiographic magnification will be evident.
2. Because the rectal and bladder shadows overlie the coccyx, it is often desirable to have the patient void and defecate before the radiographic examination.

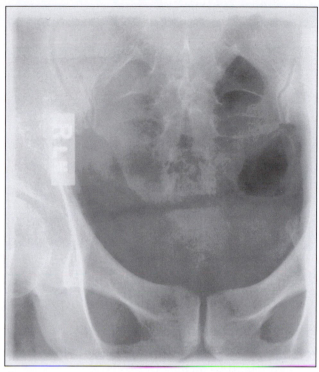

FIGURE 9.47   Coccyx; AP projection.

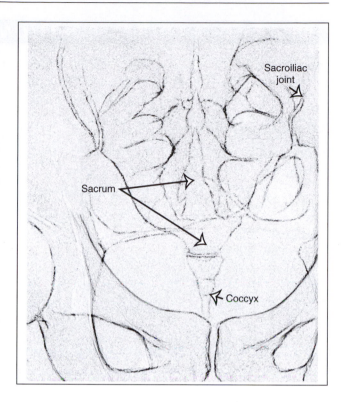

FIGURE 9.48   Coccyx; AP projection.

COCCYX—LATERAL POSITION

Exam Rationale　The lateral coccyx is taken at 90° to the AP. The most common indication for radiographic examination of the coccyx is trauma.

Technical Considerations

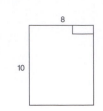

- Regular screen/film
- Grid
- kVp range: 75–80
- SID: 40 inch (100 cm)

Radiation Protection　**AEC (Phototiming)**

　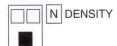 N DENSITY

Patient Position　Recumbent left lateral with knees and hips are flexed for comfort; arms are placed at right angles to the body with elbows flexed (Figure 9.49).

Part Position　Place the long axis of the spine parallel to the table; the sagittal plane should be parallel and the coronal plane perpendicular to the table; a plane approximately 5 inches (13 cm) posterior to the midaxillary line should be centered to the table.

Central Ray　Perpendicular, 1 inch (3 cm) anterior to the palpated posterior coccyx.

Patient Instructions　"Take in a breath and hold it. Don't breathe or move."

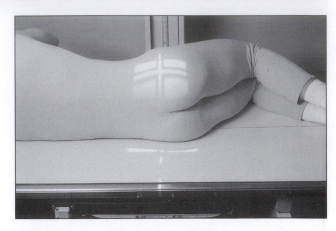

FIGURE 9.49　Coccyx; lateral projection.

Evaluation Criteria (Figures 9.50 and 9.51)

- The entire coccyx and a portion of the distal sacrum must be included.
- The acetabula should be mostly superimposed, indicating minimal rotation.

Tips

1. To obtain a more uniform density, lead blockers may be placed on the table top behind the patient to limit scatter radiation.
2. Close collimation is essential to limit scatter radiation.

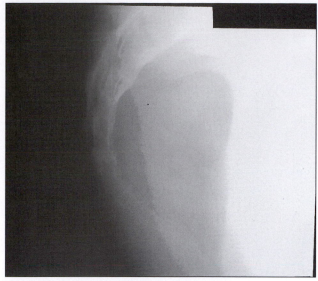

FIGURE 9.50   Coccyx; lateral projection.

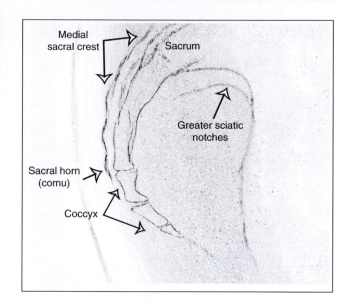

FIGURE 9.51   Coccyx; lateral projection.

Special Considerations

TRAUMA CONSIDERATIONS

Spinal trauma is common and the radiographer must give special attention to such patients. Patients with acute spinal trauma should be moved as little as possible. In general the AP and cross-table lateral are taken and reviewed by a physician before continuing with obliques or special projections (see Chapter 10).

PEDIATRIC CONSIDERATIONS

Motion is always a consideration in pediatric radiography and exposure times must be kept as low as diagnostically possible. Congenital diseases of the spine are often first diagnosed in pediatric patients. Failure of the laminae to unite, called spina bifida, may be severe and diagnosed very early in life (Figure 9.52).

GERIATRIC CONSIDERATIONS

Several major degenerative diseases affect the spine of geriatric patients. These diseases will give the patient less flexibility and mobility. The radiographer will need to adapt to this loss of vertebral motion. Several common geriatric diseases are illustrated in Figures 9.53 and 9.54.

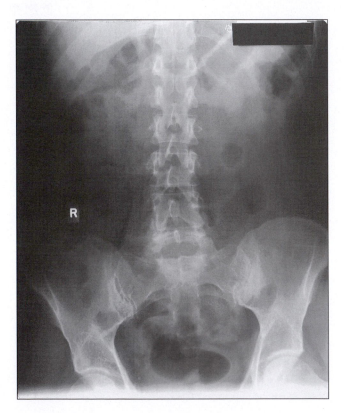

FIGURE 9.52
Spina bifida.

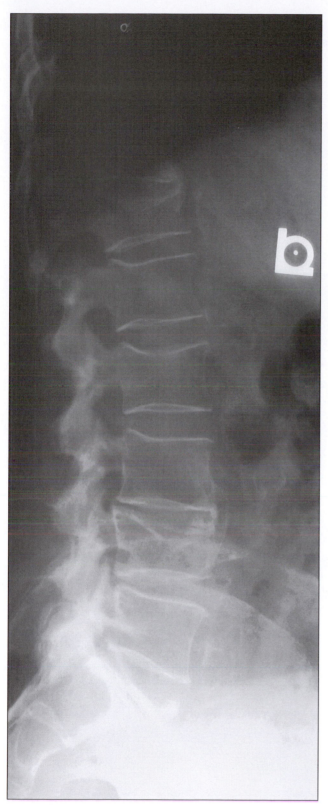

FIGURE 9.53 Osteoporosis of spine (note the pathologic fracture due to osteoporosis).

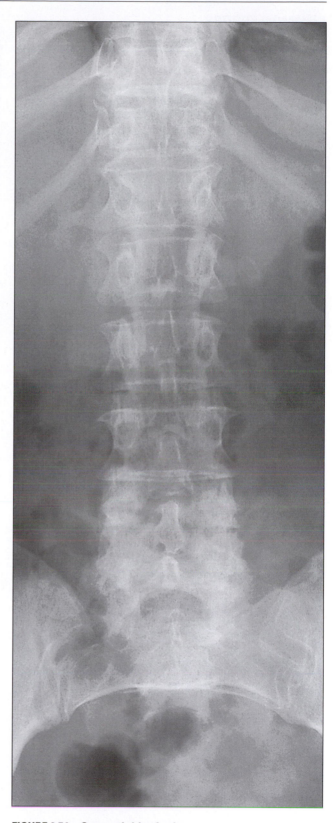

FIGURE 9.54 Osteoarthritis of spine.

COMMON ERRORS

Some common errors in lumbar spine positioning are described in the captions to Figures 9.55 through 9.58.

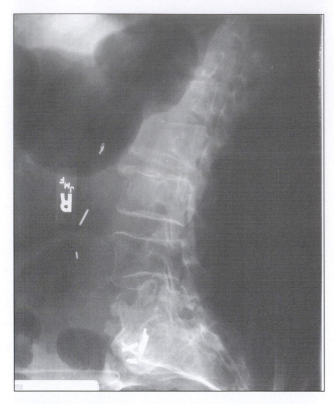

FIGURE 9.55   Too much angle on oblique lumbar spine.

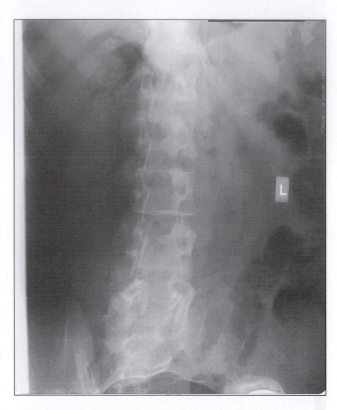

FIGURE 9.56   Not enough angle on oblique lumbar spine.

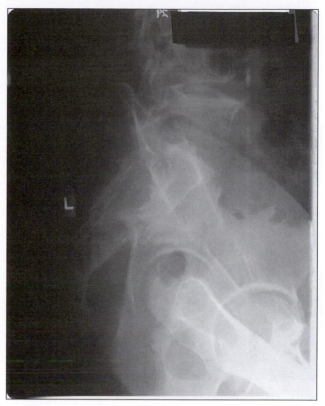

FIGURE 9.58   **Rotation on lateral sacrum or L5–S1.**

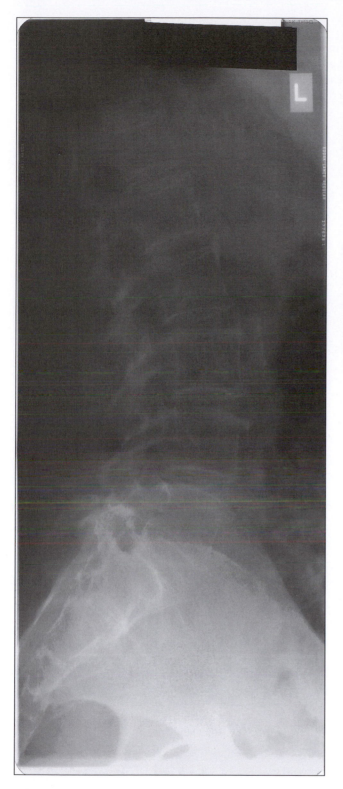

FIGURE 9.57   **Rotation on lateral lumbar spine.**

CORRELATIVE IMAGING

Bone can be imaged by a number of modalities. MRI of the lumbar spine demonstrates the spinal cord and other soft tissues surrounding the vertebrae (Figure 9.59). Myelography, or examination of the spinal cord, requires the use of contrast media (Figure 9.60). Nuclear medicine is able to visualize the physiology of bone and identify areas of increased or decreased bone cell activity (Figure 9.61).

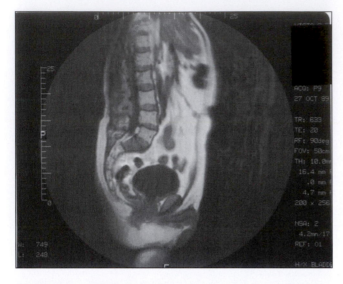

FIGURE 9.59   MRI of the lumbar spine.

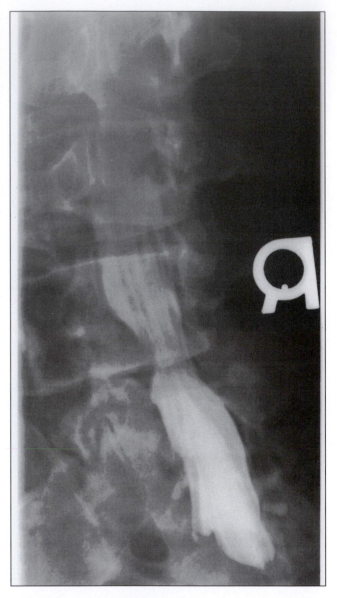

FIGURE 9.60   Lumbar myelogram.

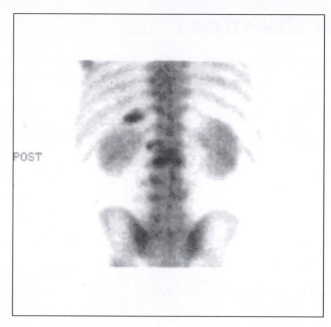

FIGURE 9.61
Nuclear medicine scan illustrating
tumor of the lumbar spine.

Review Questions

1. The inner gel-like portion of an intervertebral disk is called the:

   a. annulus fibrosis
   b. nucleus pulposis
   c. pars interarticularis
   d. promontory

2. What is the normal curvature of the lumbar spine?

   a. kyphotic
   b. lordotic
   c. scoliotic
   d. none of the above

3. What structure comprises the ear of the "Scotty dog"?

   a. inferior articulating process
   b. superior articulating process
   c. pedicle
   d. transverse process

4. The iliac crest is at the level of what lumbar vertebrae?

   a. 1–2
   b. 2–3
   c. 3–4
   d. 4–5

5. What is the name of the abnormal "swayback" curvature of the lumbar spine?

   a. kyphosis
   b. lordosis
   c. scoliosis

6. The inferior vertebral process of one vertebra and the superior vertebral process of another join to form which of the following?

   a. intervertebral arch
   b. vertebral arch
   c. zygapophyseal joint

7. On an AP projection of the lumbar spine, the central ray should be directed to:

   a. the iliac crest
   b. 2 inches superior to the iliac crest
   c. 2 inches inferior to the iliac crest
   d. symphysis pubis

8. Which projection best demonstrated zygapophyseal joints of the lumbar spine?

   a. AP
   b. oblique
   c. lateral
   d. hyperflexion lateral

9. The lateral lumbar spine should be centered:

   a. at the iliac crest
   b. at the ASIS
   c. 1.5 inches superior to the iliac crest
   d. 1.5 inches superior to the ASIS

10. What is the optimum patient rotation for an oblique lumbar spine?

    a. 15°
    b. 30°
    c. 45°
    d. 60°

11. Which position/projection best demonstrates the left intervertebral foramina of the lumbar spine?

    a. AP
    b. lateral
    c. RPO
    d. RAO

12. The LPO lumbar spine demonstrates essentially the same structures as the:

    a. RAO
    b. RPO
    c. LAO
    d. none of the above

13. When analyzing an AP projection of the coccyx, a radiographer observes the coccyx superimposed on the pubic bone. Which of the following is true?

    a. central ray should be angled more caudally
    b. central ray should be angled more cephalad
    c. oblique position should be substituted for the AP
    d. superimposition is normal for this film

14. The axial AP projection of the L5-S1 junction requires what tube angle?
    a. 10 to 15° cephalad
    b. 10 to 15° caudad
    c. 30 to 35° cephalad
    d. 30 to 35° caudad

15. Which of the following might be done to demonstrate vertebral mobility following spinal fusion?
    a. routine AP
    b. routine lateral
    c. bending exam
    d. hyperextension and hyperflexion laterals
    e. both c and d

16. Why are films taken to demonstrate scoliosis preferably done in the PA rather than the AP position?
    a. provides better detail of thoracic and lumbar vertebrae
    b. provides greater patient comfort
    c. results in less radiation to patient

17. Lumbar vertebrae do not have transverse foramina.
    a. true
    b. false

18. Oblique lumbar spine films can be taken with the patient in either the semi-supine or semi-prone position.
    a. true
    b. false

19. For an AP projection of the sacrum, the central ray should be angled cephalad and enter the body at the level of the ASIS.
    a. true
    b. false

20. On a lateral lumbar spine, the _____ plane should be parallel to the table.

21. To better open the intervertebral disk spaces on a lateral lumbar spine, the central ray may be angled _____ degrees _____ (cephalad/caudad).

22. Laterally on each side, the sacrum joins with what structure to form the sacroiliac joints?

23. For each of the following parts, list the routine positions/projections required at your clinical facility.
    a. lumbar spine
    b. sacrum
    c. coccyx

24. Special positions/projections are often required to demonstrate specific structures for certain patients. Explain why the following might be done.
    a. scoliosis series
    b. bending views

References and Recommended Reading

Ballinger, P. W. (1991). *Merrill's atlas of radiographic positions and radiologic procedures* (8th ed.). (Vol. 2). St. Louis: Mosby-Year Book.

Bontrager, K. L. (1993). *Textbook of radiographic positioning and related anatomy* (4th ed.). St. Louis: Mosby-Year Book.

Marieb, Elaine N. (1995). *Human Anatomy and Physiology* (3rd ed.). Redwood City: Benjamin/Cummings Publishing Company.

McInnes, James (1973) *Clark's Positioning in Radiography* (9th ed.). (Vol. 1). Chicago: Year Book Medical Publishers.

Meschan, I. (1975) *An Atlas of Anatomy Basic to Radiology.* Philadelphia: Lea and Febiger.

CHAPTER 10

Trauma Spine

ROBIN JONES, MS, RT(R)(ARRT)

FUNDAMENTAL PRINCIPLES

CORRELATIVE IMAGING

CERVICAL SPINE
Cross-table Lateral
AP
AP Open Mouth
Trauma Oblique

THORACIC SPINE
Cross-table Lateral
Cross-table Swimmer's Lateral
AP

LUMBAR SPINE
Cross-table Lateral
AP

OBJECTIVES

At the completion of this chapter, the student should be able to:

1. List the indications for ordering radiographs of the spine.

2. Explain the rationale for each projection used for trauma patients.

3. Describe the positioning used to visualize anatomic structures of the spine in the trauma patient.

4. Identify the location of the central ray and extent of field necessary for each projection.

5. Recommend the technical factors for producing an acceptable radiograph for each projection.

6. State the patient instructions for each projection.

7. Identify the anatomic structures that are best demonstrated on each of the trauma spine radiographs.

8. Given radiographs, evaluate positioning and technical factors.

9. Identify alternative modalities used for imaging the trauma spine.

FUNDAMENTAL PRINCIPLES

Radiologic evaluation of a patient who has sustained an injury to the spine can be challenging. Every patient with an injury to the spine will present a different set of problems for radiographers to overcome to obtain the necessary radiographs. This chapter discusses issues related to the trauma patient who has sustained an unstable injury to the spine and who cannot be moved from the spine board. Indications for plain radiographs, CT, MRI, and conventional tomography are explained.

Plain Radiographs

A patient who has endured trauma may sustain an injury to the spine. Initial evaluation of the patient takes place in the emergency room and typically includes inspection of the body, communication with the patient, palpation of the entire spine, checks for deep tendon reflexes, and evaluation of sensory responses. Indications for radiographs of the spine include: "(1) impaired consciousness, including even mild alcohol intoxication, with suspected craniofacial trauma, (2) complaints of neck or back pain, (3) evidence of significant head or facial trauma, (4) signs of focal **neurologic deficit**, (5) unexplained hypotension, (6) a suggestive mechanism of injury associated with other painful injuries, or (7) a minor mechanism of injury ('slip and fall' injuries or low-velocity motor vehicle accidents) when patient discomfort or palpable neck tenderness is greater than one would normally expect in such instances" (Rosen, 1992).

The basic views for trauma patients are two projections taken at right angles to each other. For trauma spine this would include an AP and a cross-table lateral projection. This is generally sufficient for patients who have a neurologic deficit.

However, a patient who has fewer clinical signs or symptoms may require additional views such as obliques or flexion and extension laterals. Each examination of a trauma patient will be unique and must be designed around the clinical signs and symptoms of the specific patient.

An area of special concern is the lower cervical spine area. Due to the patient's physique or injuries, it may be difficult to visualize the lower cervical spine area on the cross-table lateral film. However, all seven cervical vertebrae must be demonstrated. This may require a swimmer's position to be performed. If this radiograph does not adequately demonstrate the lower cervical vertebra, CT might be necessary.

All trauma patients are brought into the emergency room with a cervical collar. This prevents the patient from moving the neck and limits further injury to the spinal cord. A cross-table lateral projection of the cervical spine must be taken with the cervical collar in place. Specific instructions from a physician to either leave the collar on the patient or remove it should be obtained before proceeding.

An important piece of equipment for all trauma patients is the "trauma cart." This is a specially designed stretcher with a sliding tray that runs the length of the stretcher. This design enables the radiographer to place the cassette/grid in position without moving the injured patient. This is of particular importance with patients who have injuries to the spine who should not or cannot be moved.

It is especially important for radiographers to be accurate in positioning and technique when radiographing trauma patients. They should be familiar with the mobile equipment, emergency room personnel, and specific hospital policies regarding trauma patients. This will enable them to work efficiently. It is critical to get a diagnostic film on the first attempt to ensure a quick diagnosis.

In radiographing trauma patients, a common error is failure to remove artifacts from the area of interest. Even though the cervical collar must stay in place, necklaces and earrings can be carefully removed without moving the patient's neck.

CORRELATIVE IMAGING

Computed Tomography

In addition to plain films, CT plays an important role in the detection of spinal injuries. A misconception is that CT can replace plain films, but this is not the case. CT films are performed in conjunction with plain radiographs. Indications for the use of CT include:

1. Plain films do not demonstrate all the required anatomy.
2. The findings on the plain films are suspicious for spinal injury.
3. Plain films demonstrate fracture or dislocation.
4. Plain films are normal but the clinical findings are suspicious of spinal injury.

Limitations of CT include:

1. Fractures in the axial plane can be missed.
2. It may be hard to detect when the intervertebral disk spaces are widened.
3. Subluxation, dislocation, and unusual angulation of the cervical spine may be difficult to interpret.

There are several advantages of CT. The patient is able to be kept in the supine position and in traction thoughout the procedure. CT uses significantly less radiation than tomography. Axial imaging also provides accurate localization of fracture fragments in reference to the spinal cord and demonstrates hidden posterior fractures (Figures 10.1 and 10.2).

Magnetic Resonance Imaging

MRI has also become important in the detection of trauma to the nonbony structures of the spine (Figures 10.3 and 10.4). MRI visualizes the anterior, posterior, and transverse ligaments and spinal cord parenchyma in the cervical spine. Abnormalities of the ligaments can cause neurologic deficit; therefore, it becomes important in patients who have negative CT and plain films. In the lumbar spine, MRI demonstrates the neural elements, **thecal (thē′kăl) sac** and paravertebral soft tissues. For the trauma patient who is unstable, MRI may not be possible if the equipment needed by the patient cannot enter the MRI room. Also the patient may be uncooperative, which leads to unacceptable films.

Conventional Tomography

Conventional tomography still plays an important role in detecting abnormalities in patients with injuries to the spine. Tomography is excellent in the detection of atlanto-occipital (ăt-lăn′′tō-ŏk-sĭp′ĭ-tăl)

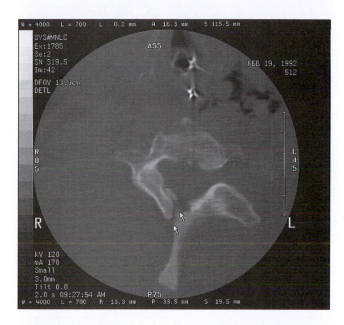

FIGURE 10.1 Lower cervical laminar fracture as indicated by the arrows.

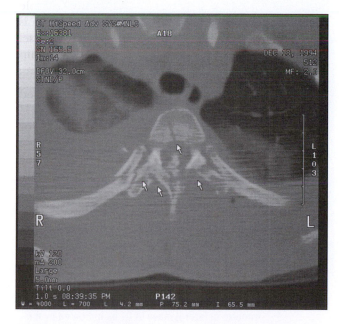

FIGURE 10.2 Sagittal fracture through the body of the thoracic vertebrae with a comminuted fracture through the posterior elements bilaterally. There are also fracture fragments located in the spinal canal.

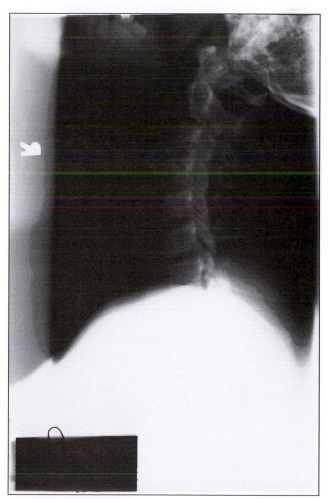

FIGURE 10.3 Widening of the spinous process between C6 and C7. An MRI was performed on this patient.

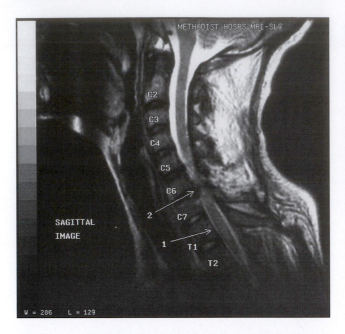

FIGURE 10.4 An MRI in the sagittal plane was performed on the same patient as in Figure 10.3. Arrow 1 is pointing to the posterior ligament (black line). Arrow 2 is pointing to the herniated disk at C6–C7 level interrupting the posterior ligament.

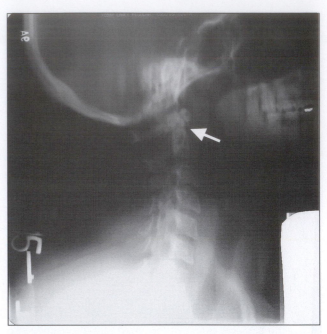

FIGURE 10.5 Conventional lateral tomogram of a fracture of C1 as indicated by the arrow.

dislocations, subluxations of the vertebral bodies, and fractures of lateral masses of C1, articular processes, vertebral bodies, and the odontoid process (Figures 10.5 and 10.6).

The position of the patient on the radiographic table makes it difficult to image the spine in the lateral position. To perform lateral images, the patient must be turned into that position, which makes it difficult when the patient has a spinal injury. However, when CT and plain films fail to detect an abnormality in a patient with clinical signs or symptoms, tomography is indicated (Figures 10.7 and 10.8).

SUMMARY

The remainder of the chapter discusses the specific positioning requirements for immobile patients with injuries to the spine. Each patient will present to the emergency room with different positioning problems associated with the injuries. It is the duty of the radiographer to creatively apply the basic procedures and principles to obtain the needed radiographs for the patient. By understanding which view demonstrates the anatomy, it will be easier to improvise.

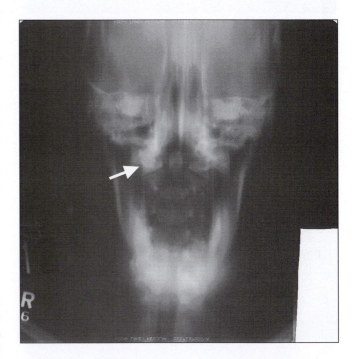

FIGURE 10.6 Same patient as Figure 10.5, AP projection; fracture of lateral mass of C1 as indicated by the arrow.

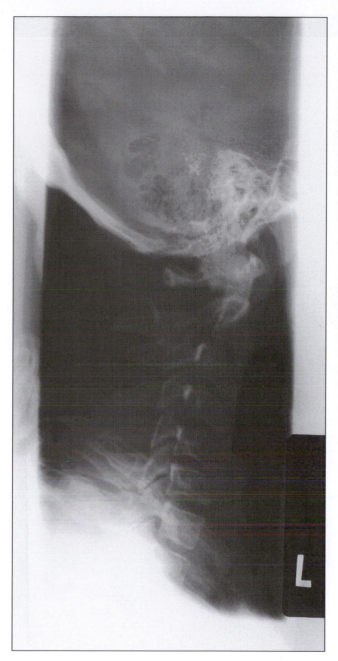

FIGURE 10.7   Patient with a fracture at C2 posterior arch with
anterior displacement of the body of C2 into C3.

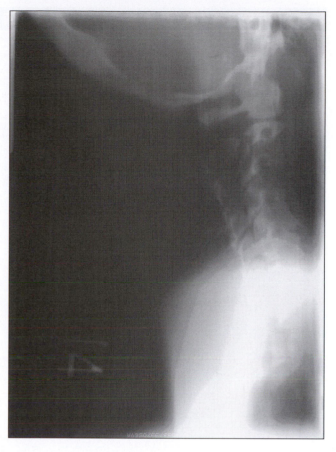

FIGURE 10.8   Same patient as Figure 10.7, with demonstration of
the fracture of C2 with conventional tomography in
the lateral position.

ALTERNATIVE POSITIONS/PROJECTIONS

CERVICAL—CROSS-TABLE LATERAL POSITION

Exam Rationale   A cross-table lateral of the cervical spine is performed on all patients who have sustained a traumatic injury to rule out the possibility of fracture or dislocation. Structures demonstrated include the bodies of all seven cervical vertebrae, the intervertebral joint spaces, articular pillars, superior and inferior articulating facets, zygapophyseal joints, and spinous processes.

Technical Considerations

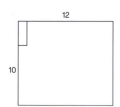

- Regular screen/film
- Grid or non-grid
- kVp range: 75–85
- SID: 72 inch (180 cm)

Radiation Protection

Patient Position   Remains recumbent on the spine board or stretcher; all potential artifacts are removed if possible, but the cervical collar is left on; the cassette/grid is placed in the vertical position with its bottom portion touching the shoulder (Figure 10.9).

Part Position   The neck remains in the cervical collar and the cervical spine is not adjusted.

Central Ray   Perpendicular to the upper margin of the thyroid cartilage; align the coronal plane, which passes through the mastoid processes, to the midline of the film.

Patient Instructions   "Take in a deep breath, let it all out. Relax your shoulders; don't breathe or move."

Evaluation Criteria (Figures 10.10 and 10.11)

- All seven cervical vertebrae should be demonstrated.
- The rami of the mandible should not be superimposed on the upper cervical vertebrae.
- The technique used should adequately show the bony structures and soft tissues.

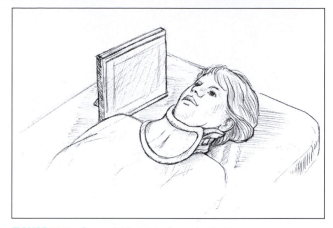

FIGURE 10.9   Cross-table lateral cervical spine.

Tips

1. The patient may need help depressing the shoulders. This can be done by:
   —Having someone pull down on the patient's arms.
   —Having the patient pull on a strap that is wrapped around the feet.
   —*These procedures should be done only with the consent of the physician and patient.*
2. The divergence of the x-ray beam can project C7 into the shoulder; therefore, it may be necessary to center at C7.
3. If all seven vertebrae are not demonstrated, it may be necessary to perform a swimmer's position (see page 378).
4. It is best to use the correct film size and collimate to the part to reduce scatter radiation.

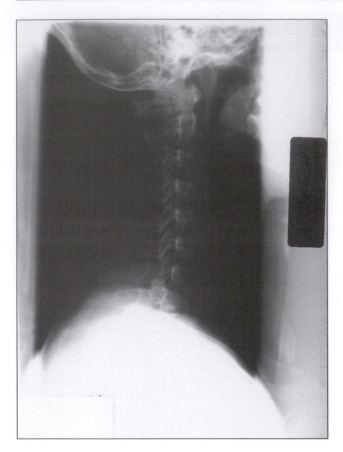

FIGURE 10.10   Cross-table lateral cervical radiograph with all seven cervical vertebrae and the first thoracic demonstrated.

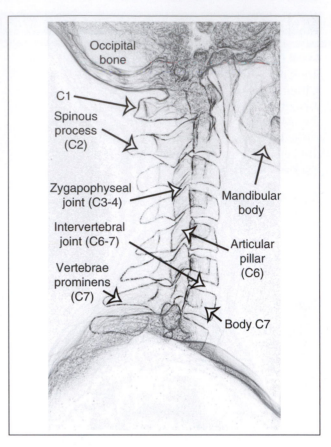

FIGURE 10.11   Cross-table lateral cervical spine.

CERVICAL—AP PROJECTION

Exam Rationale　The AP projection is done in conjunction with the lateral position for the trauma patient to rule out the possibility of a fracture or dislocation. Structures demonstrated on the AP projection include the intervertebral disk spaces, the bodies, the pedicles, spinous processes of C3–C7.

Technical Considerations

- Regular screen/film
- Grid
- kVp range: 70–80
- SID: 40 inch (100 cm)

Radiation Protection

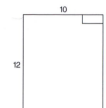

AEC (Phototiming)

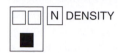

N DENSITY

Patient Position　Recumbent on the spine board. The procedure continues as in a regular cervical spine (see Chapter 7, page 347).

CERVICAL—AP OPEN MOUTH PROJECTION

Exam rationale   The AP open mouth projection is done in conjunction with the lateral position and AP projection for the trauma patient to rule out the possibility of a fracture or dislocation. Structures shown include lateral masses of C1, zygapophyseal joint space of C1–C2, odontoid process, and body of C2.

Technical Considerations

- Regular screen/film
- Grid
- kVp range: 70–80
- SID: 40 inch (100 cm)

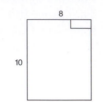

Radiation Protection

AEC (Phototiming)

☐☐ [N] DENSITY

■

Patient Position   Recumbent on the spine board. The procedure continues as in a regular cervical spine (see Chapter 7, page 347).

CERVICAL—OBLIQUE AP PROJECTION (RPO OR LPO POSITION)

Exam Rationale   The oblique projections are typically not performed as part of an initial examination of the trauma spine but may be used with patients who have injuries to areas of the body other than their spine, precluding filming in the erect position. Structures demonstrated on the oblique projections include the intervertebral foramina and pedicles farthest from the film (the up side). Both sides are examined for comparison.

Technical Considerations

- Regular screen/film
- Grid
- kVp range: 70–80
- SID: 40 inch (100 cm)

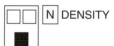

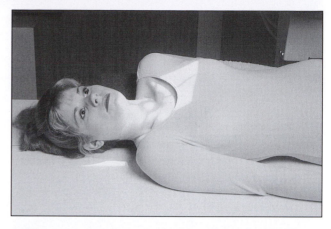

FIGURE 10.12   Oblique cervical spine with patient rotated 45°.

Radiation Protection

AEC (Phototiming)

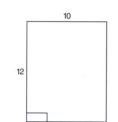

Patient Position

Recumbent (Figure 10.12)

Part Position   Adjust the entire body to form an angle of 45° with the plane of the film; the head should look straight ahead; chin should be extended slightly.

Central Ray   Angle 15° to 20° cephalic to upper margin of thyroid cartilage.

Patient Instructions   "Breathe normally but don't move."

Evaluation Criteria (Figures 10.13 and 10.14)

- Intervertebral foramina and disk spaces should be open.
- Vertebrae demonstrated are C1–C7.
- Chin should be sufficiently elevated so the mandibular rami do not overlap C1 and C2.

Tips

1. The patient can remain on the spine board. The patient can be positioned on either the trauma cart or on the radiographic table.
2. When it is not possible to rotate the patient, the x-ray tube can be angled 45° into the neck and 15° to 20° cephalic. Because there is a double angle on the tube, it is not possible to use a grid (Figure 10.15).

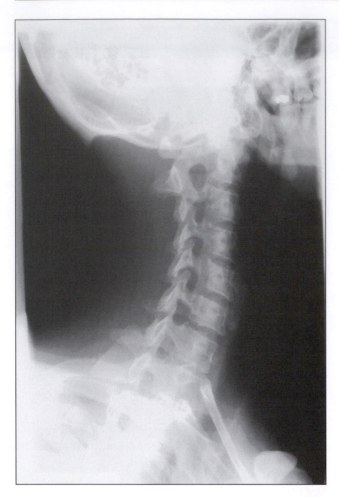

FIGURE 10.13   Oblique cervical spine with patient rotated 45°.

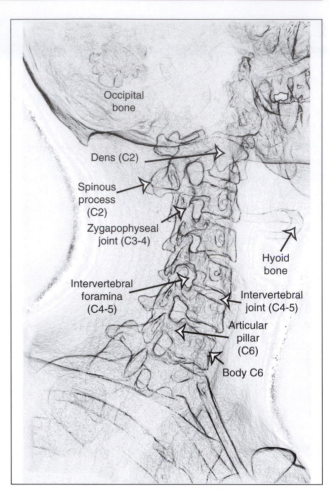

Occipital
bone

Dens (C2)

Spinous
process
(C2)

Zygapophyseal
joint (C3-4)

Hyoid
bone

Intervertebral
foramina
(C4-5)

Intervertebral
joint (C4-5)

Articular
pillar
(C6)

Body C6

FIGURE 10.14   Oblique cervical spine with patient rotated 45°.

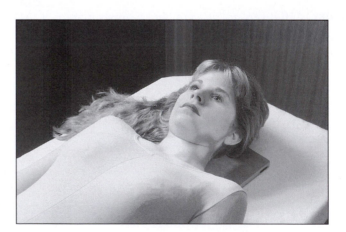

FIGURE 10.15
Oblique cervical spine with tube angled 45°.

THORACIC—CROSS-TABLE LATERAL POSITION

Exam Rationale   A cross-table lateral of the thoracic spine is performed on all patients who have sustained a traumatic injury to the thoracic spine to rule out the possibility of fracture or dislocation. Structures demonstrated include the thoracic bodies, intervertebral disk spaces, intervertebral foramina of T3–L2, and the spinous processes of the lower thoracic and upper lumbar regions.

Technical Considerations

- Regular screen/film
- Grid
- kVp range: 70–80
- SID: 40 inch (100 cm)

Radiation Protection

AEC (Phototiming)

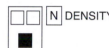

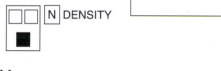

Patient Position   Recumbent on the spine board or stretcher with the midcoronal plane centered to the cassette (Figure 10.16).

Part Position   Raise the patient's arms over the head.

Central Ray   Perpendicular to T8.

Patient Instructions   "Continue to breathe normally."

Evaluation Criteria (Figures 10.17 and 10.18)

- The vertebrae from T3 to L2 should be visualized.
- Disk spaces and intervertebral foramina should be clearly demonstrated.

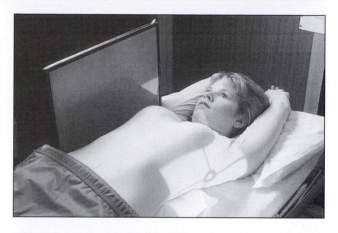

FIGURE 10.16   Cross-table lateral thoracic spine.

Tips

1. The lower margin of the film should be 1 inch (3 cm) above the lower margin of the ribs; this will place L2 at the bottom of the film.
2. Use of an upright Bucky versus a grid/cassette will produce a significantly better image (Figure 10.19).
3. Use AEC only with upright Bucky device.

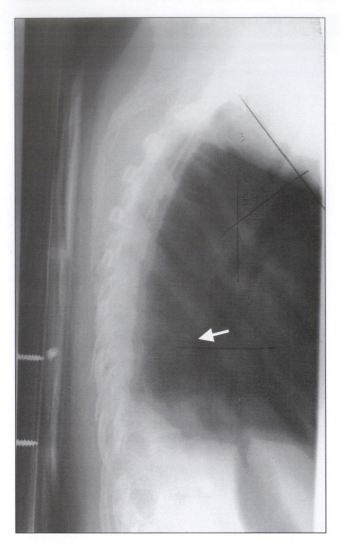

FIGURE 10.17   Cross-table lateral of the thoracic spine. There is a compression fracture of T9 as indicated by the arrow.

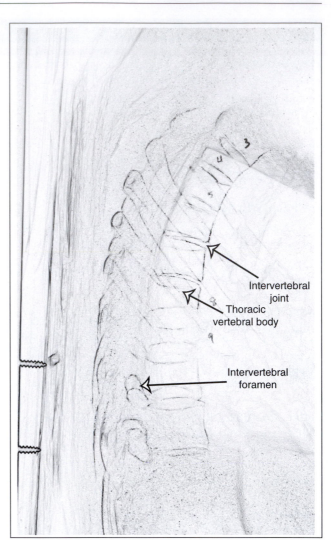

FIGURE 10.18   Cross-table lateral thoracic spine.

Intervertebral joint

Thoracic vertebral body

Intervertebral foramen

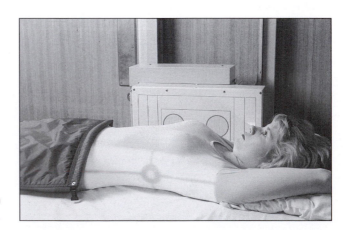

FIGURE 10.19
Cross-table lateral spine /upright Bucky.

THORACIC—CROSS-TABLE SWIMMER'S LATERAL

Exam Rationale   Structures demonstrated on the swimmer's lateral position include the bodies, intervertebral disk spaces, spinous processes, and zygapophyseal joints of upper thoracic and/or lower cervical vertebrae.

Technical Considerations

- Regular screen/film
- Grid
- kVp range: 75–85
- SID: 40 inch (100 cm)

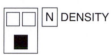

Radiation Protection   AEC (Phototiming)

   N DENSITY

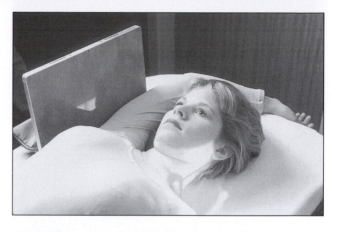

FIGURE 10.20   Cross-table lateral swimmer's lateral.

Patient Position   Recumbent on the spine board with the midaxillary line centered to the cassette (Figure 10.20).

Part Position   Raise the arm that is closest to the film and lower the arm that is farthest from the film.

Central Ray   Perpendicular to T2.

Patient Instructions   "Take in a breath and let it out. Don't breathe or move."

Evaluation Criteria (Figures 10.21 and 10.22)

- The humeral heads should not be superimposed on the vertebral bodies.
- The disk spaces between C1 and T1 and the first three to four thoracic vertebrae should be visualized.

Tips

1. If the patient cannot separate the shoulders enough, a 5° caudal angle may be used.
2. If the patient cannot raise the arm closest to the film, the other arm may be raised while depressing the arm closest to the film.
3. If the lower cervical vertebrae are of interest, the central ray should be directed to C7.

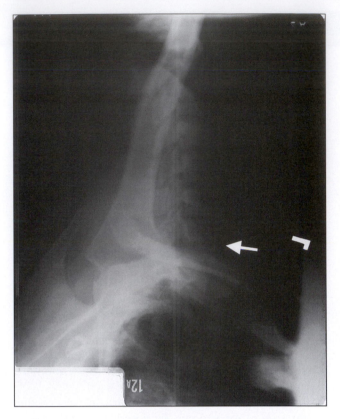

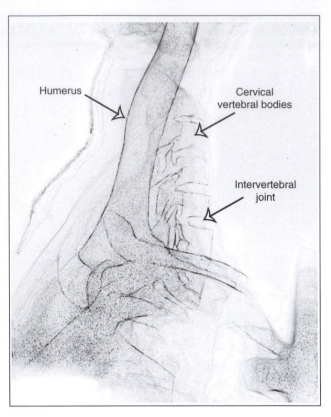

FIGURE 10.21 Swimmer's position demonstrating the lower cervical vertebrae including C7 as indicated by the arrow.

FIGURE 10.22 Cross-table swimmer's lateral.

THORACIC—AP PROJECTION

Exam Rationale   The AP projection is done in conjunction with the lateral position to rule out the possibility of fracture or dislocation. Structures demonstrated on the AP projection include the intervertebral disk spaces, the bodies, the pedicles, and spinous processes of T1–T12.

Technical Considerations

- Regular screen/film
- Grid
- kVp range: 70–80
- SID: 40 inch (100 cm)

Radiation Protection

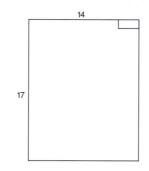

AEC (Phototiming)

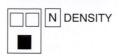 DENSITY

Patient Position   Recumbent on the spine board. The procedure continues as in a regular thoracic spine (see Chapter 8, page 372).

LUMBAR—CROSS-TABLE LATERAL POSITION

Exam Rationale   A cross-table lateral of the lumbar spine is performed on patients who have sustained a traumatic injury to the lower back to rule out the possibility of a fracture or dislocation. Structures demonstrated include the lumbar bodies, intervertebral disk spaces, intervertebral foramina, and the spinous processes of T12–S1.

Technical Considerations

- Regular screen/film
- Grid
- kVp range: 75–85
- SID: 40 inch (100 cm)

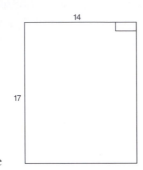

Radiation Protection

 for male patients; shielding not possible for female patients

AEC (Phototiming)

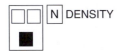 N DENSITY

Patient Position   The patient remains recumbent on the spine board or stretcher with the midcoronal plane centered to the cassette (Figure 10.23).

Part Position   Raise the patient's arms over the head.

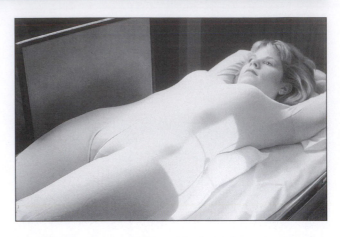

FIGURE 10.23   Cross-table lateral lumbar spine.

Central Ray   Perpendicular to L4.

Patient Instructions   "Hold your breath and don't move."

Evaluation Criteria (Figures 10.24 and 10.25)

- The vertebra from T12 to S1 should be visualized.

Tip   Use of an upright Bucky versus a grid/cassette will produce a significantly better image (Figure 10.26).

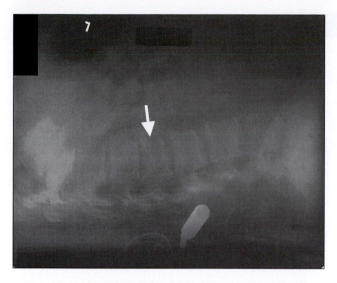

FIGURE 10.24   Cross-table lateral lumbar spine with a slight compression fracture of L1 as indicated by the arrow.

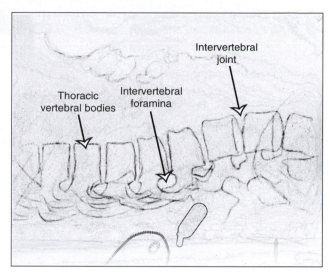

FIGURE 10.25   Cross-table lateral lumbar spine.

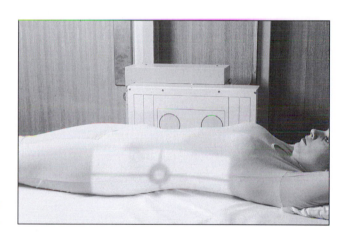

FIGURE 10.26
Cross-table lateral lumbar spine/upright Bucky.

LUMBAR—AP PROJECTION

Exam Rationale　The AP projection is performed in conjunction with the lateral position to rule out fractures and dislocations. Structures demonstrated on the AP projection include the intervertebral disk spaces, the bodies, the pedicles, spinous processes of L1–L5, and sacrum.

Technical Considerations

- Regular screen/film
- Grid
- kVp range: 70–80
- SID: 40 inch (100 cm)

Radiation Protection

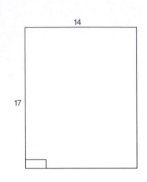

AEC (Phototiming)

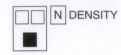

□□ N DENSITY
■

Patient Position　The procedure continues as in a routine lumbar spine (see Chapter 9, page 394).

Review Questions

1. At a minimum, trauma patients with spinal injuries require:

   a. AP and cross-table lateral positions/projections
   b. AP, oblique, and lateral positions/projections
   c. oblique positions
   d. flexion and extension positions

2. For a trauma patient, the cervical collar is removed:

   a. to remove the patient's jewelry
   b. only to take the cross-table lateral
   c. only to take the open mouth view
   d. only at the direction of the physician

3. Which of the following is an indication for radiographs of the spine?

   a. minor mechanism injury (fall)
   b. unexplained hypotension
   c. neck and back pain
   d. all of the above

4. The best imaging modality for demonstration of posterior ligaments is:

   a. CT
   b. MR
   c. plain radiography
   d. conventional tomography

5. If a cross-table lateral cervical spine radiograph does not demonstrate C6 or C7, what additional radiograph should be taken?

   a. AP projection without angle
   b. AP open mouth view
   c. swimmer's position
   d. flexion or extension lateral

6. The kVp range for a cross-table lateral cervical spine is:

   a. 65–75
   b. 75–85
   c. 85–95
   d. 95–105

7. In evaluating a radiograph of the cervical spine, the radiographer discovers 3 necklaces superimposing C5, C6, and C7. The radiographer should:

   a. pass the film
   b. remove the cervical collar and necklaces and repeat the film

   c. remove only the necklaces and repeat the film
   d. perform a swimmer's position

8. How much is the central ray angled for an AP cervical spine?

   a. 10–15
   b. 15–20
   c. 25–30
   d. 35 to 45

9. What imaging modality best demonstrates the lateral masses of C1?

   a. CT
   b. MR
   c. plain radiography
   d. conventional tomography

10. What are the breathing instructions for an AP projection of the thoracic spine?

    a. shallow breathing
    b. respiration suspended on exhalation
    c. respiration suspended on inspiration
    d. no specific breathing instructions

11. For the swimmer's position, the patient is positioned so that:

    a. both arms are pulled down toward the feet
    b. the arm closest to the film is raised above the head
    c. the arms are left in a neutral position

12. To demonstrate the intervertebral foramina of the thoracic spine, the recommended position/projection is:

    a. AP
    b. lateral
    c. oblique

13. What is the central ray location for a lateral lumbar spine?

    a. L2
    b. L3
    c. L4
    d. ASIS

14. CT can replace plain film radiography of the spine in many cases.

    a. true
    b. false

15. For the AP projection of the thoracic spine, a trauma patient is removed from the spine board.

    a. true

    b. false

16. The average kVp range for the cross-table lateral lumbar spine is 95 to 105.

    a. true

    b. false

17. If the patient cannot be rotated from the supine position for oblique cervical spine films, what modification is required?

18. What are the breathing instructions for a cross-table lateral cervical spine?

19. In evaluating an AP open mouth radiograph, the occipital bone superimposes C1. What adjustment should be made to improve the radiograph?

20. You are radiographing the thoracic spine of a trauma patient who cannot be moved. Describe how you could use an upright Bucky to perform the lateral.

References and Recommended Reading

Ballinger, P. (1995). Vertebral column. *Merrill's atlas of radiographic positions and radiologic procedures* (8th ed., Vol. 1, pp. 311–397). St. Louis: Mosby-Year Book.

Bontrager, K. (1997). Radiographic anatomy and positioning of the coccyx, sacrum and lumbar spine and radiographic anatomy and positioning of the thoracic and cervical spine. In *Radiographic positioning and related anatomy* (4th ed., pp. 243–295). St. Louis: Mosby-Year Book.

Drafke, M. (1990). *Trauma and mobile radiography*. Philadelphia: Davis.

Eisenberg, R., Dennis, C., & May, C. (1989). Vertebral column. In *Radiographic positioning* (pp. 163–205). Boston: Little, Brown.

Herman, J., & Sonntag, V. (1991). Diving accidents mechanism of injury and treatment of the patient. *Critical Care Nursing Clinics of North America, 3,* 331–337.

Herzog, R. (1991). Selection and utilization of imaging studies for disorders of the lumbar spine. *Physical Medicine and Rehabilitation Clinics of North America, 2,* 7–59.

Rogers, L. (1992). The spine. *Radiology of skeletal trauma* (2nd ed., pp. 439–579). New York: Churchill Livingstone.

Rosen, P., Barkin, R. M., Braen, G. R., Dailey, R. H., & Levy, R. C. (1992). Spinal trauma. *Emergency Medicine Concepts & Clinical Practice* (3rd. ed., pp. 386–411). St. Louis: Mosby-Year Book.

Wilberger, J. (1990). Radiologic evaluation of spinal trauma. *Topics in Emergency Medicine, 11,* 30–35.

Woodring, J., & Lee, C. (1992). The role and limitations of computed tomographic scanning in the evaluation of cervical trauma. *Journal of Trauma, 33,* 698–708.

SECTION V

SKULL RADIOGRAPHY

Introduction to Skull Radiography

TERRI LASKEY FAUBER, EdD, RT(R)(M)(ARRT)

SKULL MORPHOLOGY

CRANIAL TOPOGRAPHY, LINES, AND PLANES

PATIENT AND POSITIONING CONSIDERATIONS

OBJECTIVES

At the completion of this chapter, the student should be able to:

1. Compare and contrast cranial shapes, including differences in the degree of angle between the petrous ridges and the median plane.

2. Describe the location of cranial landmarks, lines, and planes.

3. Given radiographs, diagrams, or photographs, identify cranial landmarks, lines, and planes.

4. List the advantages and disadvantages of radiographing the cranium in the erect and recumbent positions.

5. State ways of providing reasonable comfort for all patient types during cranial radiography.

6. Describe the positioning errors that result in rotation and tilt.

7. Given radiographs, recognize and differentiate between the common positioning errors of rotation and tilt.

8. Describe special considerations when radiographing the pediatric skull.

Skull radiography offers many challenges to the radiographer. Although the thickness of the skull varies only slightly, variations in size and shape affect the radiographic demonstration of cranial structures. Knowledge of the desired anatomy and of cranial lines and planes aids in producing optimal radiographs for diagnosis.

SKULL MORPHOLOGY

The skull is classified according to its shape: **mesocephalic** (average), **brachycephalic** (short and broad), and **dolichocephalic** (long and narrow). The relation-

ship of the internal structures varies slightly with each classification. Positioning guidelines have been designed for the average or mesocephalic-shaped cranium. Adjustment in alignment of lines, planes, or tube angulation may be necessary to visualize the cranial structures for brachycephalic and dolichocephalic cranial shapes.

- **Mesocephalic**—petrous ridges form an angle of 47° with the median plane (Figure 11.1).
- **Brachycephalic**—petrous ridges form an angle of 54° with the median plane; internal structures positioned higher with reference to infraorbitomeatal line (Figure 11.2).

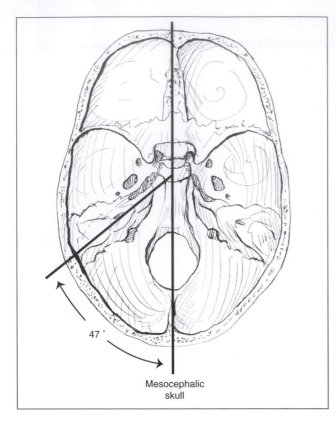

FIGURE 11.1 Mesocephalic shape.

- **Dolichocephalic**—petrous ridges form an angle of 40° with the median plane; internal structures positioned lower with reference to infraorbitomeatal line (Figure 11.3).

CRANIAL TOPOGRAPHY, LINES, AND PLANES

The following cranial topography, lines, and planes provide localization points important for positioning and centering of the cranium. Accurate adjustment or centering of these visual, palpable, and imaginary localization points will assist in producing optimal radiographs of the cranium.

Surface Landmarks Used in Skull Positioning (Figure 11.4A and B)

- **Glabella** (glă-bē´lă)—smooth flat surface just *above* the midpoint of the eyebrows
- **Acanthion** (ă-kăn´thē-ŏn)—point where the upper lip joins the base of the nose
- **Mental point**—tip of the chin
- **Superciliary** (soo´´pĕr-sĭl´ē´ă-rē) **ridge/arch**—ridge of bone at the eyebrow
- **Supraorbital groove**—depression in bone *above* the eyebrow
- **Nasion** (nā´zē-ŏn)—point where the right and left nasal bones meet

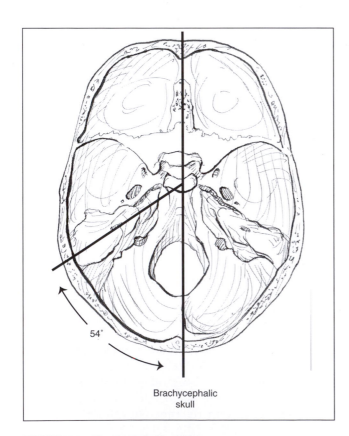

FIGURE 11.2 Brachycephalic shape.

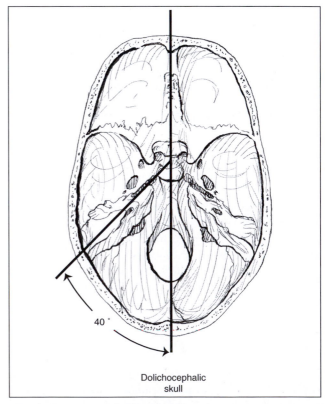

FIGURE 11.3 Dolichocephalic shape.

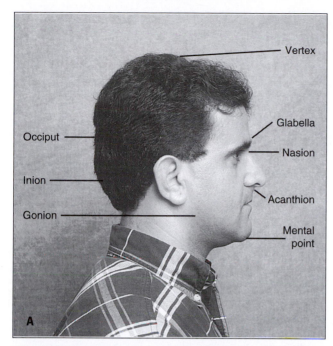

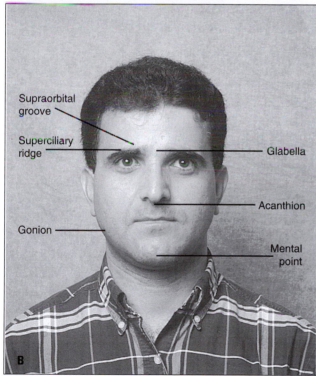

FIGURE 11.4 A and B   Cranial topography.

- **Angle of mandible/gonion** (gō´nē-ŏn)—junction of the mandibular body and ramus
- **Vertex**—most superior surface of cranium
- **Inion** (in´ē-ŏn)—external protuberance on occipital bone
- **Occiput** (ŏk´sĭ-pŭt)—most posterior surface of cranium

Base of Orbit (Figure 11.5A)

- Inner and outer **canthi**—points where the upper and lower eyelids meet (singular-**canthus**)
- Supraorbital margin (SOM)—ridge of bone *above* orbit
- Infraorbital margin (IOM)—ridge of bone *below* orbit

Ear (Figure 11.5B)

- **External auditory meatus** (EAM)—opening of the external ear canal
- **Auricle/pinna**—cartilage protecting the ear canal
- **Tragus**—cartilage flap at the opening of the EAM
- **Top of ear attachment** (TEA)—point where the auricle attaches to the cranium

Planes/Lines

These are imaginary surfaces or set of points used to adjust the position of the cranium (Figures 11.6 and 11.7).

- Midsagittal (median) plane (MSP)—divides the body into equal right and left halves
- **Interpupillary (interorbital) line**—drawn between the pupils
- **Acanthiomeatal line**—drawn between the junction of upper lip/nose and the EAM
- **Mentomeatal line** (MML)—drawn between the tip of chin and the EAM
- **Infraorbitomeatal line** (IOML)—drawn between the infraorbital margin and the EAM
- **Glabellomeatal line**—drawn between the glabella and the EAM
- **Orbitomeatal line** (OML)—drawn between the outer orbital margin and the EAM

PATIENT AND POSITIONING CONSIDERATIONS

Erect versus Recumbent

Comparable skull radiographs can be obtained in either the upright or recumbent position as long as the tube-part-film relationship is maintained. The equipment available will in part determine whether skull radiography is performed erect or recumbent. A head unit or upright Bucky device offers two advantages. The erect position is easier for the patient and, secondly, it allows for visualization of air/fluid levels with a horizontal beam.

The age and condition of the patient must be assessed and considered before attempting upright skull radiography. Pediatric patients may not be able to remain still in the upright position. Unstable or injured patients may not be able to tolerate an upright position for skull radiography.

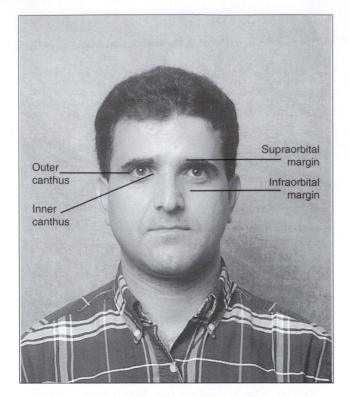

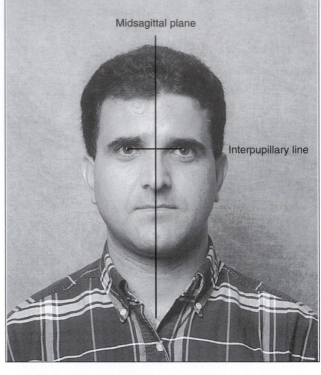

FIGURE 11.6   Positioning lines.

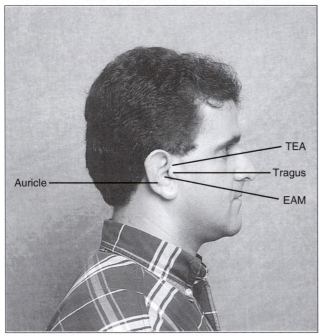

FIGURE 11.5 A and B   Cranial topography.

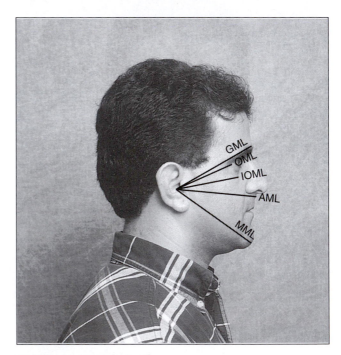

FIGURE 11.7   Positioning lines.

When performing skull radiography with the patient recumbent, it is important to maintain patient comfort with the use of positioning sponges. For example, hyposthenic or asthenic patients require a sponge under their chest for comfort during skull radiography. The sponge elevates the chest to assist in positioning and provides a cushion between the patient's chest and table. Hypersthenic patients may need to rest their head on a sponge to aid in positioning. Elevating the head will provide more flexibility to properly align the head to the film.

Every effort should be made to perform radiography of the sinuses in the upright position. This allows for the visualization of air/fluid levels within the sinuses (Figure 11.8).

Pediatric versus Adults

Pediatric patients typically have an adult size skull attached to a small body. Alternate use of flexion or extension may be needed to achieve the proper alignment of positioning lines and planes. For example, the neck of a pediatric patient may need to be extended to place the orbitomeatal line perpendicular when positioning an AP skull. Immobilization devices are often helpful in reducing motion when radiographing a pediatric skull.

Positioning Errors

When alignment of the patient's head and body is not properly maintained, positioning errors result. To prevent misalignment, the long axis of the patient's head and body must coincide with or be parallel to the midline of the table and the cervical spine must remain at the level of the foramen magnum. Asymmetry of cranial and facial features may hinder efforts to align structures during positioning. It is best to palpate landmarks such as the mastoid tips and orbital margins instead of visualizing alignment of variable facial features. Additionally, the use of an angligner or skull protractor will aid in positioning the cranium and its alignment with the cervical spine.

Common Positioning Errors

Rotation and **tilt** are the most common positioning errors during skull radiography. Motion of the head around the longitudinal axis results in rotation. On the resulting frontal image, this can be demonstrated by unequal distances between the lateral border of the orbit and edge of the cranium on the right or left sides. When the longitudinal axis of the head is no longer aligned with the longitudinal axis of the body the cranium is tilted. On a frontal projection, this is seen as unequal distance between the midline of the anatomic part and the edge of the film. Both rotation and tilt positioning errors will separate structures that should be superimposed in a lateral position. It is important to distinguish between rotation and tilt of the cranium, so when presented, the radiographer can make the appropriate adjustment (Figures 11.9 through 11.14).

Artifact Removal

Anything resulting in an artifact that could distract from the viewing of the cranial image should be removed. Obvious items such as hairpins/clips, dentures, jewelry, and eyeglasses may prevent optimal visualization of cranial structures. Less obvious artifacts are braids or other tightly bound hair that could alter the density in the area of interest.

Radiation Protection

Appropriately limiting the area of exposure by use of a collimator, cylinder, cone or diaphragm improves

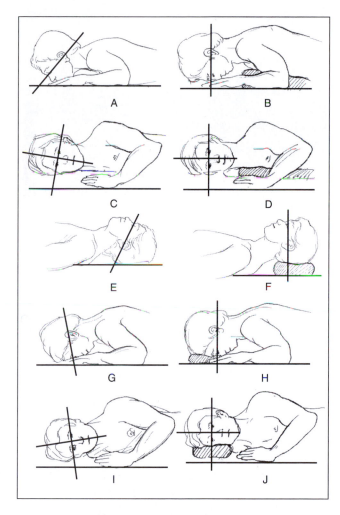

FIGURE 11.8 **(A)** Hyposthenic/asthenic patient prone.
(B) Hyposthenic/asthenic prone positioning adjustment.
(C) Hyposthenic/asthenic patient lateral.
(D) Hyposthenic/asthenic lateral positioning adjustment.
(E) Hypersthenic patient supine.
(F) Hypersthenic supine positioning adjustment.
(G) Hypersthenic patient prone.
(H) Hypersthenic prone positioning adjustment.
(I) Hypersthenic patient lateral.
(J) Hypersthenic lateral positioning adjustment.

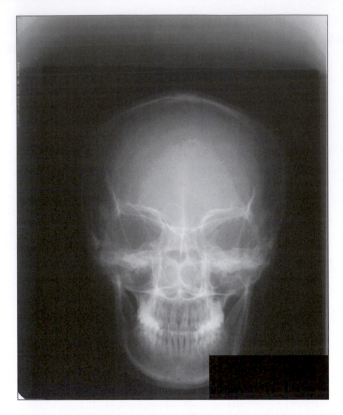

FIGURE 11.9   Frontal image with no positioning errors.

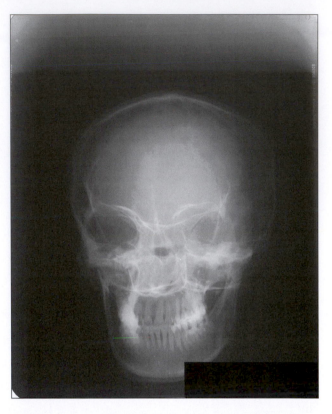

FIGURE 11.11   Frontal image with rotation positioning error.

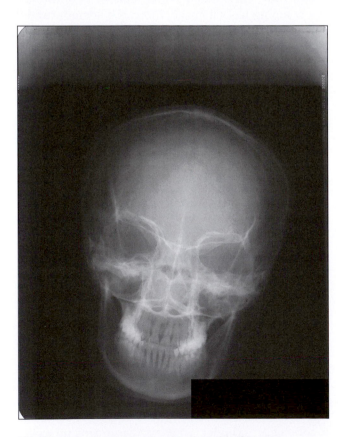

FIGURE 11.10   Frontal image with tilt positioning error.

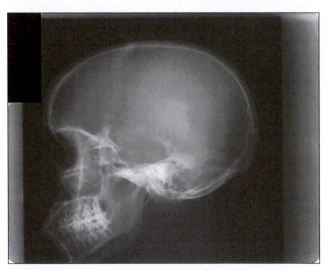

FIGURE 11.12   Lateral image with no positioning errors.

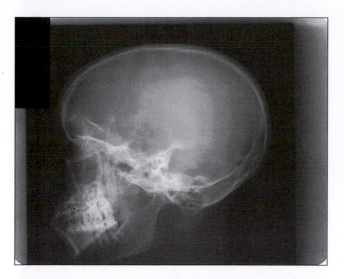

FIGURE 11.13   Lateral image with tilt positioning error.

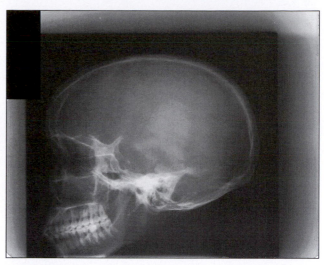

FIGURE 11.14   Lateral image with rotation positioning error.

the visibility of cranial structures while minimizing radiation exposure to areas surrounding the anatomy of interest.

Film Size

Normally the entire skull can be examined on a 10 × 12 inch (25 × 30 cm) film. Select the smallest film that would reasonably accommodate the size of the desired anatomy. In addition, when available equipment permits, two bilateral images may be placed on one appropriately sized film.

Review Questions

1. A cranial shape described as long and narrow is classified as:
   a. brachycephalic
   b. caudalcephalic
   c. dolichocephalic
   d. mesocephalic

2. Motion of the head along the longitudinal axis describes what positioning error?
   a. rotation
   b. tilt

3. When performing radiography of the head, a thin patient in the prone position can be made more comfortable by placing a small sponge under the:
   a. abdomen
   b. chest
   c. knees
   d. occiput

4. During skull radiography, the long axis of the patient's head and body should be aligned to be parallel with the midline of the table.
   a. true
   b. false

5. Because pediatric patients typically have an adult size skull, adjustments in positioning the skull are not necessary.
   a. true
   b. false

6. On a frontal projection, unequal distance between the midline of the anatomical part and the edge of the skull describes rotation.
   a. true
   b. false

7. It is not possible to get comparable skull radiographs when obtained in the recumbent versus the erect position.
   a. true
   b. false

8. It is best to use facial features to align structures during positioning of the skull.
   a. true
   b. false

9. Although skulls vary somewhat in size and shape, the relationship of internal structures does not vary.
   a. true
   b. false

10. State at least one advantage of performing skull radiography in the erect position.

11. Describe the location of the following cranial landmarks.
    a. EAM
    b. infraorbital margin
    c. acanthion

12. On the following photographs (Figures 11.15 and 11.16), write the correct name of the cranial landmark, line, or plane next to the letter.

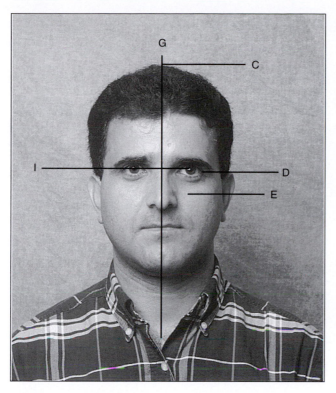

FIGURE 11.15   Frontal view.

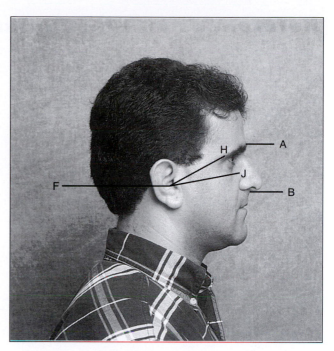

FIGURE 11.16   Lateral view.

References and Recommended Reading

Ballinger, P. W. (1995). *Merrill's atlas of radiographic positions and radiologic procedures* (8th ed.). St. Louis: Mosby-Year Book.

Bontrager, K. L. (1997). *Textbook of radiographic positioning and related anatomy* (4th ed.). St. Louis: Mosby-Year Book.

Eisenberg, R. L., Dennis, C. A., & May, C.R. (1995). *Radiographic positioning* (2nd ed.). Boston: Little, Brown.

CHAPTER 12

Basic Skull Positions/Projections

LINDA CROUCHER, MS, RT(R)(ARRT)

ANATOMY

Frontal Bone
Parietal Bones
Occipital Bone
Temporal Bones
Sphenoid Bone
Ethmoid Bone
Cranial Joints
Maxillae
Zygomatic Bones
Mandible
Nasal Bones
Lacrimal Bones
Palatine Bones
Vomer
Inferior Nasal Conchae

Orbit
Paranasal Sinuses

POSITIONING GUIDELINES

Erect Versus Recumbent
Rationale
Basic Projections/Positions

SKULL—ROUTINE POSITIONS/PROJECTIONS

Axial AP (Townes/Grashey)
PA (and Caldwell)
Lateral
Submentovertical (basilar)
Parietoacanthial (Waters)

SPECIAL CONSIDERATIONS

Correlative Imaging

OBJECTIVES

At the completion of this chapter, the student should be able to:

1. List and describe the bony anatomy of the skull.

2. List and describe the paranasal sinuses.

3. Given drawings and radiographs, locate anatomic structures.

4. Explain the general rationale for each of the five basic projections.

5. Discuss how the five basic projections form the basis for all cranial examinations.

6. Describe the basic positioning used to visualize anatomic structures of the skull.

7. List or identify the central ray location for each projection.

8. Given radiographs, evaluate positioning.

9. Describe modifications of procedures for atypical patients to better demonstrate the anatomic area of interest.

Anatomy

The skull contains twenty-two bones subdivided into cranial bones and facial bones (Color illustration 2). The eight cranial bones, which enclose and protect the brain, are the frontal, parietal (two), temporal (two), sphenoid, occipital, and ethmoid.

FRONTAL BONE (ONE)

This bone forms the forehead, the anterior portion of the cranial vault, the roof of the orbits, and a large part of the anterior portion of the cranial floor (Figures 12.1 and 12.2, 12.3 and 12.5). The frontal bone has the following features:

- *Supraorbital margin*—described in Chapter 11
- *Frontal sinuses*—found in the anterior frontal bone and discussed later in this chapter
- *Superciliary arches*—described in Chapter 11
- *Glabella*—described in Chapter 11

PARIETAL (pă-rī´ĕ-tăl) BONES (TWO)

These bones form most of the sides of the cranium and the cranial vault. They are located posterior to

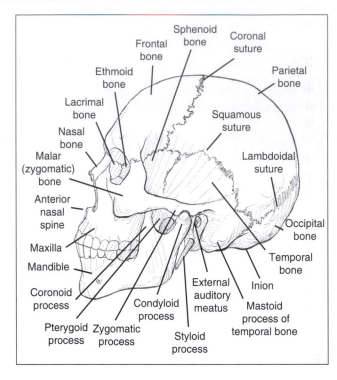

FIGURE 12.2 Skull, lateral view.

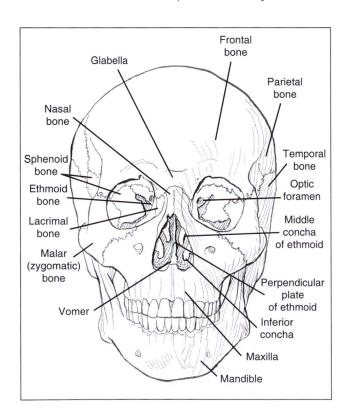

FIGURE 12.1 Skull, anterior view.

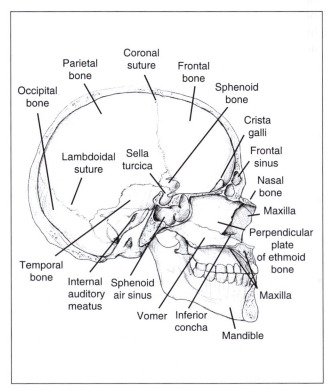

FIGURE 12.3 Skull, medial view.

the frontal bone (see Figures 12.1, 12.2, 12.3). Each articulates with the opposite parietal, the frontal bone, the occipital bone, the temporal bones, and the sphenoid bone.

OCCIPITAL (ŏk-sĭp´ĭ-tăl) BONE (ONE)

This bone forms the posterior part of the cranial vault and most of the posterior portion of the cranial floor (Figures 12.2 through 12.5). The occipital bone has the following features:

- *Foramen magnum*—large opening in the inferior portion of the occipital bone (see Figures 12.4 and 12.5) through which the spinal cord enters the cranial cavity
- *Occipital condyles*—oval processes located lateral and anterior to the foramen magnum (see Figure 12.4). They articulate with the first cervical vertebra to form the occipitoatlantal joints
- *External occipital protuberance (inion)*—a prominent projection on the posterior surface located slightly superior to the foramen magnum (see Figure 12.2)

TEMPORAL BONES (TWO)

These bones form the inferior portion of the sides of the cranium and part of the cranial floor between the sphenoid and occipital bones (see Figures 12.1 through 12.5). Features of the temporal bones include:

- *Zygomatic (zī´´gō-măt´ĭk) process*—a projection from the anterior part of the temporal bone that articulates with the zygomatic bone to form the zygomatic arch (see Figure 12.2)
- *Mandibular fossa*—depression found at the base of the zygomatic process that articulates with the mandibular condyle to form the temporomandibular joint
- *Petrous portion (**petrous pyramid**, pars petrosa)*—very dense bone, triangular in shape, that contains the structures of the middle and inner ear. The sharp superior edge is called the petrous ridge (see Figure 12.5)
- *Mastoid process*—prominent projection found posterior and inferior to the external auditory meatus (see Figure 12.2). It contains the mastoid air cells
- *Styloid processes*—slender pieces of bone that project downward from the inferior surface of the temporal bone just anterior to the mastoid processes (see Figures 12.2 and 12.4)
- *External auditory meatus (EAM)*—described in Chapter 11 (see Figure 12.2)

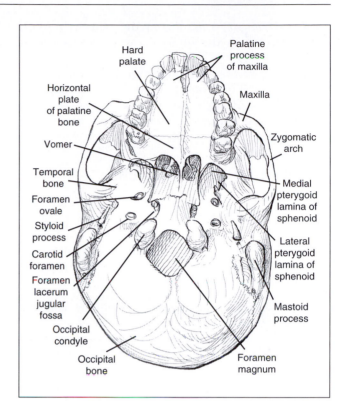

FIGURE 12.4   Skull, basal view.

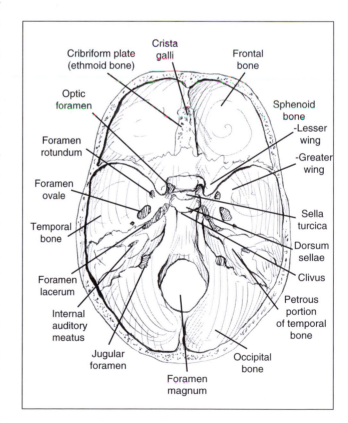

FIGURE 12.5   Skull, view from above.

- *Carotid foramen*—opening in the petrous portion through which the internal carotid artery travels (Figure 12.4)
- *Jugular foramen*—opening found in the suture between the petrous portion and the occipital bone through which the internal jugular vein and the ninth, tenth, and eleventh cranial nerves pass (see Figure 12.5)

SPHENOID (sfē´noyd) BONE (ONE)

This bone forms the portion of the cranial floor anterior to the temporal bones and posterior to the frontal bone. It is called the keystone of the cranial floor because it articulates with all other cranial bones. (Figures 12.2 through 12.7). Features of the sphenoid bone include:

- *Body*—the central portion of the bone that contains the sphenoid sinuses
- *Greater wings*—the large lateral projections from the body that form most of the posterior wall of the

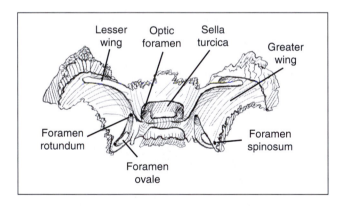

FIGURE 12.6   Sphenoid, superior view.

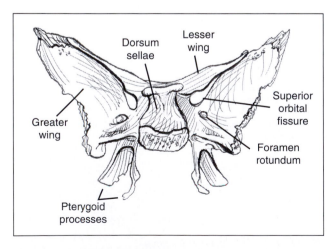

FIGURE 12.7   Sphenoid, posterior view.

orbit and a portion of the floor and sides of the cranium (see Figures 12.6 and 12.7)

- *Lesser wings*—smaller lateral projections from the superior surface of the body. They also form a portion of the posterior wall of the orbit (see Figures 12.6 and 12.7).
- *Sella turcica* (sĕl´ă tŭr´sĭ-kă)—saddle-shaped, centrally located depression on the superior surface of the body that houses the pituitary gland (hypophysis) (see Figures 12.3, 12.6, and 12.7). The posterior wall is formed by the dorsum sellae. Just posterior to the base of the dorsum sellae is a depression called the clivus (klī´vŭs), which is continuous with a similar groove at the base of the occipital bone. On the superior portion of the dorsum sellae are two lateral projections called the posterior clinoid (clī´noyd) processes.
- *Pterygoid processes* (tĕr´ĭ-goyd prŏs´ĕs-ēz)—processes that project downward from where the greater wings meet the body. They form a portion of the lateral wall of the nasal cavity (see Figures 12.4 and 12.7).
- *Optic foramen*—opening through the base of the lesser wing through which the optic nerve and the ophthalmic nerve pass (see Figures 12.5 and 12.6)
- *Inferior orbital fissure*—opening found between the greater wing of the sphenoid and the maxilla that transmits the infraorbital and zygomatic nerves and the infraorbital vessels
- *Superior orbital fissure*—slit-like opening found between the greater and lesser wings lateral to the optic foramen (see Figure 12.7)
- *Foramen rotundum*—opening found just posterior and medial to the superior orbital fissure at the base of the greater wing (see Figures 12.5 and 12.6)
- *Foramen ovale* (for-ā´mĕn ō´văl)—opening at the base of the greater wing found posterior and lateral to the foramen rotundum (see Figures 12.4 and 12.6)
- *Foramen spinosum*—small opening found posterior and lateral to the foramen ovale (see Figure 12.6)
- *Foramen lacerum* (for-ā´mĕn lă-sĕr´ŭm)—large, irregular-shaped opening found posterior and lateral to the posterior clinoid process and medial to the foramen ovale (see Figures 12.4 and 12.5)

ETHMOID (ĕth´moyd) BONE (ONE)

This light, spongy bone forms a part of the anterior cranial floor, the medial wall of the orbits, the superior portion of the nasal septum, and the lateral walls of the nasal cavity. It is located between the orbits and is inferior to the frontal bone (see Figures 12.1, 12.2, 12.5, and 12.8). Features of this bone include:

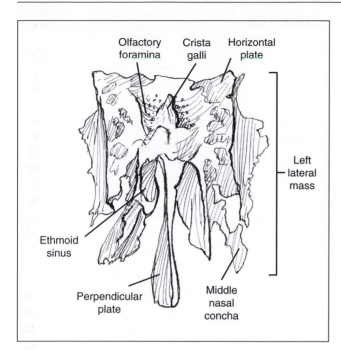

Olfactory foramina   Crista galli   Horizontal plate

Left lateral mass

Ethmoid sinus

Perpendicular plate

Middle nasal concha

FIGURE 12.8   Ethmoid, anterior view.

- *Horizontal (cribiform) plate*—transverse portion of the ethmoid that forms the roof of the nasal cavity (see Figure 12.8). The olfactory nerves pass through the many openings in it.
- *Lateral masses (labyrinths)*—project downward from the lateral borders of the horizontal plate (see Figure 12.8). Forms the medial walls of the nasal cavity and contains the air cells that make up the ethmoidal sinuses.
- *Perpendicular plate*—projects downward from the midline of the horizontal plate forming the superior part of the nasal septum (see Figure 12.3).
- *Crista galli*—triangular process that projects superiorly from the horizontal plate (see Figures 12.3, 12.5, and 12.8).
- *Superior and middle nasal conchae (turbinates)*—scroll-like projections that extend medially from the inner surfaces of the lateral masses (see Figure 12.1). They aid in cleansing and warming inhaled air.

CRANIAL JOINTS

The joints between the bones of the skull are immovable and are called **sutures**. They tend to disappear with advancing age.

- *Sagittal suture*—located midline where the parietal bones meet superiorly
- *Coronal suture*—located between the parietal bones and the frontal bone (see Figures 12.2 and 12.3)

- *Lambdoid suture* (lăm´doyd sū´chūr)—located between the parietal bones and the occipital bone (see Figures 12.2 and 12.3)
- *Squamous suture* (skwā´mŭs sū´chūr)—where the parietal and temporal bones meet (see Figure 12.2)
- *Sutural (wormian) bones*—occasionally found within the sutures
- *Bregma* (brĕg´mă)—point where the coronal suture and the sagittal suture meet
- *Lambda* (lăm´dă)—point where the lambdoid suture and the sagittal suture meet

There are fourteen immovable facial bones that help shape the face. These bones are fully developed by age 16. The facial bones are composed of the maxillae (two), the zygomatic (two), the mandible (one), the vomer (one), the inferior nasal conchae (two), the nasal (two), the palatine (two), and the lacrimal (two).

MAXILLAE (măk sĭ´lē) (TWO)

These bones make up the upper jaw. They form a portion of the floor of the orbit, part of the floor and lateral border of the nasal cavity, and the anterior portion of the hard palate (see Figures 12.1 and 12.2). They articulate with every facial bone except the mandible. Features of these bones include:

- *Alveolar* (ăl-vē´ō´lăr) *process*—inferior portion that contains the sockets that accommodate the upper teeth
- *Maxillary sinus (antrum of Highmore)*—large air-filled cavities within the bodies of the maxillae (discussed later)
- *Palatine process*—forms the anterior portion of the hard palate (see Figure 12.4)
- *Anterior nasal spine*—small pointed process found immediately below the nasal cavity where the two maxillae articulate with each other (see Figure 12.2)

ZYGOMATIC (MALAR) (zī´´gō-măt´ĭk) BONES (TWO)

These bones make up the cheek bone. They also form a portion of the floor and lateral wall of the orbit (see Figures 12.1, 12.2, and 12.4).

- *Temporal process*—part that projects posteriorly and articulates with the zygomatic process of the temporal bone. Together these two processes form the zygomatic arch.

MANDIBLE (ONE)

This bone of the lower jaw is the largest, strongest, and only movable bone in the skull (see Figures 12.1, 12.2, and 12.3). Features of this bone include:

- *Body*—curved, horizontal portion that forms the chin
- *Ramus*—process that projects upward from the posterior, lateral margin of the body
- *Mandibular condyle*—superior border of the ramus that articulates with the mandibular fossa of the temporal bone to form the temporomandibular joint
- *Coronoid process*—triangular process that projects upward and slightly forward from the anterior surface of the ramus
- *Mandibular symphysis*—where the two halves of the mandible are fused at midline
- *Alveolar process*—superior portion that contains the sockets that accommodate the lower teeth
- *Mandibular angle (gonion)*—sharp curve where the ramus meets the body

NASAL BONES (TWO)

These small bones are fused at the midline of the face to form the upper portion of the bridge of the nose (see Figures 12.1, 12.2, and 12.3). The majority of the nose is composed of cartilage.

LACRIMAL (lăk´rĭm-ăl) BONES (TWO)

These bones are found posterior and lateral to the nasal bones (see Figures 12.1 and 12.2). Each forms a part of the medial wall of the orbit and a part of the nasal cavity.

PALATINE (păl´ă-tĭn) BONES (TWO)

These bones form the posterior portion of the hard palate, a portion of the nasal cavity, and a portion of the floor of the orbit (see Figure 12.4). They resemble the letter "L."

- *Horizontal plate*—articulates with the palatine process of the maxillae to form the hard palate

VOMER (ONE)

This triangular-shaped bone forms the inferior, posterior portion of the bony nasal septum (see Figures 12.3 and 12.4).

INFERIOR NASAL CONCHAE (kŏng´kē) (TURBINATES)

These are scroll-like bones projecting medially from the lateral borders of the nasal cavity (see Figures 12.1 and 12.2). They are located immediately inferior to the middle nasal conchae of the ethmoid bone.

ORBIT

This pyramid-shaped socket contains the eyeball and its associated structures (Figure 12.9). It is composed of the following bones:

- *Roof*—portions of the frontal bone and sphenoid bones
- *Lateral wall*—portions of the zygomatic and sphenoid bones
- *Medial wall*—portions of the maxillae, lacrimal, ethmoid, and sphenoid bones
- *Floor*—portions of the maxillae, zygomatic, and palatine bones

The openings in the orbit have been discussed previously.

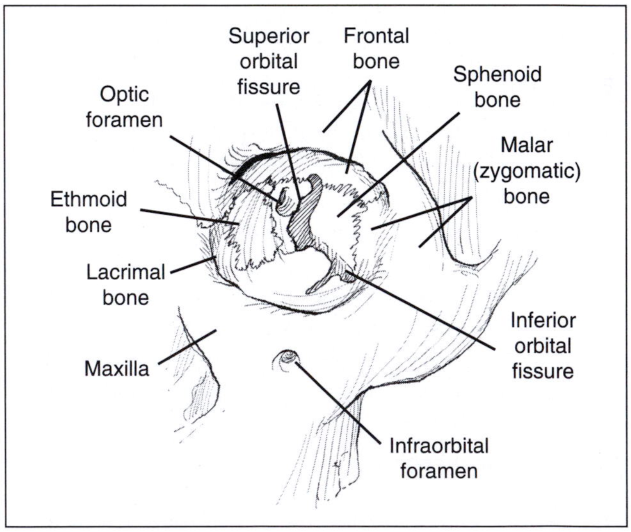

FIGURE 12.9   Orbit.

PARANASAL SINUSES

The paranasal sinuses are cavities contained within certain cranial and facial bones that are lined with mucous membranes. These cavities enlarge during childhood and adolescence and their sizes vary in adults. The sinuses communicate with the nasal cavity; therefore, secretions produced by the sinuses drain into the nasal cavity. Functions of the sinuses include: produce mucus, lighten the skull bones, add resonance to the voice, and help warm and humidify inspired air before it enters the lungs (Figures 12.10 and 12.11). There are four groups of paranasal sinuses.

Sphenoid Sinuses

This pair of sinuses is within the body of the sphenoid bone, one on each side of midline. The septum that separates the two is usually not found in the midline, making one side larger than the other. They extend backward under the sella turcica. Very small at birth, they develop largely after puberty and vary in size from person to person.

Maxillary Sinuses

These pyramid-shaped, paired cavities are found in the body of the maxillae. They, along with the sphenoid sinuses, are present at birth. The roof of the

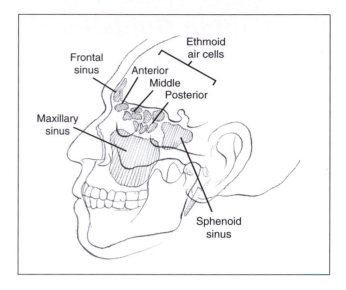

FIGURE 12.11   Sinuses, lateral view.

maxillary sinus is the floor of the orbit. It is relatively thin and if fractured can allow contents of the orbit to bulge down into the sinus. The medial wall of the sinus forms a portion of the lateral wall of the nasal cavity. The floor of the sinus is the alveolar process of the maxilla and roots of the upper teeth can be found projecting into the sinus. Inflammatory processes of the teeth can transmit inflammation to the sinus.

Frontal Sinuses

These are found at the medial end of the superciliary arches. There are two cavities separated by a septum that is rarely found at midline, causing one side to be larger than the other. They can also be separated into several intercommunicating portions. They are absent at birth and reach full size after puberty. The frontal sinuses vary greatly in size and shape in adults and may be absent.

Ethmoidal Sinuses

These are small, numerous air cells in the ethmoidal labyrinth located between the orbit and the nasal cavity. They are divided into anterior, middle, and posterior cavities. They begin to develop at birth. They, too, vary greatly in size and number in adults. Because the ethmoid and sphenoid sinuses are so closely associated, it is difficult to differentiate them.

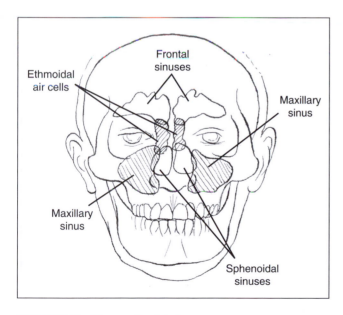

FIGURE 12.10   Sinuses, frontal view.

Positioning Guidelines

ERECT VERSUS RECUMBENT

Because of space constraints, the projections/positions of the skull will be demonstrated in *either* the upright or recumbent position. These projections can easily be performed in either position by maintaining the baselines and central rays described (Figures 12.12 and 12.13).

RATIONALE

Radiographic examinations of the cranium are used in trauma cases for determination of fractures. The sutures are observed for symmetry to differentiate normal sutures and fractures. The sinuses are evaluated for fluid, which could indicate possible fractures. One type of orbit fracture is called a "blowout" frac-

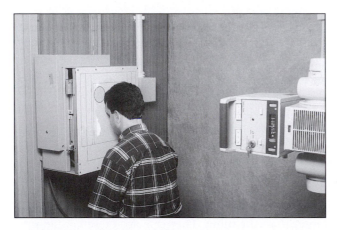

FIGURE 12.12   PA, erect.

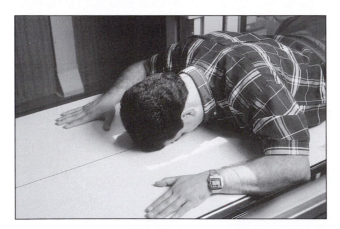

FIGURE 12.13   PA, recumbent.

ture. This occurs when the eye is struck from the front causing a fracture in the floor of the orbit, thus allowing the orbital contents to herniate through the fracture; surgical correction is usually required.

These examinations can also be used to detect **meningiomas**, to visualize thickening of the bone, and to detect metastatic disease. In children, these examinations can be used to demonstrate premature closure of sutures and to confirm suspected cases of child abuse.

Because of the curved shape of the mandible, it is not optimally demonstrated in any one projection. A complete examination includes several projections. Most fractures of the mandibular body and symphysis can be diagnosed clinically due to misalignment of the teeth; however, radiographs are necessary to determine the presence of multiple fractures. These examinations are also used to determine the presence and location of foreign bodies, dental tumors, and noncancerous abnormalities such as Paget's disease, fibrous dysplasia, and neurofibromatosis.

Temporal bone examinations are commonly performed to demonstrate inflammatory changes. Again, because of the location of the mastoid air cells, multiple projections are required. They are evaluated for symmetry of development and aeration, abnormal **sclerosis**, or bony destruction.

BASIC PROJECTIONS/POSITIONS

The table lists the basic projections/positions used in a variety of examinations of the skull and facial bones. These projections form the basis for nearly all examinations. The patient and part positioning and the baselines remain consistent throughout the various examinations. However, there are slight variations in centering. For instance, the patient is positioned with midsagittal parallel and interpupillary perpendicular to the film for all lateral projections. However, the centering point for a lateral skull is 2 inches (5 cm) superior to the EAM, for a lateral of the facial bones it is the zygoma, for sinuses it is 1 inch (3 cm) posterior to the outer canthus, and for the sella turcica it is 3/4 inch (2 cm) superior and 3/4 inch (2 cm) inferior to the EAM.

Mastery of these basic positions will give the radiographer the ability to proficiently perform a variety of cranial examinations.

ROUTINE POSITIONS/PROJECTIONS

AXIAL AP (TOWNE/GRASHEY) PROJECTION

Exam Rationale This projection demonstrates trauma or metastatic or other disease processes in examinations of the cranium, the zygomatic arches, the mandible, the temporomandibular joints, the temporal bones, and the sella turcica. The projection demonstrates a symmetrical view of the petrous portions of the temporal bone. The dorsum sella and posterior clinoids will be seen within the foramen magnum. The occipital bone is demonstrated and the lambdoidal and sagittal sutures are visualized.

Patient Position AP position with the chin tucked (Figure 12.14).

Part Position Chin depressed to place OML perpendicular to the film; MSP is perpendicular to the film to avoid rotation or tilt.

Central Ray 30° caudal angle; entrance or exit points vary depending on the examination/anatomy to be demonstrated.

Evaluation Criteria (Figures 12.15 and 12.16)

- The specific anatomy to be demonstrated should be well visualized.
- The petrous ridges should be symmetrical.
- The distance from the lateral border of the foramen magnum to the lateral border of the cranium should be equal on each side to demonstrate the absence of rotation.

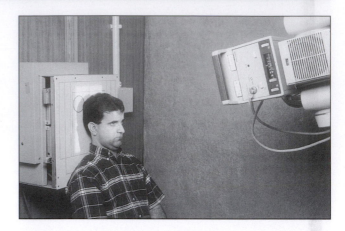

FIGURE 12.14   Axial AP (Towne/Grashey).

Tip If the patient is unable to depress the chin enough to place the OML perpendicular to the film, the IOML should be perpendicular to the film. The angle of the central ray is increased to 37°.

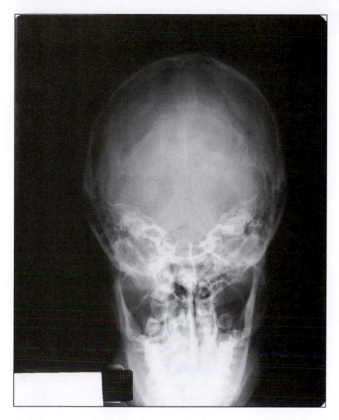

FIGURE 12.15   **Axial AP (Towne/Grashey).**

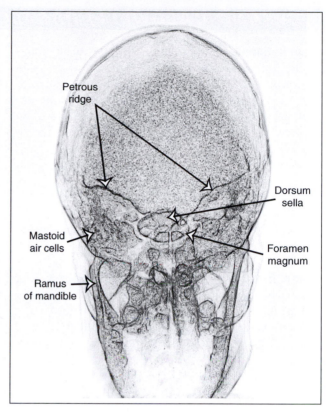

FIGURE 12.16   **Axial AP (Towne/Grashey).**

PA (AND CALDWELL) PROJECTION

Exam Rationale   Examinations of the facial bones, orbits, and sinuses use this projection/method for the determination of fractures and disease processes. Structures that may be demonstrated include the frontal bone, nasal septum, zygomatic bones, orbital rim, and the frontal and ethmoid sinuses.

Patient Position   PA position with the forehead and nose touching the cassette holder (Figure 12.17).

Part Position   MSP perpendicular to the film to avoid rotation or tilt; flexion of the neck adjusted to place OML perpendicular to the film.

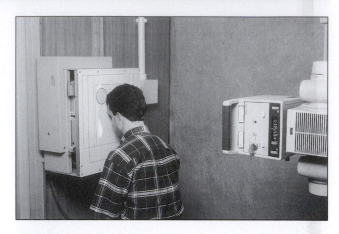

FIGURE 12.17   PA.

Central Ray   If the frontal bone is of primary interest, a perpendicular central ray is used. To visualize the orbital structures without petrous ridge obstruction, the central ray is angled 15° caudally (Caldwell method). Entrance and exit points will depend on the anatomy to be demonstrated (Figure 12.18).

Evaluation Criteria (Figures 12.19 through 12.22)

- Equal distance from the lateral border of the orbit to the lateral border of the skull on each side confirms the absence of rotation.
- Petrous portion of the temporal bone fills the orbit when a perpendicular central ray is used.
- With the Caldwell method, the petrous ridges are demonstrated in the lower third of the orbit.

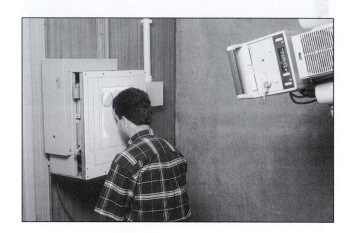

FIGURE 12.18   PA Caldwell.

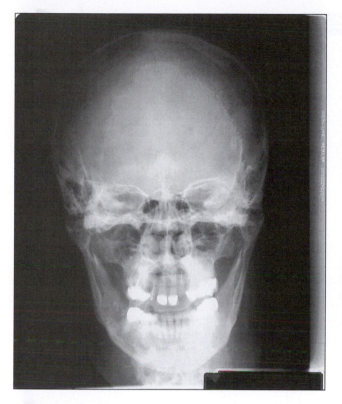

FIGURE 12.19   PA.

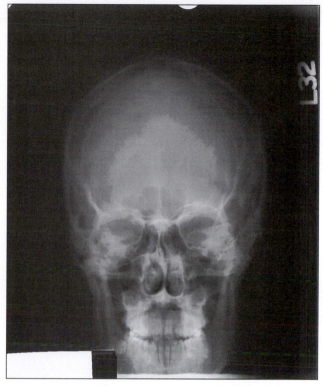

FIGURE 12.21   PA Caldwell.

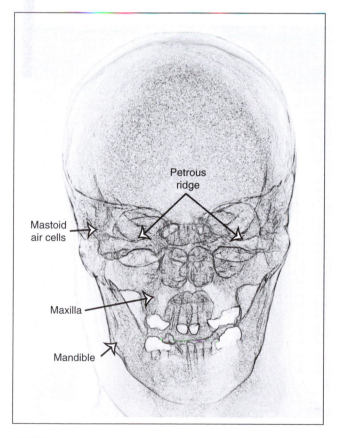

FIGURE 12.20   PA.

Petrous ridge

Mastoid air cells

Maxilla

Mandible

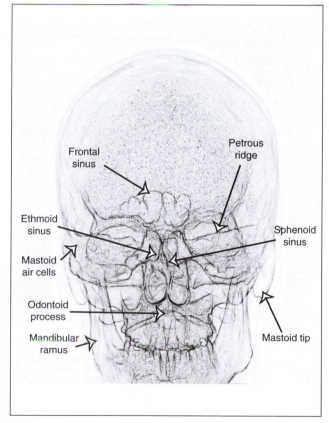

FIGURE 12.22   PA Caldwell.

Frontal sinus

Petrous ridge

Ethmoid sinus

Mastoid air cells

Sphenoid sinus

Odontoid process

Mandibular ramus

Mastoid tip

LATERAL POSITION

Exam Rationale The lateral position is used in examinations of the cranium, facial bones, nasal bones, sinuses, and sella turcica. Adaptations of the lateral position incorporating rotation, tilt, or central ray angles are used to demonstrate the mandible, temporomandibular joints, and temporal bones. As with the other positions/projections, it is used to detect fractures and disease processes.

Patient Position Positioning of the patient depends on the equipment used. With a head unit, the film holder can usually be placed above the shoulder with the patient facing forward (Figure 12.23). At an upright Bucky or recumbent on the table, for patient comfort and ease of positioning, the patient should be placed in an RAO or LAO position placing the side of the head against the holder (Figure 12.24). The trauma patient is usually radiographed in the supine position with a horizontal beam (see Chapter 14).

Part Position MSP parallel to the cassette; interpupillary line perpendicular to the cassette; IOML parallel to the transverse axis of the cassette.

Central Ray Perpendicular to the film; entrance or exit points depend on the anatomy to be demonstrated.

Evaluation Criteria (Figures 12.25 and 12.26)

- Structures to be demonstrated should be well visualized.
- Mandibular rami and orbital roofs should be superimposed to confirm the absence of rotation or tilt.

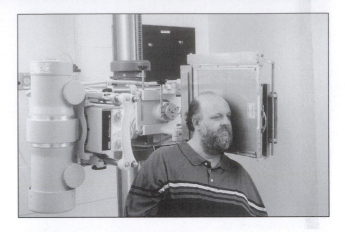

FIGURE 12.23   Lateral at head unit.

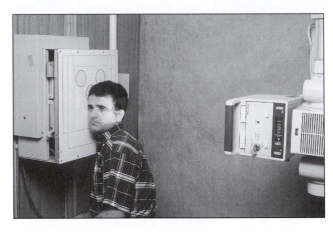

FIGURE 12.24   Lateral at upright Bucky.

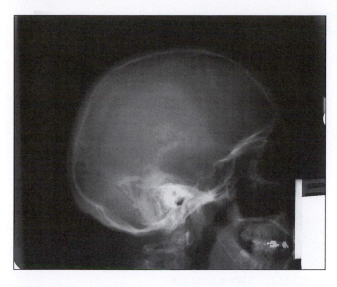

FIGURE 12.25   Lateral.

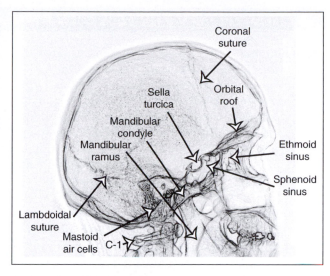

FIGURE 12.26   Lateral.

SUBMENTOVERTICAL (BASILAR) (SMV) PROJECTION

Exam Rationale This projection demonstrates the base of the skull and is known as the basal or basilar projection. It demonstrates fractures and disease processes in examinations of the cranium, zygomatic arches, paranasal sinuses, and temporal bones. It also demonstrates such structures as the petrous pyramids, the mastoid processes, basal foramina, the mandible, the foramen magnum, the occipital bone, and the sphenoid and ethmoid sinuses.

Patient Position The use of the head unit greatly facilitates the ease of positioning the patient for this projection. For patients who have limited extension of the neck, the Bucky can be angled to allow the vertex to rest on the film. If the equipment does not allow angulation of the cassette, the patient should extend the neck as much as possible if in an erect position (Figure 12.27). If in a recumbent position, sponges or pillows can be placed under the shoulders to allow for extension (Figure 12.28).

Part Position MSP perpendicular to the film to alleviate rotation or tilt; IOML parallel to the film.

Central Ray Perpendicular to the IOML. If the patient is unable to place IOML parallel to the film, it is important that the central ray be angled to place it perpendicular to IOML. The entrance point will depend on the anatomy to be demonstrated.

Evaluation Criteria (Figures 12.29 and 12.30)

- Appropriate structures should be well demonstrated.
- Mandibular symphysis should superimpose the anterior frontal bone to indicate adequate extension of the neck or tube angle.
- To confirm the absence of rotation, the distance from the mandibular condyles to the lateral border of the skull should be equal on both sides.

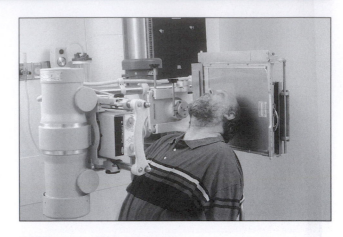

FIGURE 12.27   SMV at head unit.

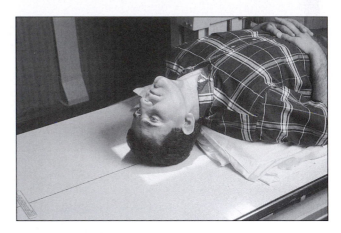

FIGURE 12.28   SMV recumbent.

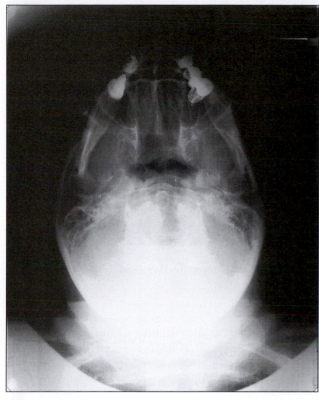

FIGURE 12.29   SMV.

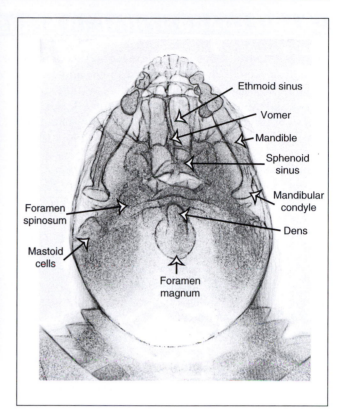

FIGURE 12.30   SMV.

PARIETOACANTHIAL (WATERS) PROJECTION

Exam Rationale   This projection is used to demonstrate fractures or disease processes in examinations of the facial bones, nasal bones, orbits, and paranasal sinuses. Demonstrated anatomy includes the orbital floor, the bony nasal septum, and the maxillary sinuses.

Patient Position   PA with the chin touching the Bucky; the nose does not touch the Bucky (Figure 12.31).

Part Position   Film is centered to the acanthion; the MSP is perpendicular to the film to avoid rotation or tilt; extension of the neck is adjusted to place OML at a 37° angle to the plane of the film.

Central Ray   Perpendicular to the plane of the film exiting at the acanthion.

Evaluation Criteria (Figures 12.32 through 12.35)

- Petrous ridges should be projected immediately below the maxillary sinuses.
- Increased extension of the head will demonstrate the petrous ridges well below the maxillary sinuses causing distortion of the sinuses.
- Decreased extension will place the petrous ridges within the maxillary sinuses.
- The absence of rotation is demonstrated by an equal distance from the orbit to the lateral border of the skull on each side.

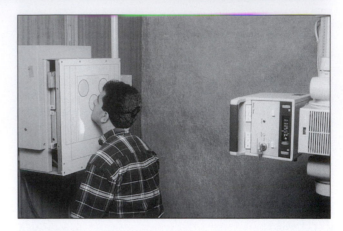

FIGURE 12.31   Parietoacanthial (Waters).

Tip   Hints such as the distance of the nose from the film and perpendicular MML are sometimes offered, but it is best to use an "angligner," a "skull protractor," or other degree-calibrated accessory to ensure consistently accurate positioning.

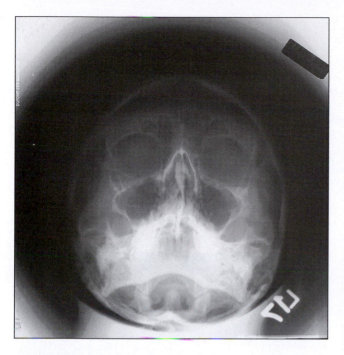

FIGURE 12.32   Parietoacanthial (Waters).

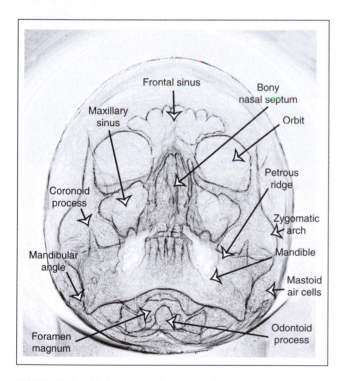

FIGURE 12.33   Parietoacanthial (Waters).

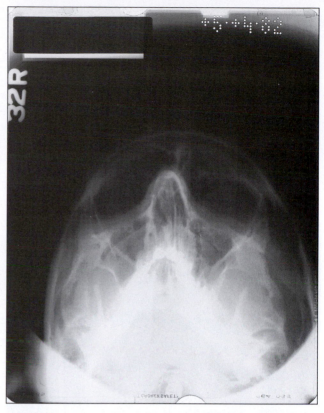

FIGURE 12.34   Parietoacanthial (Waters) with overextension.

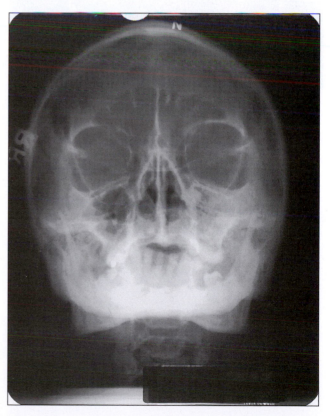

FIGURE 12.35   Parietoacanthial (Waters) with underextension.

Special Considerations

CORRELATIVE IMAGING

Conventional radiography of the skull is now primarily performed to detect the effects of trauma and confirm the presence of certain disease processes such as inflammation (e.g., **sinusitis**) and bony abnormalities such as **Paget's (păj´ĕt) disease**. However, disease processes of the brain and abnormalities of the brain due to trauma are better evaluated by CT and MRI. CT frequently is the examination of choice in suspected cases of **subdural** or **epidural hematomas** and intracranial **hemorrhage** (Figure 12.36). MRI has become the preferred method to demonstrate central nervous system diseases such as **multiple sclerosis** and **Alzheimer's disease**, tumors, and abnormalities of the posterior fossa and the brainstem (Figure 12.37).

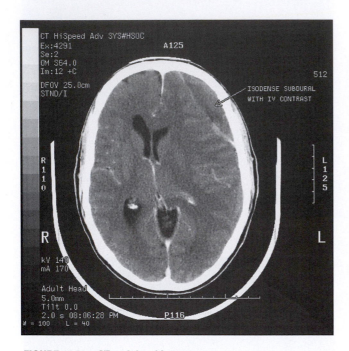

FIGURE 12.36   CT, subdural hematoma.

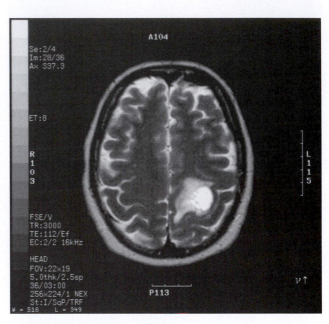

FIGURE 12.37   MRI, tumor.

Review Questions

1. The sagittal suture joins the _____ bones of the skull.

   a. temporal
   b. frontal
   c. parietal
   d. occipital

2. The _____ bone articulates with the vertebral column.

   a. temporal
   b. parietal
   c. mandible
   d. occipital

3. The _____ bone contains the inner ear.

   a. temporal
   b. sphenoid
   c. occipital
   d. ethmoid

4. The central ray for an axial AP projection of the skull uses what angle?

   a. perpendicular
   b. 30° caudal to the OML
   c. 30° caudal to the IOML
   d. 30° caudal to the glabellomeatal line

5. When performing a PA projection of the skull, the _____ line should be perpendicular to the film.

   a. glabellomeatal
   b. OML
   c. IOML
   d. acanthiomeatal

6. In which of the following projections would the midsagittal plane be parallel to the film?

   1. PA
   2. parietoacanthial
   3. axial AP
   4. lateral
   a. 1 only
   b. 4 only
   c. 1 and 2
   d. 1, 3, and 4

7. On a PA projection of the skull with a perpendicular central ray, the petrous ridges will be demonstrated :

   a. filling the orbital shadow
   b. in the lower third of the maxillary sinuses
   c. immediately below the maxillary sinuses
   d. significantly below the maxillary sinuses

8. On a properly positioned parietoacanthial (Waters) view, the petrous ridges:

   a. fill the orbital shadows
   b. are projected in the lower half of the maxillary sinuses
   c. are projected immediately below the maxillary sinuses
   d. are projected significantly below the maxillary sinuses

9. The routine submentovertical projection places the _____ line parallel to the film.

   a. glabelloalveolar
   b. OML
   c. IOML
   d. acanthiomeatal

10. When performing the parietoacanthial view, the OML is placed at an angle of _____ to the plane of the film.

    a. 25
    b. 30
    c. 37
    d. 45

11. The PA Caldwell with a 15° caudal angle will demonstrate the petrous ridges:

    a. filling the orbital shadow
    b. in the lower third of the orbital shadow
    c. in the lower third of the maxillary sinuses
    d. immediately below the maxillary sinuses

12. Although the centering point varies, positioning is the same for both a lateral skull and lateral facial bones.

    a. true
    b. false

13. When performing an axial AP projection of the skull in cases where the patient cannot depress the chin enough to place the OML perpendicular to the film, a comparable image can be obtained by increasing the usual caudal angle.

a. true
b. false

14. When properly positioned, the parietoacanthial projection will project the petrous ridges within the maxillary sinuses.

a. true
b. false

15. The mandibular rami would be superimposed on a properly positioned lateral of the cranium.

a. true
b. false

16. The submentovertical projection uses a central ray that is perpendicular to the IOML.

a. true
b. false

17. Name the two major bones on either side of the squamous suture; the coronal suture.

18. What bone contains the foramen magnum?

19. What is the name of the point where the coronal and sagittal sutures meet?

20. Which cranial/facial bones contain the paranasal sinuses?

21. List at least two functions of the sinuses.

22. Name the bone that transmits the olfactory nerves that convey the sense of smell.

23. Name the only movable facial bone.

24. Portions of what two bones form the zygomatic arch?

25. What bone contains the sella turcica?

References and Recommended Reading

Anthony, C., & Thibodeau, G. (1983). *Textbook of anatomy and physiology* (11th ed.) St. Louis: Mosby.

Ballinger, P. W. (1995). *Merrill's atlas of radiographic positions and radiologic procedures* (8th ed.) St. Louis: Mosby Year-Book.

Basmajian, J. (1982). *H. A. Cates' Primary anatomy* (8th ed.) Baltimore: Waverly Press.

Bontrager, K. L. (1993). *Textbook of radiographic positioning and related anatomy* (3rd ed.) St. Louis: Mosby-Year Book.

Mader, S. (1994). *Understanding human anatomy & physiology* (2nd ed.) Dubuque, IA: Wm. C. Brown.

Moore, K. (1980). *Clinically oriented anatomy.* Baltimore: Waverly Press.

Rogers, A. (1992). *Textbook of anatomy.* New York: Churchill Livingstone.

Ryan, S. P., & McNicholas, M. M. J. (1994). *Anatomy for diagnostic imaging.* Philadelphia: Saunders.

Spence, A. (1990). *Basic human anatomy* (3rd ed.) Redwood City, CA: Benjamin/Cummings.

CHAPTER 13

Skull and Facial Bones

LINDA CROUCHER, MS, RT(R)(ARRT)

SKULL—ROUTINE POSITIONS/PROJECTIONS

Axial AP
PA
Lateral
Submentovertical

FACIAL BONES (SURVEY)—ROUTINE POSITIONS/ PROJECTIONS

PA (Caldwell)
Parietoacanthial (Waters)
Lateral

NASAL BONES—ROUTINE POSITIONS/ PROJECTIONS

PA Caldwell
Parietoacanthial (Waters)
Lateral
Superoinferior (axial)

ORBITS—ROUTINE POSITIONS/PROJECTIONS

PA
Modified Parietoacanthial (Modified Waters)
Lateral
Parieto-orbital Oblique (Rhese)

ORBITS—ALTERNATE POSITIONS/PROJECTIONS

Orbitoparietal Oblique (Reverse Rhese)

ZYGOMATIC ARCHES—ROUTINE POSITIONS/ PROJECTIONS

Axial AP (Townes/Grashey)
Submentovertical

ZYGOMATIC ARCHES—ALTERNATE POSITIONS/ PROJECTIONS

Axial Oblique (May)

MANDIBLE—ROUTINE POSITIONS/PROJECTIONS

Axial AP (Townes/Grashey)
PA
Axiolateral

TEMPOROMANDIBULAR JOINTS—ROUTINE POSITIONS/PROJECTIONS

Axiolateral Transcranial (Schuller)
Transcranial Lateral
Pantomography

PARANASAL SINUSES—ROUTINE POSITIONS/ PROJECTIONS

PA Caldwell
Parietoacanthial (Waters)
Lateral
Submentovertical
Axial Transoral (Pirie)

TEMPORAL BONES—ROUTINE POSITIONS/ PROJECTIONS

Axial AP (Townes/Grashey)
Axiolateral Oblique (Law)
Posterior Profile (Stenvers/Arcelin)
Axioposterior Oblique (Mayer)
Submentovertical

**SELLA TURCICA—ROUTINE POSITIONS/
PROJECTIONS**

Axial AP (Townes/Grashey)
Lateral

**SELLA TURCICA—ALTERNATE POSITIONS/
PROJECTIONS**

Axial PA (Haas)

OBJECTIVES

At the completion of this chapter, the student should be able to:

1. Given radiographs, locate anatomic structures and landmarks.

2. Explain the rationale for each projection.

3. Describe the positioning used to visualize anatomic structures of the skull and facial bones.

4. List or identify central ray location and identify the extent of field necessary for each projection.

5. Recommend the technical factors for producing an acceptable radiograph.

6. State the patient instructions for each projection.

7. Given radiographs, evaluate positioning and technical factors.

8. Describe modifications of procedures for atypical or impaired patients to better demonstrate the anatomic area of interest.

ROUTINE AND ALTERNATIVE POSITIONS/PROJECTIONS

SKULL—AXIAL AP (TOWNE/GRASHEY) PROJECTION

Exam Rationale This projection demonstrates the occipital bone, the petrous ridges, the mastoid air cells, and the foramen magnum with the dorsum sella and posterior clinoid processes projected within its shadow. It is used to rule out fractures and disease processes.

Technical Considerations

- Regular screen/film
- Grid
- kVp range: 70–80
- SID: 40 inch (100 cm)

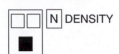

Radiation Protection

AEC (Phototiming)

 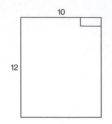 N DENSITY

Patient Position Facing the tube; all potential artifacts removed (Figure 13.1).

Part Position As in Axial AP in Chapter 12; MSP is perpendicular to the midplane of the cassette; film is centered to the foramen magnum with the top of the cassette at the top of the patient's head; chin is depressed to place OML perpendicular to the film.

Central Ray 30° caudal to OML.

Patient Instructions "Hold your breath and don't move."

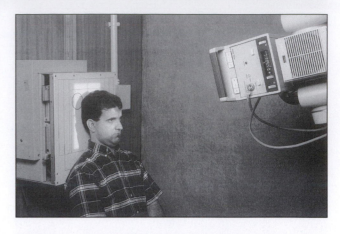

FIGURE 13.1 AP axial (Towne/Grashey) skull.

Evaluation Criteria (Figures 13.2 and 13.3)

- Entire skull is demonstrated.
- The dorsum sella and posterior clinoids should be seen within the foramen magnum.
- The petrous pyramids should be symmetrical to evidence no rotation.
- The distance from the lateral border of the skull to the foramen magnum should be equal on each side to evidence no rotation.

Tip If the patient is unable to depress the chin enough to place OML perpendicular to the film, place the IOML perpendicular to the film and increase the central ray to 37° caudal.

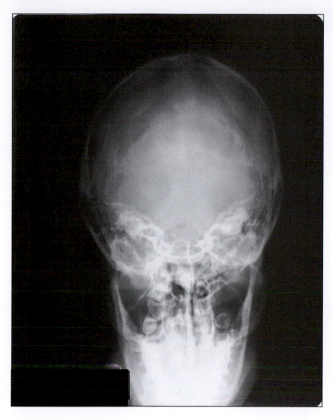

FIGURE 13.2 AP axial (Towne/Grashey) skull.

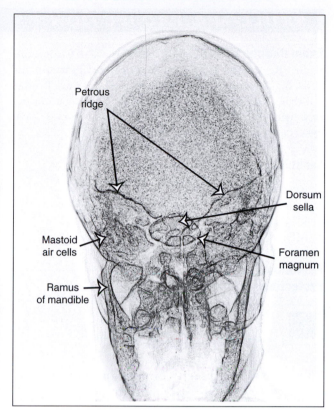

FIGURE 13.3 AP axial (Towne/Grashey) skull.

Petrous ridge

Dorsum sella

Mastoid air cells

Foramen magnum

Ramus of mandible

SKULL—PA PROJECTION

Exam Rationale   This projection is used to demonstrate the frontal bone, the frontal and ethmoid air cells, facial bones, orbital margin, and the mandibular condyles and rami. It is frequently used in conjunction with other modalities to confirm disease processes as well as in trauma situations.

Technical Considerations

- Regular screen/film
- Grid
- kVp range: 70–80
- SID: 40 inch (100 cm)

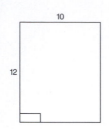

Radiation   AEC
Protection   (Phototiming)

 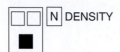 N DENSITY

Patient Position   Facing the film; all potential artifacts removed (Figure 13.4).

Part Position   As in PA projection in Chapter 12; cassette is centered to the nasion with the top of the film approximately 1 1/2 inches (4 cm) above the vertex of the skull; MSP is perpendicular to the midline of the cassette; OML is perpendicular to the film.

Central Ray   Perpendicular to the film exiting at the nasion.

Patient Instructions   "Hold your breath and don't move."

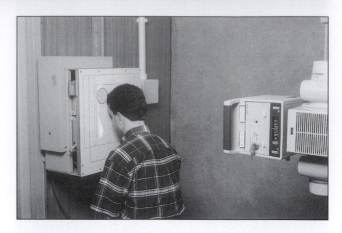

FIGURE 13.4   PA skull.

Evaluation Criteria (Figures 13.5 and 13.6)

- Entire skull is demonstrated.
- The distance from the lateral border of the skull to the lateral border of the orbit should be equal on each side to evidence no rotation.
- The petrous pyramids will fill the entire orbit.

Tip   Some department protocols use a PA Caldwell in which case the central ray is directed 15° caudally. This would project the petrous pyramids into the lower third of the orbits.

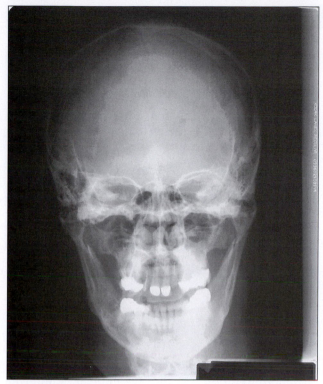

FIGURE 13.5   PA skull.

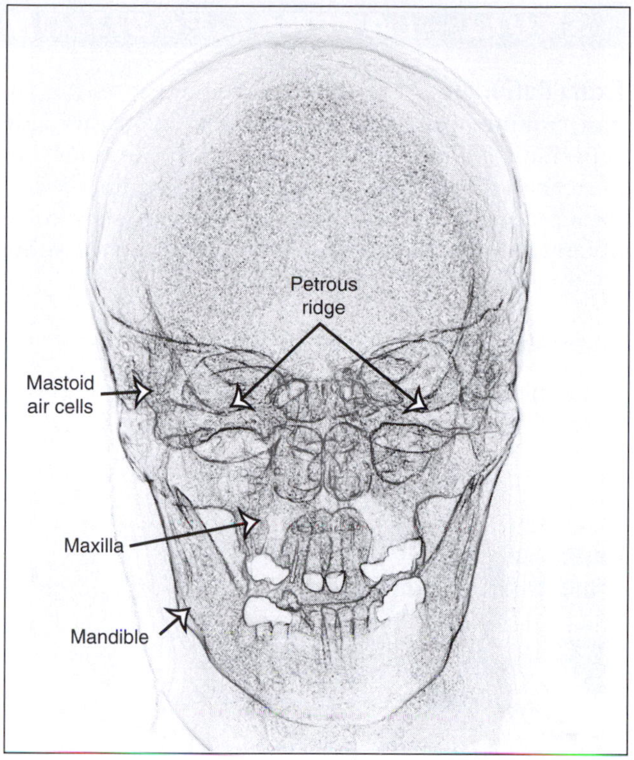

Petrous
ridge

Mastoid
air cells

Maxilla

Mandible

FIGURE 13.6   PA skull.

SKULL—LATERAL POSITION

Exam Rationale This position demonstrates the lateral cranium closest to the film with the other side superimposed, the sella turcica, and the anterior and posterior clinoid processes. To determine fracture localization, both right and left laterals should be obtained. It will also demonstrate upper cervical spine alignment.

Technical Considerations

- Regular screen/film
- Grid
- kVp range: 70–80
- SID: 40 inch (100 cm)

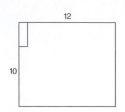

Radiation Protection

AEC (Phototiming)

 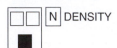 N DENSITY

Patient Position In lateral position; all potential artifacts removed (Figure 13.7).

Part Position As in lateral in Chapter 12; EAM is centered to the midline of the cassette with the top of the film approximately 2 inches (5 cm) above the vertex of the skull; MSP is parallel to the cassette, interpupillary line is perpendicular to the cassette; IOML is parallel to the transverse axis of the cassette.

Central Ray Perpendicular to the film entering 2 inches (5 cm) superior to the EAM.

Patient Instructions "Hold your breath and don't move."

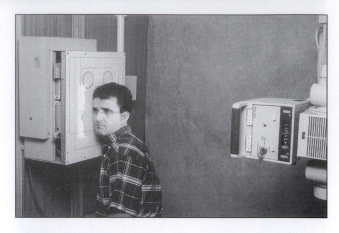

FIGURE 13.7   Lateral skull.

Evaluation Criteria (Figures 13.8 and 13.9)

- The entire skull should be demonstrated.
- Superimposition of the mandibular rami, the orbital roofs, and the external auditory canals indicates no rotation or tilt.
- The sella turcica should be seen in profile (indicates no rotation or tilt).

Tips

1. If recumbent, place the patient in the RAO position for the right lateral and the LAO position for the left lateral.
2. A cross-table lateral should be used for patients with trauma or cervical spine injury. This would demonstrate fluid levels that would indicate a basal fracture (see Chapter 14).

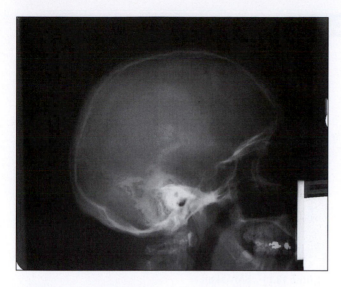

FIGURE 13.8   Lateral skull.

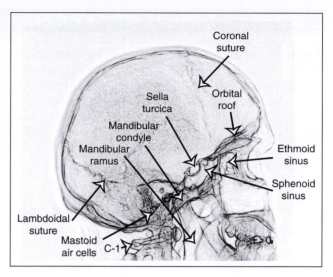

FIGURE 13.9   Lateral skull.

SKULL—SUBMENTOVERTICAL (BASILAR) PROJECTION

Exam Rationale   This projection is used to demonstrate the petrous pyramids, the mastoid processes, the foramina ovale and spinosum, the mandible, the sphenoid and ethmoid sinuses, the foramen magnum, the zygomatic arches, the nasal passages, and the occipital bone.

Technical Considerations

- Regular screen/film
- Grid
- kVp range: 70–80
- SID: 40 inch (100 cm)

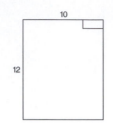

Radiation Protection   **AEC (Phototiming)**

   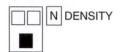

Patient Position   Facing the tube; all potential artifacts removed (Figure 13.10).

Part Position   As in SMV in Chapter 12; patient's neck is extended until the head is resting on the vertex; cassette is centered to the level of the sella turcica; MSP is perpendicular to the midplane of the cassette; IOML parallel to the cassette.

Central Ray   Perpendicular to the IOML entering between the angles of the mandible.

Patient Instructions   "Hold your breath and don't move."

Evaluation Criteria (Figures 13.11 and 13.12)

- Entire skull is demonstrated.
- The mandibular symphysis should superimpose the anterior frontal bone (indicates adequate extension or tube angle).

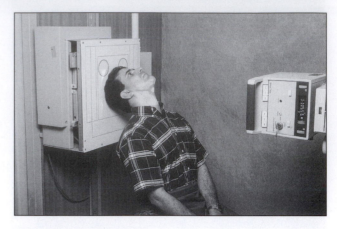

FIGURE 13.10   SMV skull.

- The mandibular condyles should be demonstrated anterior to the petrous pyramids (indicates adequate extension or tube angle).
- The distance from the lateral border of the skull to the mandibular condyles should be equal on each side (indicates no rotation).
- The petrous ridges should be symmetrical (indicates no rotation).

Tips

1. Work quickly because this position is uncomfortable for the patient.
2. The preferred position is erect; if recumbent, place pillows or sponges under the shoulders (see Chapter 12).
3. If unable to place the IOML parallel to the film, the central ray should be perpendicular to the IOML.

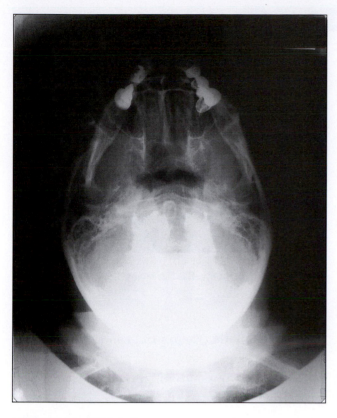

FIGURE 13.11   SMV skull.

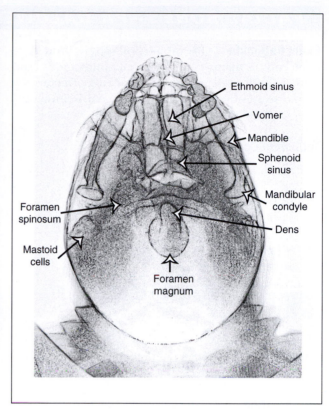

FIGURE 13.12   SMV skull.

FACIAL BONES—PA CALDWELL PROJECTION

Exam Rationale   This projection is performed to demonstrate fractures of the facial bones and is especially helpful to determine alveolar ridge fractures. It demonstrates the orbital rim, the nasal septum, and the mandibular condyles.

Technical Considerations

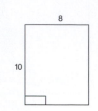

- Regular screen/film
- Grid
- kVp range: 70–80
- SID: 40 inch (100 cm)

Radiation Protection   **AEC (Phototiming)**

    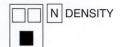 N DENSITY

Patient Position   Facing the film; all potential artifacts removed (Figure 13.13).

Part Position   As in PA Caldwell in Chapter 12; cassette is centered to the nasion; MSP is perpendicular to the midline of the cassette; OML is perpendicular to the film.

Central Ray   15° caudal to nasion.

Patient Instructions   "Hold your breath and don't move."

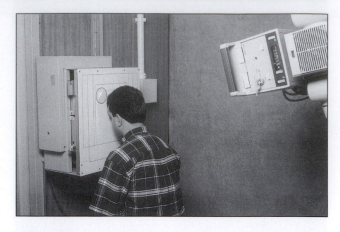

FIGURE 13.13   PA Caldwell facial bones.

Evaluation Criteria (Figures 13.14 and 13.15)

- No rotation.
- The petrous pyramids will fill the lower one-third of the orbit.

Tip   Some department protocols call for a perpendicular central ray in which case the petrous pyramids would fill the orbits.

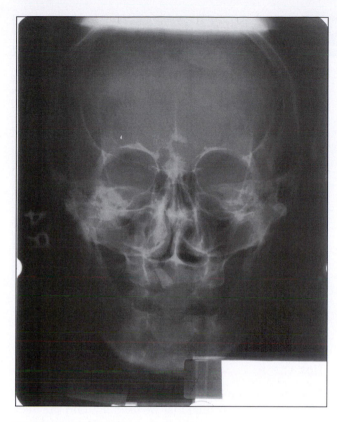

FIGURE 13.14   **PA Caldwell facial bones.**

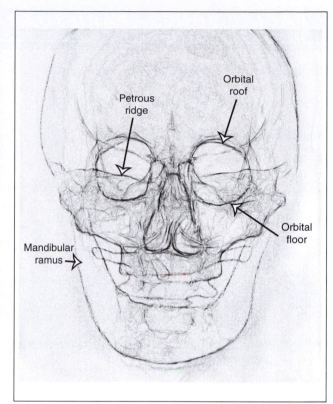

FIGURE 13.15   **PA Caldwell facial bones.**

FACIAL BONES—PARIETOACANTHIAL (WATERS) PROJECTION

Exam Rationale   This projection is especially good for demonstrating fractures of the orbit and depressed fractures of the nasal wings.

Technical Considerations

- Regular screen/film
- Grid
- kVp range: 70–80
- SID: 40 inch (100 cm)

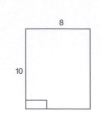

Radiation Protection   AEC (Phototiming)

   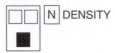 N DENSITY

Patient Position   Facing the film; all potential artifacts removed (Figure 13.16).

Part Position   As in parietoacanthial in Chapter 12; the neck is extended and the chin placed on the Bucky; the cassette is centered to the acanthion; MSP is perpendicular to the midline of the cassette; OML forms a 37° angle to the film.

Central Ray   Perpendicular to the film exiting at the acanthion.

Patient Instructions   "Hold your breath and don't move."

Evaluation Criteria (Figures 13.17 and 13.18)

- No rotation as evidenced by an equal distance from the orbit to the lateral border of the skull on both sides.
- Petrous ridges should be projected immediately below the maxillary sinuses.

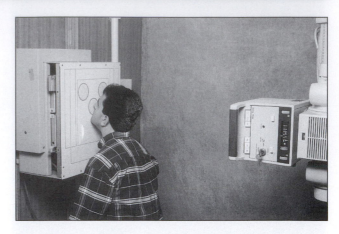

FIGURE 13.16   Parietoacanthial (Waters) facial bones.

Tips

1. To better demonstrate the orbital floor, the modified parietoacanthial may be used. Extend the neck and place the chin on the cassette holder; center the film to the acanthion; adjust the flexion of the neck to place OML at a 55° angle to the plane of the film. The petrous ridges would be demonstrated immediately below the inferior border of the orbits. (See modified Waters for orbits, on page 514).
2. Use of **stereoscopy** in this projection is especially helpful to demonstrate subtle fractures of the zygoma.

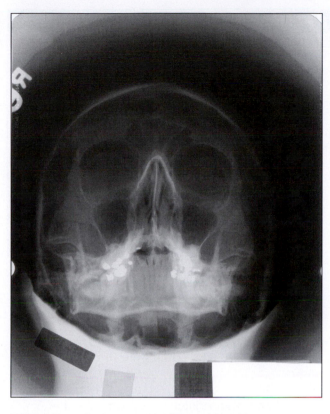

FIGURE 13.17   Parietoacanthial (Waters) facial bones.

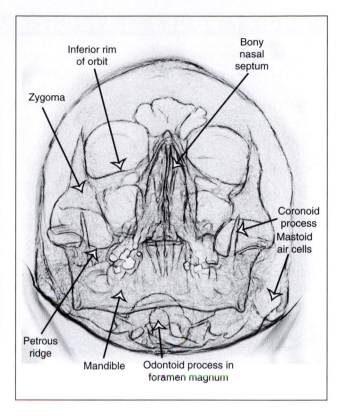

FIGURE 13.18   Parietoacanthial (Waters) facial bones.

FACIAL BONES—LATERAL POSITION

Exam Rationale This position is used to demonstrate the facial bones of the side closest to the film with the opposite side superimposed. It is useful for demonstrating depressed fractures of the frontal sinus. It also demonstrates the orbital roof, sella turcica, and mandible.

Technical Considerations

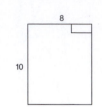

* Regular screen/film
* Grid
* kVp range: 70–80
* SID: 40 inch (100 cm)

Radiation Protection AEC (Phototiming)

  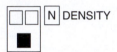 N DENSITY

Patient Position In lateral position; all potential artifacts removed (Figure 13.19).

Part Position As in lateral in Chapter 12; cassette is centered to the zygoma; MSP is parallel to the film; interpupillary line is perpendicular to the film; IOML is parallel to the transverse axis of the cassette.

Central Ray Perpendicular to the film entering at the zygoma.

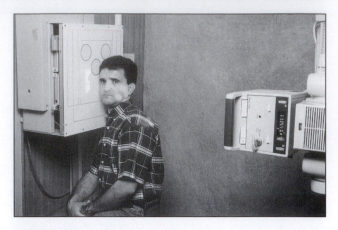

FIGURE 13.19　**Lateral facial bones.**

Patient Instructions "Hold your breath and don't move."

Evaluation Criteria (Figures 13.20 and 13.21)

* Includes all facial bones.
* True lateral as evidenced by:
  —Superimposition of the mandibular rami.
  —Superimposition of the orbital roofs.
  —No rotation seen in the sella turcica.

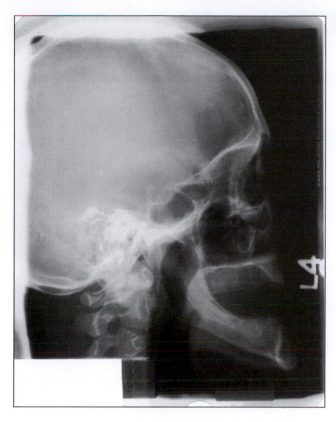

FIGURE 13.20   Lateral facial bones.

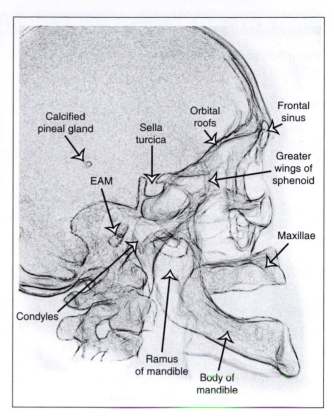

FIGURE 13.21   Lateral facial bones.

NASAL BONES—PA CALDWELL PROJECTION

Exam Rationale   This projection best demonstrates the bony nasal septum.

Technical Considerations

- Regular screen/film
- Grid
- kVp range: 70–80
- SID: 40 inch (100 cm)

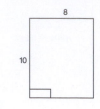

**Radiation   AEC
Protection   (Phototiming)**

 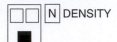 N DENSITY

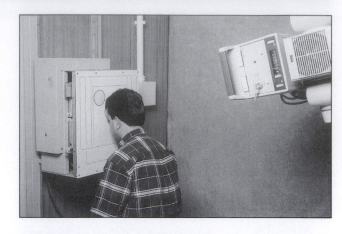

FIGURE 13.22   PA Caldwell nasal bones.

Patient Position   Facing the film; all potential artifacts removed (Figure 13.22).

Part Position   As in PA Caldwell in Chapter 12; cassette is centered to the nasion; OML is perpendicular to the film; MSP is perpendicular to the midline of the cassette.

Central Ray   15° caudal to nasion.

Patient Instructions   "Hold your breath and don't move."

Evaluation Criteria (Figures 13.23 and 13.24)

- The petrous ridges are projected in the lower one-third of the orbit.
- No rotation as evidenced by an equal distance from the crista galli to the lateral border of the orbit on each side.

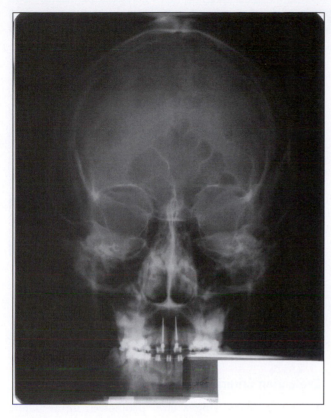

FIGURE 13.23   PA Caldwell nasal bones.

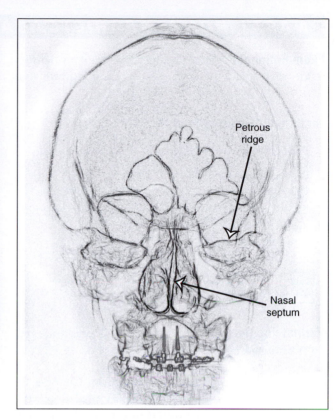

FIGURE 13.24   PA Caldwell nasal bones.

NASAL BONES—PARIETOACANTHIAL (WATERS)

Exam Rationale This projection is used to demonstrate displacement of the bony nasal septum and depressed fractures of the nasal wings.

Technical Considerations

- Regular screen/film
- Grid
- kVp range: 70–80
- SID: 40 inch (100 cm)

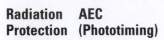

Radiation Protection   **AEC (Phototiming)**

     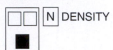 N DENSITY

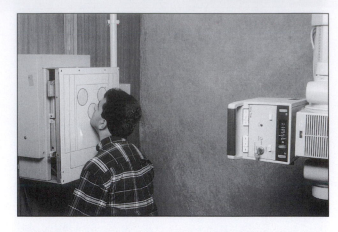

FIGURE 13.25 Parietoacanthial (Waters) nasal bones.

Patient Position Facing the film; all potential artifacts removed (Figure 13.25).

Part Position As in parietoacanthial in Chapter 12; the neck is extended and the chin placed on the Bucky; the cassette is centered to the acanthion; MSP is perpendicular to midline of cassette; OML forms a 37° angle to the film.

Central Ray Perpendicular to the film exiting at the acanthion.

Patient Instructions "Hold your breath and don't move."

Evaluation Criteria (Figures 13.26 and 13.27)

- The petrous ridges are projected immediately below the maxillary sinuses.
- No rotation as evidenced by equal distance from the orbit to the lateral border of the skull on each side.

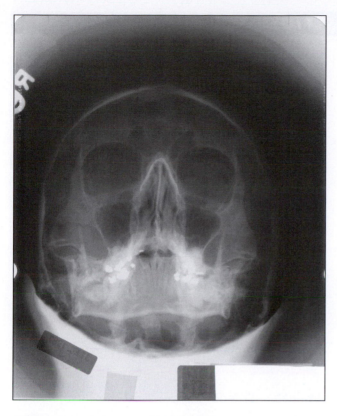

FIGURE 13.26 Parietoacanthial (Waters) nasal bones.

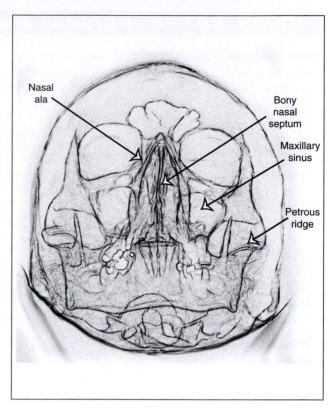

FIGURE 13.27 Parietoacanthial (Waters) nasal bones.

NASAL BONES—LATERAL POSITION

Exam Rationale This position is used to demonstrate the nasal bones and soft tissue structures of the nose. It is the best position to demonstrate nondisplaced, linear fractures of the nasal bones. Both laterals are normally done for comparison.

Technical Considerations

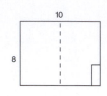

- Detail screen/film
- Non-grid
- kVp range: 60–65
- SID: 40 inch (100 cm)

Radiation Protection

  Manual Timing Recommended

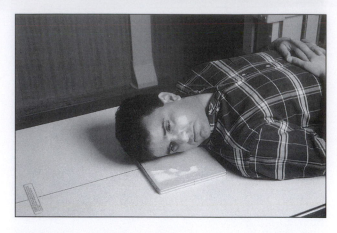

FIGURE 13.28   Lateral nasal bones.

Patient Position In lateral position; all potential artifacts removed (Figure 13.28).

Part Position As in the lateral in Chapter 12; side of the head against the film; centered to the nasal bones; MSP is parallel and interpupillary line perpendicular to the film; IOML is parallel to the transverse axis of the cassette.

Central Ray Perpendicular to the film at a point 1/2 inch (1 cm) inferior and posterior to the nasion.

Patient Instructions "Hold your breath and don't move."

Evaluation Criteria (Figures 13.29 and 13.30)

- The frontonasal suture, the nasal bones, the anterior nasal spine, and the soft tissue should be included.
- There should be no rotation.

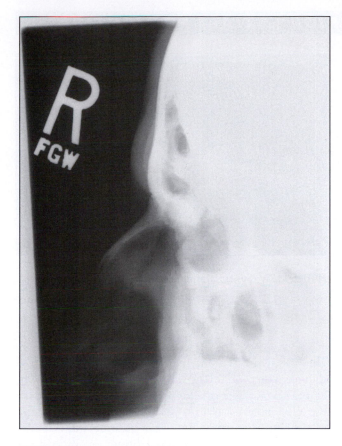

FIGURE 13.29   **Lateral nasal bones.**

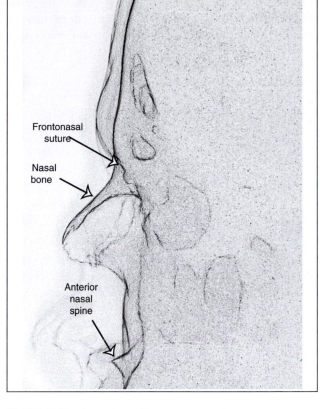

FIGURE 13.30   **Lateral nasal bones.**

NASAL BONES—SUPEROINFERIOR (AXIAL) PROJECTION

Exam Rationale This projection demonstrates medial or lateral displacement of nasal bone fractures.

Technical Considerations

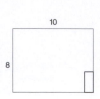

- Detail screen/film
- Non-grid
- kVp range: 58–60
- SID: 40 inch (100 cm)

Radiation Protection

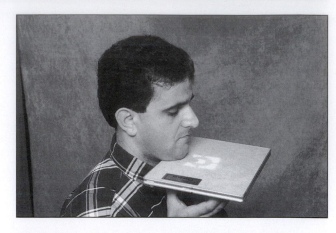

FIGURE 13.31   Superoinferior (axial) nasal bones, erect.

Patient Position Seated in a chair (Figure 13.31).

Part Position Patient holds the cassette in a horizontal position under the chin; adjust the flexion or extension of the head to place the glabelloalveolar line perpendicular to the plane of the film.

Central Ray Perpendicular to the film along the glabelloalveolar line.

Patient Instructions "Hold your breath and don't move."

Evaluation Criteria (Figures 13.32 and 13.33)

- Demonstrates the nasal bones.
- Soft tissue should also be demonstrated.

Tip With the patient in the supine position, place the cassette under the chin in a vertical position; adjust the flexion or extension of the head to place the glabelloalveolar line perpendicular to the plane of the film (Figure 13.34). This position will not adequately demonstrate the nasal bones on individuals with a prominent forehead or chin or protruding front teeth. If intraoral film is available, place it in the mouth and position the patient and central ray as described above.

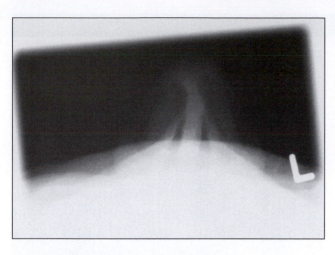

FIGURE 13.32   Superoinferior nasal bones.

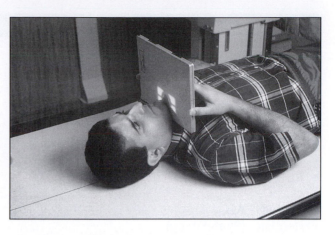

FIGURE 13.34   Superoinferior (axial) nasal bones, recumbent.

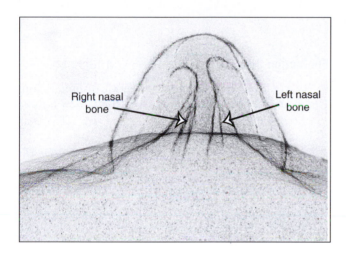

Right nasal bone

Left nasal bone

FIGURE 13.33   Superoinferior nasal bones.

ORBITS—PA PROJECTION

Exam Rationale This projection demonstrates the upper two-thirds of the orbit.

Technical Considerations

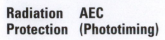

- Regular screen/film
- Grid
- kVp range: 70–80
- SID: 40 inch (100 cm)

Radiation Protection   AEC (Phototiming)

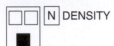
N DENSITY

Patient Position Facing the film; all potential artifacts removed (Figure 13.35).

Part Position As in the PA projection in Chapter 12; cassette is centered to the orbits; MSP is perpendicular to the midpoint of the cassette; OML is perpendicular to the film.

Patient Instructions "Hold your breath and don't move."

Central Ray Perpendicular to the film.

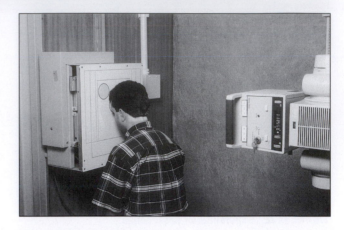

FIGURE 13.35   PA orbit.

Evaluation Criteria (Figures 13.36 and 13.37)

- No rotation as evidenced by equal distance from the lateral border of the orbit to the lateral border of the skull on each side.
- Petrous ridges fill the orbit.

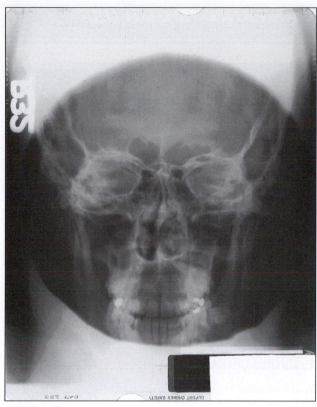

FIGURE 13.36   PA orbit.

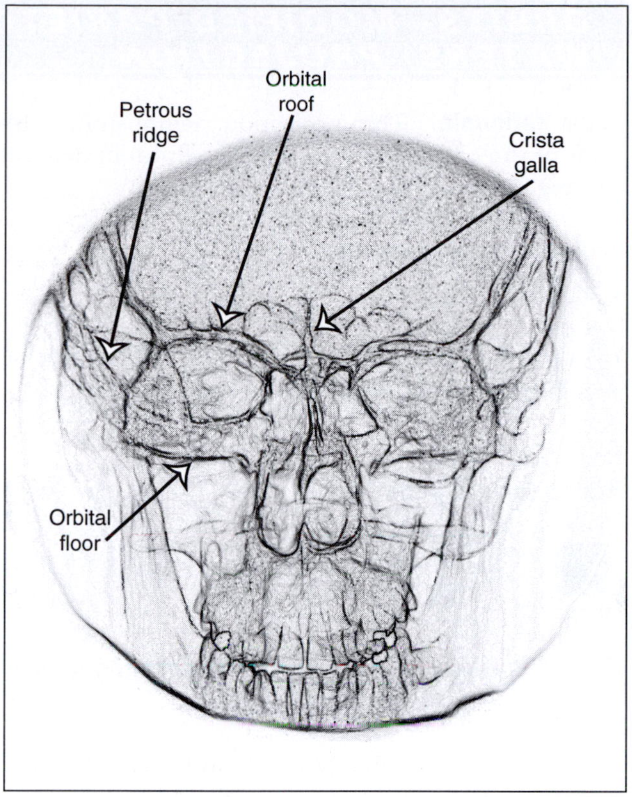

Petrous
ridge

Orbital
roof

Crista
galla

Orbital
floor

FIGURE 13.37   PA orbit.

ORBITS—MODIFIED PARIETOACANTHIAL (MODIFIED WATERS) PROJECTION

Exam Rationale This projection demonstrates the floor of the orbits and is especially helpful in demonstrating "blowout" fractures.

Technical Considerations

- Regular screen/film
- Grid
- kVp range: 70–80
- SID: 40 inch (100 cm)

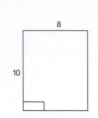

Radiation Protection

AEC (Phototiming)

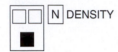 N DENSITY

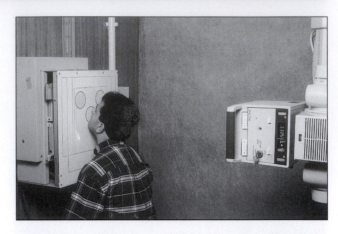

FIGURE 13.38 Modified parietoacanthial (modified Waters) orbit.

Patient Position Facing the film; all potential artifacts removed (Figure 13.38).

Part Position Extend the neck and place the chin on the Bucky; cassette is centered to the level of the acanthion; MSP is centered to the film; OML forms a 55° angle with the plane of the film.

Central Ray Perpendicular to the film exiting at the acanthion.

Patient Instructions "Hold your breath and don't move."

Evaluation Criteria (Figures 13.39 and 13.40)

- The entire orbital rim and the maxillae should be demonstrated.
- No rotation as evidenced by an equal distance from the lateral orbital border to the lateral border of the skull on each side.
- The petrous ridges are projected into the maxillary sinuses.

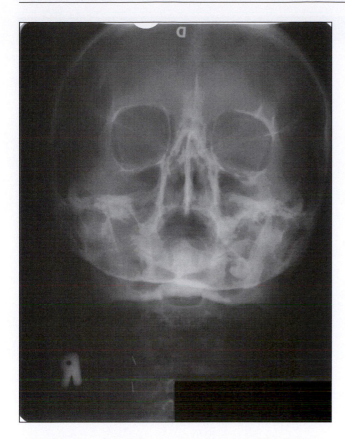

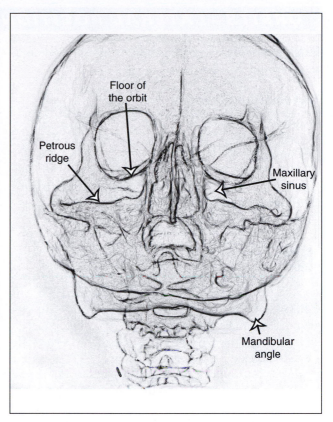

FIGURE 13.39 Modified parietoacanthial (modified Waters) orbit.

FIGURE 13.40 Modified parietoacanthial (modified Waters) orbit.

ORBITS—LATERAL POSITION

Exam Rationale   This position is used to demonstrate foreign bodies.

Technical Considerations

- Regular screen/film
- Grid
- kVp range: 70–80
- SID: 40 inch (100 cm)

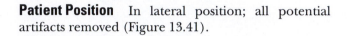

Radiation   AEC
Protection   (Phototiming)

 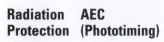 N DENSITY

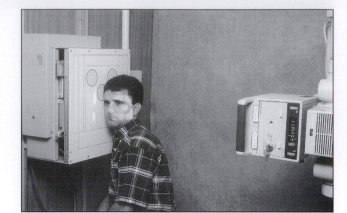

FIGURE 13.41   Lateral orbit.

Patient Position   In lateral position; all potential artifacts removed (Figure 13.41).

Part Position   As in lateral in Chapter 12; cassette is centered to the orbit; MSP is parallel and interpupillary line is perpendicular to the film.

Patient Instructions   "Hold your breath and don't move."

Central Ray   Perpendicular to the film.

Evaluation Criteria (Figures 13.42 and 13.43)

- Superimposition of both orbits.

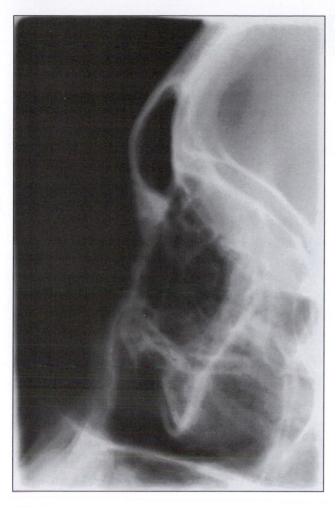

FIGURE 13.42   Lateral orbit.

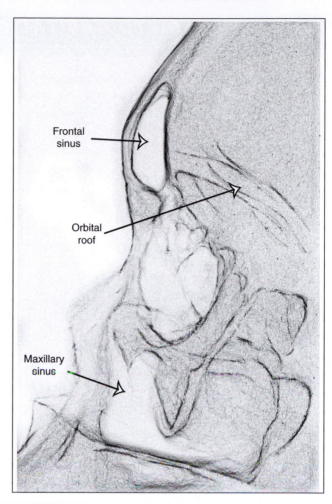

Frontal
sinus

Orbital
roof

Maxillary
sinus

FIGURE 13.43   Lateral orbit.

ORBITS—PARIETO-ORBITAL OBLIQUE (RHESE) PROJECTION

Exam Rationale   This projection demonstrates the optic foramen. Enlargement or erosion is usually associated with tumor; narrowing could indicate abnormal bone growth. Normally both sides are taken for comparison.

Technical Considerations

- Regular screen/film
- Grid
- kVp range: 70–80
- SID: 40 inch (100 cm)

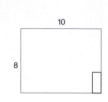

Radiation Protection

AEC (Phototiming)

   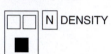 N DENSITY

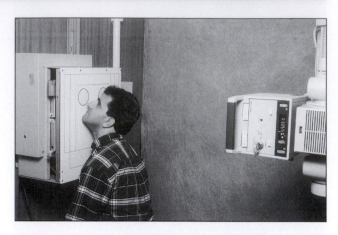

FIGURE 13.44   Parieto-orbital oblique (Rhese) orbit.

Patient Position   Facing the film; all potential artifacts removed (Figure 13.44).

Part Position   Center affected orbit to midline of the grid and center the film to the orbit; patient's zygoma, nose, and chin rest on the table; MSP forms a 53° angle to the film; acanthiomeatal line is perpendicular to the plane of the film.

Central Ray   Perpendicular to the film exiting through the affected orbit.

Patient Instructions   "Hold your breath and don't move."

Evaluation Criteria (Figures 13.45 and 13.46)

- The entire orbit should be included.
- The optic foramen should be projected in the lower, outer quadrant of the orbit.
- The optic foramen should be found at the end of the sphenoid ridge.

Tips

1. It is important to collimate to the orbit to maximize detail.
2. If the optic foramen does not lie in the lower quadrant, the acanthiomeatal line is not perpendicular to the film; if it does not lie in the outer quadrant, the MSP is not at a 53° angle to the film.

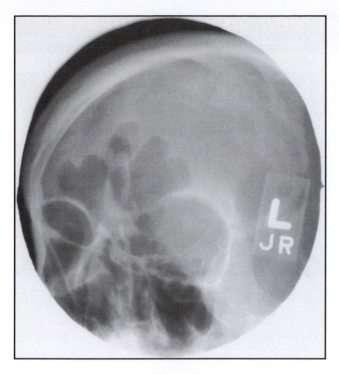

FIGURE 13.45   Parieto-orbital oblique (Rhese) orbit.

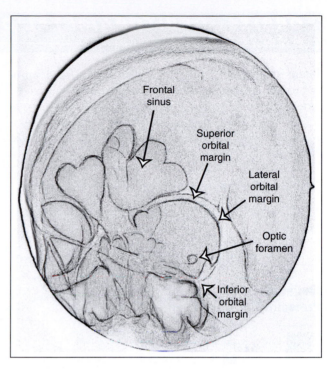

FIGURE 13.46   Parieto-orbital oblique (Rhese) orbit.

Frontal sinus

Superior orbital margin

Lateral orbital margin

Optic foramen

Inferior orbital margin

ORBITS—ORBITOPARIETAL OBLIQUE (REVERSE RHESE) PROJECTION

Exam Rationale This projection is used to demonstrate the optic foramen for patients who cannot be examined in the upright or prone positions. Enlargement or erosion is usually associated with tumor; narrowing could indicate abnormal bone growth. Normally both sides are taken for comparison.

Technical Considerations

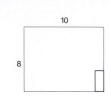

- Regular screen/film
- Grid
- kVp range: 70–80
- SID: 40 inch (100 cm)

**Radiation AEC
Protection (Phototiming)**

 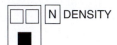

Patient Position Facing the tube; all potential artifacts removed (Figure 13.47).

Part Position Rotate the head toward the unaffected side so that MSP forms a 53° angle to the plane of the film; acanthiomeatal line is perpendicular to the plane of the film; affected orbit (uppermost) is centered to the grid and the film.

Central Ray Perpendicular to the film entering the uppermost orbit.

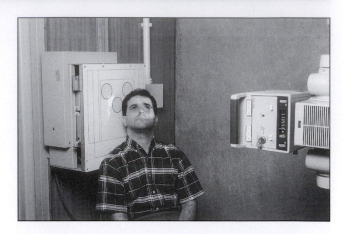

FIGURE 13.47   Orbitoparietal oblique (reverse Rhese) orbit.

Patient Instructions "Hold your breath and don't move."

Evaluation Criteria (Figures 13.48 and 13.49)

- Include the entire orbit.
- Optic foramen should lie in the lower, outer quadrant of the orbit at the end of the sphenoid ridge.

Tip This position will demonstrate increased magnification and increased radiation dose to the eye when compared to the parieto-orbital position.

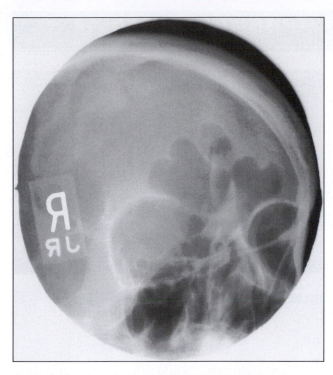

FIGURE 13.48 Orbitoparietal oblique (reverse Rhese) orbit.

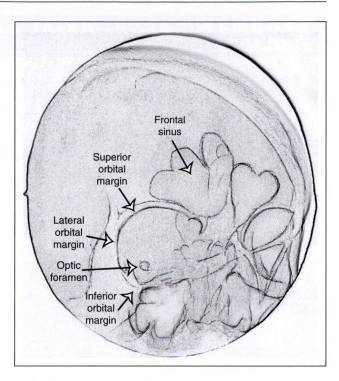

FIGURE 13.49 Orbitoparietal oblique (reverse Rhese) orbit.

ZYGOMATIC ARCH—AXIAL AP (TOWNE/GRASHEY) PROJECTION

Exam Rationale   This projection is used to demonstrate the zygomatic arches free of superimposition. It is normally used to demonstrate fracture.

Technical Considerations

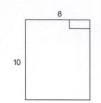

- Regular screen/film
- Grid
- kVp range: 60–70
- SID: 40 inch (100 cm)

Radiation   AEC
Protection (Phototiming)

 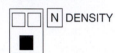 N DENSITY

Patient Position   Facing the tube; all potential artifacts removed (Figure 13.50).

Part Position   As in axial AP in Chapter 12; cassette is centered to the level of the mandibular angles; MSP is perpendicular to the center of the grid; OML is perpendicular to the plane of the film.

Central Ray   30° caudal entering the glabella.

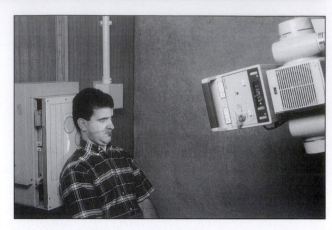

FIGURE 13.50   Axial AP zygomatic arch.

Patient Instructions   "Hold your breath and don't move."

Evaluation Criteria (Figures 13.51 and 13.52)

- Zygomatic arches projected free of the mandible.
- No rotation demonstrated as evidenced by the symmetrical demonstration of the zygomatic arches.

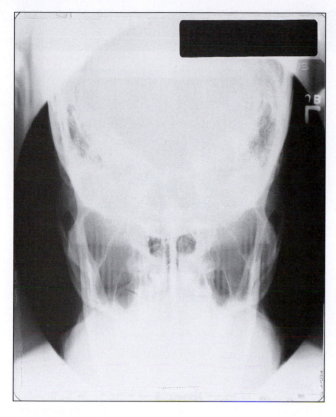

FIGURE 13.51   Axial AP zygomatic arch.

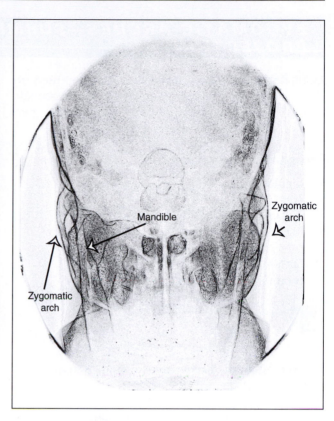

FIGURE 13.52   Axial AP zygomatic arch.

ZYGOMATIC ARCHES—SUBMENTOVERTICAL (SMV) PROJECTION

Exam Rationale This projection can be used to demonstrate the lateral margins of the zygomatic arches free of superimposition. It is usually performed to identify fractures.

Technical Considerations

- Regular screen/film
- Grid
- kVp range: 60–70
- SID: 40 inch (100 cm)

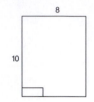

Radiation Protection

AEC (Phototiming)

 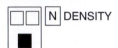 N DENSITY

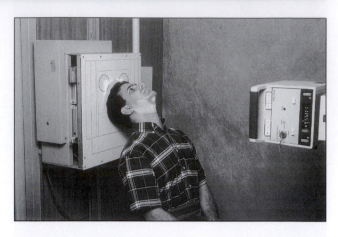

FIGURE 13.53 SMV zygomatic arch.

Patient Position Facing the tube; all potential artifacts removed (Figure 13.53).

Part Position As in SMV in Chapter 12; patient's neck is extended until head is resting on the vertex; cassette is centered to a level 1 inch (3 cm) posterior to the outer canthus; MSP is perpendicular to the plane of the film; IOML is parallel to the cassette.

Central Ray Perpendicular to IOML entering midway between the zygomatic arches.

Patient Instructions "Hold your breath and don't move."

Evaluation Criteria (Figures 13.54 and 13.55)

- The zygomatic arches should be projected free of superimposition.
- No rotation is demonstrated.

Tips

1. Due to the difficulty of maintaining this position, do this projection as quickly as possible.
2. Decreasing the mAs approximately 50% from the SMV to demonstrate the base of the cranium should demonstrate the arches with the proper density.

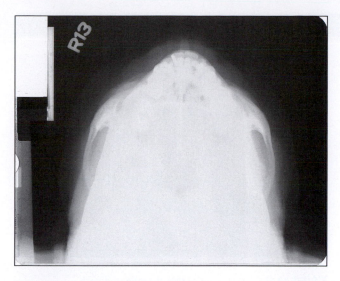

FIGURE 13.54   SMV zygomatic arch.

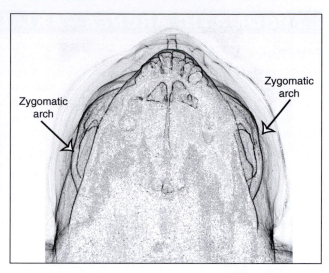

FIGURE 13.55   SMV zygomatic arch.

ZYGOMATIC ARCHES—AXIAL OBLIQUE (MAY) POSITION

Exam Rationale This position is used to demonstrate a unilateral zygomatic arch projected free from superimposition. It is particularly helpful with patients who have flat cheekbones or a depressed fracture of the zygomatic arch. Both sides are usually done for comparison.

Technical Considerations

- Regular screen/film
- Grid
- kVp range: 60–70
- SID: 40 inch (100 cm)

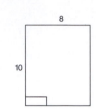

Radiation Protection   AEC (Phototiming)

 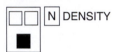 N DENSITY

Patient Position Facing the film; all potential artifacts removed (Figure 13.56).

Part Position Extend the neck and place the vertex of the head on the cassette holder; center the affected zygomatic arch to the center of the grid; center the film to a point approximately 3 inches (8 cm) inferior to the zygomatic bone; IOML as close to parallel to the film as possible; tilt the head 15° away from the affected side.

Central Ray Angle the tube caudally to place the central ray perpendicular to the IOML; center the central ray to the affected zygomatic arch (approximately 1 inch [3 cm] posterior to the outer canthus); center the cassette to the central ray.

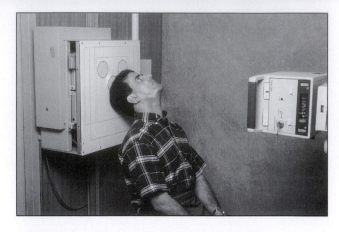

FIGURE 13.56   Oblique axial (May) zygomatic arch.

Patient Instructions "Hold your breath and don't move."

Evaluation Criteria (Figures 13.57 and 13.58)

- Affected zygomatic arch projected free of superimposition.

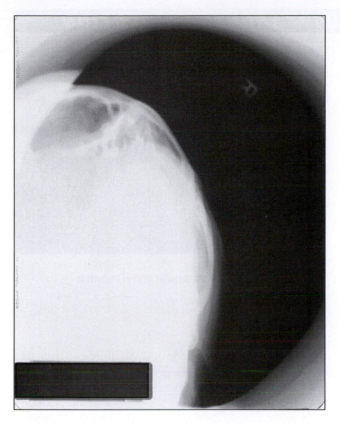

FIGURE 13.57   Oblique axial (May) zygomatic arch.

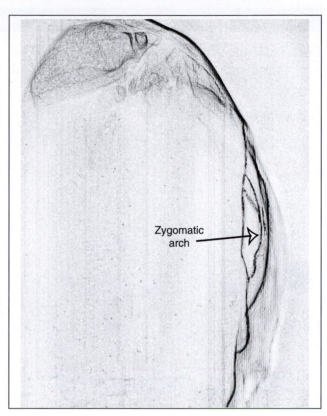

FIGURE 13.58   Oblique axial (May) zygomatic arch.

MANDIBLE—AXIAL AP (TOWNE/GRASHEY) PROJECTION

Exam Rationale This projection demonstrates the mandibular rami, the mandibular condyles, and the temporomandibular fossae.

Technical Considerations

- Regular screen/film
- Grid
- kVp range: 70–80
- SID: 40 inch (100 cm)

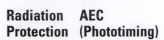
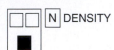

Radiation Protection   AEC (Phototiming)

N DENSITY

Patient Position Facing the tube; all potential artifacts removed (Figure 13.59).

Part Position As in AP axial in Chapter 12; OML and MSP are perpendicular to the film.

Central Ray 35° caudally entering the glabella.

Patient Instructions "Hold your breath and don't move."

Evaluation Criteria (Figures 13.60 and 13.61)

- The condyloid processes and mandibular rami are demonstrated without rotation as evidenced by symmetrical views of the rami.

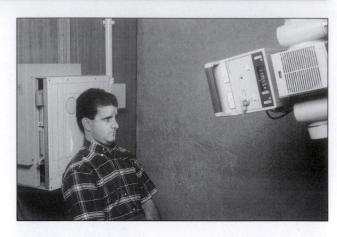

FIGURE 13.59   Axial AP (Towne/Grashey) mandible.

Tip If unable to place the OML perpendicular to the film, place the IOML perpendicular to the film and increase the central ray angle by 7°.

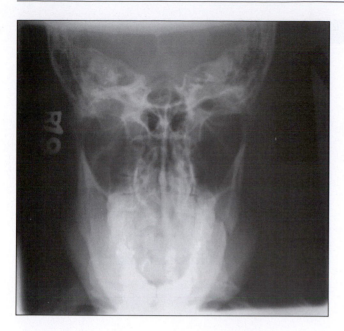

FIGURE 13.60   Axial AP (Towne/Grashey) mandible.

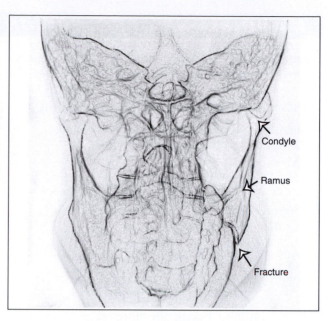

FIGURE 13.61   Axial AP (Towne/Grashey) mandible.

MANDIBLE—PA PROJECTION

Exam Rationale This projection is used to demonstrate the mandibular rami and body.

Technical Considerations

- Regular screen/film
- Grid
- kVp range: 70–80
- SID: 40 inch (100 cm)

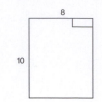

Radiation Protection   AEC (Phototiming)

     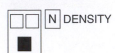 N DENSITY

Patient Position Facing the film; all potential artifacts removed (Figures 13.62 and 13.63).

Part Position As in PA projection in Chapter 12; MSP is perpendicular to the midline of the grid; OML is perpendicular to film; cassette is centered to the level of the lips.

Central Ray Perpendicular to the film exiting at the lips.

Patient Instructions "Hold your breath and don't move."

Evaluation Criteria (Figures 13.64 through 13.67)

- The entire mandible should be included.
- No rotation as evidenced by symmetrical visualization of the rami.

Tip To demonstrate the mentum, place the nose and chin on the table top with the MSP perpendicular to the midline of the grid.

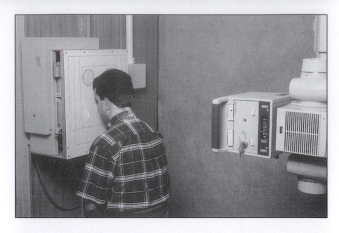

FIGURE 13.62   PA mandible.

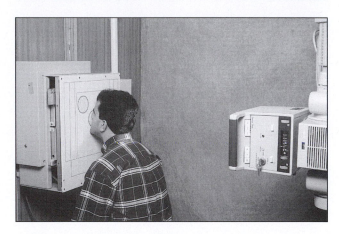

FIGURE 13.63   PA mandible, mentum.

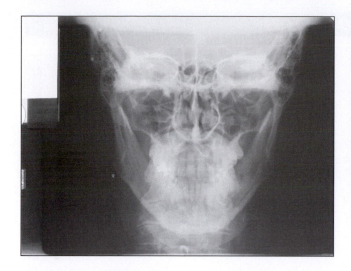

FIGURE 13.64 PA mandible.

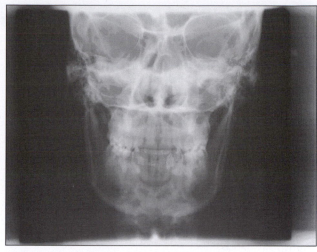

FIGURE 13.66 PA mandible, mentum.

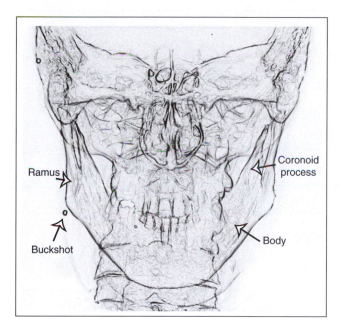

FIGURE 13.65 PA mandible.

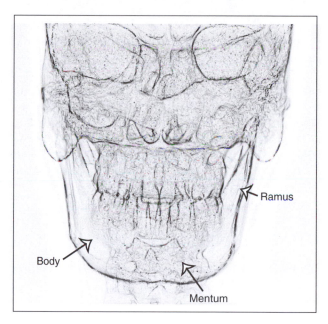

FIGURE 13.67 PA mandible, mentum.

MANDIBLE—AXIOLATERAL POSITION

Exam Rationale This position demonstrates the temporomandibular joint (TMJ), condyle, coronoid process, ramus, body, and mentum of the side of the mandible closest to the film. Both sides are taken for comparison.

Technical Considerations

- Regular screen/film
- Grid
- kVp range: 70–80
- SID: 40 inch (100 cm)

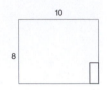

Radiation Protection   AEC (Phototiming)

   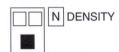 N DENSITY

Patient Position In lateral position; all potential artifacts removed (Figures 13.68, 13.69, and 13.70).

Part Position Head in a lateral position with side of interest closest to the film; extend the chin to prevent superimposition on the cervical spine; to demonstrate the ramus, the head should be in a true lateral position; to demonstrate the body, rotate the head approximately 30° toward the film; to demonstrate the mentum, rotate the head approximately 45° toward the film.

Central Ray 25° to 35° cephalic to the area of interest.

Patient Instructions "Hold your breath and don't move."

Evaluation Criteria (Figures 13.71 through 13.74)

- Area of interest is well demonstrated.
- No superimposition of the opposite side of the mandible.

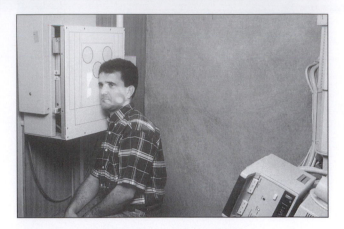

FIGURE 13.68   Axiolateral mandible, lateral.

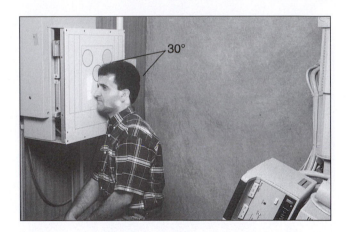

FIGURE 13.69   Axiolateral mandible, 30° rotation.

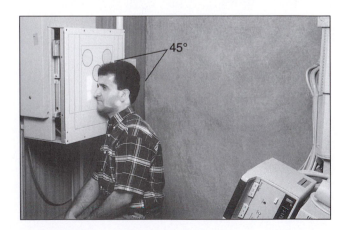

FIGURE 13.70   Axiolateral mandible, 45° rotation.

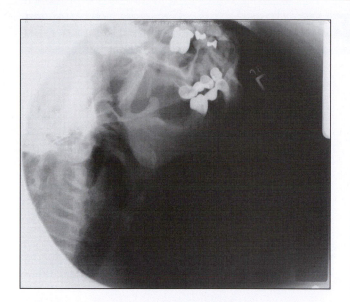

FIGURE 13.71   Axiolateral mandible, lateral.

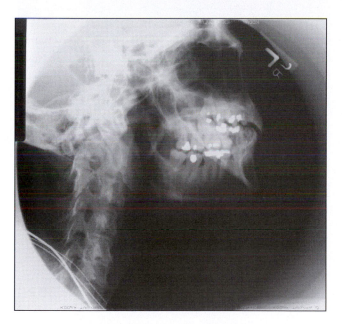

FIGURE 13.72   Axiolateral mandible, 30° rotation.

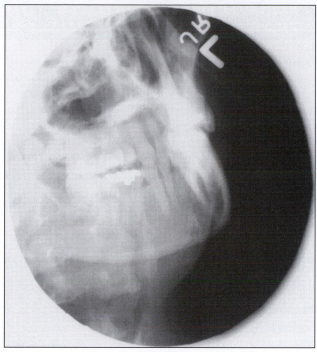

FIGURE 13.73   Axiolateral mandible, 45° rotation.

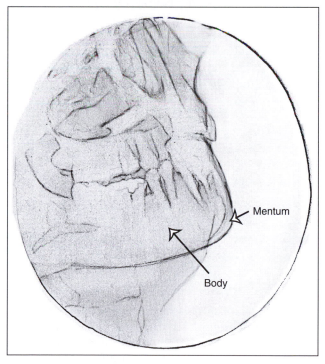

FIGURE 13.74   Axiolateral mandible.

TEMPOROMANDIBULAR JOINTS—AXIOLATERAL TRANSCRANIAL (SCHULLER) PROJECTION

Exam Rationale This projection better demonstrates the TMJ closest to the film. The configuration of the condyle and mandibular fossa and the direction and amount of movement is demonstrated. In cases of trauma, the position can illustrate dislocation or small fractures of the cortex of the condyle. Both sides are usually taken in both the open and closed mouth positions.

Technical Considerations

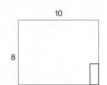

- Regular screen/film
- Grid
- kVp range: 70–80
- SID: 40 inch (100 cm)

Radiation Protection   AEC (Phototiming)

 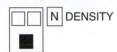

Patient Position In the lateral position; all potential artifacts removed (Figure 13.75).

Part Position As in the lateral in Chapter 12; cassette is centered to the TMJ; MSP is parallel to the film; interpupillary line is perpendicular to the film; IOML is parallel to the transverse axis of the film.

Central Ray 25° to 30° caudal centered to the center of the film.

Patient Instructions

- Closed mouth: "With your mouth closed, hold your breath and don't move."
- Open mouth: "Open your mouth, hold your breath and don't move."

Evaluation Criteria (Figures 13.76 through 13.79)

- With the mouth closed, the mandibular condyle will be visualized within the mandibular fossa.
- With the mouth open, the mandibular condyle will move inferior and anterior and will be demonstrated inferior to the articular tubercle.

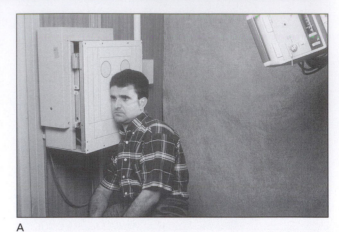

A

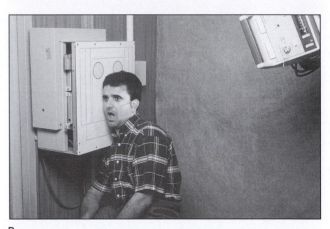

B

FIGURE 13.75   Axiolateral transcranial (Schuller) TMJ. (A) Closed mouth. (B) Open mouth.

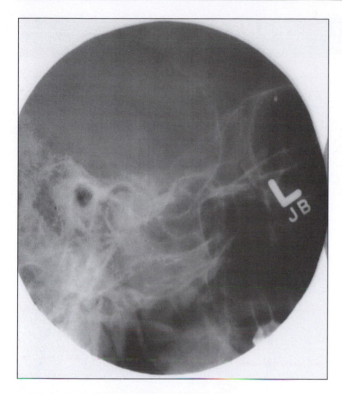

FIGURE 13.76   Axiolateral transcranial (Schuller) TMJ, closed mouth.

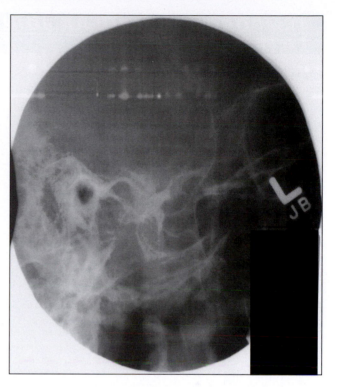

FIGURE 13.78   Axiolateral transcranial (Schuller) TMJ, open mouth.

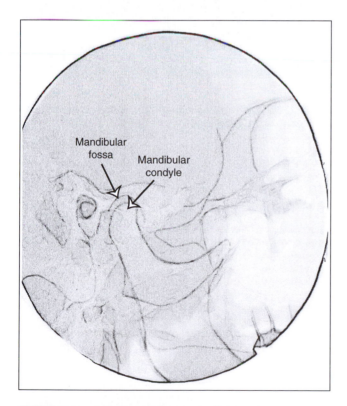

FIGURE 13.77   Axiolateral transcranial (Schuller) TMJ, closed mouth.

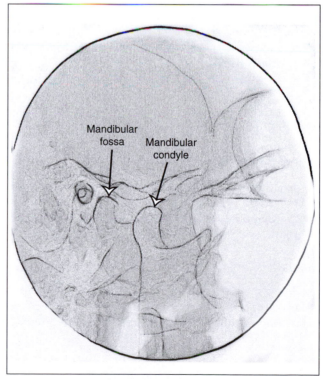

FIGURE 13.79   Axiolateral transcranial (Schuller) TMJ, open mouth.

TEMPOROMANDIBULAR JOINTS—TRANSCRANIAL LATERAL POSITION

Exam Rationale This position best demonstrates the TMJ closest to the film. The configuration of the condyle and mandibular fossa and the direction and amount of movement is demonstrated. The position also illustrates dislocation or small fractures of the cortex of the condyle. Both sides are usually taken in both the open and closed mouth positions.

Technical Considerations

- Regular screen/film
- Grid
- kVp range: 70–80
- SID: 40 inch (100 cm)

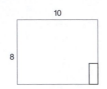

Radiation Protection

AEC (Phototiming)

 N DENSITY

Patient Position In a lateral position; all potential artifacts removed (Figure 13.80).

Part Position With the side to be demonstrated closest to the film, rest the cheek against the cassette holder; cassette is centered to the TMJ; rotate the head toward the film until MSP forms a 15° angle to the film; acanthiomeatal line is parallel to the transverse axis of the film.

Central Ray 15° caudal exiting through the TMJ.

Patient Instructions

- Closed mouth: "With your mouth closed, hold your breath and don't move."
- Open mouth: "Open your mouth, hold your breath, and don't move.

Evaluation Criteria (Figures 13.81 through 13.84)

- Closed mouth position demonstrates the mandibular condyle in the mandibular fossa.
- In open mouth position condyle will move inferior and anterior.

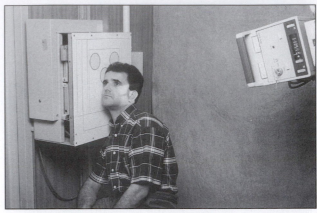

A

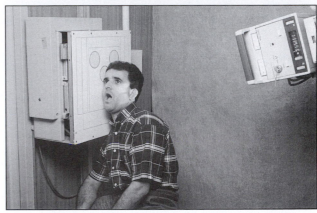

B

FIGURE 13.80   Lateral transcranial TMJ. **(A)** Closed mouth. **(B)** Open mouth.

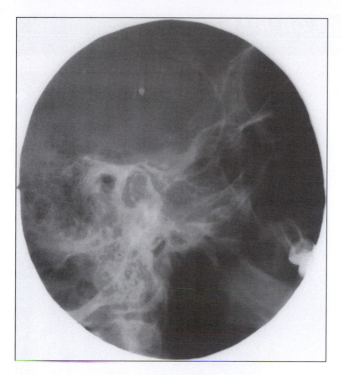

FIGURE 13.81   Lateral transcranial TMJ, closed mouth.

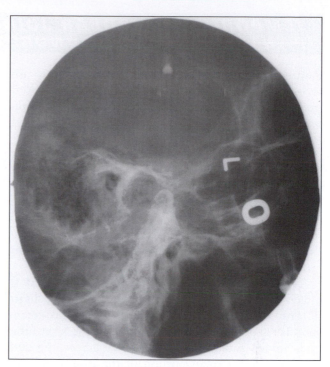

FIGURE 13.83   Lateral transcranial TMJ, open mouth.

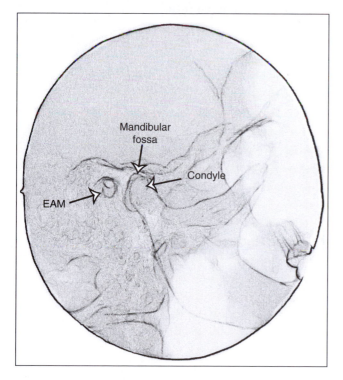

FIGURE 13.82   Lateral transcranial TMJ, closed mouth.

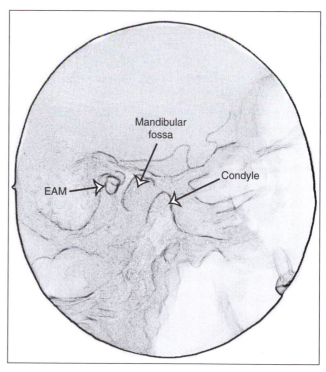

FIGURE 13.84   Lateral transcranial TMJ, open mouth.

TEMPOROMANDIBULAR JOINTS OR MANDIBLE— PANTOMOGRAPHY (PANOREX)

Pantomography and panoramic tomography are techniques used to produce a radiograph of a curved surface. The entire mandible and the TMJs are demonstrated on one film. It demonstrates fractures and mandibular or dental tumors.

The patient is seated with the head placed in the head holder and with the bite device between the upper and lower teeth. This centers the patient's head and aligns the upper and lower central incisors. The MSP is perpendicular and the occlusal plane is parallel to the floor. The patient remains stationary while the x-ray tube and film rotate in the same direction around the head (Figure 13.85).

The film is placed in a flexible cassette and is attached to a holder or drum that has a narrow slit in it. The x-ray beam is tightly collimated and corresponds to the slit in the film holder. As the x-ray tube and holder rotate, the film moves across the slit, exposing only a small portion of the film at a time. The resultant radiograph demonstrates the entire curved mandible laid out across the film.

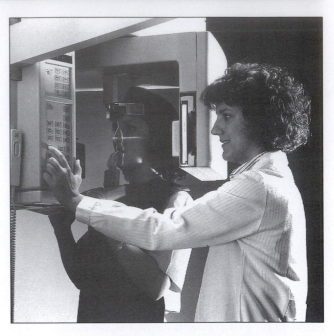

FIGURE 13.85   **Panorex (Courtesy of DENTSPLY International Inc., GENDEX Corporation, Midwest Dental Products Corporation).**

Evaluation Criteria (Figures 13.86 and 13.87)

- The entire mandible and TMJs should be demonstrated.
- An exaggerated smile indicates the occlusal plane is too low; a frown indicates the occlusal plane is too high.
- The spine should not overlap the ramus.
- There should be an even density throughout.

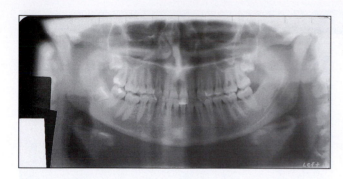

FIGURE 13.86   Panorex.

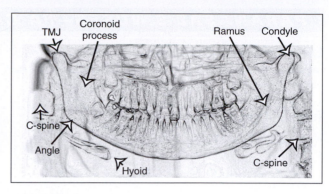

FIGURE 13.87   Panorex.

PARANASAL SINUSES—PA CALDWELL PROJECTION

Exam Rationale This projection best demonstrates inflammatory changes in the frontal sinuses and the ethmoid sinuses.

Technical Considerations

- Regular screen/film
- Grid
- kVp range: 70–80
- SID: 40 inch (100 cm)

Radiation Protection

AEC (Phototiming)

 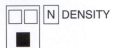 N DENSITY

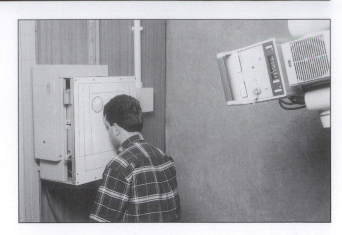

FIGURE 13.88 PA Caldwell sinuses.

Patient Position Facing the film; all potential artifacts removed (Figure 13.88).

Part Position As in the PA Caldwell in Chapter 12; cassette is centered to the nasion; MSP is perpendicular to the midpoint of the grid; OML is perpendicular to the film.

Central Ray 15° caudal exiting at the nasion.

Patient Instructions "Hold your breath and don't move."

Evaluation Criteria (Figures 13.89 and 13.90)

- The petrous ridges are demonstrated in the lower third of the orbits.
- The frontal sinuses are situated above the fronto-nasal suture.

- The anterior ethmoid sinuses are demonstrated immediately lateral to the nasal bones and directly below the frontal sinuses.
- No rotation is evident.

Tip To use a horizontal beam, tilt the film holder 15° with the superior edge toward the patient. Rest the nose and forehead on the holder and adjust the MSP perpendicular and OML perpendicular to the film (Figure 13.91).

This projection can be used to demonstrate the floor of the **antra** in those cases where it is difficult to demonstrate in other projections.

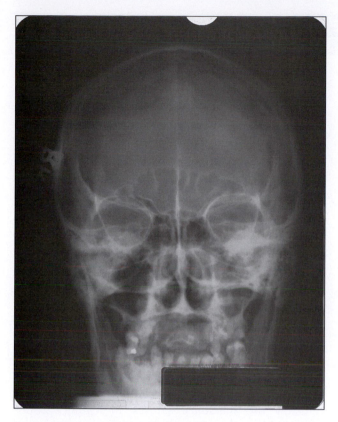

FIGURE 13.89   **PA Caldwell sinuses.**

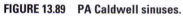

FIGURE 13.91   **PA sinuses with horizontal beam.**

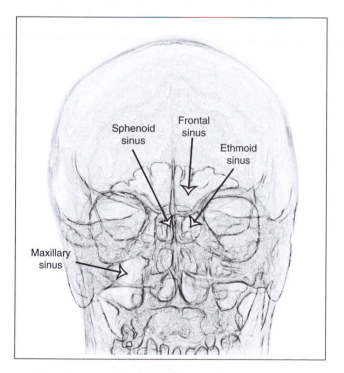

FIGURE 13.90   **PA Caldwell sinuses.**

PARANASAL SINUSES—PARIETOACANTHIAL (WATERS) PROJECTION

Exam Rationale   This projection is used to demonstrate sinusitis of the maxillary sinuses, which are the most commonly infected. Retention cysts and nasal deviation can also be demonstrated.

Technical Considerations

- Regular screen/film
- Grid
- kVp range: 70–80
- SID: 40 inch (100 cm)

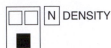

Radiation Protection   **AEC (Phototiming)**

   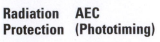 N DENSITY

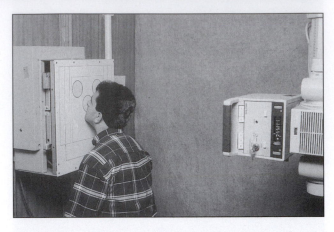

FIGURE 13.92   Parietoacanthial (Waters) sinuses.

Patient Position   Facing the film; all potential artifacts removed (Figure 13.92).

Part Position   As in the parietoacanthial in Chapter 12; cassette is centered to the level of the acanthion; MSP is perpendicular to the midpoint of the grid; OML forms an angle of 37° to the plane of the film.

Central Ray   Perpendicular to the film exiting at the acanthion.

Patient Instructions   "Hold your breath and don't move."

Evaluation Criteria (Figures 13.93 and 13.94)

- The petrous ridges are projected immediately below the maxillary sinuses indicating proper extension.
- No rotation as evidenced by equal distance from the lateral border of the skull to the orbit on each side.

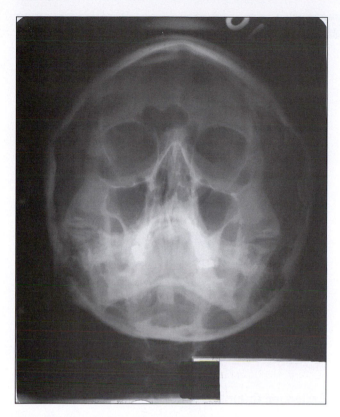

FIGURE 13.93   Parietoacanthial (Waters) sinuses.

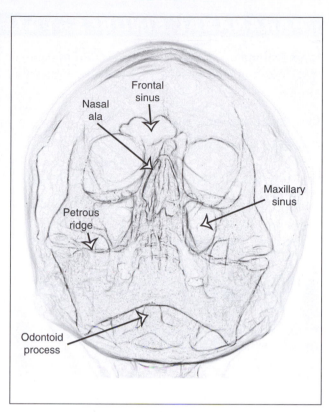

FIGURE 13.94   Parietoacanthial (Waters) sinuses.

PARANASAL SINUSES—LATERAL POSITION

Exam Rationale This is the best position to demonstrate the sphenoid sinuses; it also demonstrates the frontal, maxillary, and ethmoid sinuses.

Technical Considerations

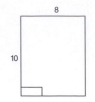

- Regular screen/film
- Grid
- kVp range: 70–80
- SID: 40 inch (100 cm)

Radiation Protection   AEC (Phototiming)

 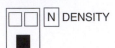 N DENSITY

Patient Position In lateral position; all potential artifacts removed (Figure 13.95).

Part Position As in the lateral in Chapter 12; side of interest closest to the film; cassette is centered to a point 1/2 to 1 inch (1–3 cm) posterior to the outer canthus; MSP is parallel to the film; interpupillary line is perpendicular to the film; IOML is parallel to the transverse axis of the film.

Central Ray Perpendicular to the film entering 1/2 to 1 inch (1–3 cm) posterior to the outer canthus.

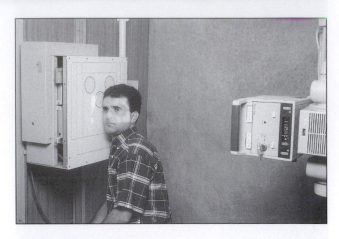

FIGURE 13.95   Lateral sinuses.

Patient Instructions "Hold your breath and don't move."

Evaluation Criteria (Figures 13.96 and 13.97)

- All sinuses should be visualized.
- No rotation as evidenced by superimposition of the mandibular rami and orbital roofs and the sella turcica is seen without rotation.

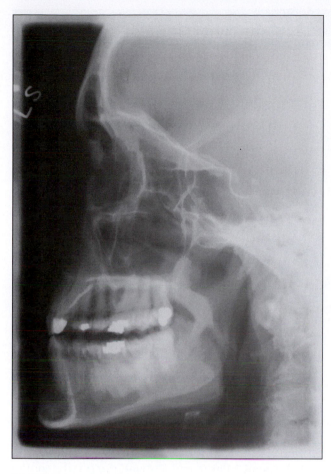

FIGURE 13.96 Lateral sinuses.

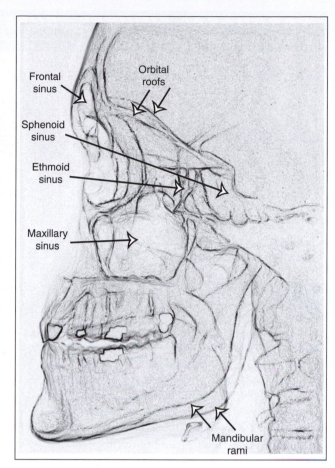

Frontal
sinus

Orbital
roofs

Sphenoid
sinus

Ethmoid
sinus

Maxillary
sinus

Mandibular
rami

FIGURE 13.97 Lateral sinuses.

PARANASAL SINUSES—SUBMENTOVERTICAL PROJECTION

Exam Rationale　This projection best demonstrates the sphenoid sinuses, the ethmoid sinuses, and the nasal passages.

Technical Considerations

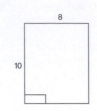

- Regular screen/film
- Grid
- kVp range: 70–80
- SID: 40 inch (100 cm)

Radiation Protection　AEC (Phototiming)

 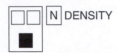 N DENSITY

Patient Position　Facing the tube; all potential artifacts removed (Figure 13.98).

Part Position　As in the SMV in Chapter 12; vertex of the head is resting on the cassette holder; cassette is centered to the level of the sella turcica; MSP is perpendicular to the midpoint of the grid; IOML is parallel to the plane of the film.

Central Ray　Perpendicular to the IOML entering midway between the angles of the mandible approximately 2 inches (5 cm) inferior to the mandibular symphysis.

Patient Instructions　"Hold your breath and don't move."

Evaluation Criteria (Figures 13.99 and 13.100)

- The mandibular symphysis is superimposed on the anterior frontal bone indicating adequate extension or tube angle.
- There is no rotation as evidenced by symmetrical petrous ridges and equal distance between the mandible and the lateral border of the skull.

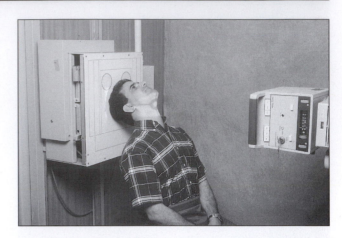

FIGURE 13.98　SMV sinuses.

Tip　For the patient who is unable to assume this position, the verticosubmental is an option. With the patient seated at the end of the table, the cassette is placed on an angle sponge. The patient's chin rests on the cassette and the head is adjusted to place the MSP perpendicular to the film and the IOML parallel to the film. The central ray is perpendicular to the IOML (Figure 13.101).

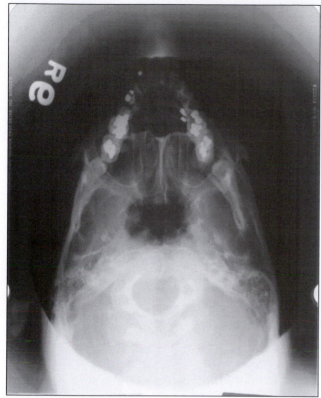

FIGURE 13.99   SMV sinuses.

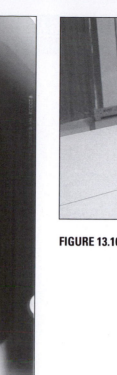

FIGURE 13.101   Verticosubmental sinuses.

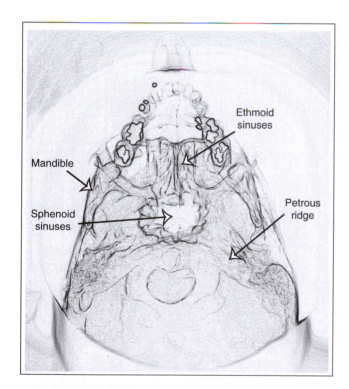

FIGURE 13.100   SMV sinuses.

PARANASAL SINUSES—AXIAL TRANSORAL (PIRIE) PROJECTION

Exam Rationale   This projection demonstrates the sphenoid sinuses projected through the open mouth. The maxillary sinuses and nasal fossae are also visualized.

Technical Considerations

- Regular screen/film
- Grid
- kVp range: 70–80
- SID: 40 inch (100 cm)

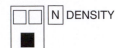

Radiation Protection

AEC (Phototiming)

    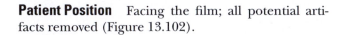 N DENSITY

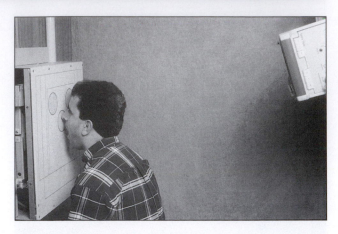

FIGURE 13.102   Axial transoral (Pirie) sinuses.

Patient Position   Facing the film; all potential artifacts removed (Figure 13.102).

Part Position   Place the nose and chin on the cassette holder; the mouth is open and centered to the film; MSP is perpendicular to the film and centered to the grid.

Central Ray   At a 30° caudal angle along a line extending from the sella turcica to the center of the open mouth.

Patient Instructions   "Hold your breath and don't move."

Evaluation Criteria (Figures 13.103 and 13.104)

- Sphenoid sinuses demonstrated through the open mouth.

Tips

1. The sella turcica is located at a level 3/4 inch (2 cm) anterior and 3/4 inch (2 cm) superior to the external auditory meatus.
2. It is especially important to clean the Bucky surface in the presence of the patient before positioning.

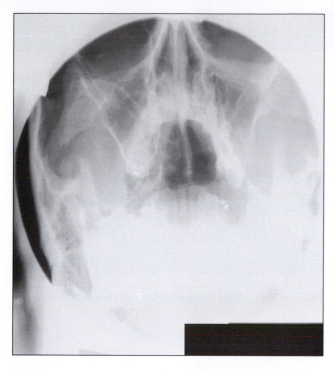

FIGURE 13.103   Axial transoral (Pirie) sinuses.

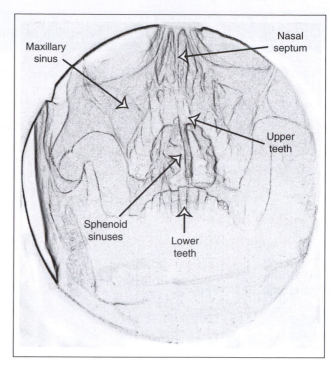

FIGURE 13.104   Axial transoral (Pirie) sinuses.

TEMPORAL BONES—AXIAL AP (TOWNE/GRASHEY) PROJECTION

Exam Rationale This projection demonstrates a symmetrical image of the petrous portion of the temporal bone, the internal auditory canals, the arcuate eminences, labyrinths, mastoid antrum, and middle ear.

Technical Considerations

- Regular screen/film
- Grid
- kVp range: 70–80
- SID: 40 inch (100 cm)

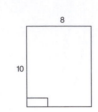

Radiation Protection

AEC (Phototiming)

   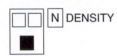

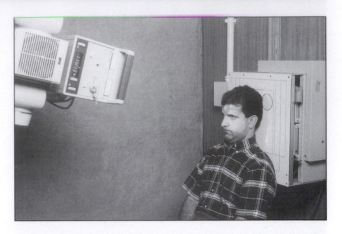

FIGURE 13.105   Axial AP (Towne/Grashey) temporal bones.

Patient Position Facing the tube; all potential artifacts removed (Figure 13.105).

Part Position As in the AP axial in Chapter 12; MSP is perpendicular to the midpoint of the film; OML is perpendicular to the film.

Central Ray At a 30° caudal angle exiting through the external auditory meatus.

Patient Instructions "Hold your breath and don't move."

Evaluation Criteria (Figures 13.106 and 13.107)

- The petrous ridges and mastoid air cells should be included.
- No rotation as evidenced by:
  —Symmetrical petrous ridges
  —Equal distance from lateral border of foramen magnum to lateral border of skull
- Dorsum sella and posterior clinoids should be visualized within the foramen magnum.

Tip If it is not possible to place the OML perpendicular to the film, the IOML can be placed perpendicular to the film, and the central ray angle is increased to 37°.

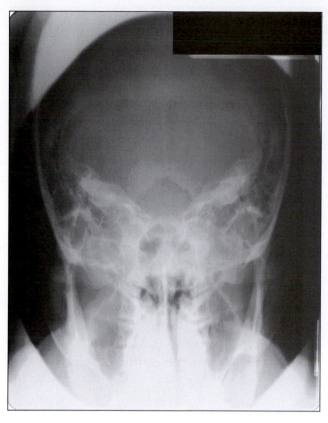

FIGURE 13.106 Axial AP (Towne/Grashey) temporal bones.

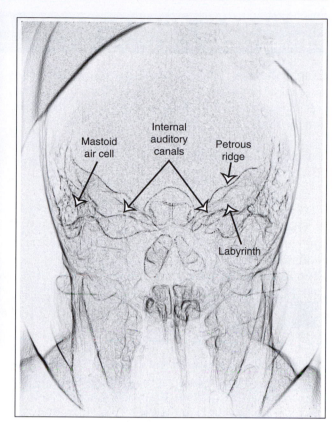

FIGURE 13.107 Axial AP (Towne/Grashey) temporal bones.

TEMPORAL BONES—AXIOLATERAL OBLIQUE (LAW) POSITION

Exam Rationale This position demonstrates the mastoid air cells and the internal auditory canal of the side closest to the film. Both sides should be done for comparison.

Technical Considerations

- Regular screen/film
- Grid
- kVp range: 70–80
- SID: 40 inch (100 cm)

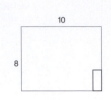

Radiation Protection

AEC (Phototiming)

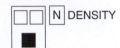 N DENSITY

Patient Position In a lateral position; all potential artifacts removed. The auricle of the ear should be taped forward to prevent superimposition of it over the mastoid air cells (Figure 13.108).

Part Position Place head in lateral position and then rotate the face toward the film so the MSP is 15° to the plane of the film; center the film approximately 1 inch (3 cm) posterior to the EAM closest to the film.

Central Ray 15° caudal entering approximately 2 inches (5 cm) posterior and 2 inches (5 cm) superior to the uppermost EAM.

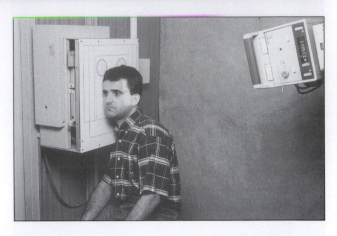

FIGURE 13.108 Axiolateral oblique (Law) temporal bones.

Patient Instructions "Hold your breath and don't move."

Evaluation Criteria (Figures 13.109 and 13.110)

- The mastoid air cells of interest are located in the center of the film without superimposition of the opposite side.
- The internal and external meatuses are superimposed.
- The TMJ is located anterior to the mastoid air cells.
- The auricle of the ear should not superimpose the mastoid air cells.

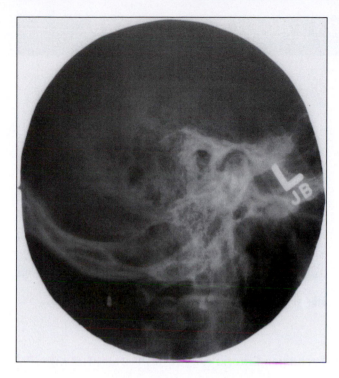

FIGURE 13.109   **Axiolateral oblique (Law) temporal bones.**

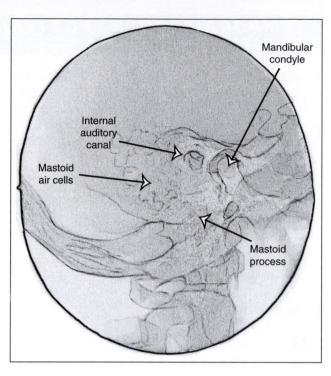

FIGURE 13.110   **Axiolateral oblique (Law) temporal bones.**

TEMPORAL BONES—POSTERIOR PROFILE (STENVERS) POSITION

Exam Rationale This position demonstrates the dependent petrous portion parallel to the film. The petrous ridge, the mastoid air cells, the tip of the mastoid, the mastoid antrum, the labyrinth, and the internal auditory canal are visualized. Both sides should be done for comparison.

Technical Considerations

- Regular screen/film
- Grid
- kVp range: 70–80
- SID: 40 inch (100 cm)

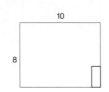

10

8

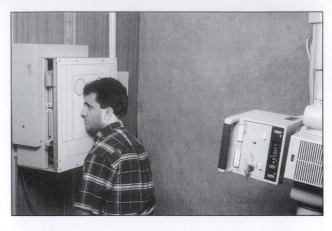

FIGURE 13.111   Posterior profile (Stenvers) temporal bones.

Radiation Protection　　AEC (Phototiming)

　　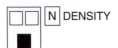 N DENSITY

Patient Position Facing the film; all potential artifacts removed (Figure 13.111).

Part Position Rest the patient's head on the forehead, nose, and zygoma; center the film 1 inch (3 cm) anterior to the external auditory canal closest to the film; IOML is parallel to the transverse axis of the film; MSP forms an angle of 45° to the film.

Central Ray 12° cephalad entering approximately 2 inches (5 cm) posterior to the uppermost EAM.

Patient Instructions "Hold your breath and don't move."

Evaluation Criteria (Figures 13.112 and 13.113)

- The petrous ridge and mastoid process of the side of interest is included.
- The internal auditory canal and bony labyrinths are demonstrated below the petrous ridge.
- The mandibular ramus and condyle are superimposed on the cervical spine.

Tip For patients who cannot be placed in a prone position, the anterior profile (Arcelin method) can be used. Center the MSP to the midpoint of the film; rotate the head 45° away from the side of interest; place IOML perpendicular to the film; angle the central ray 10° caudal, entering approximately 1 inch (3 cm) anterior and slightly above the uppermost EAM (Figure 13.114).

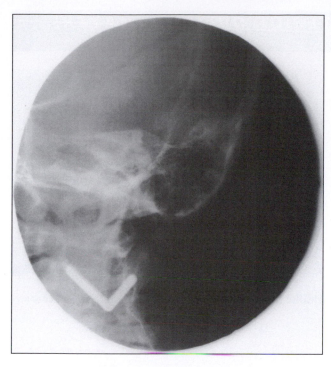

FIGURE 13.112   Posterior profile (Stenvers) temporal bones.

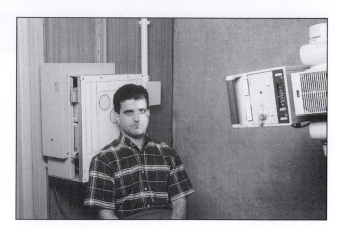

FIGURE 13.114   Anterior profile (Arcelin) temporal bones.

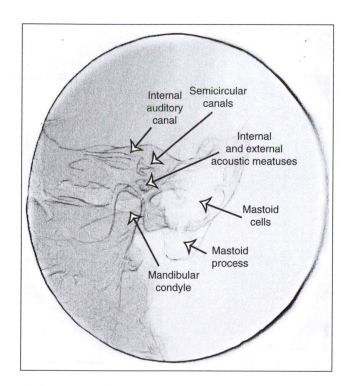

FIGURE 13.113   Posterior profile (Stenvers) temporal bones.

TEMPORAL BONES—AXIOPOSTERIOR OBLIQUE (MAYER) POSITION

Exam Rationale An axial oblique position of the mastoid air cells is demonstrated. The external auditory meatus, the mastoid antrum, and bony labyrinth are visualized. Both sides should be done for comparison.

Technical Considerations

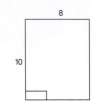

- Regular screen/film
- Grid
- kVp range: 70–80
- SID: 40 inch (100 cm)

Radiation Protection **AEC (Phototiming)**

 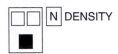

Patient Position Facing the tube; all potential artifacts removed (Figure 13.115).

Part Position With the back of the patient's head against the cassette holder, rotate the head 45° toward the side of interest; the chin is depressed to place the IOML parallel to the transverse axis of the film.

Central Ray 45° caudal exiting through the EAM of interest.

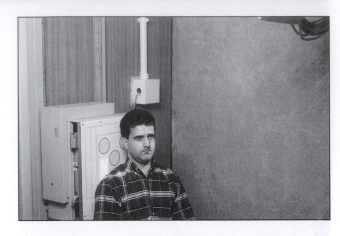

FIGURE 13.115 Axioposterior oblique (Mayer) temporal bones.

Patient Instructions "Hold your breath and don't move."

Evaluation Criteria (Figures 13.116 and 13.117)

- The mastoid air cells of the side of interest are located in the center of the film.
- The external auditory meatus is demonstrated anterior to the petrosa.
- The TMJ is anterior to the EAM.

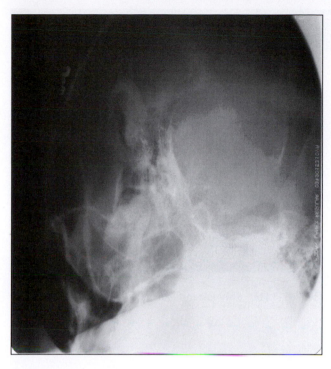

FIGURE 13.116 Axioposterior oblique (Mayer) temporal bones.

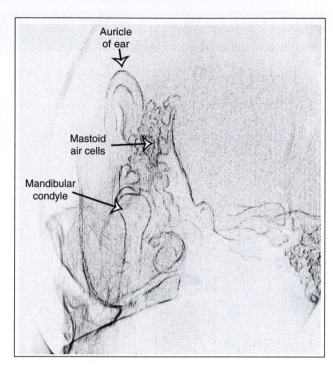

FIGURE 13.117 Axioposterior oblique (Mayer) temporal bones.

TEMPORAL BONES—SUBMENTOVERTICAL (SMV) PROJECTION

Exam Rationale   This projection demonstrates symmetrical petrosa, the auditory canals, the mastoid processes, the labyrinths, and the tympanic cavities.

Technical Considerations

- Regular screen/film
- Grid
- kVp range: 70–80
- SID: 40 inch (100 cm)

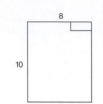

Radiation Protection

AEC (Phototiming)

 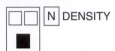

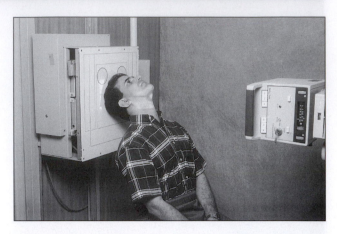

FIGURE 13.118   SMV temporal bones.

Patient Position   Facing the tube; all potential artifacts removed (Figure 13.118).

Part Position   As in the SMV in Chapter 12; patient's neck is extended until the head is resting on the vertex; cassette is centered to the level of the mandibular angles; IOML is parallel to the film.

Patient Instructions   "Hold your breath and don't move."

Central Ray   Perpendicular to IOML entering midway between the mandibular angles.

Evaluation Criteria (Figures 13.119 and 13.120)

- The mandibular condyles should be demonstrated anterior to the petrous ridges and the external auditory canals.
- The distance from the lateral border of the mandibular condyle to the lateral border of the cranium should be equal on both sides demonstrating no rotation.
- The petrosa should be symmetrical.

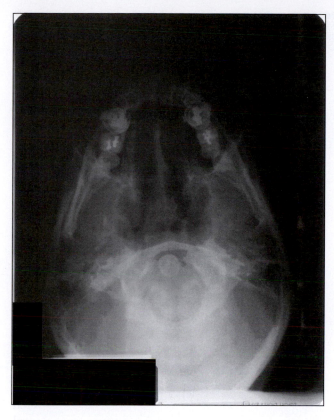

FIGURE 13.119   SMV temporal bones.

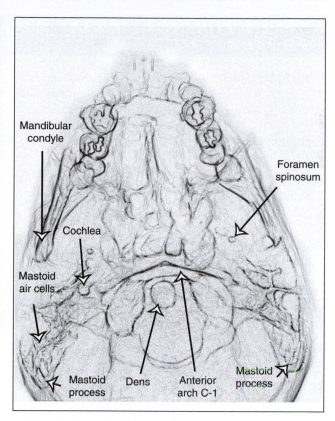

FIGURE 13.120   SMV temporal bones.

SELLA TURCICA—AXIAL AP (TOWNE/GRASHEY) PROJECTION

Exam Rationale This projection demonstrates the dorsum sella, anterior and posterior clinoids, the petrous pyramids, and the foramen magnum.

Technical Considerations

- Regular screen/film
- Grid
- kVp range: 70–80
- SID: 40 inch (100 cm)

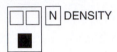

Radiation Protection   AEC (Phototiming)

  □ □ N DENSITY

Patient Position Facing the tube; all potential artifacts removed (Figure 13.121).

Part Position As in the AP axial in Chapter 12; MSP is perpendicular to the midpoint of the film; IOML is perpendicular to the film; center the cassette to coincide with the central ray.

Central Ray 30° caudal if the anterior clinoids are of interest or 37° caudal if the dorsum sella and posterior clinoids are of interest. The central ray should exit through the foramen magnum.

Patient Instructions "Hold your breath and don't move."

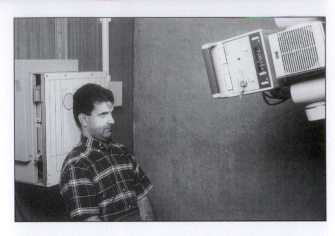

FIGURE 13.121   Axial AP (Towne/Grashey) sella turcica.

Evaluation Criteria (Figures 13.122 through 13.125)

- No rotation as evidenced by symmetrical petrous ridges.
- 30° caudal angle:
  —The dorsum sella and anterior clinoids are projected through the occipital bone and are visualized above the foramen magnum.
- 37° caudal angle:
  —The dorsum sella and posterior clinoids are projected through the foramen magnum.

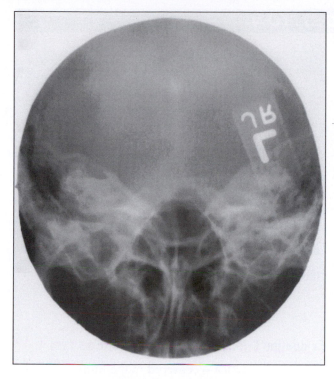

FIGURE 13.122   Axial AP (30°) sella turcica.

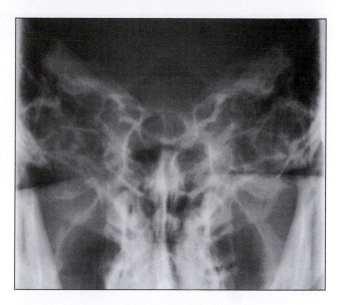

FIGURE 13.124   Axial AP (37°) sella turcica.

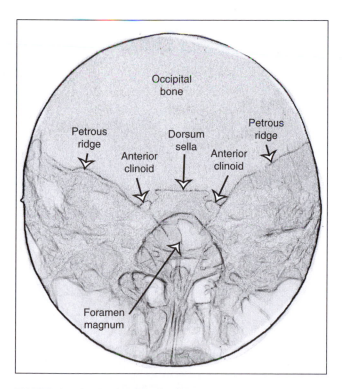

FIGURE 13.123   Axial AP (30°) sella turcica.

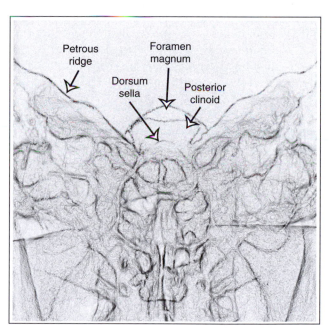

FIGURE 13.125   Axial AP (37°) sella turcica.

SELLA TURCICA—LATERAL POSITION

Exam Rationale This position demonstrates a lateral view of the sella turcica, the anterior and posterior clinoids, the dorsum sella, and the clivus.

Technical Considerations

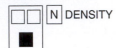

- Regular screen/film
- Grid
- kVp range: 70–80
- SID: 40 inch (100 cm)

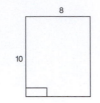

	8
10	

Radiation Protection · AEC (Phototiming)

☐ ☐ N DENSITY
■

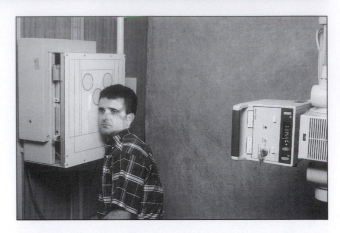

FIGURE 13.126   Lateral sella turcica.

Patient Position In lateral position; all potential artifacts removed (Figure 13.126).

Part Position As in the lateral in Chapter 12; cassette is centered to a point 3/4 inch (2 cm) anterior and 3/4 inch (2 cm) superior to the EAM; MSP is parallel to the film; interpupillary line is perpendicular to the film; IOML is parallel to the transverse axis of the film.

Central Ray Perpendicular to the film entering 3/4 inch (2 cm) anterior to and 3/4 inch (2 cm) superior to the EAM.

Patient Instructions "Hold your breath and don't move."

Evaluation Criteria (Figures 13.127 and 13.128)

- The sella turcica is centered to the film.
- No rotation is visualized as evidenced by superimposition of the anterior clinoids and of the posterior clinoids.
- Sella turcica is seen in profile.

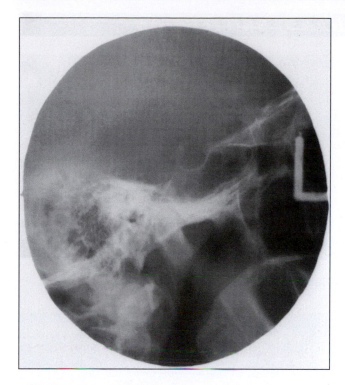

FIGURE 13.127   Lateral sella turcica.

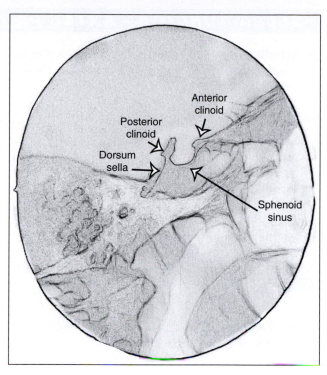

FIGURE 13.128   Lateral sella turcica.

SELLA TURCICA—AXIAL PA (HAAS) PROJECTION

Exam Rationale This is an alternate projection for demonstrating the dorsum sella, posterior clinoids, foramen magnum, and petrous ridges.

Technical Considerations

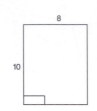

- Regular screen/film
- Grid
- kVp range: 70–80
- SID: 40 inch (100 cm)

Radiation Protection   AEC (Phototiming)

 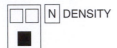 N DENSITY

Patient Position Facing the film; all potential artifacts removed (Figure 13.129).

Part Position Patient's forehead and nose rest against the cassette holder; cassette is centered 1 inch (3 cm) superior to the superciliary arch; MSP is perpendicular to the midline of the film; OML is perpendicular to the film.

Central Ray 25° cephalic entering 1 1/2 inch (4 cm) inferior to the inion.

Patient Instructions "Hold your breath and don't move."

Evaluation Criteria (Figures 13.130 and 13.131)

- The dorsum sellae and the posterior clinoids should be demonstrated within the shadow of the foramen magnum.
- No rotation should be demonstrated.
- Symmetrical petrous pyramids are visualized.

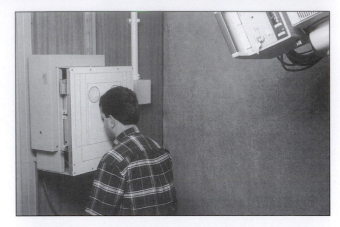

FIGURE 13.129   Axial PA (Haas) sella turcica.

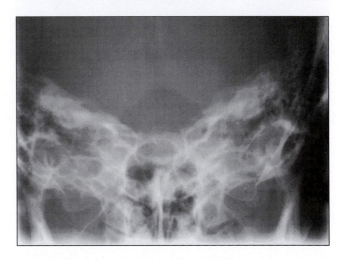

FIGURE 13.130   Axial PA (Haas) sella turcica.

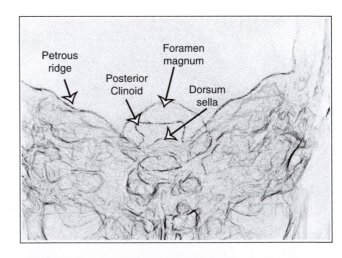

FIGURE 13.131   Axial PA (Haas) sella turcica.

13

Review Questions

1. In the axial AP projection of the skull, which of the following is best demonstrated?

   a. frontal bone
   b. frontal sinuses
   c. occipital bone
   d. sphenoid bone

2. In the axial AP projection of the skull, the central ray is angled _____.

   a. 30° caudad to the OML
   b. 30° cephalad to the OML
   c. 30° caudad to the IOML
   d. 30° cephalad to the IOML

3. On a properly positioned axial AP projection of the skull, the dorsum sella should be seen:

   a. not at all
   b. within the foramen magnum
   c. on either side of the foramen magnum
   d. just below the foramen magnum

4. For a PA projection of the skull, the central ray is directed to exit at the:

   a. hairline
   b. lips
   c. mentum
   d. nasion

5. Which of the following statements is true for the lateral skull?

   1. MSP is perpendicular to the film
   2. interpupillary line is perpendicular to the film
   3. central ray is perpendicular to the film

   a. 1 only
   b. 2 only
   c. 1 and 3
   d. 2 and 3

6. Of the following positions/projections, which demonstrates the foramina ovale and spinosum, the petrous ridges, and the sphenoid sinuses?

   a. axial AP
   b. PA
   c. parietoacanthial
   d. SMV

7. When performing the parietoacanthial (Waters), the _____ line forms an angle of 37° with the plane of the film.

   a. acanthiomeatal
   b. glabellomeatal
   c. IOML
   d. OML

8. In the parieto-orbital oblique (Rhese) to demonstrate the optic foramen, the MSP forms an angle of _____ to the film.

   a. 30°
   b. 37°
   c. 53°
   d. 60°

9. For a parieto-orbital oblique (Rhese) of the optic foramen, the head should rest on the:

   a. forehead
   b. forehead, cheek, and nose
   c. cheek, nose, and chin
   d. chin

10. The parieto-orbital oblique (Rhese) uses which baseline?

    a. acanthiomeatal
    b. glabellomeatal
    c. IOML
    d. OML

11. A properly positioned parieto-orbital oblique will demonstrate the optic foramen in the _____ quadrant of the orbit.

    a. upper, outer
    b. lower, outer
    c. upper, inner
    d. lower, inner

12. In which of the following positions/projections is the OML perpendicular to the film?

    a. lateral
    b. parietoacanthial
    c. PA
    d. SMV

13. Which projection would best demonstrate the zygomatic arch?

    a. PA
    b. lateral
    c. SMV
    d. axial AP

14. In the axiolateral of the mandible, the central ray is angled:

    a. cephalad
    b. caudad
    c. not at all

15. The patient should be in which of the following positions for radiography of the paranasal sinuses?

    a. erect
    b. lordotic
    c. recumbent
    d. Trendelenburg

16. Which position/projection best demonstrates the sphenoid sinuses?

    a. PA Caldwell
    b. axial AP
    c. submentovertical
    d. parietoacanthial (Waters)

17. Which of the following will best demonstrate the maxillary sinuses?

    a. PA Caldwell
    b. parietoacanthial (Waters)
    c. axiolateral oblique (Law)
    d. axial transoral (Pirie)

18. On a parietoacanthial (Waters) of the sinuses, the petrous ridges should:

    a. fill in the orbital shadow
    b. be projected in the lower third of the maxillary sinuses
    c. be projected just below the maxillary sinuses
    d. not be seen

19. For which of the following is the MSP perpendicular to the plane of the film?

    1. lateral skull
    2. lateral sinuses
    3. PA Caldwell skull
    4. axial AP zygomatic arches

    a. 1 and 2
    b. 3 and 4
    c. 1 and 3
    d. 2 and 4

20. The posterior profile (Stenvers) to demonstrate the temporal bone uses a _____ central ray.

    a. 12° cephalad
    b. 12° caudad
    c. 15° cephalad
    d. 15° caudad

21. Which of the following statements concerning the axiolateral oblique (Law) is true?

    1. MSP is 15° toward the film
    2. central ray is 15° cephalad
    3. auricle of the ear should be taped forward

    a. 1 only
    b. 2 only
    c. 1 and 3
    d. 1, 2, and 3

22. The PA Caldwell uses a 15° cephalad central ray.

    a. true
    b. false

23. When positioning for a recumbent lateral skull, the patient should be semi-prone.

    a. true
    b. false

24. The preferred position for any SMV projection is recumbent.

    a. true
    b. false

25. For a PA projection of the mandible, the central ray is directed perpendicular to exit at the lips.

    a. true
    b. false

26. In the superoinferior projection of the nasal bones, the _____ line is perpendicular to the film.

27. Panoramic tomography is used to demonstrate the _____ and the _____ .

28. Lateral transcranial temporomandibular joints (Schuller) are done in both the _____ and_____ positions.

29. For an axial transoral (Pirie) radiograph of the sinuses, the _____ and the _____ rest on the cassette.

30. The axiolateral oblique (Law) of the temporo-mandibular bones demonstrates what structure?

31. Indicate the centering point for each of the following.

    a. lateral skull
    b. lateral facial bones
    c. lateral nasal bones
    d. lateral sinuses
    e. lateral sella turcica

32. Explain the modification of the parietoacanthial (Waters) projection used to demonstrate the floor of the orbit.

33. When doing a parieto-orbital oblique (Rhese), describe the adjustment that should be made if the optic foramen is demonstrated in the upper outer quadrant of the orbital shadow.

34. For the axiolateral mandible, the head begins in the lateral position. Describe the modification required to demonstrate the following.

    a. body of the mandible

    b. mentum

References and Recommended Reading

Anthony, C., & Thibondeau, G. (1983). *Textbook of anatomy and physiology* (11th ed.) St. Louis: Mosby.

Ballinger, P. W. (1995). *Merrill's atlas of radiographic positions and radiologic procedures* (8th ed.) St. Louis: Mosby Year-Book.

Basmajian, J. (1982). *H. A. Cates' primary anatomy* (8th ed.) Baltimore: Waverly Press.

Bontrager, K. L. (1993). *Textbook of radiographic positioning and related anatomy* (3rd ed.) St. Louis: Mosby-Year Book.

Eisenberg, R., Dennis, C., & May, C. (1989). *Radiographic positioning.* Boston: Little, Brown.

Mader, S. (1994). *Understanding human anatomy & physiology* (2nd ed.) Dubuque, IA: Wm. C. Brown.

Moore, K. (1980). *Clinically oriented anatomy.* Baltimore: Waverly Press.

Rogers, A. (1992). *Textbook of anatomy.* New York: Churchill Livingstone.

Ryan, S. P., & McNicholas, M. M. J. (1994). *Anatomy for diagnostic imaging.* Philadelphia: Saunders.

Spence, A. (1990). *Basic human anatomy* (3rd ed.) Redwood City, CA: Benjamin/Cummings.

CHAPTER 14

Trauma Head Positioning

TERRI LASKEY FAUBER, EdD, RT(R)(M)(ARRT)

TRAUMA SKILLS

PATIENT ASSESSMENT

FUNDAMENTAL PRINCIPLES

TRAUMA SKULL
AP
Axial AP (Grashey/Townes)
Lateral

OBJECTIVES

At the completion of this chapter, the student should be able to:

1. Describe the circumstances and patient conditions that would necessitate a trauma skull series.

2. Explain the rationale for each projection used for trauma patients.

3. List or discuss the skills the radiographer should possess to perform trauma radiography.

4. Describe the positioning and cassette placement used to visualize anatomic structures in the skull of the trauma patient and describe how these differ from routine projections.

5. Identify the location of the central ray and the extent of the field necessary for producing each projection.

6. Recommend the technical factors for producing an acceptable radiograph for each projection and discuss differences from routine studies.

7. State the patient instructions for each projection.

8. Given radiographs, evaluate positioning and technical factors.

Radiography of the injured or unstable patient offers many challenges. Preparation, creative thinking, and determination will aid the radiographer in the task of producing diagnostic images.

TRAUMA SKILLS

According to Drafke (1990), the radiographer needs to be mentally prepared for trauma radiography in terms of planning, organization, and nonverbal communication. Because time is critical, planning skills are important in arranging the most efficient method of completing the radiographic examinations. The radiographer needs to anticipate the coordination and flow of the examination. Organization skills are then needed to prepare and collect the necessary supplies (such as immobilization devices, positioning sponges, cassette holders, and shielding devices) and equipment to perform bedside radiography in the emergency room or on an unstable patient in the radiographic room. In addition, the radiographer must be aware of any nonverbal communication from the patient that could affect the progress of the examination. Responding appropriately to cues as a result of the patient's psychological state, (confusion, anxiety, or agitation) and physical status (respiration, skin color, or wounds) is critical to the successful completion of the examination. Also, the radiographer must refrain from unintentionally responding to the severity of the patient's injury. Adverse reactions in facial expressions or body language may indicate the degree of injury to the patient. Nonverbal and verbal communication must convey a sense of compassion and confidence in completing the task at hand.

PATIENT ASSESSMENT

It is important for the radiographer to be able to assess the patient's condition and circumstances to determine whether a routine or a trauma series is indicated. The radiographer needs to particularly assess the following:

- Level of consciousness—whether the patient is alert, drowsy, or unresponsive
- Mobility—whether the patient can adequately move or physically attain routine positions
- Severity of injury—whether the injury to the skull is critical enough to warrant a trauma skull series

Following patient assessment, the radiographer must use sound judgment to produce diagnostic images of the skull while providing quality patient care. The radiographer must determine whether the degree of consciousness, mobility, or injury could jeopardize successful completion of a routine study. The decision to proceed with a trauma skull series must be made considering the patient's best interest and circumstances surrounding the examination.

FUNDAMENTAL PRINCIPLES

Always, if there is any concern about cervical spine injury, trauma skull films should not be attempted until a lateral cervical spine radiograph has been completed and interpreted by a physician.

When performing trauma radiography, two basic principles should be kept in mind. First, it is important to obtain two views 90° apart. For most situations this will include an AP and lateral. If true AP and lateral projections cannot be obtained, then two projections as close to 90° apart should be attempted.

The second principle concerns the alignment between the central ray, the part being radiographed, and the film. As with routine skull radiography, the relationship between these three variables must be maintained. The radiographer must be creative in adjusting the standard routines to maintain these relationships.

ALTERNATIVE POSITIONS/PROJECTIONS

Part	Alternative	Page
Skull	AP	572
(trauma)	Axial AP (Grashey/Townes)	574
	Lateral	576

TRAUMA SKULL—AP PROJECTION

Exam Rationale   This projection is used to evaluate the condition or status of the cranial bones in patients who have experienced trauma or are in unstable condition. Structures demonstrated are the frontal and parietal bones. It is comparable to a routine PA projection.

Technical Considerations

- Regular screen/film
- Grid
- kVp range: 70–80
- SID: 40 inch (100 cm)

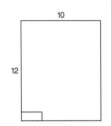

Radiation Protection

AEC (Phototiming)

 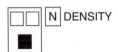 N DENSITY

Patient Position   Supine on stretcher or table (Figure 14.1).

Part Position   With minimal movement of the patient, place the cassette under the patient's head or in the table Bucky to position the top of the cassette slightly above the top of the patient's head and perpendicular to the MSP; adjust the patient's head to place the OML perpendicular to the cassette.

Patient Instructions   "Stop breathing and don't move."

Central Ray   Perpendicular to the film, entering at the nasion.

Evaluation Criteria (Figures 14.2 and 14.3)

- Entire cranium is demonstrated.
- No rotation or tilt as evidenced by equal distance between lateral border of orbit and edge of skull on each side and equal distance between midpoint of cranium and edge of film on each side.

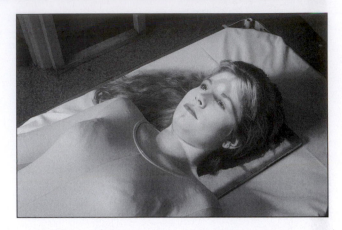

FIGURE 14.1   Trauma head positioning, AP projection.

- Petrous ridges fill the orbits.
- Sufficient density to visualize the frontal bone.
- No motion.

Tips

1. When the patient's condition will not allow movement of the head, angle the central ray until it is parallel to the OML.
2. Pediatric patients may require extension of the neck to place OML perpendicular to the cassette.

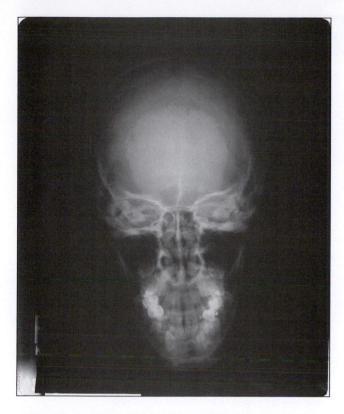

FIGURE 14.2   **AP projection of trauma skull.**

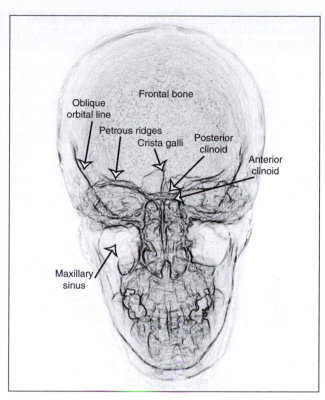

Frontal bone

Oblique
orbital line

Petrous ridges

Crista galli

Posterior
clinoid

Anterior
clinoid

Maxillary
sinus

FIGURE 14.3   **AP projection of trauma skull.**

TRAUMA SKULL—AXIAL AP (GRASHEY/TOWNES) PROJECTION

Exam Rationale   This projection is used to evaluate the condition or status of the cranial bones in patients of unstable condition or who have experienced trauma. Structures demonstrated are the occipital bone, petrous ridges, and dorsum sellae and posterior clinoid processes projected within the shadow of the foramen magnum.

Technical Considerations

- Regular screen/film
- Grid
- kVp range: 70–80
- SID: 40 inch (100 cm)

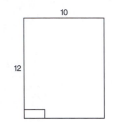

Radiation   AEC
Protection   (Phototiming)

     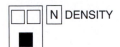 N DENSITY

Patient Position   Supine on stretcher or table (Figure 14.4).

Part Position   With minimal movement of the patient, place the cassette under the patient's head or in the table Bucky to place the top of the cassette at the top of the patient's head and perpendicular to the MSP; adjust the patient's head to place the OML perpendicular to the cassette.

Central Ray   30° caudad to enter the upper forehead and exit the foramen magnum.

Patient Instructions   "Stop breathing and don't move."

Evaluation Criteria (Figures 14.5 and 14.6)

- Entire skull, including occipital and parietal bones, is demonstrated.
- No rotation or tilt as evidenced by equal distance between foramen magnum and edge of skull on

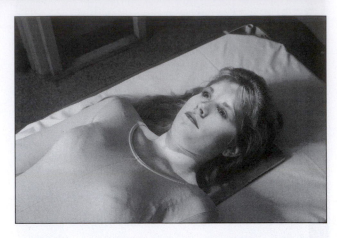

FIGURE 14.4   Trauma head positioning, Axial AP projection.

each side, and equal distance between midpoint of cranium and edge of film on each side.
- Petrous ridges superior to mastoids.
- Dorsum sellae and posterior clinoid processes projected through shadow of foramen magnum.
- Sufficient density to visualize the occipital bone.
- No motion.

Tips

1. When the patient's condition will not allow movement of the head, increase the central ray angle (not to exceed 45°), to compensate for the angle between the OML and the vertical. For example, if the OML is angled 7° from the vertical (IOML perpendicular), increase the central ray angle to 37°, the angle between the OML and CR should always be 30°.
2. Pediatric patients may require extension of the neck to place OML perpendicular to the cassette.

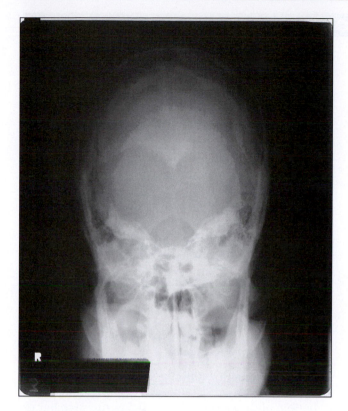

FIGURE 14.5 Axial AP projection of trauma skull.

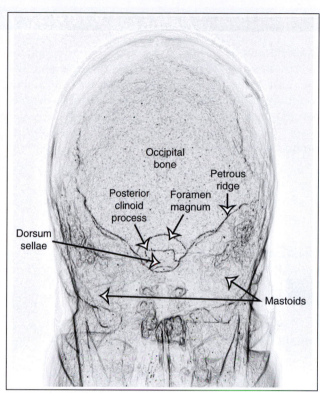

FIGURE 14.6 Axial AP projection of trauma skull.

TRAUMA SKULL—LATERAL POSITION

Exam Rationale   This position is used to evaluate the condition or status of the cranial bones in patients who have experienced trauma or who are in unstable condition. The parietal bone closest to the cassette is best demonstrated.

Technical Considerations

- Regular screen/film
- Grid
- kVp range: 60–70
- SID: 40 inch (100 cm)

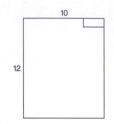

Radiation Protection

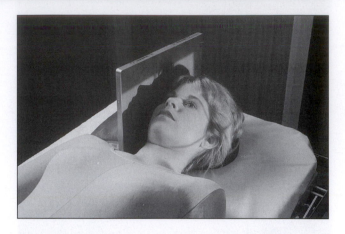

FIGURE 14.7   Trauma head positioning, lateral position.

Patient Position   Supine on stretcher or table (Figure 14.7).

Part Position   With minimal movement of the patient, elevate the head on a radiolucent support; place the cassette vertical and in contact with the side of interest and parallel to the MSP; adjust the patient's head to place the interpupillary line perpendicular and IOML parallel to the cassette.

Central Ray   Horizontal; perpendicular to cassette to enter 2 inches (5 cm) superior to the EAM.

Patient Instructions   "Stop breathing and don't move."

Evaluation Criteria (Figures 14.8 and 14.9)

- Entire cranium is demonstrated.
- No rotation as evidenced by mandibular rami, orbital roofs, sphenoid wings, and external auditory canals superimposed.
- Sella turcica in profile without rotation.
- Sufficient density to visualize parietal bone.
- No motion.

Tips (Figure 14.10 A, B, and C)

1. When the patient's condition will not allow the head to be elevated on a radiolucent sponge, place the bottom of the cassette slightly below the stretcher or table and occiput region. If this cannot be done, place the cassette vertical on stretcher or table and center the central ray 2 inches (5 cm) superior to and slightly *posterior* to EAM, open collimation to include the entire cranium. This off-centering will allow for the divergent beam to project the occipital region onto the film.

2. When doing only one lateral view, the side of the skull presenting the greatest injury should be radiographed.

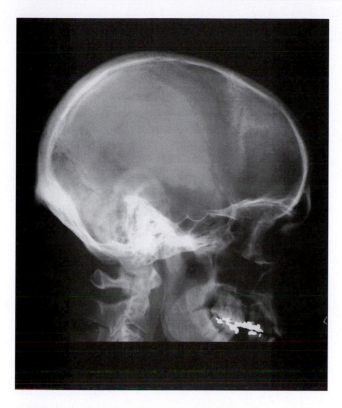

FIGURE 14.8   Lateral position of trauma skull.

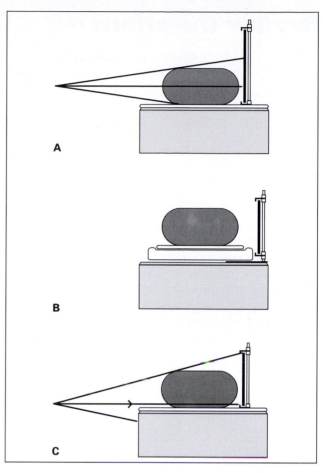

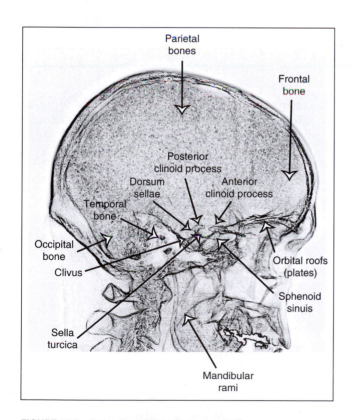

Parietal
bones

Frontal
bone

Posterior
clinoid process

Dorsum
sellae

Anterior
clinoid process

Temporal
bone

Occipital
bone

Clivus

Orbital roofs
(plates)

Sphenoid
sinuis

Sella
turcica

Mandibular
rami

FIGURE 14.9   Lateral position of trauma skull.

FIGURE 14.10   (A) Divergence of the x-ray beam projects structures on, or close to, the tabletop below the film. (View from end of table.) (B) A method for positioning the edge of the film below the patient for a horizontal beam projection. (View from end of table.) (C) Centering the beam closer to the tabletop can help overcome the problem of divergent x-rays projecting structures. (See Figure 14.10 A.) (View from end of table.) (Courtesy of Drafke, M. W. (1990). *Trauma and mobile radiography* (pp. 131–134). Philadelphia: F. A. Davis).

Review Questions

1. Which of the following is a skill needed by a radiographer in performing a trauma skull series?

   a. organization
   b. nonverbal communication
   c. ability to assess patient's condition
   d. a and c only
   e. all of the above

2. Which of the following statements best describes an important radiographic principle?

   a. Only one good image is needed for an accurate diagnosis.
   b. Any two projections that can be obtained are sufficient for an accurate diagnosis.
   c. A full routine series must be accomplished for a trauma examination.
   d. Two projections/positions taken 90° apart are required for an accurate diagnosis.

3. Which of the following statements accurately describes the relationship between the central ray, the part, and the cassette/film for an AP projection of the skull?

   a. central ray perpendicular to IOML and cassette/film
   b. central ray horizontal and perpendicular to cassette/film
   c. central ray parallel to OML and perpendicular to cassette/film
   d. central ray angled 30° to IOML

4. Of the following, which best describes the central ray location for an AP projection of the skull?

   a. central ray is perpendicular to nasion
   b. central ray is perpendicular to forehead
   c. central ray is directed to nasion at a 15° caudal angle
   d. central ray is directed to nasion at a 15° cephalad angle

5. Of the following, which best describes the centering for an axial AP (Grashey/Townes) projection?

   a. central ray enters the upper forehead and exits the foramen magnum
   b. central ray enters two inches superior to the EAM
   c. central ray enters the nasion
   d. central ray enters the foramen magnum and exits the nasion

6. On a properly positioned AP projection of the skull, where would the petrous ridges be projected?

   a. in the lower one-third of the orbit
   b. below the inferior orbital ridge
   c. to fill the orbits
   d. below the maxillary sinuses

7. For each of the following, list the anatomy demonstrated.

   a. AP skull
   b. axial AP skull (Grashey/Townes)
   c. lateral skull

8. List at least two patient conditions that would require a trauma skull series.

9. Discuss the importance of the radiographer's assessment of and interaction with the trauma patient.

10. Under what circumstance would preliminary radiographs be necessary before performing any trauma skull views?

11. With regard to Figure 14.11, how would you correct the demonstrated error if

    a. the patient can be moved

    b. the patient cannot be moved

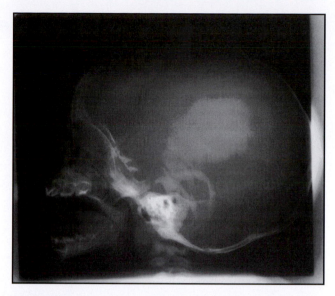

FIGURE 14.11

References and Recommended Reading

Ballinger, P. W. (1995). *Merrill's atlas of radiographic positions and radiologic procedures* (8th ed.). St. Louis: Mosby-Year Book.

Bontrager, K. L. (1993). *Textbook of radiographic positioning and related anatomy* (3rd ed.). St. Louis: Mosby-Year Book.

Drafke, M. W. (1990). *Trauma and mobile radiography.* Philadelphia: Davis.

Eisenberg, R. L., Dennis, C. A., & May, C. R. (1995). *Radiographic positioning* (2nd ed.). Boston: Little, Brown.

SECTION VI

DIGESTIVE SYSTEM
and
URINARY TRACT

Upper Gastrointestinal Tract

MARY LORTISCH, EdD, RT(R)(ARRT), FASRT

OBJECTIVES

At the completion of this chapter, the student should be able to:

1. List and describe the anatomy of the upper gastro-intestinal (GI) tract.
2. Describe the physiology of the upper GI tract.
3. Given drawings and radiographs, locate anatomic structures and landmarks of the upper GI tract.
4. Explain the rationale for each projection.
5. Explain the patient preparation for each examination.
6. Describe the positioning used to visualize anatomic structures of the upper GI tract.
7. List and/or identify the central ray location and identify the extent of field necessary for each projection.

8. Explain the protective measures that should be taken for each examination.
9. Recommend the technical factors for producing an acceptable radiograph for each projection.
10. State the patient instructions for each projection.
11. Given radiographs, evaluate positioning and technical factors.
12. Describe modifications of procedures for atypical or impaired patients to better demonstrate the anatomic area of interest.

Anatomy and Physiology

The GI tract, also called the digestive system and/or alimentary canal, includes structures from the mouth to the anus (Figure 15.1, Color illustration7). The GI tract can further be divided into upper and lower portions. The upper GI tract includes the mouth, esophagus, and stomach. Although technically a part of the lower GI tract, the small bowel is generally radiographed in conjunction with the upper GI tract, so it is presented in this chapter. The lower GI tract includes the cecum, colon, rectum, and anal canal, which are discussed in Chapter 16. Accessory organs that contribute to the digestive process include the teeth; the parotid, submaxillary and sublingual salivary glands; the liver; the pancreas; and the spleen, some of which are described in Chapter 17 (Figure 15.2). The primary and accessory organs of the GI tract have the purposes of ingestion, digestion, and absorption and elimination of food products or nutritive substances.

MOUTH

The **mouth** is the beginning of the GI tract and is where mastication (chewing) of food occurs. Deglutition (dē´´gloo-tĭsh´ŭn) (swallowing) occurs at the back of the **pharynx** (făr´ĭnks) (throat), the common area where air passes from the nasal cavity to the **trachea** (trā´ke-ă) (windpipe) and food passes from the mouth to the **esophagus** (ē-sŏf´ă-gŭs). The trachea is anterior to the esophagus. When swallowing occurs, a specialized flap of skin called the **epiglottis** (ĕp´´ĭ-glŏt´ĭs), covers the trachea so food can pass into the esophagus and not enter the respiratory system (Figure 15.3).

ESOPHAGUS

The esophagus is a muscular tube, approximately 10 inches (25 cm) long, that extends from the pharynx to the entrance of the **stomach**. Masticated food is

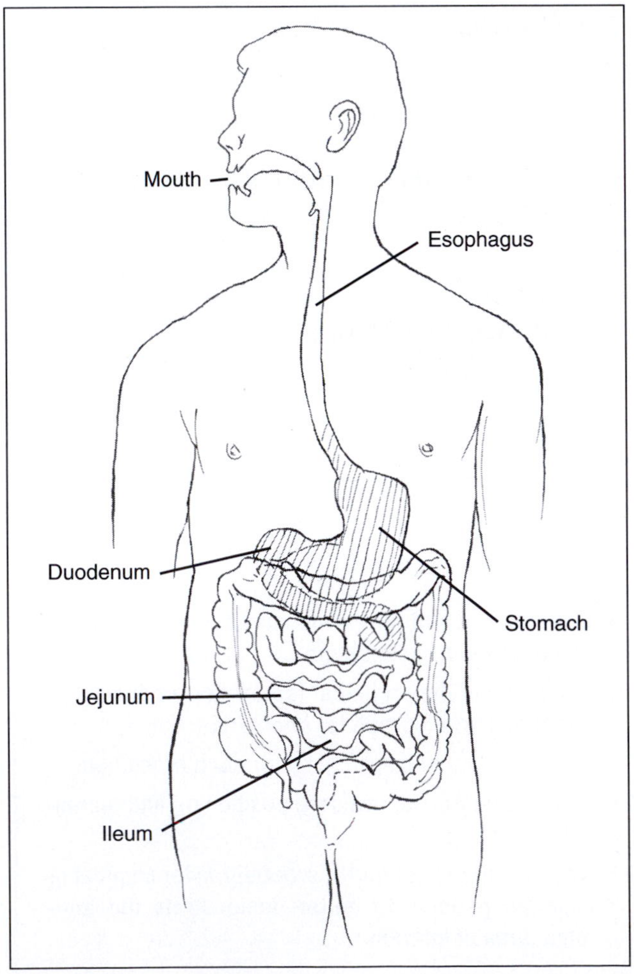

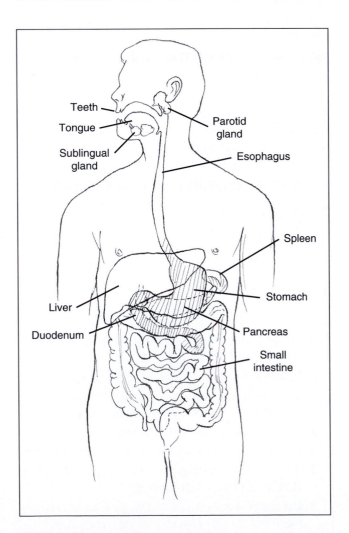

FIGURE 15.1   Upper GI tract.

FIGURE 15.2   Accessory organs anatomy.

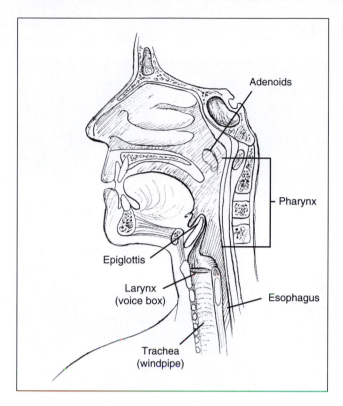

FIGURE 15.3   Pharynx cross-sectional view.

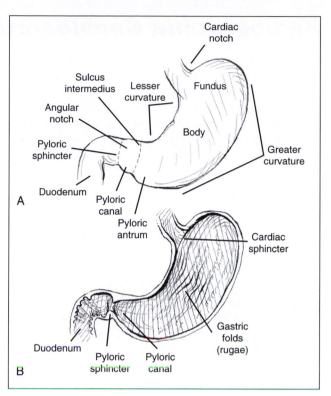

FIGURE 15.4   Stomach: (A) external, (B) internal.

propelled through the esophagus and throughout the entire GI tract by involuntary, wave-like contractions called **peristalsis** (pĕr-ĭ-stăl´sĭs). The esophagus enters the stomach at the **cardiac orifice** (kăr´dē-ăk or´ĭ-fĭs) and is surrounded by a muscular ring called the **cardiac sphincter** (kăr´dē-ăk sf ĭngk´tĕr) (Figure 15.4).

STOMACH

The stomach, approximately the size of a large fist, is the most expanded portion of the GI tract, and can hold up to 1 1/2 quarts of material. The position of the stomach varies according to body habitus (see Chapter 1) as well as respiratory phase, amount of material in the organ, and general body position. The primary function of the stomach is digestion. The main parts of the stomach are the fundus, body, greater and lesser curvatures, pylorus (pī-lor´ŭs), and pyloric sphincter. The stomach is lined with soft mucosa, which lays in folds called **rugae** (roo´gē). Digestive enzymes and hydrochloric acid are produced in the stomach's mucosa. The stomach prepares food, now called **chyme** (kīm), chemically and mechanically for digestion and moves it, by peristalsis, toward the narrow end of the stomach, called the pylorus. The pyloric sphincter allows small portions of chyme to enter the **duodenal bulb** (dū-ō-dē´năl bŭlb) and travel on through the **duodenum** (dū´´ō-dē´nŭm).

SMALL INTESTINE

Further digestion with absorption occurs in the small intestine, which is approximately 20 feet long. It consists of three segments: the duodenum, the jejunum, and the ileum. The first segment, the duodenum, is approximately 1 foot long. Digestion in this segment is aided by bile from the liver and gallbladder as well as enzymes from the pancreas. The next small intestine segment, called the **jejunum** (jē-jū´nŭm), is about 8 feet long and connects with the third and final small intestine segment, the **ileum** (ĭl´ē-ŭm), which is 11 feet long. The loops of small bowel occupy the center of the abdomen and lie largely within the curves of the large intestine. The entire length of the small intestine is lined with **villi**, which absorb the nutrients of the digested food into the bloodstream through their microscopic blood network. The remaining chyme, which is waste material high in water content, passes through the **terminal ileum** at the **ileocecal valve** (ĭl´ē-ō-sē´kăl vălv) into the cecum of the large intestine. From there, water is absorbed and the waste hardens to form feces (fē-sēz) (stools) that are passed through the large intestine and eliminated through the anus.

Depending on the quantity and consistency of food ingested, the stomach may take 2 to 6 hours to empty. After ingestion, food may begin to reach the ileocecal valve in as little as 3 hours or as much as 8 hours, with the rectum ready to evacuate feces in 12 to 24 hours.

Radiographic Considerations

Imaging of the GI tract demonstrates anatomy, function, foreign bodies, and pathology, including ulcers, tumors, and diaphragmatic hernias. The most common examinations of the GI tract include esophagrams or barium swallows, upper gastrointestinal series (upper GI or UGI), and small bowel or small bowel follow-through (SBFT).

PATIENT PREPARATION

In preparation for an upper GI study, the patient is usually kept NPO (nothing by mouth) after midnight the night before the examination, so the stomach will be empty of food and liquids. In the case of small bowel studies, the patient may be instructed to stop food and drink after the dinner meal. Department protocols vary, but many also call for refraining from the use of gum and tobacco products due to their effects on salivary and gastric secretions. Large amounts of fluid in the stomach will result in dilution of the contrast media, which can interfere with the study.

Before beginning the radiographic procedure, the radiographer should obtain a brief medical history and ensure that appropriate preparation procedures were followed. The patient should remove all clothing except shoes and socks, and dress in a patient gown. The radiographer should explain all aspects of the procedure, including the expected length. This is particularly important in small-bowel studies, which can take several hours.

CONTRAST MEDIA

Structures of the digestive system are not clearly visible on plain radiographs. Contrast media must be used to outline the structures and to examine function. The contrast of choice for the upper GI tract is barium sulfate, a barium compound available in many forms (Figure 15.5).

One form is a powder that has to be mixed with water to form a suspension. Because it is a suspension, the barium may tend to flocculate or clump out. Adding stabilizing agents may help, but constant stirring and mixing are needed. Barium products are also available in prepackaged solutions of different concentrations. Esophagrams may require a very thick barium paste (Esophotrast) to examine the esophagus and the swallowing process, as well as a thinner barium solution. Upper GI studies may be done as sin-

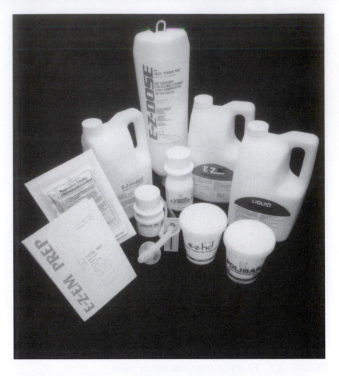

FIGURE 15.5   Current variety of barium products (Courtesy of E-Z-EM Company, Westbury, NY).

gle-contrast examinations, using only barium, or as double-contrast examinations using both a relatively thick barium and granules or powder added to produce carbon dioxide. The barium coats the gastric mucosa, and the gas distends the stomach. Air-contrast or double-contrast studies are useful in detecting lesions in the gastric mucosa (Figures 15.6 and 15.7). Most barium products also contain flavoring additives to make them more palatable.

For patients who have had stomach surgery or who might have a perforation, a water-soluble iodinated contrast (Gastrographin) may be used to examine the GI tract. If a barium sulfate contrast is used and a perforation is present, barium that leaked out into the abdominal cavity would not be absorbed and would have to be surgically removed. If the water-soluble contrast escapes into the abdominal or thoracic cavity, the body can absorb it.

Patients may also be given an injection of an antispasmodic drug (e.g., ProBanthine) to slow or dull the peristaltic activity in the GI tract if it is inhibiting the procedures.

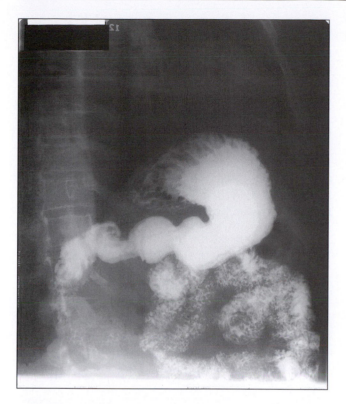

FIGURE 15.6   Single-contrast upper GI.

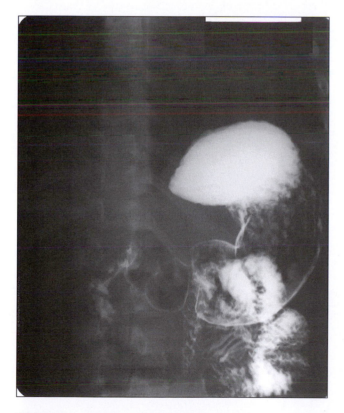

FIGURE 15.7   Double-contrast upper GI.

Other forms of barium products used in upper GI studies include barium tablets or capsules and small pieces of cotton soaked in barium, ingested to detect foreign bodies. Barium may be administered through bottles to pediatric patients or through feeding tubes to some adult patients.

After ingesting a barium contrast, patients should be offered a cleansing agent (castor oil, Milk of Magnesia, etc.) or given instructions about the need to drink plenty of fluids to assist in moving the barium through the digestive system in a timely fashion. Barium products not evacuated from the digestive system can harden and cause obstructive problems.

ROOM PREPARATION

Imaging of the upper GI tract is performed in a room with both radiographic and fluoroscopic capabilities. Spot filming devices vary from roll or cut 100- to 105-mm film to digital images. Video recording devices may also be utilized. Auxiliary equipment may include compression devices, sponges, and lead and protective apparel. All of the necessary materials, including the appropriate barium preparation, should be in the room or immediately available. The table should be in the upright position and the control panel set for fluoroscopy (Figure 15.8).

PROCEDURE

The fluoroscopic procedure begins with the table in an upright position. The radiologist generally observes and images the patient's swallowing process. The table is then lowered to a horizontal position and further imaging of the stomach and duodenum occurs. Before the study ends, the head of the table

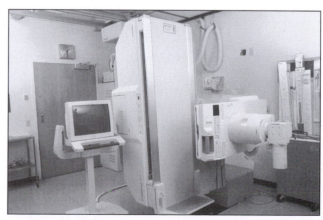

FIGURE 15.8   Fluoroscopic room ready for upper GI study.

may be lowered approximately 30° to further check for **esophageal reflux** (ē-sŏf´´ă-jē´ăl rē´flŭks) and **hiatal hernias** (hī-ā´tăl hĕr´nē-ă). During fluoroscopy, the room lighting may be dimmed to better visualize the imaging monitors. After fluoroscopic imaging is completed, overhead filming occurs. Additional films taken at intervals ranging from 15 minutes to several hours may be required to evaluate the entire small bowel.

TECHNICAL CONSIDERATIONS

Upper GI tract examinations require the use of higher kVp and lower mA as compared to standard radiography. This allows for adequate penetration of the barium. For fluoroscopy, suggested kVp ranges from 90 to 125 with mA ranges from 0.5 to 5. Suggested kVp ranges for overhead films with barium are 90 to 125 kVp with a fixed rate of 90 being the standard. Milliampere-seconds (mAs) varies from 4 to 200, depending on the size of the patient.

RADIATION PROTECTION

Fluoroscopic procedures produce higher radiation exposure rates than standard radiography. Gonadal shielding should be used both during fluoroscopy and for overhead filming whenever possible.

ROUTINE AND ALTERNATIVE POSITIONS/PROJECTIONS

Part	Routine	Page	Alternative	Page
Esophagus	AP/PA	590		
	Lateral	592		
	Oblique	594		
			Lateral neck	596
Stomach	Preliminary AP	598		
	PA/AP	598		
	Oblique	600		
	Lateral	602		
Small bowel	PA/AP	604		
	Ileocecal valve spot filming	606		

ESOPHAGRAM—AP PROJECTION

Exam Rationale   The radiographic examination of the esophagus attempts to image the swallowing process and the route of transmission for ingested material to the stomach. Common clinical indications are dysphagia, mediastinal pain, esophageal reflux, dyspepsia, dysphonia, a feeling of stricture or not being able to clear one's throat, and obstruction of food.

Technical Considerations

- Regular film/screen
- Bucky/grid
- kVp range: 75–85
- SID: 40 inch (100 cm)

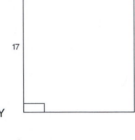

Radiation Protection   AEC (Phototiming)

 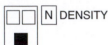 N DENSITY

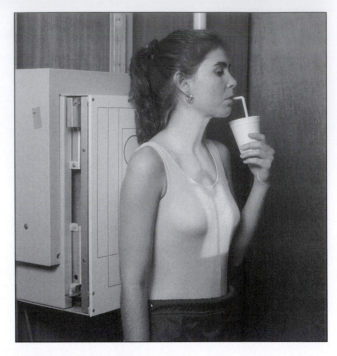

FIGURE 15.9   AP esophagus.

Patient Position   Back against the upright Bucky with the MSP parallel to the long axis of the film; no rotation of the shoulders or pelvis; head may be turned to the side to aid in swallowing of contrast during filming (Figure 15.9).

Central Ray   Perpendicular to the film at the level of T-6.

Patient Instructions   "Drink through the straw."

Evaluation Criteria (Figures 15.10 and 15.11)

- Demonstrates the entire esophagus.
- No rotation of the body.
- Short scale of contrast to enhance visualization of the esophagus.

Tips

1. To ensure a contrast-filled esophagus, instructions to the patient must be very clear. Take time for explanation and check the patient's comprehension.
2. The PA projection may be used and gives similar results.
3. This may also be done in the recumbent position.

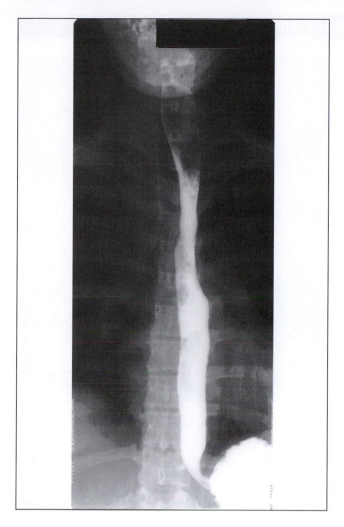

FIGURE 15.10   AP esophagus.

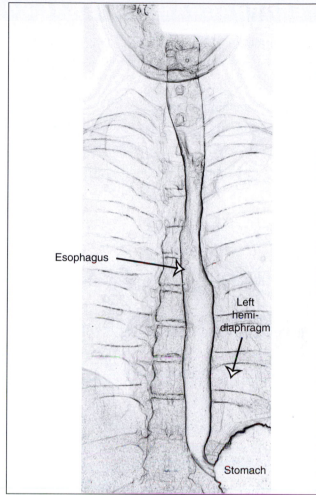

FIGURE 15.11   AP esophagus.

ESOPHAGRAM—LATERAL POSITION

Exam Rationale This position demontrates the esophagus free from superimposition of the thoracic spine and heart. The left lateral is usually done.

Technical Considerations

- Regular film/screen
- Bucky/grid
- kVp range: 80–90
- SID: 40 inch (100 cm)

Radiation Protection   AEC (Phototiming)

     N DENSITY

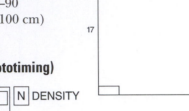

Patient Position Left lateral with the arms up and out of the way of the chest (Figure 15.12).

Central Ray Perpendicular to the film at the level of T6 and 1 inch (3 cm) anterior to the midcoronal plane.

Patient Instructions "Drink through the straw."

Evaluation Criteria (Figures 15.13 and 15.14)

- Should demonstrate entire esophagus filled with contrast.
- Little or no rotation of the thoracic cavity.
- Arms should not superimpose the esophagus.
- Short scale of contrast to enhance visualization of esophagus.

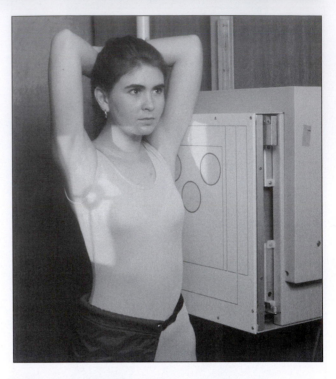

FIGURE 15.12   Lateral esophagus.

Tip

1. To ensure a contrast-filled esophagus, instructions to the patient must be very clear. Take time for explanation and check the patient's comprehension.
2. This may also be done in the recumbent position.

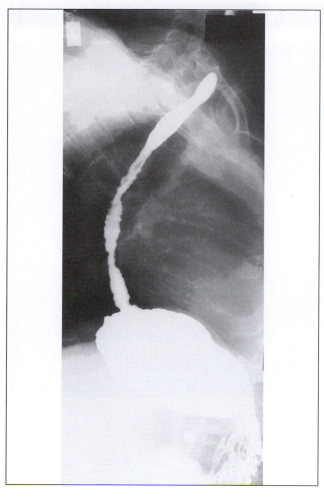

FIGURE 15.13 Lateral esophagus.

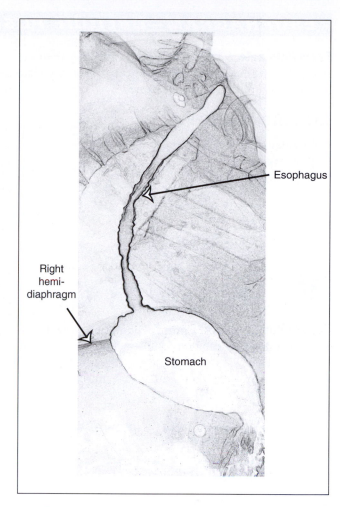

FIGURE 15.14 Lateral esophagus.

ESOPHAGRAM—OBLIQUE POSITION

Exam Rationale The oblique positions demonstrate the esophagus between the vertebrae and heart. One or both obliques may be done.

Technical Considerations

- Regular film/screen
- Bucky/grid
- kVp range: 80–90
- SID: 40 inch (100 cm)

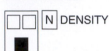

Radiation Protection   AEC (Phototiming)

      N DENSITY

Patient Position RAO (approximately 40°) with the right arm down by the body and the left arm up by the elevated shoulder; MSP 2 inches (5 cm) to left of spinous processes is centered to the midline of the upright Bucky (Figure 15.15).

Central Ray Two to 3 inches (5–8 cm) lateral to the MSP at the level of T6.

Patient Instructions "Drink through the straw."

Evaluation Criteria (Figures 15.16 and 15.17)

- Entire contrast-filled esophagus should be visible and demonstrated between the thoracic spine and the heart for the RAO.
- Hips and shoulders should be in the same plane.
- Short scale of contrast to enhance visualization of the esophagus.

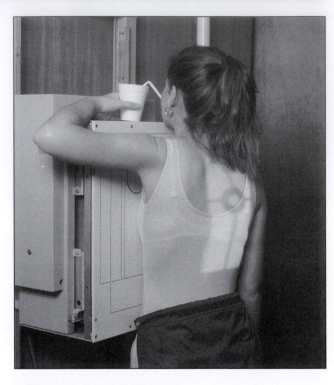

FIGURE 15.15   RAO esophagus.

Tips

1. An LPO will produce a comparable image and may be indicated by department protocol or patient condition.
2. An angle sponge may be used to obtain proper obliquity and patient cooperation when this is done in the recumbent position.

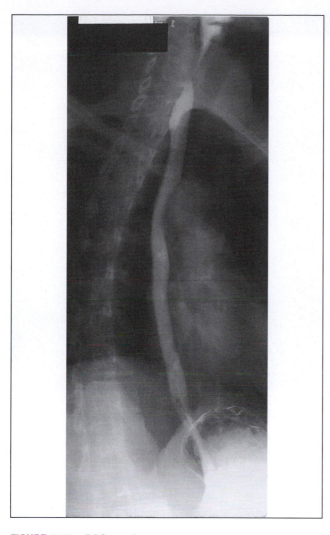

FIGURE 15.16   RAO esophagus.

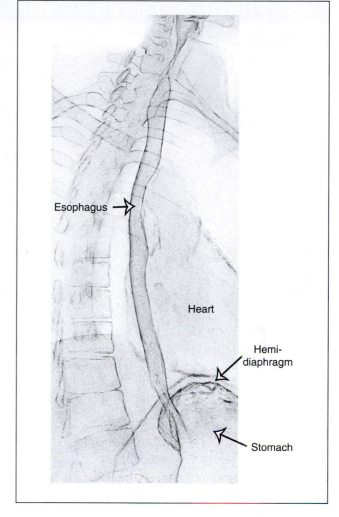

Esophagus

Heart

Hemi-
diaphragm

Stomach

FIGURE 15.17   RAO esophagus.

ESOPHAGUS—LATERAL SOFT TISSUE POSITION

Exam Rationale This position demonstrates the pharynx and upper esophagus and may be done to visualize opaque foreign bodies, lesions, or calcifications.

Technical Considerations

- Regular film/screen
- Bucky/grid
- kVp range: 60–65
- SID: 40 inch (100 cm)

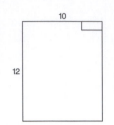

Radiation Protection

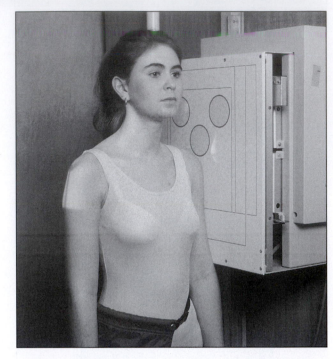

FIGURE 15.18 Lateral neck.

Patient Position Erect in the left lateral position; chin is slightly extended; midsagittal and interpupillary lines are perpendicular to the film; midcoronal plane is centered to the midline of the film (Figure 15.18).

Central Ray Perpendicular to the film at the level of C4.

Patient Instructions "Close your mouth and breathe through your nose. Breathe in and hold it."

Evaluation Criteria (Figures 15.19 and 15.20)

- Sides of the mandible superimposed.
- Limited or no rotation.
- Soft tissues demonstrated.

Tip This may also be done with the patient in a left lateral recumbent position.

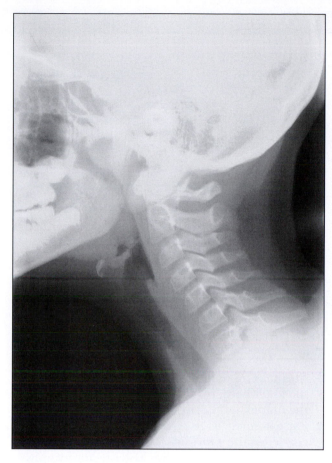

FIGURE 15.19   Soft tissue lateral neck.

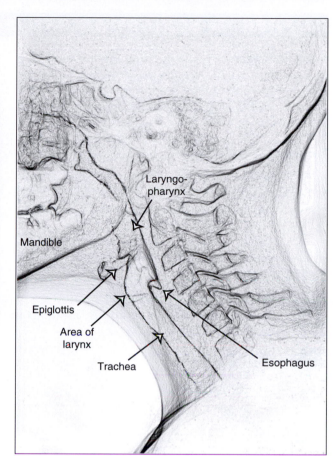

FIGURE 15.20   Lateral neck.

UPPER GI SERIES—AP PROJECTION

Exam Rationale   This projection can be used as a preliminary film to overview the area and check for adequate preparation or, after administration of contrast, to demonstrate the entire stomach and the duodenal loop.

Technical Considerations

- Regular film/screen
- Bucky/grid
- kVp range: preliminary—70–75; opacified—90–95
- SID: 40 inch (100 cm)

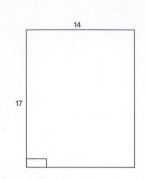

Radiation Protection

   Yes if protocol allows; most protocols require visualization of the entire abdomen.

AEC (Phototiming)

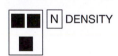   N DENSITY

Patient Position   Supine with the MSP parallel to the long axis of the table (Figure 15.21).

Central Ray   Perpendicular to the film with the central ray entering the patient on the midline at the level of L1.

Patient Instructions   "Take in a breath, let it all out. Don't breathe or move."

Evaluation Criteria (Figures 15.22 and 15.23)

- Spine straight.
- No rotation of iliac crests or rib cage.
- Diaphragm elevated to demonstrate gastric area.
- Centered to body to demonstrate gastric area.
- No abdominal or respiratory motion.
- Barium will appear in the fundus and upper body, air in the lower body, pylorus, and duodenum.

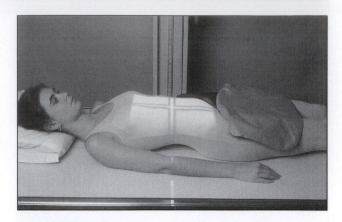

FIGURE 15.21   AP (preliminary or afterfilm).

Tips

1. This may be done PA; this would show barium in the lower body, pylorus, and duodenum with air in the fundus and upper body of stomach.
2. For extremely large patients, two 14 × 17 (36 × 43 cm) crosswise films may be used and centered to include anatomy from the axilla to the symphysis pubis.
3. A sponge may be placed under the knees to lessen back strain and place the back in contact with the table.
4. This may be done erect.
5. By observing the location of anatomic structures during the fluoro procedure, the radiographer can gain insight into the location of the stomach relative to other landmarks.

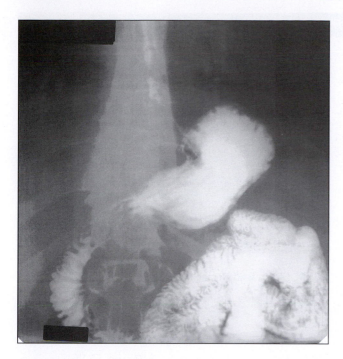

FIGURE 15.22 AP upper GI.

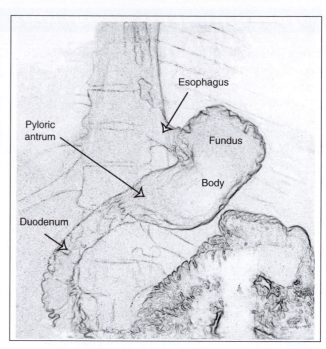

FIGURE 15.23 AP upper GI.

UPPER GI SERIES—OBLIQUE POSITION

Exam Rationale The obliques are performed to demonstrate the stomach, especially the fundus and the duodenal loop. The duodenal bulb is also projected free of superimposition of the pylorus.

Technical Considerations
Note: Due to body habitus and the position of the stomach, filming may also use 10 × 12 crosswise (25 × 30 cm) or 11 × 14 (28 × 36 cm) lengthwise or crosswise film sizes.

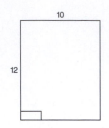

- Regular film/screen
- Bucky/grid
- kVp range: 90–95
- SID: 40 inch (100 cm)

Radiation Protection

  (but not to obscure digestive anatomy)

AEC (Phototiming)

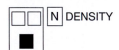 N DENSITY

Patient Position RAO—rotated approximately 45° (Figure 15.24).

Central Ray RAO—perpendicular to the film at the level of ASIS on the left side (side up) of the patient at a point midway between the vertebral column and the lateral border of the body.

Patient Instructions "Take in a breath; let it all out. Don't breathe or move."

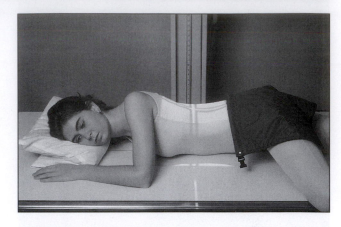

FIGURE 15.24   RAO stomach.

Evaluation Criteria (Figures 15.25 and 15.26)

- Entire stomach is visualized; fundus is well seen.
- Duodenal bulb is shown without superimposition of the pylorus.
- Duodenal loop is shown in profile.
- Contrast is adequately penetrated.
- Air is in the fundus and barium is in the body, pylorus, and duodenum.

Tips

1. An LPO will demonstrate the same anatomy and may be indicated by patient condition.
2. Obliquity can vary from 30° to 60°, with thinner patients requiring less rotation.
3. Sponges may be used to achieve correct positioning angles.

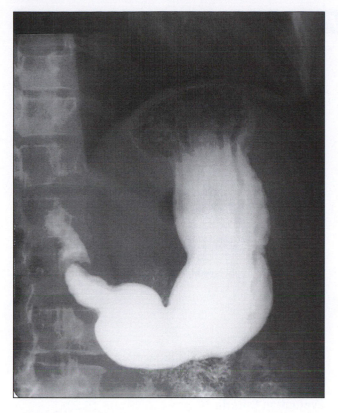

FIGURE 15.25   RAO stomach.

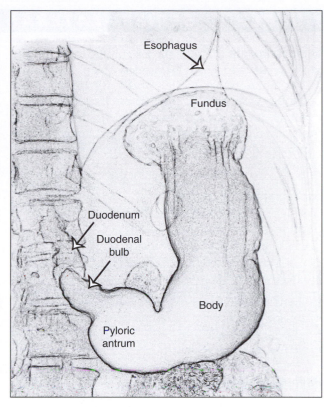

FIGURE 15.26   RAO stomach.

UPPER GI SERIES—LATERAL POSITION

Exam Rationale   The right lateral affords a look at the anterior and posterior aspects of the stomach as well as an unobstructed view of the pylorus, duodenal bulb, and loop. Visualization of the duodenal loop is essential due to the anatomic location of the head of the pancreas nestled in the C-shaped loop and the joining of the second segment of the small intestine, the jejunum.

Technical Considerations

Note: Due to body habitus and the position of the stomach, filming may also use 10 × 12 (25 × 30 cm) crosswise or 11 × 14 (28 × 36 cm) lengthwise or crosswise film sizes.

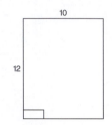

- Regular film/screen
- Bucky/grid
- kVp range: 90–95
- SID: 40 inch (100 cm)

Radiation Protection

   (but not to obscure digestive anatomy)

AEC (Phototiming)

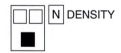 DENSITY

Patient Position   Right lateral recumbent; for average patients center at a point midway between the midcoronal plane and the anterior surface of the body to the midline of the table (Figure 15.27).

Central Ray   Perpendicular at a point midway between the midcoronal plane and the anterior surface of the body to the center of the film.

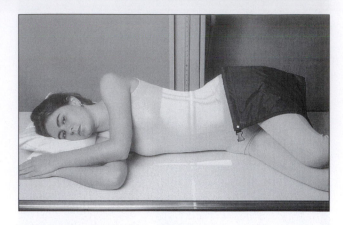

FIGURE 15.27   Right lateral stomach.

Patient Instructions   "Take a deep breath, let it all out. Don't breathe or move."

Evaluation Criteria   (Figures 15.28 and 15.29)

- Patient is in a true lateral position, no rotation.
- Visualization of the entire stomach and the duodenal loop.
- Contrast is adequately penetrated.

Tips

1. Placing small sponges between the knees and elbows of the patient may create more stable positioning and less opportunity for movement. Some very thin patients may also benefit from a small sponge placed under the right iliac crest.
2. For larger patients, watching the fluoroscopy monitor to locate the stomach in relation to a landmark (vertebral level, ribs, etc.) will be helpful in positioning the patient for overhead films.

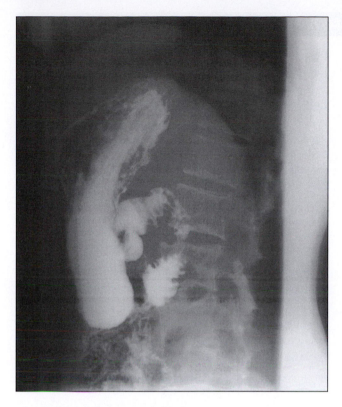

FIGURE 15.28   Right lateral stomach.

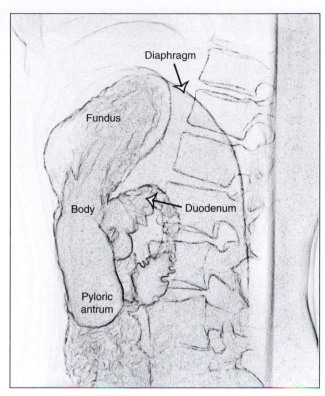

FIGURE 15.29   Right lateral stomach.

SMALL BOWEL—PA PROJECTION

Exam Rationale   Radiographic examination of the small bowel attempts to image the route taken by food products through the duodenum, jejunum, and the ileum into the cecum. If a small-bowel study follows an upper GI, additional contrast is administered and monitored until it reaches the cecum of the colon. Contrast may be administered orally or by means of intubation. The intubation process is a barium enema of the small intestine and is called enteroclysis. Enteroclysis procedures are not very common because they are lengthy rather unpleasant for the patient. The small bowel can be imaged with the patient in the supine or prone position. Filming occurs at 15-minute to 1-hour intervals and may continue for several hours.

Technical Considerations
Note: Film may be crosswise as patient habitus dictates.

- Regular film/screen
- Bucky/grid
- kVp : 90
- SID: 40 inch (100 cm)

Radiation Protection

For male patients, gonadal shielding is not possible for female patients.

AEC (Phototiming)

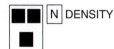 DENSITY

Patient Position   Prone or supine with MSP centered to the midline of the table.

Central Ray   Radiographs will occur at different time intervals. For early imaging, the central ray should be directed at the L1 level on the MSP to the center of the film. For later imaging, the central ray should be directed at the level of the iliac crests on the MSP to the center of the film.

Patient Instructions   "Take in a breath, let it all out. Don't breathe or move."

Evaluation Criteria (Figures 15.30, 15.31, and 15.32)

- Abdomen straight, no rotation or motion.
- Lower portion of stomach may be visualized on early filming.
- Small intestine is visible.
- Contrast is adequately penetrated.

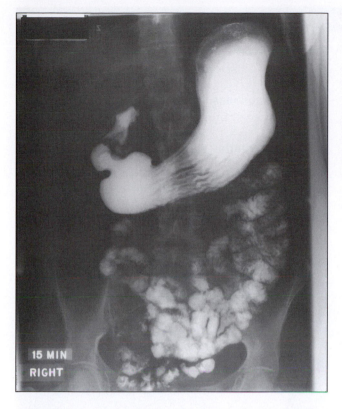

FIGURE 15.30   Fifteen-minute radiograph of small-bowel study.

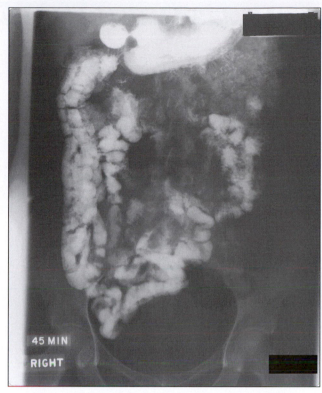

FIGURE 15.32   Forty-five-minute radiograph of small-bowel study.

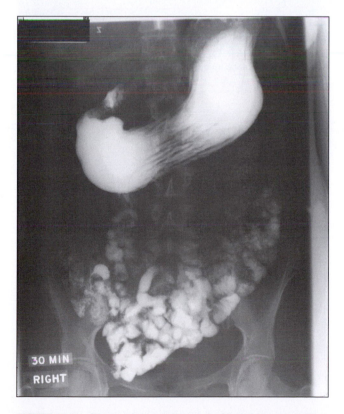

FIGURE 15.31   Thirty-minute radiograph of small-bowel study.

SMALL BOWEL—ILEOCECAL VALVE

Exam Rationale   When the barium contrast reaches the cecum of the large intestine, the radiologist may choose to demonstrate the terminal area of the ileum by using one of two filming methods: a PA projection with compression or fluoroscopic spot filming.

Technical Considerations
(for fluoroscopic spot filming)

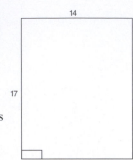

* Regular film/screen
* Bucky/grid
* kVp range: 90–95
* Fluoroscopic kVp: 80
* SID: 40 inch (100 cm) unless fluoroscopic spot filming

Radiation Protection

    (if small bowel anatomy is not obscured)

AEC (Phototiming)

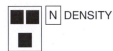   N DENSITY

Patient Position   Prone with the MSP centered to the table. A small sponge or paddle device is placed under the patient, in the lower right quadrant, at approximately the lower level of the sacroiliac joint.

Central Ray   Perpendicular to the film centered at the level of the iliac crests on the MSP.

Patient Instructions   "Take in a breath, let it all out. Don't breathe or move."

Evaluation Criteria (Figure 15.33)

* Terminal ileum visible.
* Compression, if used, visible.
* Contrast is adequately penetrated.

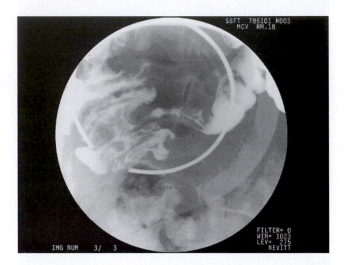

FIGURE 15.33   Spot film of terminal ileum.

Special Considerations

SELECTED PATHOLOGY

Esophageal varices are swollen and twisted veins around the distal esophagus that are often a complication of liver disease and can lead to esophageal hemorrhage (Figure 15.34).

Esophageal reflux occurs when previously ingested digestive contents are regurgitated through the cardiac sphincter to the distal end of the esophagus, causing irritation. If the condition persists over a long period of time, further lesions may develop.

An *ulcer* is an open sore in the epithelial lining of the digestive system. Gastric and duodenal ulcers are specific forms of ulcers that are also called peptic ulcers (Figure 15.35). A perforating ulcer is one that creates a hole through the lining of the organ.

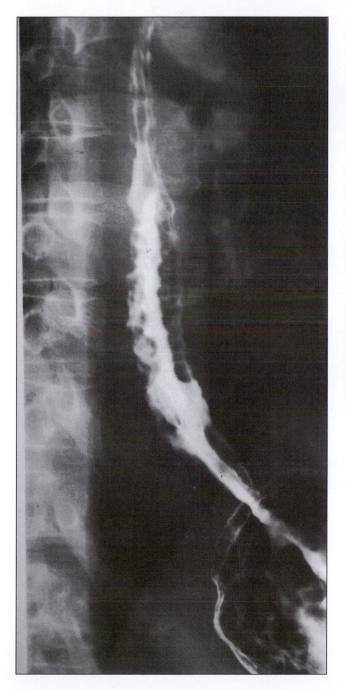

FIGURE 15.34 Esophageal varices.

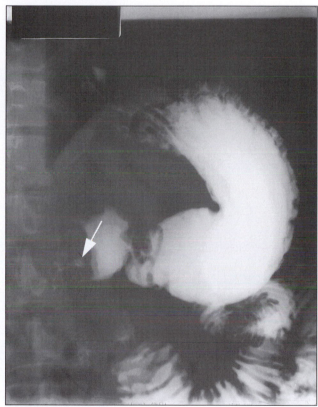

FIGURE 15.35 Duodenal ulcer.

Pyloric stenosis is an abnormal condition of narrowing of the pyloric canal that prevents or hinders digested food from leaving the stomach. Dilation or surgery may be treatment options (Figure 15.36).

Crohn's disease is a chronic inflammatory condition that can affect the entire digestive system but most commonly affects the terminal ileum. The inflammation results in diarrhea, fever, and cramping. The etiology is unknown. Treatment may include medications for symptom relief or, in more extensive conditions, surgical intervention (Figure 15.37).

Hiatal hernia occurs when the distal esophagus is not properly anchored and the upper portion of the stomach may herniate or protrude through the esophageal opening into the diaphragm. This hernia is often associated with esophageal reflux (Figure 15.38).

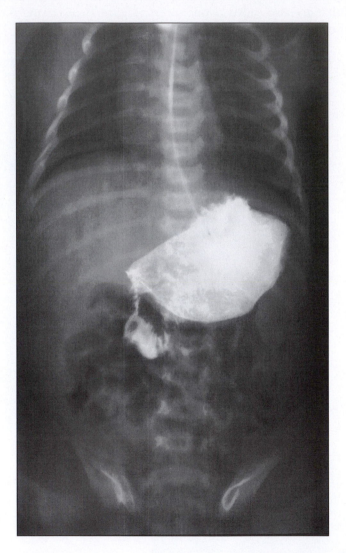

FIGURE 15.36
Pyloric stenosis.

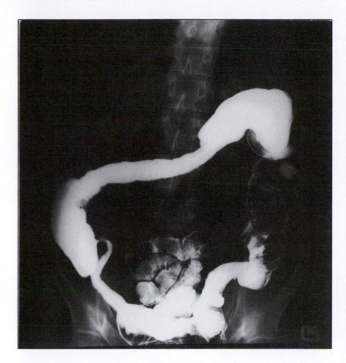

FIGURE 15.37   Crohn's disease.

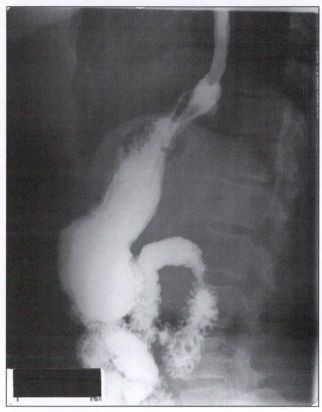

FIGURE 15.38   Hiatal hernia.

Review Questions

1. The esophagus is _____ to the trachea.
   a. anterior
   b. posterior
   c. lateral
   d. medial

2. In the hypersthenic body type, the stomach lies:
   a. at the level of the iliac crest
   b. below the level of the iliac crest
   c. higher and more transverse than in a sthenic patient

3. Hydrochloric acid and digestive enzymes are produced in the:
   a. gastric mucosa
   b. pyloric sphincter
   c. terminal ileum
   d. villi

4. The contrast medium of choice for upper GI imaging is:
   a. air
   b. barium sulfate
   c. Gastrographin
   d. iodinated solutions

5. Water-soluble contrast are indicated for patients with suspected:
   a. gallstones
   b. hemorrhoids
   c. perforated stomach
   d. ulcer

6. What is the name for the condition in which digestive contents pass through or re-enter the cardiac sphincter to the distal esophagus, causing irritation.
   a. diverticula
   b. esophageal reflux
   c. hiatal hernia
   d. ulcer

7. Which of the following is a common clinical indication for an esophagram?
   a. chest pain
   b. constipation
   c. difficulty swallowing
   d. indigestion

8. On the AP projection of the stomach, barium is visualized in the:
   a. fundus and upper body
   b. lower body
   c. pylorus and duodenum

9. For an oblique stomach, the average patient is rotated _____ from the prone position.
   a. 30°
   b. 45°
   c. 60°
   d. 90°

10. Imaging of the upper GI tract can be done with the patient in the recumbent or erect position.
    a. true
    b. false

11. An upper GI series always includes a small bowel follow-through.
    a. true
    b. false

12. The small bowel can be imaged in the supine or prone position.
    a. true
    b. false

13. To adequately penetrate the barium during an upper GI exam, the kVp should be set _____ (higher/lower) than the usual 70 kVp.

14. The _____ position will produce an image comparable to that of the standard RAO of the stomach.

15. For a complete small bowel study, images of the abdomen are taken until the barium reaches the _____ .

16. What structure serves as the beginning of the GI tract?

17. What is the name of the wave-like contractions that propel food through the digestive tract?

18. What is the central ray location for an AP projection of the esophagus?

19. What position/projection of the upper GI tract is taken to provide a preliminary evaluation and to assess patient preparation for the procedure?

20. What are the instructions to the patient as you prepare to make the exposure for an AP or lateral esophagus?

References and Recommended Reading

Adler, A. M., & Carlton, R. R. (1994). *Introduction to radiography and patient care.* Philadelphia: Saunders.

Ballinger, P. W. (1995). *Merrill's atlas of radiographic positions and radiologic procedures.* (8th ed., Vol. 2). St. Louis: Mosby-Year Book.

Chabner, D. E. (1996). *The language of medicine.* (5th ed.). Philadelphia: Saunders.

Dowd, S. B., & Wilson, B. G. (1995). *Encyclopedia of radiographic positioning* (Vol. 2). Philadelphia: Saunders.

Halpert, R. D., & Goodman, P. (1993). *Gastrointestinal radiology.* St. Louis: Mosby-Year Book.

Margulis, A. R., & Burhenne, J. H. (Eds.). (1984). *Alimentary tract radiology* (3rd ed., Vol. 1). St. Louis: Mosby.

O'Toole, M., (Ed.). (1992). *Miller-Keane encyclopedia & dictionary of medical, nursing, & allied health* (5th ed.). Philadelphia: Saunders.

Sheldon, H. (1992). *Boyd's introduction to the study of disease* (11th ed.). Philadelphia: Lea & Febiger.

Thompson, M. A., Hattaway, M. P., Hall, J. D., & Dowd, S. B. (1994). *Principles of imaging science and protection.* Philadelphia: Saunders.

CHAPTER 16

Lower Gastrointestinal Tract

JOANNE S. GREATHOUSE, EdS, RT(R)(ARRT), FASRT

MICHAEL MADDEN, PhD, RT(R)(ARRT)

MARY J. HAGLER, MHA, BA, RT(R)(ARRT)(N)(M)

ANATOMY AND PHYSIOLOGY

Cecum

Appendix

Colon

GENERAL CONSIDERATIONS

Barium Enema

BARIUM ENEMA—ROUTINE POSITIONS/ PROJECTIONS

PA/AP

Axial PA/AP

Obliques

Lateral Decubiti

Lateral Rectum

AP/PA Postevacuation

BARIUM ENEMA—ALTERNATE POSITIONS/ PROJECTIONS

Axial Oblique

Axial Rectosigmoid Junction (Chassard-Lapine)

Defecogram

SPECIAL CONSIDERATIONS

Pediatric Considerations

Geriatric Considerations

Common Errors

Selected Pathology

Correlative Imaging

OBJECTIVES

At the completion of this chapter, the student should be able to:

1. List and describe the anatomy of the large intestine.

2. Explain the physiology of the lower digestive tract.

3. Given drawings and radiographs, locate anatomic structures of the lower digestive tract.

4. Explain the rationale for each projection.

5. Explain the patient preparation required for each examination.

6. Describe the positioning used to visualize anatomic structures of the large intestine.

7. List or identify the central ray location and identify the extent of field necessary for each projection.

8. Recommend the technical factors for producing an acceptable radiograph for each projection.

9. State the patient instructions for each projection.

10. Given radiographs, evaluate positioning and technical factors.

11. Describe modifications of procedures for atypical or impaired patients to better demonstrate the anatomic area of interest.

Anatomy and Physiology

The large intestine is the lower portion of the digestive tract. Among its functions are the elimination of feces and some absorption of water, inorganic salts, amino acids, and vitamin K. It extends from the terminus of the ileum to the anus and is about 5 feet (1.5 meters) long. It consists of the following regions: cecum, colon, rectum, and anal canal. The large intestine surrounds the more centrally located small intestine. Structurally, the large intestine has the following distinctive features as compared to the small intestine: greater size, more fixed in position, longitudinal muscles bands called **taeniae coli**, folds in the wall called **haustrations**, and numerous small fat-filled sacs called **epiploic appendages** (Figures 16.1 and 16.2).

CECUM (sē´kŭm)

The first segment of the large intestine forms a large blind pouch in the right iliac fossa. The cecum is the widest part of the large intestine, approximately 2 1/2 inches (6 cm) in length and 3 inches (7.5 cm) in diameter, and is continuous with the last segment of the small intestine, the ileum. The passageway between the large and small bowel is regulated by the ileocolic or ileocecal valve, which is located superior to the cecum. The valve consists of two lips on either side of the opening creating membranous ridges in the cecum, the **frenula** of the valve. This valve slows the passage of and prevents backflow of intestinal contents. A second opening in the cecum, located just an inch (2 cm) or less below the ileocecal valve, is the opening of the appendix (Figure 16.3).

APPENDIX

More traditionally described as the vermiform appendix, it is a narrow, worm-shaped tube, which originates from the posteromedial wall of the cecum. The length and the location of the appendix are highly variable; however, the length averages approximately 3 1/2 inches (9 cm) and the location of the base can be

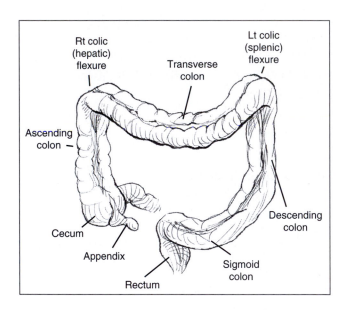

FIGURE 16.1   Frontal view of large intestine.

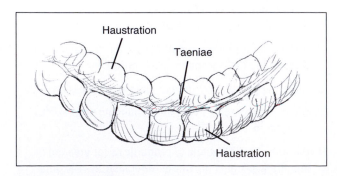

FIGURE 16.2   Haustra.

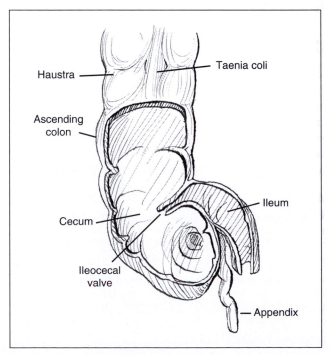

FIGURE 16.3   Ileocecal valve.

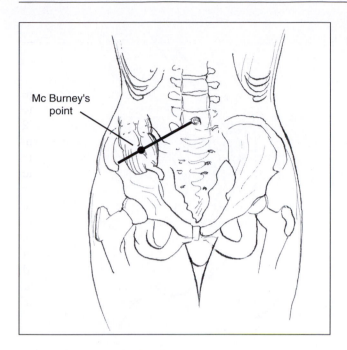

FIGURE 16.4   McBurney's point.

approximated with **McBurney's point**. McBurney's point (Figure 16.4) is a useful surgical approximation for the location of the appendix. To locate this point, draw a line between the umbilicus and the anterior superior iliac spine. McBurney's point is located at a point one-third of the distance along the line starting from the anterior superior iliac spine.

COLON

The colon is a term often interchanged with the large intestine; however, this is inaccurate because the colon is only one of the regions within the large intestine. The colon begins at the ileocecal valve at the superior margin of the cecum and terminates at the rectum. The colon can be divided into four parts: ascending, transverse, descending, and sigmoid.

Ascending
Beginning at the cecum, the ascending colon ascends to the inferior surface of the right lobe of the liver. This region of the colon is about 6 inches (15 cm) long and is narrow as compared to the cecum. In the abdominal cavity, the ascending colon is located posteriorly near the musculature of the posterior abdominal wall and the lateral part of the right kidney.

Right Colic (kŏl′ĭk) Flexure
At its most superior point, the ascending colon bends sharply to the left creating the right colic or hepatic

flexure just below the right lobe of the liver. At this flexure, the colon turns downward and forward giving rise to the next region of the colon, the transverse. Due to this orientation, the right colic flexure is not completely visualized from the anterior aspect, but is better demonstrated with an oblique view from the anterior right side.

Transverse
This section is the longest, approximately 20 inches (50 cm), and most movable segment of the colon and passes across the abdomen between the right and left colic flexures. In its course across the abdomen, the location of the transverse colon is highly variable and is generally described as either U-shaped or V-shaped depending on its shape. Also, the location of the mid-transverse colon has been found to vary as much as 7 inches (17 cm) in individuals between upright and recumbent positions.

Left Colic Flexure
At this junction between the transverse and descending colon, the colon bends inferiorly near the lower spleen. The left colic flexure lies at a higher level and more posterior than the right and is attached to the diaphragm. Similar to the right colic flexure, the flexure is not completely visualized from the true anterior aspect, but is better demonstrated with an oblique view from the anterior left side.

Descending
This region is approximately half the length of the transverse colon, 9 inches (25 cm) long, and extends from the left colic flexure to the pelvic brim or lesser pelvis. As it descends, the descending colon is posteriorly situated near the abdominal wall and the pelvis.

Sigmoid (sĭg′moyd)
This S-shaped continuation of the colon within the lesser pelvis originates at the pelvic brim from the descending colon and terminates in the midline at the third sacral segment, where it joins the rectum. The length of this region is highly variable but averages approximately 16 inches (40 cm).

Rectum
The continuation of the sigmoid colon, the rectum, begins at the level of the third sacral segment and descends to a level slightly below the tip of the coccyx. In the adult, the rectum is approximately 5 inches (12 cm) long. Its upper part is about the same diameter as the sigmoid colon. The dilated region anterior to the coccyx is called the rectal ampulla. As the rectum descends, it demonstrates two posteroanterior curvatures: the upper portion curves anteriorly while

the lower portion curves posteriorly to the anal opening. Clinically, the direction of these curvatures must be considered when an enema tip is inserted into the rectum (Figure 16.5).

Anal Canal

The anal canal originates as the rectal ampulla narrows due to the underlying sphincter musculature and descends posteriorly to the external anal opening. The canal ranges from 1 to 2 inches (2.5–4.0 cm) in length and has a shorter anterior wall. The rectum and anal canal are surrounded by a network of veins, the **rectal plexus**, that are dilated and sacculated. In the clinical condition of **hemorrhoids**, these veins become enlarged and protrude into the rectum and anal canal, and in some cases, may be seen in the anal opening.

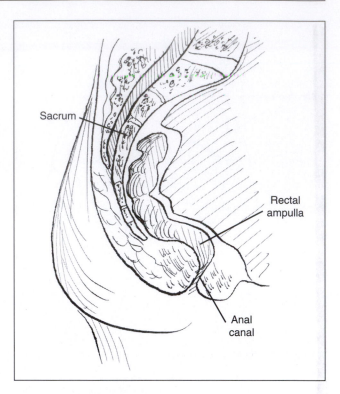

FIGURE 16.5   Lateral view of rectum.

General Considerations

BARIUM ENEMA (OR LOWER GI SERIES)

This examination is done to study the structure and function of the large intestine. It requires administration of contrast material and may be done using one of the following methods:

1. Single contrast, using only barium sulfate (Figure 16.6)
2. Double contrast, using both barium sulfate and air (Figure 16.7):
   • A single-stage procedure, in which the radiologist instills barium and air during a single filling procedure
   • A two-stage procedure, in which the barium is partially or completely evacuated before the air is instilled

Indications/Contraindications

The primary indications for a barium enema include **colitis**, **diverticulosis/diverticulitis**, **intussusception**, **volvulus**, and possible **neoplastic disease**. The primary contraindication is a recent biopsy because this can weaken the bowel wall and predispose it to perforation during the study.

Patient Preparation

Preparation of the patient for a barium enema is intensive. Department protocols vary considerably, so the radiographer should be familiar with the protocol of the institution in which he is practicing. Although the specific protocols differ significantly, the goal for all is a complete cleansing of the large bowel. The protocol usually combines some or all of the following elements: dietary restrictions, **cathartics** (ka-thar'tik)/ **laxatives**, and cleansing enemas.

Because improper cleansing can result in a less than adequate examination or yield an inaccurate diagnosis, patient instructions are critical. Both staff and patients must understand the preparation protocol and be rigorous in its implementation. A scout film is taken before beginning a barium enema procedure to evaluate the adequacy of patient preparation.

There are some contraindications to routine bowel preparation. In patients with gross hemorrhage, severe diarrhea, and some other conditions, the preparation may need to be modified by the physician, who must understand the desired rigorous bowel cleansing.

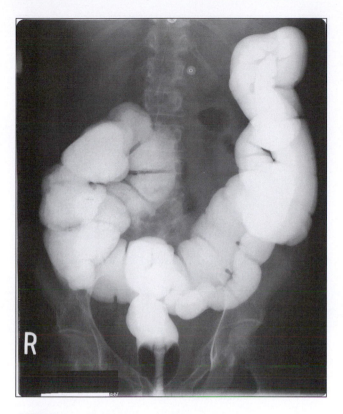

FIGURE 16.6   **Single-contrast enema.**

Contrast Media

The contrast material used for most barium enemas is a suspension of barium sulfate. Although some barium enema preparations include ingredients that help resist precipitation, all of the preparations are suspensions rather than solutions. Thus, it is important to frequently shake the enema bag to ensure adequate mixing.

The most common gaseous medium used in examination of the lower GI tract is air because of its ready availability. It is also possible to use carbon dioxide. Its primary advantage is quicker absorption following the procedure.

In cases where perforation is suspected or where the patient is likely to be scheduled for surgery after an examination of the lower GI tract, a water-soluble medium is indicated. It can be administered in the same fashion as barium or air (Figure 16.8).

Barium Enema Apparatus

Barium enema preparations come in a variety of forms. Premixed liquids are available or an institution can mix its own barium; these need only be poured into a disposable enema bag. Also available are enema bags that contain barium powder; water is added and the bag shaken to complete the enema preparation (Figure 16.9).

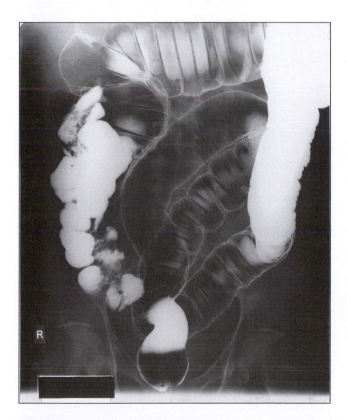

FIGURE 16.7   **Double-contrast enema.**

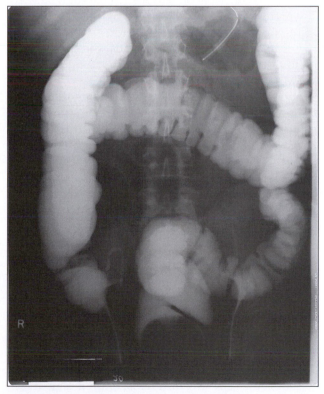

FIGURE 16.8   **Water-soluble enema.**

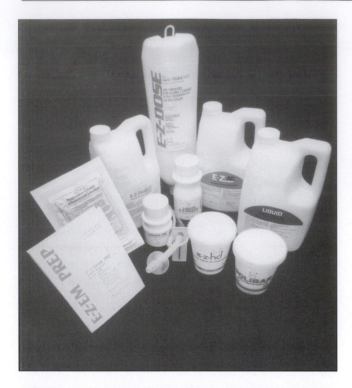

FIGURE 16.9   Barium enema preparations (Courtesy of E-Z-EM Company, Westbury, NY).

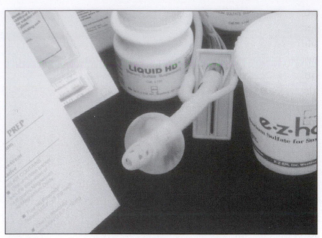

FIGURE 16.10   Enema tip (Courtesy of E-Z-EM Company, Westbury, NY).

The specific type of barium preparation and its concentration will vary depending on the radiologist's preference. Typically, double-contrast studies use a higher density preparation. Most bags hold 3000 mL of fluid, although the actual amount prepared and administered varies.

There is considerable debate regarding the appropriate temperature for the enema preparation. Some experts recommend a warm temperature, either room temperature or between 102° and 105°F. They believe this is easier for the patient to retain and minimizes cramping. Others recommend using cold water for the enema or even refrigeration overnight of the enema preparation, asserting that the colder temperature has a soothing, anesthetic effect.

The enema tip may come already attached to the end of the enema tubing or may come separately and need to be attached to the distal end of the tubing by the radiographer (Figure 16.10). There are three primary types of enema tips available:

1. Simple enema tip
2. Retention tip
3. Air contrast retention tip

All enema tips are disposable and designed for one-time use. The retention tip has a rubber balloon at its distal end which, when placed in the rectum, can be inflated to aid a patient who has difficulty retaining the enema. The air-contrast retention tip has the same balloon as a retention tip but also has a separate tube for the instillation of air.

Room Preparation

The fluoroscopic room should be ready for the procedure before the patient enters. The table should be placed in the horizontal position and cleaned before each patient. All of the required materials, including barium preparations, lead aprons and gloves, and cassettes should be in the room or immediately available. It is also important to have available a bedpan, extra patient gowns, and towels. The control panel should be set for fluoroscopy and the timer set for the maximum 5 minutes. Once begun, the examination needs to proceed as quickly and efficiently as possible, so adequate preparation should be made for any possible contingency or unexpected emergency.

Procedure Preparation

Once the room is ready, the patient may be brought into the room. The patient should have been instructed to remove all clothing and put on a hospital gown. It is preferable for the patient to be given disposable slippers rather than wearing shoes and socks.

This procedure is uncomfortable and often embarrassing for the patient, so it is imperative to begin by fully explaining the procedure and reassuring the patient that his modesty will be protected throughout. The patient should be told about the rotation of the body, which will be required to adequately visualize all portions of the large intestine, about the need for the series of radiographs that will be taken after the radiologist leaves the room and before the barium can be evacuated, and the need for his cooperation throughout the entire procedure. The radiographer should also obtain a brief history from the patient.

Enema Tip Insertion

The patient should be placed on the table and instructed to lie on the left side and lean forward. The knees should be flexed with the right leg in front of the left (**Sims' position**). Before inserting the rectal tube, barium mixture should be run through the tubing to displace the air. The IV pole should be placed so that the enema bag is 24 to 36 inches (60–75 cm) above the level of the rectum.

Wearing gloves, the radiographer should place a generous amount of lubricant on the tip. Opening the back of the patient's gown to expose only the anal region, the radiographer should grasp the right buttocks with the heel of the hand to expose the anus. The patient should exhale as the tip is inserted into the rectum in a forward direction approximately 1 1/2 inches (4 cm). After the initial insertion, the tip should be directed superiorly to follow the normal curvature of the rectum. The tip should be inserted no more than a total of 3 to 4 inches (7.5 to 10 cm); doing so is not only unnecessary but also risks injury to the rectum (Figure 16.11).

The tip should never be forcefully inserted; if the radiographer experiences difficulty with insertion, assistance from the patient or the radiologist should be sought.

If a retention tip is being used, some departments allow the radiographer to give one or two pumps of air to slightly inflate the balloon. The retention tip should be fully inflated, however, only by the radiologist under fluoroscopic guidance. After insertion of the tip, it should be held in position while the patient turns to the supine or prone position in preparation for fluoroscopy. Care should be taken that the tubing is adequately adjusted to allow for the free flow of the barium mixture.

Fluoroscopic/Filming Procedures

Once preparations are complete, the radiologist is called to the room and introduced to the patient. During the procedure, the radiographer's responsibilities are to follow the radiologist's instructions, assist and support the patient as necessary, and change the spot film cassettes. The radiographer will also control the flow of the enema as directed by the radiologist. To ensure that instructions are accurately heard and followed, the radiographer should respond "on" and "off" to the directions of the radiologist to start or stop the flow of barium during the procedure.

After the completion of the fluoroscopic portion of the examination and before the patient is allowed to evacuate the barium and air, several overhead radiographs of the large intestine are taken. Department protocols or even preferences of different radiologists in a single department vary considerably. Most departments will include some of the positions/projections described in the following pages. Obviously, filming should proceed as rapidly as possible.

If a simple enema tip is used, it is generally more comfortable for the patient to have the tip removed before overhead filming. A retention catheter is left in place until the patient is in place on the commode or bedpan, although it is possible to unhook the enema tubing from the retention catheter (being sure the retention catheter is appropriately clamped off). If the tip is left in place during filming, care should be taken as the patient changes position, so the tip is not inadvertently pulled out.

Technical Considerations The use of high kVp technique (100–120 kVp) is recommended with the use of high-density contrast media. For air-contrast studies or studies using water-soluble contrast, a mid-range kVp (80–90) should be used.

Gonadal shielding is not possible for female patients undergoing examination of the lower digestive tract. Gonadal shielding is always recommended

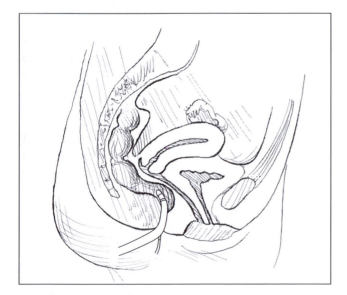

FIGURE 16.11 Enema tip placement.

for male fluoroscopy patients. However, due to the placement of the enema tip, this type of shielding may hinder the examination. A shadow shield is ideal for radiographic imaging of the large intestine in male patients. It is also possible to reduce male gonadal dose by consistently keeping the primary beam above the level of the symphysis pubis.

Follow-up   Once overhead filming is complete, the patient should be escorted to the bathroom or be provided with a bedpan. The retention catheter is removed only after the patient is on the commode or bedpan. Air should be released from the balloon before removal of the tip.

After evacuation of the barium, most department routines call for a postevacuation radiograph to determine the extent of evacuation. If sufficient evacuation is not demonstrated on the first postevacuation film, it may be necessary for the patient to return to the bathroom for further evacuation and a second postevacuation film.

ROUTINE AND ALTERNATIVE POSITIONS/PROJECTIONS

Part	Routine	Page	Alternative	Page
Large Intestine	PA/AP	622		
	Axial PA/AP	624		
	Obliques	626		
	Lateral decubitus	628		
	Lateral rectum	630		
			Axial oblique	632
			Axial rectosigmoid (Chassard-Lapine)	634
			Defecogram	636

LARGE INTESTINE—PA/AP PROJECTION

Exam Rationale This projection is used in one or more of the following ways: as a preliminary film to check for adequate bowel cleansing, as a pre-evacuation film to demonstrate all of the barium-filled large intestine, or as a postevacuation film to demonstrate the extent of bowel emptying.

Technical Considerations

- Regular screen/film
- Grid
- kVp range:
  —Opacified: 100–120 (single contrast); 80–90 (double contrast)
  —Preliminary or postevacuation: 80–90
- SID: 40 inch (100 cm)

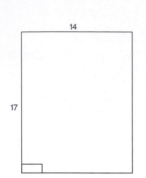

Radiation Protection   See pages 619-620.

AEC (Phototiming)

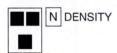

Patient Position Supine or prone with the MSP centered to the midline of the table (Figure 16.12).

Part Position Adjust so there is no rotation of the body.

Central Ray Perpendicular to iliac crest.

Patient Instructions "Blow your breath out. Don't breathe or move."

Evaluation Criteria (Figures 16.13 and 16.14)

- Should demonstrate entire large intestine.
- There should be no rotation as evidenced by symmetry of hips and wings of ilium.

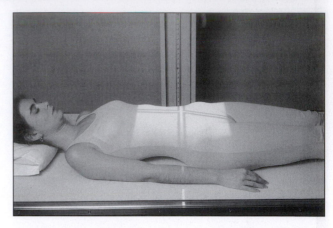

FIGURE 16.12   AP colon.

Tips

1. For a hypersthenic or asthenic patient, the central ray should be adjusted 1 inch (3 cm) higher or lower respectively.
2. For a patient with a large, wide colon, it may be necessary to use two 14 × 17 (36 × 43 cm) films crosswise to include all of the colon (Figure 16.15).
3. Do not ask the patient to take in a deep breath and let it out. This may relax the abdominal muscles and result in poor retention of the barium.

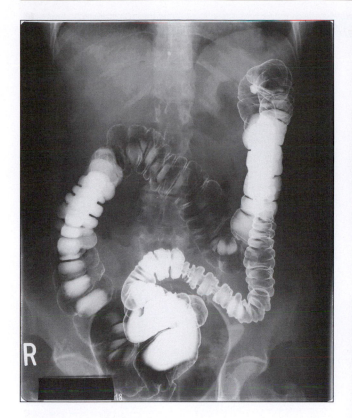

FIGURE 16.13 AP colon.

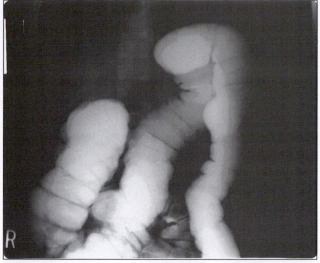

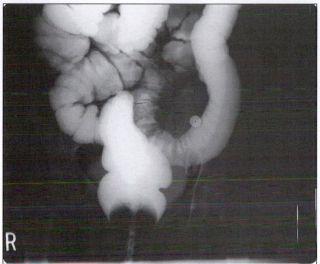

FIGURE 16.15 AP colon with two transverse films.

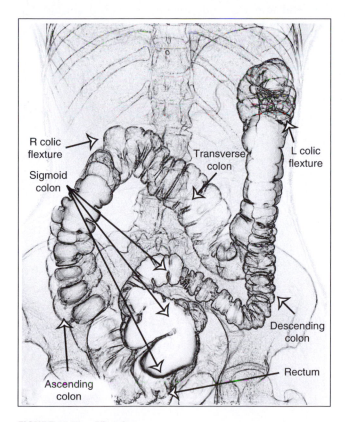

FIGURE 16.14 AP colon.

LARGE INTESTINE—AXIAL PA/AP PROJECTION

Exam Rationale This projection gives an elongated view of the rectosigmoid area of the colon.

Technical Considerations

- Regular screen/film
- Grid
- kVp range: 100–200 (single contrast); 90–100 (double contrast)
- SID: 40 inch (100 cm)

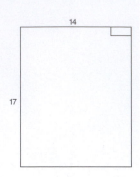

Radiation Protection

See pages 619-620.

AEC (Phototiming)

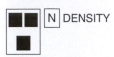 N DENSITY

Patient Position Supine or prone with the MSP centered to the midline of the table (Figure 16.16).

Part Position Adjust so there is no rotation of the body.

Central Ray

- Supine: 2 inches (5 cm) inferior to the ASIS at a 30° to 40° cephalic angle.
- Prone: To exit at the level of the ASIS with a 30° to 40° caudal angle.

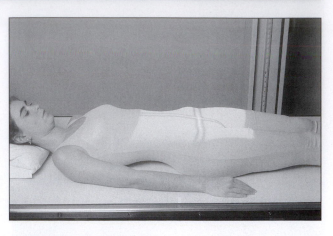

FIGURE 16.16   Axial AP colon.

Patient Instructions "Blow your breath out. Don't breathe or move."

Evaluation Criteria (Figures 16.17 and 16.18)

- Should be no rotation as evidenced by symmetrical appearance of hips.
- Rectal and sigmoid portions of colon should be elongated and less superimposed than on PA or AP.
- Not necessary to include transverse colon and flexures.

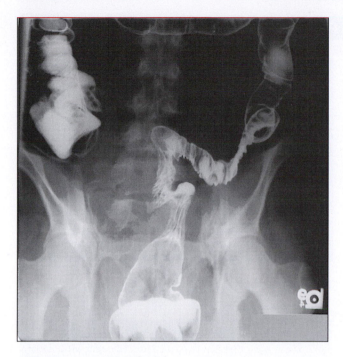

FIGURE 16.17   Axial AP colon.

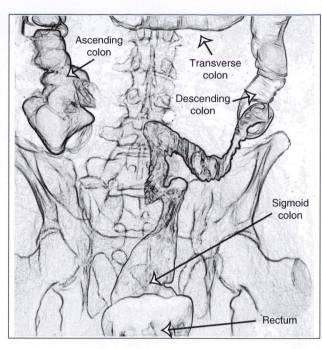

FIGURE 16.18   Axial AP colon.

LARGE INTESTINE—OBLIQUE POSITION

Exam Rationale　The RAO (or LPO) demonstrates the right colic (hepatic) flexure and the ascending colon. The LAO (or RAO) demonstrates the left colic (splenic) flexure and the descending colon.

Technical Considerations

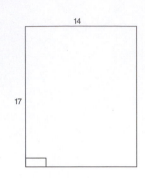

- Regular screen/film
- Grid
- kVp range: 100–200 (single contrast); 80–90 (double contrast)
- SID: 40 inch (100 cm)

Radiation Protection
See pages 619-620.

AEC (Phototiming)

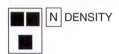 N DENSITY

Patient Position　Supine or prone with the MSP centered to the midline of the table (Figures 16.19 and 16.20).

Part Position　Rotate the body 35° to 45° from the supine or prone position.

Central Ray　Perpendicular at the level of the iliac crest about 1 inch (3 cm) anterior to the MSP.

Patient Instructions　"Take in a deep breath, let it all out. Don't breathe or move."

Evaluation Criteria (Figures 16.21 through 16.24)

- Entire colon should be included.
- RAO (LPO) should demonstrate ascending colon and right colic flexure.
- LAO (RPO) should include descending colon and left colic flexure.

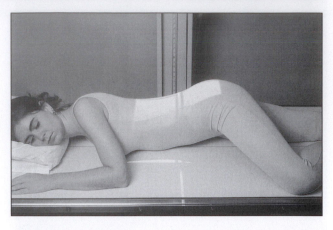

FIGURE 16.19　RAO colon.

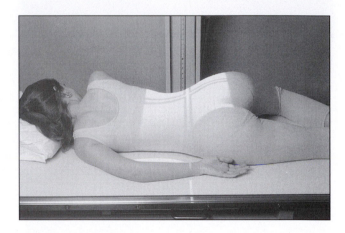

FIGURE 16.20　LAO colon.

Tips

1. For a hypersthenic or asthenic patient, the central ray should be adjusted 1 inch (3 cm) higher or lower, respectively.
2. For a patient with a large, wide colon, it may be necessary to use two 14 × 17 (36 × 43 cm) films crosswise to include all of the colon.

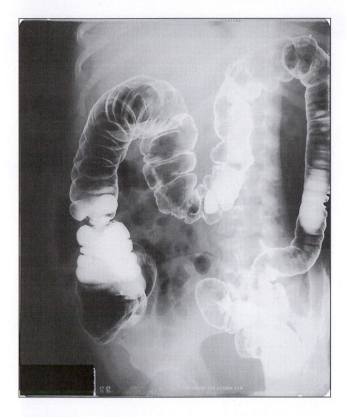

FIGURE 16.21   LAO colon.

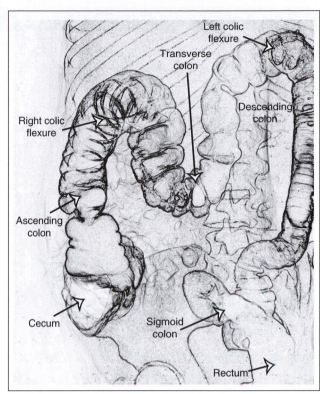

FIGURE 16.23   LAO colon.

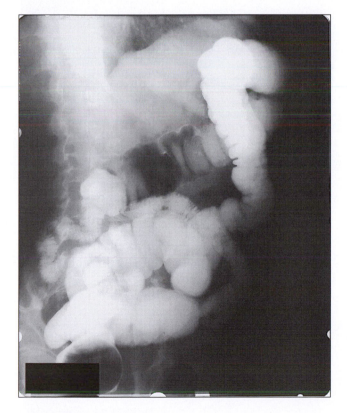

FIGURE 16.22   RAO colon.

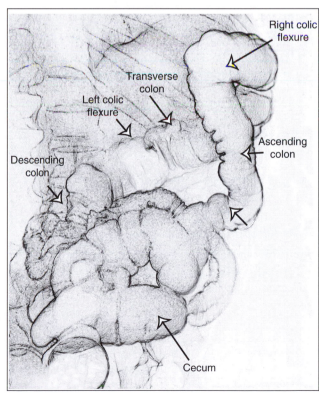

FIGURE 16.24   RAO colon.

LARGE INTESTINE—LATERAL DECUBITUS POSITION

Exam Rationale　The right and left lateral decubiti are done in conjunction with a double-contrast barium enema to demonstrate the entire contrast-filled colon. These projections are particularly useful in the evaluation of polyps. Both sides are typically done, with the "up" side (air-filled) portion best demonstrated.

Technical Considerations

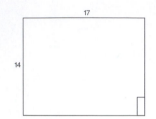

- Regular screen/film
- Grid
- kVp range: 80–90 (double contrast)
- SID: 40 inch (100 cm)

Radiation Protection　See pages 619-620.

AEC (Phototiming)

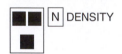 N DENSITY

Patient Position　Left lateral and right lateral recumbent positions with iliac crest centered to the midline of the table or film holder; patient's knees should be flexed to aid in maintaining the position (Figures 16.25 and 16.26).

Part Position　Adjust so there is no rotation of the body.

Central Ray　Horizontal: perpendicular to the iliac crest.

Patient Instructions　"Blow your breath out. Don't breathe or move."

Evaluation Criteria (Figures 16.27 through 16.30)

- Should demonstrate entire large intestine.
- There should be no rotation as evidenced by symmetry of wings of ilium.

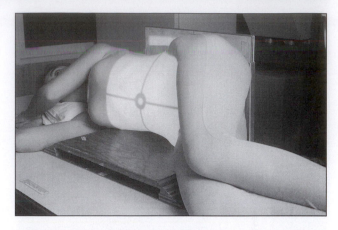

FIGURE 16.25　Right lateral decubitus colon.

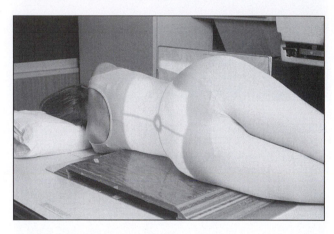

FIGURE 16.26　Left lateral decubitus colon.

Tips

1. To ensure visualization of "down" side, patient should be slightly elevated with some type of radiolucent support.
2. Projections may be done with patient facing either toward or away from the film holder; facing away from the film is generally more comfortable for the patient.
3. Use AEC only with upright Bucky device.

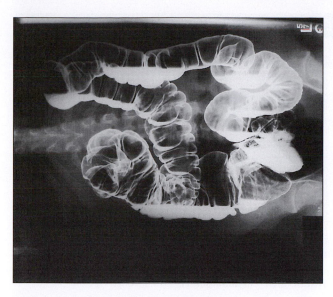

FIGURE 16.27   **Right lateral decubitus colon.**

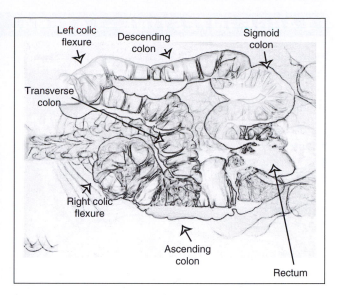

FIGURE 16.29   **Right lateral decubitus colon.**

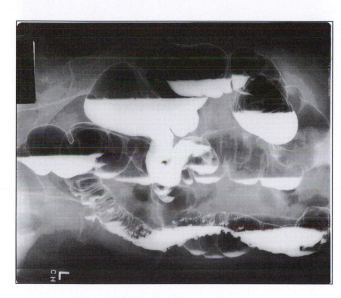

FIGURE 16.28   **Left lateral decubitus colon.**

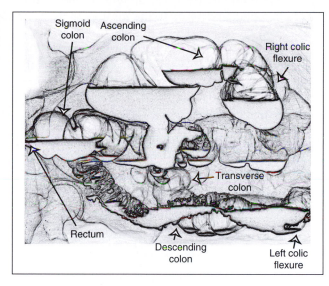

FIGURE 16.30   **Left lateral decubitus colon.**

LARGE INTESTINE—LATERAL RECTUM

Exam Rationale   The lateral position demonstrates the rectum and rectosigmoid areas.

Technical Considerations

- Regular screen/film
- Grid
- kVp range: 100–125
- SID: 40 inch (100 cm)

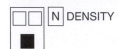

Radiation Protection
See pages 619-620.

AEC (Phototiming)

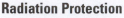 N DENSITY

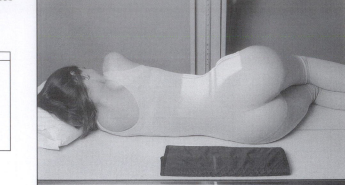

FIGURE 16.31   Lateral rectum.

Patient Position   Lateral recumbent position with midaxillary plane centered to the midline of the table (Figure 16.31).

Part Position   Adjust so there is no rotation of the body.

Central Ray   Perpendicular to iliac crest.

Patient Instructions   "Blow your breath out. Don't breathe or move."

Evaluation Criteria (Figures 16.32 and 16.33)

- Rectosigmoid area should be in center of film.
- There should be no rotation as evidenced by super-imposition of the hips and femurs.

Tips

1. Although the left lateral is more commonly used, either a right or left lateral may be done.
2. Tight collimation is essential to minimize scatter radiation. The placement of a lead strip behind the patient's buttocks will also help reduce scatter.

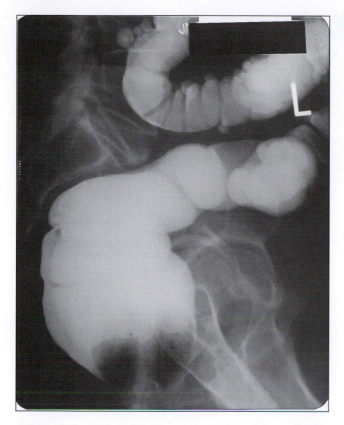

FIGURE 16.32   Lateral rectum.

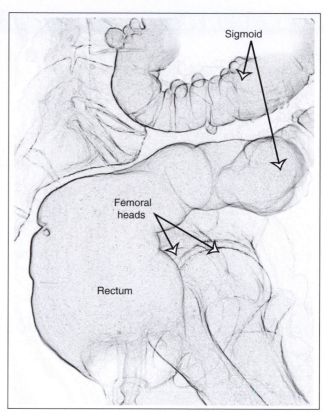

FIGURE 16.33   Lateral rectum.

LARGE INTESTINE—OBLIQUE AXIAL POSITION

Exam Rationale   These projections provide an elongated view of the rectosigmoid portion of the colon with less superimposition than on other views.

Technical Considerations

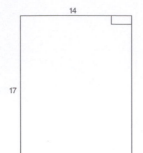

- Regular screen/film
- Grid
- kVp range: 100–200 (single contrast); 80–90 (double contrast)
- SID: 40 inch (100 cm)

Radiation Protection
See pages 619-620.

AEC (Phototiming)

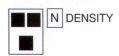 N DENSITY

Patient Position   Supine or prone with the MSP centered to the midline of the table (Figures 16.34 and 16.35).

Part Position   Rotate the body 30° to 40° from the supine or prone position.

Central Ray

- Supine: 2 inches (5 cm) inferior to the ASIS and 2 inches (5 cm) anterior to the MSP at a 30° to 40° cephalic angle.
- Prone: At the level of the ASIS and 2 inches (5 cm) anterior to the MSP at a 30° to 40° caudal angle.

Patient Instructions   "Blow your breath out. Don't breathe or move."

Evaluation Criteria (Figures 16.36 through 16.39)

- Should have sufficient obliquity of patient and angulation of the central ray to elongate the rectosigmoid area and to minimize superimposition.

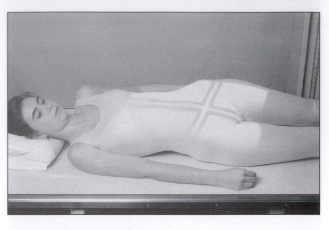

FIGURE 16.34   RPO oblique axial.

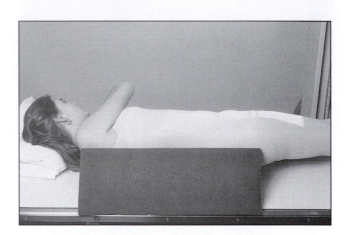

FIGURE 16.35   LPO oblique axial.

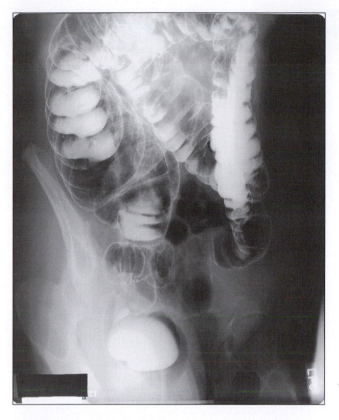

FIGURE 16.36   RPO oblique axial.

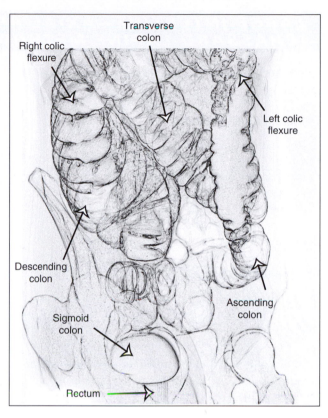

FIGURE 16.38   RPO oblique axial.

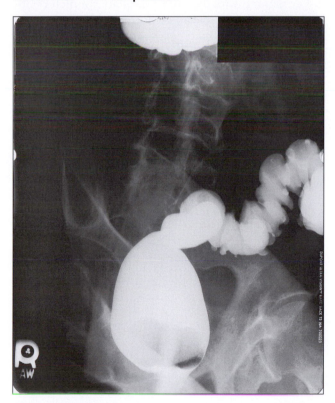

FIGURE 16.37   LPO oblique axial.

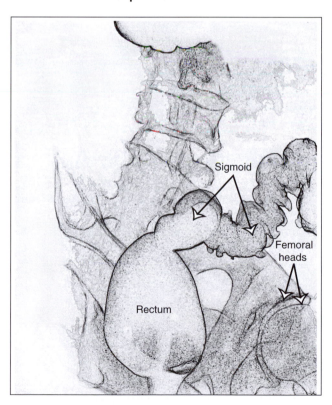

FIGURE 16.39   LPO oblique axial.

LARGE INTESTINE—AXIAL RECTOSIGMOID PROJECTION (CHASSARD-LAPINE METHOD)

Exam Rationale This projection demonstrates the rectosigmoid portion of the colon.

Technical Considerations

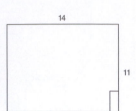

- Regular screen/film
- Grid
- kVp range: 110–125 (single contrast)
- SID: 40 inch (100 cm)

Radiation Protection See pages 619-620.

AEC (Phototiming)

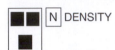

Patient Position Seated at the end of, but well back on, the table, with feet separated and supported on foot stool (Figure 16.40).

Part Position The patient leans forward as far as possible and grasps the ankles; the spine should be as close to parallel with the table as possible.

Central Ray Perpendicular through a line midway between the greater trochanters.

Patient Instructions "Blow your breath out. Don't breathe or move."

Evaluation Criteria (Figures 16.41 and 16.42)

- Rectosigmoid area should be centered to the film.
- Sigmoid portion should appear in profile with minimal superimposition.
- Lumbosacral region and barium should be adequately penetrated.

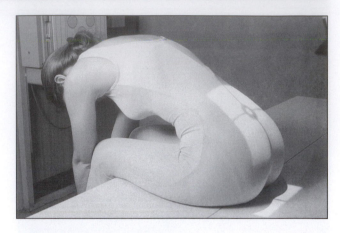

FIGURE 16.40   Chassard-Lapine.

Tips

1. This projection is not routinely done on younger patients because of the inability to shield the gonads and the large radiation exposure.
2. For patients with less than adequate sphincter control, this projection can be done after partial evacuation of the barium.

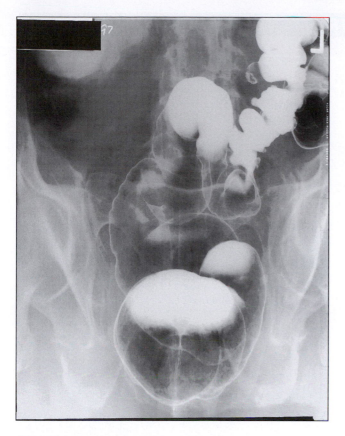

FIGURE 16.41   Chassard-Lapine.

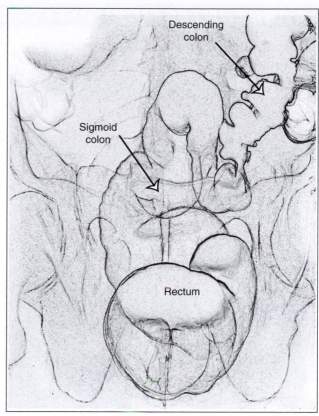

FIGURE 16.42   Chassard-Lapine.

LARGE INTESTINE—DEFECOGRAM

Procedure Rationale This procedure is done with patients who have problems with defecation, due to rectal intussusception, rectal prolapse, or rectoceles. Filming is done during the act of defecation, using special apparatus.

Patient Preparation No preparation of the patient is required.

Procedure With the patient in a lateral recumbent position on a stretcher, an injector is used to instill a thick barium paste either directly into the rectum or into a rectal tube that has been inserted into the rectum. After the barium is instilled, the patient is quickly moved to a specially constructed, radiolucent commode placed in front of a fluoroscopic unit. With the patient in the lateral position, the anorectal area is centered to the exposed field (Figure 16.43).

Using a spot filming device or a video recorder, images are made while the patient defecates, usually in both straining and relaxed stages. A lateral rectum projection is usually done as a postevacuation film (Figures 16.44 and 16.45).

This examination is extremely uncomfortable and embarrassing for the patient. The procedure must be thoroughly explained before beginning, and the patient's modesty should be vigilantly protected.

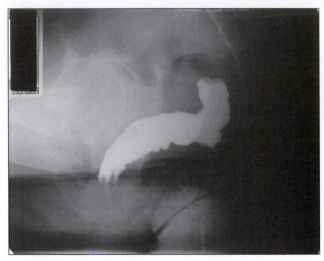

FIGURE 16.44 Defecogram.

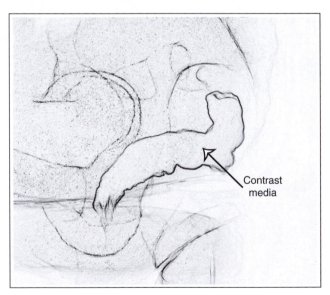

FIGURE 16.45 Defecogram.

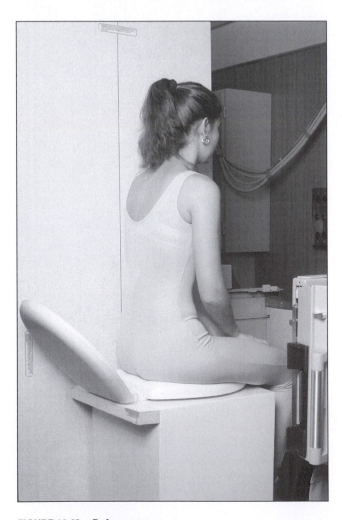

FIGURE 16.43 Defecogram.

Special Considerations

PEDIATRIC CONSIDERATIONS

Less stringent bowel preparation is needed for pediatric patients. A circumcision board or Octastop restraint board can be invaluable during a barium enema procedure on younger children. The octagonal restraint device has the advantage of allowing easy rotation of the child into various degrees of obliquity (Figures 16.46 and 16.47).

GERIATRIC CONSIDERATIONS

As patients age, muscle control decreases. Thus, it is important for older patients to clearly understand the barium enema procedure and the need for their cooperation in retaining the enema. If the patient is concerned about the ability to retain the enema, a retention tip should be used.

Due to reduced mobility and flexibility, geriatric patients may have difficulty in moving quickly from one position to another. Assistance in slow, gentle movements is required, even given the urgency to complete filming.

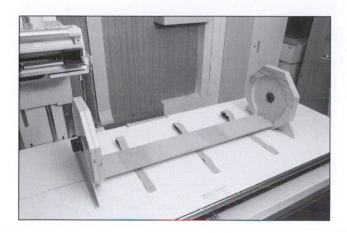

FIGURE 16.46   Octastop board.

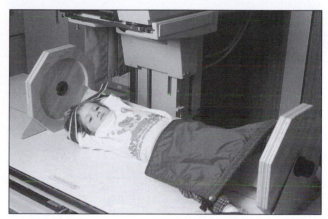

FIGURE 16.47   Octastop board with pediatric patient.

COMMON ERRORS

- Insufficient angle on PA axial projection fails to adequately elongate rectosigmoid area of colon and to minimize overlap (Figure 16.48).
- Inadequate exposure factors; barium is not adequately penetrated (Figure 16.49).
- Overpenetration on double-contrast enema (Figure 16.50).
- Clipping of the flexures is another common error. The radiographer can often avoid this error by observing the spot filming during fluoroscopy, gaining information about the position of the flexures.

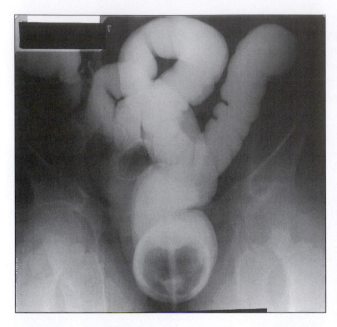

FIGURE 16.48   Insufficient angle on PA axial.

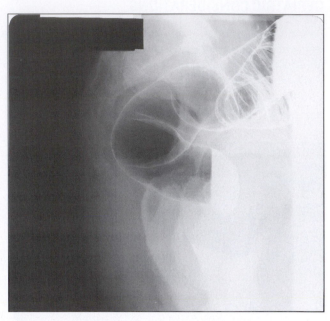

FIGURE 16.49   Inadequate technique to penetrate barium.

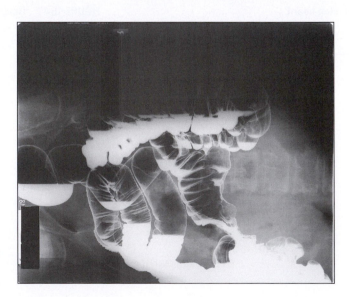

**FIGURE 16.50
Overexposure on
double-contrast enema.**

SELECTED PATHOLOGY

Diverticulosis (dĭ´´vĕr-tĭk´´ū-lō´sĭs) is a condition of multiple pouch-like herniations of the mucosal wall of the large intestine. The number of diverticula increase with age and are most more frequently seen in patients with low-fiber diets. Although diverticulosis is asymptomatic and the patient is usually unaware of the condition, these individuals are more predisposed to diverticulitis, or inflammation of the diverticula (Figure 16.51).

Intussusception (ĭn´´tū-sū-sĕp´shŭn) is found predominantly in pediatric patients; the large bowel invaginates or telescopes on itself. Radiographically, the location of the pathology within the large intestine appears much like a coiled spring inside the colon, the coiled-spring sign. Intussusception of the bowel is a life-threatening condition that is frequently treated with hydrostatic reduction, which is most often performed with a modified barium enema (Figure 16.52).

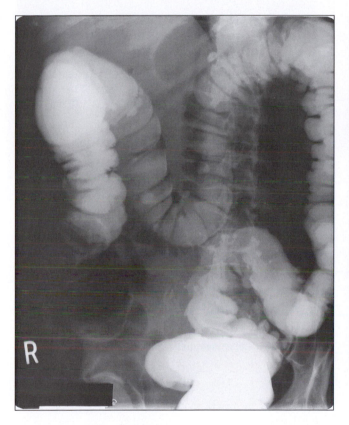

FIGURE 16.51 Diverticulosis.

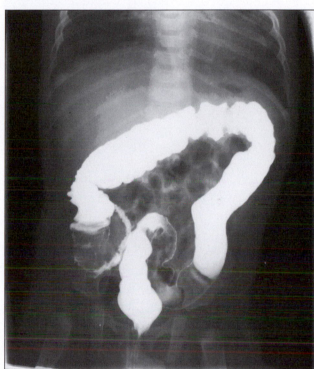

FIGURE 16.52 Intussusception.

Volvulus (vŏl′vū-lŭs) occurs most frequently in the sigmoid colon when the bowel twists on itself resulting in blockage of the large intestine. Although this condition is life-threatening, the use of a sigmoidoscope can usually reduce the blockage (Figure 16.53).

CORRELATIVE IMAGING

CT is often used as a follow-up to a barium enema examination that demonstrates a space-occupying lesion (Figure 16.54). Use of CT in confirmed pathologies of the large intestine verifies the size, shape, and extent of the space-occupying lesion.

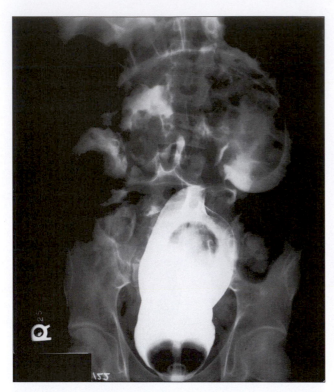

FIGURE 16.53   Volvulus.

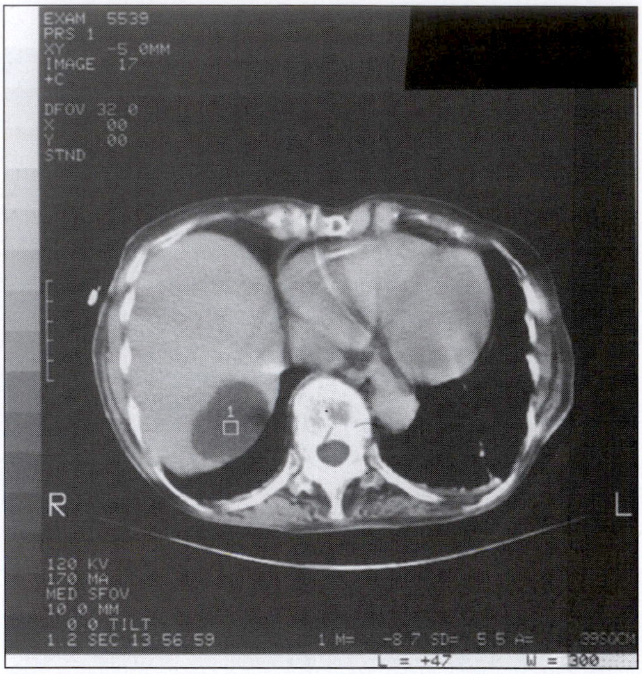

FIGURE 16.54   CT demonstrating lesion.

Review Questions

1. The location of the cecum is best described as:

    a. adjacent to the descending colon
    b. adjacent to the transverse colon
    c. superior to the ileocecal valve
    d. inferior to the ileocecal valve

2. What is the name of the S-shaped portion of the colon that terminates at the rectum?

    a. anus
    b. ascending
    c. sigmoid
    d. transverse

3. Which of the following is a common indication for a barium enema?

    1. colitis
    2. diverticulosis
    3. severe diarrhea

    a. 1 only
    b. 2 only
    c. 1 and 2
    d. 2 and 3
    e. 1, 2, and 3

4. Routine preparation for a lower GI series includes which of the following?

    a. NPO the night before the examination
    b. no smoking or gum chewing on the morning of the examination
    c. cathartic the evening before the examination
    d. all of the above

5. Which of the following would contraindicate the use of barium in radiographic examination of the large intestine?

    a. colitis
    b. diverticulitis
    c. perforation of the bowel wall
    d. volvulus

6. Which of the following positions/projections would best demonstrate the hepatic flexure?

    a. AP projection
    b. RAO position
    c. LAO position
    d. left lateral position

7. The oblique axial views of the colon are done to primarily demonstrate the:

    a. ascending colon
    b. descending colon
    c. sigmoid colon
    d. transverse colon

8. Lateral decubiti films are particularly useful in the evaluation of:

    a. appendicitis
    b. diarrhea
    c. polyps
    d. volvulus

9. Which of the following technical factors would not usually be considered for an oblique of the large intestine during a single contrast barium enema?

    a. 14 × 17 (35 × 43 cm) lengthwise
    b. SID: 72 inch
    c. kVp in the range of 100–120
    d. more than one of the above

10. The right colic flexure is the most superior portion of the large intestine.

    a. true
    b. false

11. Gonadal shielding is possible for male patients during a lower GI series.

    a. true
    b. false

12. When using a retention tip, the radiographer should fully inflate the balloon as soon as the tip is properly inserted.

    a. true
    b. false

13. Number the following from 1 to 4 based on when they should occur during an examination of the lower intestine.

    a. _____ enema tip insertion
    b. _____ patient preparation
    c. _____ explanation of procedure to patient
    d. _____ room preparation

14. The large intestine extends from the terminal end of the _____ to the _____ .

15. The large intestine has sacculations known as _____ folds.

16. The rectum is found between the _____ and the _____ .

17. The junction between the ascending and transverse portions of the colon is called the _____ flexure. The junction between the transverse and descending portions of the colon is called the _____ flexure.

18. Although protocols for patient preparation for lower GI studies vary from institution to institution, the goal of them all is _____ .

19. In the PA projection of the large intestine on an average patient, the central ray should be directed to the _____ . For a hypersthenic patient, the central ray is adjusted _____; for an asthenic patient, the central ray is adjusted _____.

20. On a lateral rectum, the _____ area should be centered to the film.

21. What structure regulates the passageway between the small and large bowel?

22. What kVp range is recommended for:
a. air contrast BE studies
b. single contrast BE studies

23. If you are performing a PA projection of the large intestine on a very large patient, what film size would you use?

24. The patient is placed in what position to facilitate insertion of an enema tip?

25. Before making an exposure of a lateral decubitus of the large intestine, what verbal instructions would you give to the patient?

References and Recommended Reading

Anderson, J. E. (1983). *Grant's atlas of anatomy* (8th ed.). Baltimore: Williams & Wilkins.

Ballinger, P. W. (1995). *Merrill's atlas of radiographic positions and radiologic procedures* (8th ed.). St. Louis: Mosby-Year Book.

Bates, B. (1983). *A guide to physical examination* (3rd ed.). Philadelphia: Lippincott.

Bo, W., Wolfman, N., Krueger, W., & Meschan, I. (1990). *Basic atlas of sectional anatomy with correlated imaging* (2nd ed.). Philadelphia: Saunders.

Bontrager, K. L. (1993). *Textbook of radiographic positioning and related anatomy* (3rd ed.). St. Louis: Mosby-Year Book.

Cahil, D. R., & Orland, M. J. (1984). *Atlas of human cross-sectional anatomy.* Philadelphia: Lea & Febiger.

Dorland's illustrated medical dictionary (28th ed.). (1995). Philadelphia: Saunders.

Eisenberg, R. L. (1992). *Clinical imaging: An atlas of differential diagnosis* (2nd ed.). Gaithersburg, MD: Aspen.

Eisenberg, R., & Dennis, C. (1990). *Comprehensive radiographic pathology.* St. Louis: Mosby.

Gardner, E., Gray, D. J., & O'Rahilly, R. (1975). *Anatomy: A regional study of human structure* (4th ed.). Philadelphia: Saunders.

Gray, H. (1995). In C. D. Clements (Ed.). *Anatomy of the human body* (30th ed.). Philadelphia: Lea & Febiger.

Halpert, R. D., & Goodman, P. (1993). *Gastrointestinal radiology: The requisites.* St. Louis: Mosby.

Hollinshead, W. H., & Rosse, C. (1985). *Textbook of anatomy* (4th ed.). New York: Harper & Row.

International Anatomical Nomenclature Committee. (1989). *Nomina anatomica* (6th ed.). Baltimore: Waverly Press.

Juhl, J. H. (1981). *Paul and Juhl's essentials of roentgen interpretation* (4th ed.). Philadelphia: Harper & Row.

Laudicina, P. F. (1989). *Applied pathology for radiographers.* Philadelphia: Saunders.

Mace, D. M., & Kowalczyk, N. (1995). *Radiographic pathology for technologists* (2nd ed.). St. Louis: Mosby-Year Book.

Meschan, I. (1975). *An atlas of anatomy basic to radiology.* Philadelphia: Lea & Febiger.

Norkin, C., & LeVange, P. (1983). *Joint structure & function: A comprehensive analysis.* Philadelphia: Davis.

Pansky, B. (1996). *Review of gross anatomy* (6th ed.). New York: Macmillan.

Robins, S. L., & Vinay, K. (1987). *Basic pathology* (4th ed.). Philadelphia: Saunders.

Snell, R. S. (1992). *Clinical anatomy for medical students* (4th ed.). Boston: Little, Brown.

Tortora, G. R., & Anagnostakos, N. P. (1984). *Principles of anatomy and physiology* (4th ed.). New York: Harper & Row.

Williams, P. L., & Warwick, R. (Eds.). (1980). *Gray's anatomy* (36th ed.). Philadelphia: Saunders.

Woodburne, R. T. (1983). *Essentials of human anatomy* (7th ed.). New York: Oxford University Press.

Woodburne, R. T., & Burkel, W. E. (1988). *Essentials of human anatomy* (8th ed.). New York: Oxford University Press.

CHAPTER 17

Hepatobiliary System

ANITA MARIE SLECHTA, MS, BSRT, (R)(M)(ARRT)

OBJECTIVES

At the completion of this chapter, the student should be able to:

1. List and describe the basic anatomic components of the hepatobiliary system.

2. Given drawings and radiographs, locate anatomic structures and landmarks.

3. Describe the expected location of the gallbladder for each of the four body habitus classifications.

4. Describe the physiology of the hepatobiliary system, including its role in digestion and the production of bile.

5. List the most common clinical indications for imaging the hepatobiliary system.

6. Explain why it is necessary to use radiographic contrast media to image the hepatobiliary system.

7. Describe patient preparation for each hepatobiliary procedure for both typical and atypical patients.

8. Describe the positioning used for an oral cholecystogram (OCG).

9. List or identify the central ray location and identify the extent of field necessary for each projection.

10. Explain the protective measures appropriate for each examination.

continued

11. Recommend the technical factors for producing an acceptable radiograph for each routine OCG projection.

12. State the instructions given to the patient before and during an OCG procedure.

13. Explain the rationale for each of the following:

   a. Non-fat or low-fat diet 24 hours before an OCG

   b. Oral contrast administration 10 to 12 hours before an OCG

   c. Fat meal after contrast-filled radiographs of the hepatobiliary system

   d. Radiographs of the hepatobiliary system after a fat meal

   e. Upright and decubitus projections of the gallbladder

14. Given radiographs, evaluate positioning and technical factors.

15. State the purpose of postoperative cholangiogram.

16. State the goal of endoscopic retrograde cholangiopancreatography (ERCP).

17. Describe the procedure for percutaneous transhepatic cholangiography (PTC).

Anatomy and Physiology

LIVER

The liver is the largest organ in the body. It comprises 2.5% of the body's weight, weighing over 3 lb, and is located in the RUQ of the abdomen. The liver has four lobes. The largest, right lobe is at least six times as large as the next biggest left lobe. The right and left lobes are separated by the falciform (făl´sĭ-form) ligament (Figure 17.1). The two inferior lobes are called the quadrate (kwŏd´rāt) and caudate (kaw´dāt). The shape of the liver conforms to its surrounding anatomy as the superior portion domes under the diaphragm and then curves down the right side of the abdominal wall. The anterior surface also has the smooth curve of the body wall, whereas the inferior and posterior surfaces have depressions molded around the stomach, kidney, duodenum, large bowel, and gallbladder. The actual shape of the liver varies from person to person, although the shape is unrelated to function. Only disease and blockage affect liver function.

The biliary ducts (collecting system) begin with very small collecting ducts in the liver parenchyma (păr-ĕn´kĭ-mă). These small ducts drain **bile** and form a network of larger and larger collecting ducts, which eventually empty into the left and right hepatic ducts. The left and right hepatic ducts leave the liver inferiorly and join to become one large hepatic duct that continues inferiorly (Figure 17.2). The hepatic duct joins with the gallbladder's cystic duct and becomes the common bile duct, which is about 3 inches (8 cm) long as it continues inferiorly to the duodenum. At the terminal end of the common bile duct is a circular band of muscle (**sphincter of Oddi** [ŏd´ē]) and an opening into the duodenum, which forms the greater duodenal papilla called the **papilla or ampulla of**

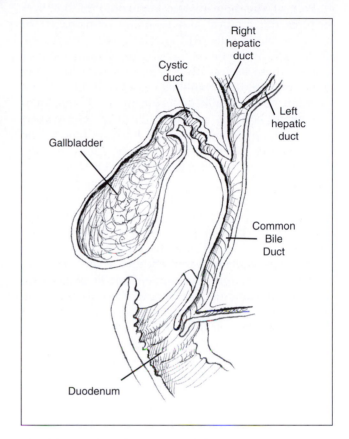

FIGURE 17.2 Biliary ducts and the gallbladder.

Vater (fā´tĕrz). When the sphincter of Oddi is constricted, the bile cannot empty into the duodenum and is shunted back into the gallbladder for storage and concentration. In about 95% of the population, the common bile duct and the pancreatic duct enter the duodenum at the same papilla (Agur, 1991). Of these, 60% anastomose and form an enlarged sac-like dilatation or ampulla (hepatopancreatic ampulla) before entering the duodenum (Bontrager, 1993).

The liver has over 200 vital functions that involve aspects of metabolic regulation; hematologic regulation; detoxification of poisons; digestion of nutrients; monitoring of blood metabolites; storing of vitamins, glycogen, and iron for future use; and production of bile, a digestive enzyme and waste product.

The liver is able to monitor and regulate blood and nutrients because of its unique dual blood supply. The first source of blood is the hepatic artery, which brings oxygen and nutrients to the liver cells. The second source of entering blood is the portal system, which brings the nutrient-rich venous blood from the small bowel. It is at this first stop that the liver inventories,

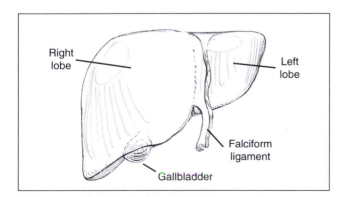

FIGURE 17.1   Liver, right and left lobes, falciform ligament, gallbladder orientation.

detoxifies, extracts, and monitors the nutrient-rich blood and makes adjustments as needed.

Part of the hematologic regulation of the liver involves the removal and recycling of damaged or aged red blood cells (RBCs). The phagocytic (fāg´´ō-sĭt´ĭk) cells in the blood-forming tissues and the liver remove these useless RBCs. The process of recycling some of the RBC building blocks results in the breakup of the heme molecule in the hemoglobin (hē´´mō-glō´bĭn). As a result bilirubin (bĭl-ĭ-roo´bĭn) (the yellow pigment) is spilled into the blood. The liver removes this bilirubin, converts it into the bile, and excretes it for elimination from the body in the feces. If the RBC destruction is too rapid or the biliary ducts or liver are damaged, the bilirubin cannot be removed from the blood and it backs up into the interstitial fluids, creating a condition known as **jaundice** (jawn´dĭs). Jaundice is the yellowing of all body tissues, most easily seen in the whites of the eyes.

Part of the liver's involvement in fat metabolism uses dietary cholesterol or creates cholesterol for bile production. The Greek prefix chole- means bile, so cholesterol is bile fat or lipid. Bile lipids derived from cholesterol are collectively called bile salts. The bile salts aid in the digestion of dietary fats by emulsifying or breaking up the ingested fat into small, evenly dispersed globules that can be digested by the pancreatic digestive enzymes. Ninety percent of these bile salts are reabsorbed by the intestine for use by the liver again.

Bile that is secreted by the liver is stored in the gallbladder for modification until it is needed in fat digestion. The modification is made possible by the gallbladder's mucous membrane lining that reabsorbs the water and concentrates the bile up to five times its original strength. If there is too much fat from years of a high-fat diet or if the concentration is too high, a precipitation of stones may result (**choleliths** [kō´lē-lĭth] or gallstones). The most common stone is the cholesterol gallstone, and the most common reason for ordering a study of the hepatobiliary system is to search for gallstones. The size and shape of a stone determine if it can leave the gallbladder and enter the common bile duct.

GALLBLADDER

The gallbladder is a muscular pear-shaped sac. It has a neck, a body, and a fundus, which holds a maximum of 40 to 50 mL of bile (see Figure 17.2). The gallbladder is usually situated obliquely under the right lobe of the liver with the fundus projecting anterolaterally. Its position varies greatly in different body habitus because the liver molds to the different body shapes and the gallbladder conforms to the liver (Figure 17.3). The hypersthenic individual's liver is normally

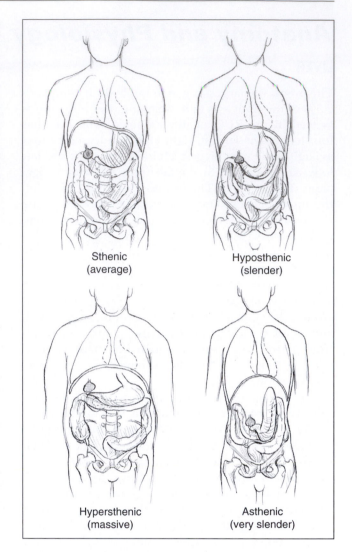

Sthenic (average)　　　　Hyposthenic (slender)

Hypersthenic (massive)　　　　Asthenic (very slender)

FIGURE 17.3　**Position of gallbladder in different body habitus.**

located high in the RUQ, whereas the asthenic individual's gallbladder is found on the upper border of the RLQ nearer the midline. In the average body habitus, sthenic and hyposthenic, the gallbladder is found in the middle of the RUQ.

The gallbladder stores bile until the sphincter of Oddi relaxes and the gallbladder contracts, pushing the bile into the duodenum. The trigger for contraction is a hormone called **cholecystokinin** (CCK) (kō´´lē-sĭs´´tō-kī´nĭn). CCK is secreted by the intestinal wall in response to the **chyme** that enters the intestine. The more dietary fat in the chyme, the more CCK released and the more emptying or contraction of the gallbladder. If a person has small stones, they may enter the common bile duct on contraction and cause blockage and pain. If there are large stones, the contracting gallbladder around them will also result in RUQ pain.

Radiographic Considerations

The radiographic examination of the hepatobiliary system attempts to image the transport and storage of bile. The mechanical or pathologic obstruction of this system will result in the congestion of bile in the liver and a general backup of bile products in the blood. The goal of radiographic imaging of this system is to pinpoint the cause of a suspected obstruction. The most common radiographic procedure of the hepatobiliary system is the oral cholecystogram (kō′′lē-sĭs′′tō′grăm) (OCG). The Greek prefix chole- means bile, and the Greek term cyst- means sac or bladder. An OCG is a study of the bile sac with a radiographic contrast media taken orally the day before the examination. The number of OCG examinations has dropped sharply over the last several years as sonography has become an effective tool in the diagnosis of gallstones. The use of the intravenous radiographic contrast media for imaging of the biliary ducts and gallbladder (intravenous cholecystography or IVCG) has all but disappeared over the same time period because of the high reaction rate and the effective use of fiberoptic cannulation and instillation of contrast into the bile ducts (ERCP, endoscopic retrograde cholangiopancreatography).

The radiographic investigation and documentation of gallstone removal occurs with the direct instillation of contrast into a biliary duct through the drainage tube during surgery (operative cholangiography [kō-lăn′′jē-ŏg′ră-fē) or following surgery (T-tube cholangiography). The Greek term angio- means vessel; therefore the cholangiogram is a study of the bile vessels. In cases of severe obstruction where access to the biliary tract is needed, a needle puncture through the liver and into the biliary tree followed by radiographic imaging of instilled contrast is conducted (percutaneous transhepatic cholangiography, PTC).

CLINICAL INDICATIONS AND CONTRAINDICATIONS

The most common clinical indication for a radiographic study of the hepatobiliary system is **dyspepsia** (dĭs-pĕp′sē-ă) and RUQ pain (especially after eating) caused by suspected choleliths. Women have gallstones twice as often as men, and obesity predisposes individuals to gallstones. Additional indications include jaundice, suspected obstruction from a pathologic lesion, and postoperative follow-up.

Contraindications for OCG and IVCG are an elevated bilirubin (> 2 mg/dL), which indicates that bile transport or production is impeded. Persistent diarrhea or vomiting, which curtails the absorption of oral contrast media, and allergy to radiographic contrast media are also contraindications. Patients with contraindications are referred for sonographic hepatobiliary studies.

CONTRAST MEDIA

The gallbladder and biliary ducts do not provide enough subject contrast with the surrounding liver to be imaged radiographically without the administration of a radiographic contrast media. Although cholesterol gallstones provide an increased radiographic density and calcium-laden gallstones provide an area of decreased radiographic density on plain films, the actual gallbladder and biliary tract are not visualized.

The contrast media used in OCG are different from most iodinated contrast media in that they are not injected or instilled into the vasculature or duct system. These contrast media are administered orally and absorbed through the intestinal wall into the bloodstream. The first stop for this venous portal blood is the liver, where it is removed for excretion in the bile. To achieve maximum concentration and opacification of the gallbladder the contrast must be ingested 10 to 12 hours before the scheduled radiographs for concentration in the gallbladder, and the gallbladder must not be stimulated to contract and spill out the contrast-laden contents. If the gallbladder is not opacified, the patient should be questioned in detail about any gastric disturbances or anything taken by mouth after the contrast media. Whether or not the patient followed the instructions, if the liver function is normal, a repeat examination with an additional dose of contrast media is routinely scheduled. No more than two doses (6 g) of contrast within 24 hours should be administered.

The contrast used is organically bound iodinated salts (either Ipodate sodium or Ipodate calcium). The rate of uptake by the liver and excretion into the bile varies between the two salts, with the calcium suspensions collecting in the biliary ducts in as little as 30 minutes. Both salts require 1 to 3 hours for maximum opacification of the biliary ducts. Maximum opacity of the gallbladder is attained 10 to 12 hours after ingestion of either contrast medium.

Both compounds are tolerated well. As with intravenous contrast media, a history of allergies or known reactions to products containing iodine implies a potential risk for reaction to these oral compounds. It is therefore prudent to question all patients about allergy and radiographic contrast history. Most radiology departments request that the patient fill out an allergy questionnaire and sign a consent form after review of the information about risks of radiographic contrast media. If the patient has a known allergy to radiographic contrast media, a sonogram of the gall-bladder will be performed in lieu of the OCG.

PATIENT PREPARATION

Patient preparation for the OCG on an otherwise healthy adult may include bowel cleansing routines with laxatives two evenings before the examination and cleansing enemas the day of the examination. Laxatives must be taken a day before the oral contrast media administration so that the contrast pills are not cleansed away with the laxatives. Many institutions do not require bowel cleansing because of the need for the patient to strictly follow the directions, and, because the gallbladder is somewhat mobile, various upright, decubitus, and oblique projections often shift the superimposed unprepared bowel out of view.

Although bowel cleansing is the most variable part of the preparation for an OCG, the remaining preparation is fairly standard. The patient has a low-fat or non-fat meal the evening before the examination and takes six tablets of contrast media with a small amount of water 3 to 4 hours after the last meal (10–12 hours before the examination). The patient must then be NPO until after the examination. Any food or water may stimulate the gallbladder to contract and spill the contrast before the radiographic examination. If the patient vomits after the contrast is ingested, the contrast media may be lost. If the patient has vomited after ingesting the contrast media, a scout abdomen is often taken at the originally scheduled examination time in the hope that the gallbladder is opacified. If there is no scout radiograph or if it does not image an opacified gallbladder, the patient is rescheduled and given a second dose of contrast media.

RADIOGRAPHS

If the gallbladder opacified well and there are no apparent stones on the initial films, a fat meal may be given to the patient to stimulate CCK production with resulting contraction of the gallbladder and relaxation of the sphincter of Oddi. There are commercially available fat meals, or simply a cup of cream may be given to the patient. Radiographs taken 15 to 30 minutes following the fatty meal will visualize the biliary tract as the contrast is pushed out of the contracting gallbladder and into the duodenum. In this manner the OCG may also serve as a cholangiogram. If there are stones, a postfat meal is generally not done because this may cause an obstruction and patient distress. Historically, the postfat cholangiogram has not enhanced the diagnostic information in the OCG and is rarely done today.

PROCEDURE PREPARATION

The technologist:

1. Prepares the room for a scout film or fluoroscopy, depending on department protocol.
2. Has the patient remove all undergarments and dress in a radiolucent patient gown.
3. Obtains a clinical history from the patient and details of the success the patient had complying with the examination preparation.
4. Takes scout radiograph and checks for opacified gallbladder.

ORAL CHOLECYSTOGRAM (OCG) ROUTINE POSITIONS/ PROJECTIONS

ORAL CHOLECYSTOGRAM—PA SCOUT

Exam Rationale   The scout film is taken to locate the gallbladder and check patient preparation and concentration of the contrast media in the gallbladder.

Technical Considerations

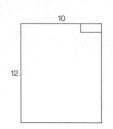

- Regular film/screen
- Bucky/grid
- kVp range: 70–75 (ideally < 75 for contrast media)
- SID: 40 inch (100 cm)

Radiation Protection

   (do not obscure RUQ)

AEC (Phototiming)

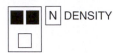 N DENSITY

Patient Position   Prone with the MSP parallel to the long axis of the table (Figure 17.4).

Central Ray   Perpendicular to the film through the center of the RUQ or 3 inches (8 cm) to the right of the spine and 4 inches (10 cm) superior to the iliac crest.

Patient Instructions   "Take in a breath; let it out. Don't breathe or move."

Evaluation Criteria (Figures 17.5 and 17.6)

- Entire gallbladder and area with biliary ducts is imaged.
- No rotation of the abdomen as evidenced by symmetrical appearance of the transverse spinous processes.

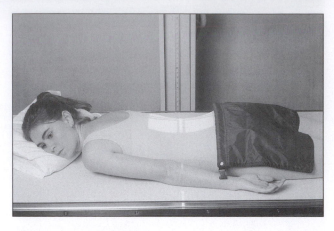

FIGURE 17.4   PA scout OCG.

- No abdominal or respiratory motion.
- Sufficient radiographic density and short scale of contrast to well delineate the gallbladder from surrounding anatomy and possible choleliths.

Tips

1. Evaluate body habitus by looking at the patient's bone structure and not the soft tissue.
2. Once the scout has been evaluated for gallbladder location, mark the patient's skin for future centering.
3. The hypersthenic (broad) individual's gallbladder is normally located high in the RUQ. The asthenic (long) individual's gallbladder is found on the upper border of the RLQ and midline (see Figure 17.3).

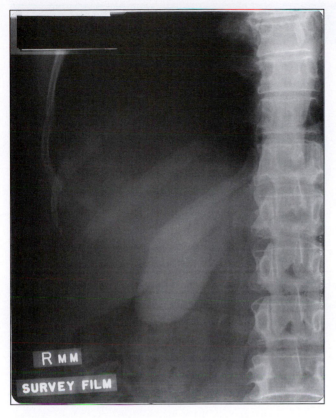

FIGURE 17.5   PA scout OCG.

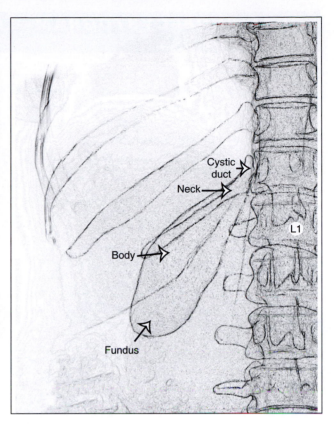

FIGURE 17.6   PA scout OCG.

ORAL CHOLECYSTOGRAM—LEFT ANTERIOR OBLIQUE POSITION

Exam Rationale   The oblique provides another perspective of the gallbladder. It eliminates or minimizes self-superimposition. The LAO also places the typical gallbladder closest and most parallel to the film, thereby minimizing shape distortion.

Technical Considerations

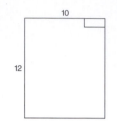

- Regular film/screen
- Bucky/grid
- kVp range: 70–75 (mAs may need to be increased as much as 40% from AP technique depending on how much abdomen falls into the field of view.)
- SID: 40 inch (100 cm)

Radiation Protection

    (do not obscure RUQ)

AEC (Phototiming)

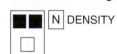   N DENSITY

Patient Position   From the prone position, the patient's right side is rotated up 15° to 40°; center the right side of the patient to the film with the MSP parallel to the long axis of the table (Figure 17.7).

Central Ray   Perpendicular through the gallbladder as identified on the scout film.

Patient Instructions   "Take in a breath; let it out. Don't breathe or move."

Evaluation Criteria (Figures 17.8 and 17.9)

- Entire gallbladder and area with biliary ducts is imaged.
- Gallbladder is elongated as compared to PA and has a minimum of self-superimposition.

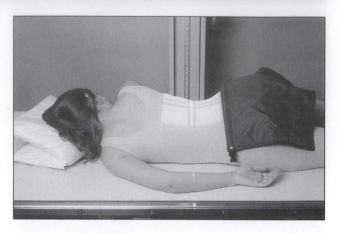

FIGURE 17.7   LAO OCG.

- No abdominal or respiratory motion.
- Sufficient radiographic density and short scale of contrast to well delineate the gallbladder from surrounding anatomy and possible choleliths.

Tips

1. A clean radiolucent sponge placed under the abdomen may decrease the chance of abdominal motion on the radiograph. However, an unclean sponge may introduce artifacts.
2. The degree of obliquity depends on the patient's anatomy. Thinner, asthenic patients need more rotation; broader, hypersthenic patients need less rotation.

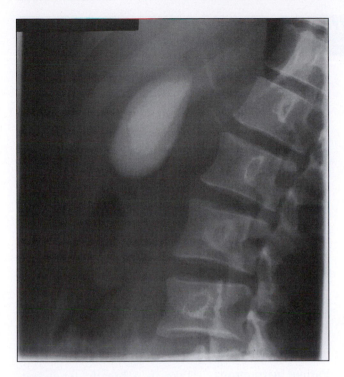

FIGURE 17.8　LAO OCG.

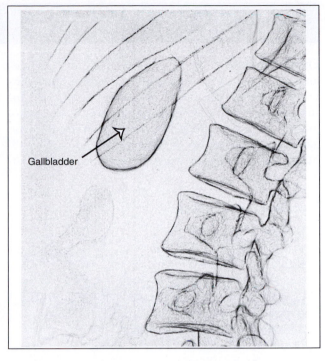

Gallbladder

FIGURE 17.9　LAO OCG.

ORAL CHOLECYSTOGRAM—RIGHT LATERAL DECUBITUS POSITION

Exam Rationale The decubitus position provides another perspective of the gallbladder and allows layering of stones as the heavy stones settle out and stones lighter than bile float together for better radiographic demonstration. The decubitus will allow the gallbladder to fall out laterally, realigning the gallbladder away from any superimposed bowel gas pattern.

Technical Considerations

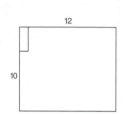

- Regular film/screen
- Bucky/grid
- kVp range: 70–75 (mAs may need to be increased as much as 40% from AP technique depending on how much abdomen falls into the field of view.)
- SID: 40 inch (100 cm)

Radiation Protection

 (do not obscure RUQ)

AEC (Phototiming)

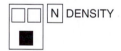 DENSITY

Patient Position Right lateral recumbent on a stretcher on a radiolucent sponge with back against an upright Bucky; neither the pelvis nor chest should be rotated; film is centered to the right side of the body (Figure 17.10).

Central Ray Perpendicular, 1 inch (3 cm) lateral to the position of the gallbladder, as determined on the PA scout.

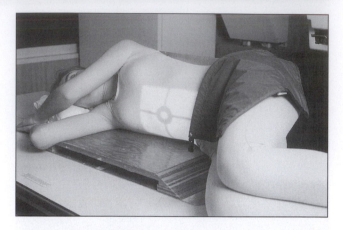

FIGURE 17.10　Right lateral decubitus OCG.

Patient Instructions "Take in a breath; let it out. Don't breathe or move."

Evaluation Criteria (Figures 17.11 and 17.12)

- Entire gallbladder and area with biliary ducts is imaged.
- No rotation of the abdomen as evidenced by symmetrical appearance of transverse spinous processes.
- No abdominal or respiratory motion.
- Sufficient radiographic density and short scale of contrast to well delineate the gallbladder from surrounding anatomy and possible choleliths.

Tips

1. The gallbladder moves easily on thinner patients within the abdominal viscera and will fall out laterally, requiring that the patient be built up on a radiolucent sponge.
2. Secure the stretcher with locks on all four wheels.

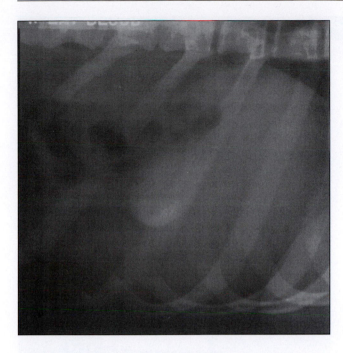

FIGURE 17.11 **Right lateral decubitus OCG.**

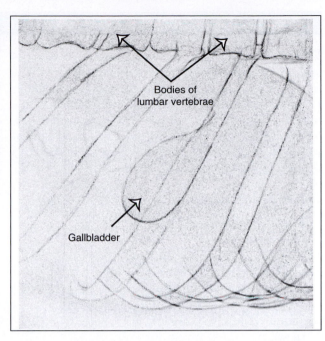

FIGURE 17.12 **Right lateral decubitus OCG.**

ORAL CHOLECYSTOGRAM—UPRIGHT PA PROJECTION

Exam Rationale The upright position provides another perspective of the gallbladder. It allows heavier stones to settle out in the fundus for better radiographic demonstration. Additionally, the upright will allow the gallbladder to move into a different position and potentially shift the superimposed unprepared bowel out of view or into a different area of the gallbladder.

Technical Considerations

- Regular film/screen
- Bucky/grid
- kVp range: 70–75 (mAs may need to be increased as much as 40% from AP technique depending on how much abdomen falls into the field of view.)
- SID: 40 inch (100 cm)

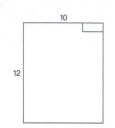

Radiation   AEC
Protection   (Photetiming)

      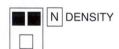

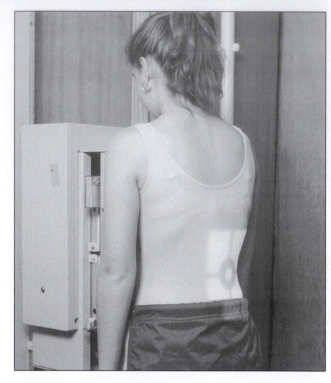

FIGURE 17.13   Upright PA OCG.

Patient Position PA erect; MSP parallel to the long axis of the table (Figure 17.13).

Central Ray 2 to 4 inches (5–10 cm) below the gallbladder, as located from the scout film.

Patient Instructions "Take in a breath; let it out. Don't breathe or move."

Evaluation Criteria (Figures 17.14 and 17.15)

- Entire gallbladder and area with biliary ducts is imaged.
- No rotation of the abdomen as evidenced by symmetrical appearance of transverse spinous processes.

- No abdominal or respiratory motion.
- Sufficient radiographic density and short scale of contrast to well delineate the gallbladder from surrounding anatomy and possible choleliths.

Tip The gallbladder moves easily within the abdominal viscera and will drop 2 to 4 inches (5–10 cm) when the patient is in the upright position.

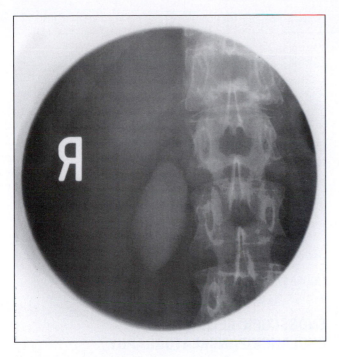

FIGURE 17.14   **Upright PA OCG.**

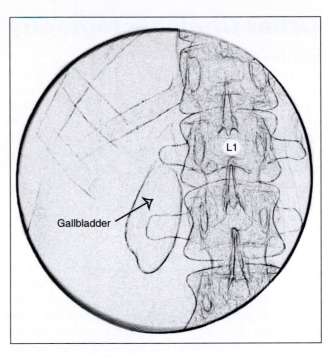

FIGURE 17.15   **Upright PA OCG.**

Other Cholecystography

Operative

Removal of the gallbladder (cholecystectomy) is the preferred procedure for chronic choleliths. During surgery to remove the gallbladder and stones, residual stones left in the biliary duct are a common occurrence. In order for the surgeon to evaluate the presence of residual stones without the added and risky surgical exploration of the biliary ducts, an operative cholangiogram is done. Water soluble urographic contrast media is instilled directly into the biliary tree through a small catheter placed in the cystic duct. Films are taken and evaluated during surgery for any remaining removable stones. The surgeon must make sure that there are no air bubbles in the contrast or catheter so that air bubble artifacts are not imaged. The technologist should set up the room for the cholangiogram prior to surgery, ensuring that the film-holder's grid lead strips are aligned perpendicular to the long axis of the table. It is sometimes necessary to angle the tube or tilt the table to eliminate the superimposition of the spine and the biliary ducts. Placement of the grid in this fashion will permit the proper angulation without grid cutoff. The operative cholangiogram also allows evaluation of biliary duct strictures and neoplastic obstructions.

POSTOPERATIVE (T TUBE)

If the surgeon is concerned about postoperative residual stones or the postoperative status of the biliary tract, a drainage tube may be placed in the biliary tract during surgery and clamped off outside of the body. The term T tube refers to the shape of the drainage tube that gives access to the biliary tree for postoperative cholangiogram in the radiology department (Figure 17.16). The T tube or postoperative cholangiogram occurs 1 to 3 days after surgery and is normally done by the radiologist under fluoroscopy. The technologist is responsible for setting up the equipment, preparing the contrast, changing the spot films, and monitoring the patient. The contrast used in both the operative and postoperative cholangiogram is a water-soluble urographic contrast agent (see Chapter 18).

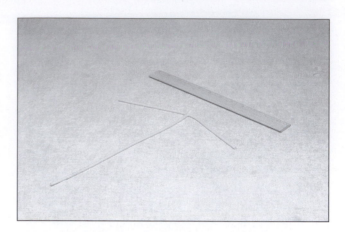

FIGURE 17.16   T tube.

ENDOSCOPIC RETROGRADE CHOLANGIOPANCREATOGRAPHY

Thorough investigation of the biliary ducts and pancreatic ducts is accomplished with ERCP. The patient is kept NPO before the procedure and is mildly sedated. Under fluoroscopic control, a fiberoptic scope is passed through the patient's esophagus and stomach into the duodenum. A gastroenterologist normally conducts the examination and locates the ampulla of Vater in the duodenum (Figure 17.17). A

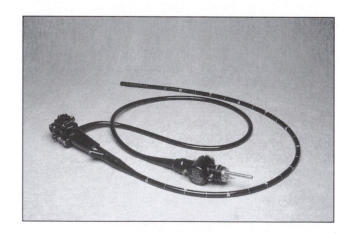

FIGURE 17.17   ERCP endoscope.

small catheter is passed through the ampulla and digestive enzymes can be collected for analysis before the direct retrograde instillation of radiographic contrast media and filming. ERCPs also demonstrate biliary stones and strictures and are helpful in evaluating pancreatic duct patency. Strictures or obstructions in the distal common bile duct or at the ampulla of Vater will interfere with the cannulation done in ERCP and may require the more invasive PTC procedure.

PERCUTANEOUS TRANSHEPATIC CHOLANGIOGRAPHY

Obstructive jaundice is the main indication for PTC. Obstructive jaundice usually results in dilated biliary ducts, which makes the needle puncture less difficult. The patient is given a local anesthetic at the puncture site and prepared for a sterile procedure. A fine needle (Chiba needle) (Figure 17.18) is passed percutaneously through the right flank and the liver into a biliary duct. The radiologist performs the placement under fluoroscopic control. Once the needle is in

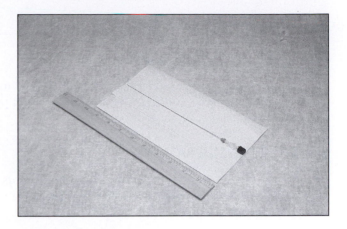

FIGURE 17.18   Chiba needle.

position, the biliary tract can be evaluated with the instillation of contrast and subsequent filming. After imaging, a guidewire can be passed through the needle for drainage, catheter placement, or stone removal apparatus.

Special Considerations

PEDIATRIC CONSIDERATIONS

The patient preparations and oral contrast media tend to dehydrate the patient as compared to the NPO preparation for a sonographic study. Consequently, pediatric patients are routinely sent to ultrasound for the hepatobiliary study.

GERIATRIC CONSIDERATIONS

The oral contrast media causes diarrhea in some patients. These gastric disturbances along with the added dehydration of the contrast media also result in ultrasound being the preferred preliminary study of the hepatobiliary system for geriatric patients.

SELECTED PATHOLOGY

Choleliths or gallstones form in the gallbladder when the bile salts are concentrated in the bile above normal limits. This high concentration may cause the cholesterol to precipitate out and form small stone nuclei that continue to aggregate with other bile salt constituents and form stones that can be imaged radiographically or sonographically. Although most of the gallstones are composed of cholesterol, some stones also contain calcium salts and are therefore visualized on a radiograph without any contrast media (Figure 17.19).

CORRELATIVE IMAGING

Sonography is now used as the primary preliminary examination of the hepatobiliary system. Suspected gallstones or biliary tract disease are readily assessed by ultrasound with the added bonus of being able to visualize the head of the pancreas and liver in the same examination (Figure 17.20).

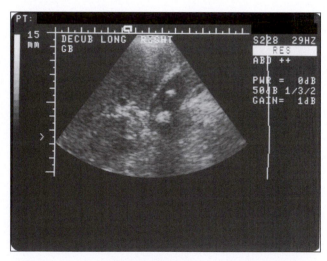

FIGURE 17.20 Sonogram of gallbladder with gallstones.

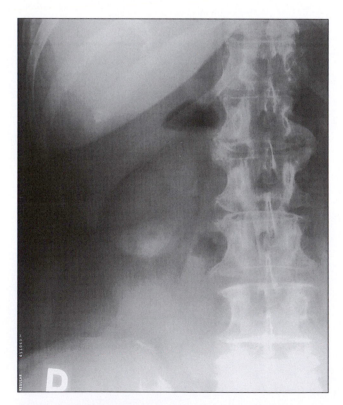

FIGURE 17.19 Radiograph of gallbladder with gallstones.

Review Questions

1. The liver is located in the _____ of the abdomen and has _____ lobes.

   a. RUQ, 3
   b. RUQ, 4
   c. LUQ, 3
   d. LUQ, 4

2. When bile is pushed out of the gallbladder, it first passes through the:

   a. common bile duct
   b. cystic duct
   c. pancreatic duct
   d. sphincter of Oddi

3. Bile is needed in the digestion of:

   a. carbohydrates
   b. fat
   c. glycogen
   d. vitamins

4. Bile is stored in the _____ until it is needed for digestion.

   a. duodenum
   b. gallbladder
   c. liver

5. The most common clinical indication for an OCG is:

   1. vomiting
   2. diarrhea
   3. chest pain
   4. RUQ pain

   a. 1 only
   b. 4 only
   c. 1 and 3
   d. 2 and 4

6. To achieve maximum concentration of contrast in the gallbladder, the contrast material should be ingested _____ before the scheduled radiographs are taken.

   a. immediately
   b. 1 to 2 hours
   c. 4 to 6 hours
   d. 10 to 12 hours

7. The contrast material used for an OCG is:

   a. iodinated urographic contrast
   b. iodinated calcium salts
   c. iodinated sodium salts
   d. both b and c
   e. all of the above

8. The most common position for imaging the gallbladder which places it closest and most parallel to the film is an _____ of the RUQ.

   a. LAO
   b. LPO
   c. RAO
   d. RPO

9. The rationale for decubitus or upright films of the gallbladder is:

   a. to provide another perspective of the gallbladder
   b. to layer any gallstones
   c. to eliminate bowel superimposition
   d. both a and b
   e. all of the above

10. During a PA scout cholecystogram on a sthenic patient, the central ray is directed:

    1. 3 inches to the left of the spine
    2. 3 inches to the right of the spine
    3. 4 inches superior to the iliac crest
    4. 4 inches superior to the ASIS

    a. 1 and 3
    b. 1 and 4
    c. 2 and 3
    d. 2 and 4

11. Which of the following examinations is designed to visualize the hepatic ducts?

    1. intravenous cholecystogram
    2. post fatty meal oral cholecystogram
    3. ERCP
    4. PTC

    a. 1, 2, and 3
    b. 2, 3, and 4
    c. 3 and 4
    d. 1, 2, 3, and 4

12. A T tube is used for _____ of the biliary tract and is used during a _____ .

    a. drainage, post-operative
    b. drainage, ERCP
    c. dilatation, post-operative
    d. dilatation, ERCP

13. Patient preparation for an OCG usually includes the administration of laxatives the evening before the study.

    a. true
    b. false

14. The liver converts bilirubin into bile.

    a. true
    b. false

15. The optimal kVp for a radiographic contrast study such as an OCG is below 75 kVp.

16. Pediatric and geriatric patients nearly always tolerate an OCG well.

17. When the _____ is constricted, bile cannot empty into the duodenum and is shunted back into the gallbladder.

18. For the oblique position of the gallbladder, the patient should be rotated _____ to _____ degrees from the _____ .

19. The central ray on an upright PA gallbladder is typically _____ (higher/lower) than on the recumbent PA.

20. During PTC, a Chiba needle is passed through the _____ into a _____ .

21. Why are there significantly fewer OCG studies now versus several years ago?

22. Describe the position of the gallbladder in:

    a. a hypersthenic patient
    b. an asthenic patient

References and Recommended Reading

Agur, A. (1991). *Grant's atlas of anatomy* (9th ed., p. 120). Baltimore: Williams & Wilkins.

Ballinger, P. W. (1991). *Merrill's atlas of radiographic positions and radiologic procedures* (8th ed., Vol. 2). St. Louis: Mosby-Year Book.

Bontrager, K. L. (1997). *Textbook of radiographic positioning and related anatomy* (3rd ed., p. 485). St. Louis: Mosby-Year Book.

Friedman, A. (Ed.). (1987). *Golden's diagnostic radiology: Radiology of the liver, biliary tract, pancreas and spleen.* Baltimore: Williams & Wilkins.

Laudicina, P., & Wean, D. (1994). *Applied angiography for radiographers.* Philadelphia: Saunders.

Martini, F. (1992). *Fundamentals of anatomy and physiology* (2nd ed.) Upper Saddle River, NJ: Prentice Hall.

Novelline, R., & Squire, L. F. (1987). *Living anatomy—A working atlas using computed tomography, magnetic resonance and angiography images.* St. Louis: Mosby.

Solomon, E. P., & Davis, P. W. (1978). *Understanding human anatomy and physiology.* New York: McGraw-Hill.

Sutton, D. (1994). *Radiology and imaging for medical students* (6th ed.). New York: Churchhill Livingstone.

CHAPTER 18

Urinary System

ANITA MARIE SLECHTA, MS, BSRT, (R)(M)(ARRT)

OBJECTIVES

At the completion of this chapter, the student should be able to:

1. List and describe the basic anatomic components of the urinary system and identify the basic parenchymal unit of the kidney.

2. Given drawings and radiographs, locate anatomic structures.

3. Describe the physiology of the urinary system and describe its role in maintaining the body's homeostasis.

4. List four common clinical indications for imaging the urinary system.

5. Explain why it is necessary to use radiographic contrast media to image the urinary system.

6. List the two main categories of radiographic contrast media used in intravenous urography and the factors determining their use.

continued

7. State the main difference between the contrast used in intravenous urography and retrograde cystography.

8. Discuss adverse patient reactions to radiographic contrast and list the medical responses necessary for each.

9. Describe preparation for each urinary procedure for both typical and atypical patients.

10. Describe the positioning used in imaging of the urinary system.

11. List or identify the central ray location and identify the extent of field necessary for each projection.

12. Explain the protective measures appropriate for each examination.

13. Recommend the technical factors for producing an acceptable radiograph during each urinary procedure.

14. Identify the normal postinjection sequencing of radiographs during imaging of the urinary system.

15. Identify the hypertensive postinjection sequencing of radiographs during imaging of the urinary system.

16. State the instructions given to the patient before and during each urinary imaging procedure.

17. Explain the rationale for the following procedures/projections in urinary system imaging.

   a. Postinjection sequencing of radiographs following contrast media injection
   b. 30° RPO or LPO projections of the kidneys
   c. Nephrotomograms
   d. Upright projections
   e. Postvoid projections

18. Given radiographs, evaluate positioning and technical factors.

19. Describe modifications of procedures for atypical or impaired patients to better demonstrate the anatomic area of interest.

Anatomy and Physiology

The urinary system has a vital excretory function that assists in maintaining **homeostasis** in the body. The urinary system eliminates organic (nitrogenous) wastes and maintains the water and electrolyte balance in the body. If the billions of cells in the body were to function without this waste removal, the cells would suffocate as cellular wastes build up. The urinary system is often classified under the category *genitourinary*. However the Latin prefix genito means of birth and refers solely to the reproductive organs. Because several of the reproductive organs share areas of the body with the urinary system, a disorder in one system may create problems in another. An example is enlargement of the male prostate gland, which results in difficulty in urinating. However, this chapter is dedicated solely to the imaging of the urinary system.

The urinary system consists of two kidneys, two ureters (ū´rĕ-ter), a bladder, and a urethra (ū-rē´thră) (Figure 18.1). The kidneys are the filters of the system and also reabsorb water and electrolytes to achieve optimal fluid balance for the body. Urine, the waste product filtrate, is initially collected in the kidneys and then channeled through tubes called ureters to the bladder. The bladder acts as a storage container, so that elimination can occur occasionally rather than continuously. When the bladder is full, the urethra conducts the urine to the external environment through a process called urination or **micturition** (mĭk-tū-rĭ´shŭn).

KIDNEYS

The kidneys are shaped like kidney beans with a concave curve medially and a convex curve laterally. They are approximately 4 inches (10 cm) long, 2 inches (5.5 cm) wide, and 1 inch (3 cm) thick. Medially, the concave surface seems to fold into a long narrow depression or "pocket" called the **hilus** (hī´lŭs). The hilus is where the ureters and the renal arteries and veins enter and exit the kidney (Figure 18.2). The kidneys are retroperitoneal organs lying lateral to each side of the vertebral column. The left kidney is normally situated slightly higher than the right kidney. The top of the left kidney is found at T12 and extends to L3. The right kidney is positioned about an inch (1–2 cm) below the left due to the volume of the liver on the right side. The kidneys are rotated 30° from the coronal plane, with the lateral border posterior to the medial border (Figure 18.3). This rotation becomes important when doing oblique radiographs. Because the kidney is rotated 30° with the patient in the AP position, the technologist rotates the patient 30° to place the kidney parallel to the film and image it with less distortion. With the patient in the RPO or LPO position, the kidney away from the film is parallel to the film.

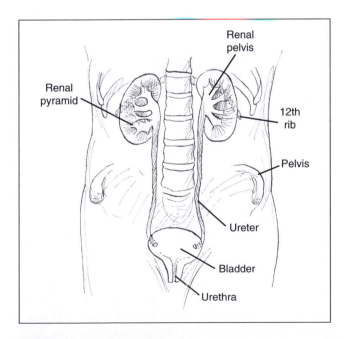

FIGURE 18.1   Urinary system.

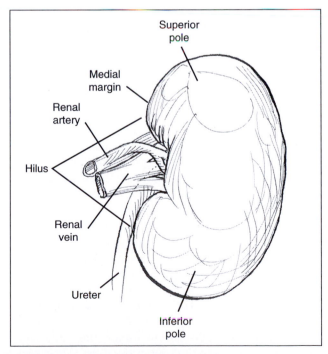

FIGURE 18.2   Gross anatomy of the kidney.

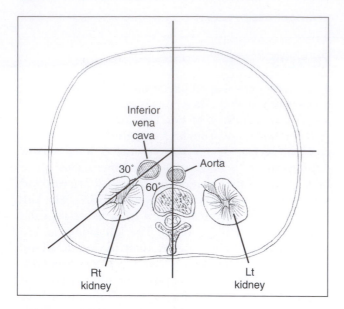

FIGURE 18.3 **Cross section of kidney.**

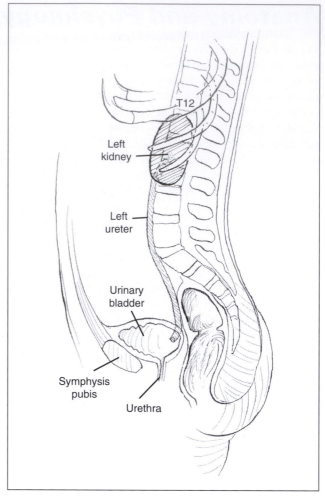

FIGURE 18.4 **Lateral abdomen.**

In a lateral projection of the abdomen, the kidneys lie against the posterior abdominal muscle wall (Figure 18.4). The ureters exit the kidneys and travel anteriorly and inferiorly.

The kidney is surrounded by a tough fibrous and dense adipose capsule, thereby creating enough subject contrast between the kidney and surrounding muscle to visualize the kidney's silhouette on a plain abdomen radiograph. The kidneys are suspended by fibers attached to adjacent structures. This suspension system protects the kidneys from normal jarring and allows their mobility during respiration. This mobility is important because the kidneys sit below and are attached to the constantly moving diaphragm. If these connections break due to trauma or disease, then a "loose" or "free-floating" kidney exists, which may result in a twisting or contortion of the renal vessels and ureters. An upright radiograph will determine if the kidney's mobility is beyond normal limits and is therefore part of most urinary radiographic examinations. Additionally, even normal kidney mobility requires that, for consistency, all radiographs in a study of the urinary system be taken at the same state of respiration, preferably on expiration.

Internally the kidney has two regions: (1) the **cortex**, which is a peripheral ring of parenchymal (păr-ĕn´kĭ-măl) tissue, and (2) the **medulla** (mĕ-dŭl´lă), which is an internal band of densely packed collecting ducts (Figure 18.5, Color illustration 4). The medulla is sectioned into six to eighteen lobes or pyramids. The apex of each pyramid, called the papilla, points toward the renal hilus and empties urine into the contiguous calyces (kā´ĕ-sēz). The calyces then empty urine into the renal pelvis.

The parenchyma or working/filtering unit of the kidney is the **nephron** (nĕf´rŏn) unit (Figure 18.6, Color illustration 4). It is the nephron unit that removes waste from the blood and reabsorbs fluid and electrolytes during the concentration of urine. The nephron is composed of the renal corpuscle (also known as *Bowman's capsule*), **glomerulus** (glō-mĕr´ū-lŭs), convoluted tubules, the loop of Henle, and collection ducts. Blood enters the renal corpuscle through afferent arterioles and leaves via efferent arterioles. Once the blood enters the corpuscle it is filtered by a capillary network called the glomerulus. Nitrogenous wastes, small ions, and water are removed from the blood and enter the nephron collecting system. Water and electrolytes are reabsorbed back into the bloodstream as this filtrate passes through the convoluted tubules and loop of Henle, thereby maintaining the volume and electrolyte balance of the blood. When a radiopaque contrast media

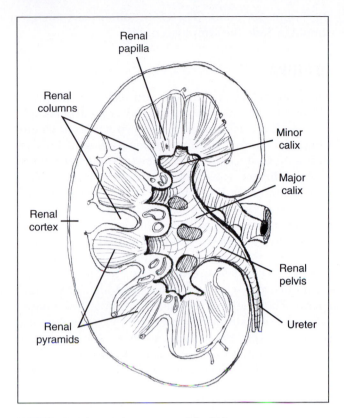

FIGURE 18.5   Internal structures of the kidney.

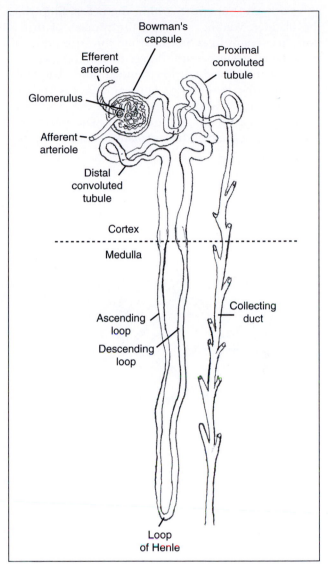

FIGURE 18.6   A nephron unit.

is injected into the bloodstream, it enters the renal corpuscle and is distributed in this capillary network. This "lights up" the parenchyma on a radiograph, hence the term radiographic nephrogram. The urine that leaves the nephron's collecting ducts in the medulla drains into the renal calyces and then flows into the renal pelvis. The Greek term pyelo- means pelvis and therefore a pyelogram (pī′ĕ-lō-grăm) is a study of the renal pelvis, the first major collecting area for urinary wastes.

URETERS

The pelvis continues out of the hilus and becomes a ureter at the *ureteropelvic* (ū-rē′′tĕr-ō-pĕl′vĭk) *junction.* The ureters are 10 to 12 inch (25 to 30 cm) long tubes that have a thin muscle wall that massages the urine away from the kidney through peristalsis. The ureters are also retroperitoneal as they travel inferiorly to the bladder along the anterior surface of the psoas muscles. Because of the ureters' small diameter (1/2 inch [1 cm] or less), they are a common site for the lodgement of renal stones. This obstruction of urine flow is very painful and commonly occurs where urine leaves the kidney, at the ureteropelvic junction, or where the ureter enters the bladder—the ureterovesical (ū-rē′′tĕr-ō-vĕs′ĭ-kăl) junction.

The ureters enter the bladder laterally and posteriorly. This entrance point allows the ureter to enter at an angle that elongates the ureterovesical junction and provides a longer muscle flap to act as a sphincter, which prevents **reflux** (backflow of urine into the kidney).

BLADDER

The **trigone** (trī′gōn) is a triangular-shaped muscle mass at the floor of the bladder. The three corners of the trigone are the two ureterovesical junctions and the urethrovesical junction (orifice [or′ĭ-fĭs] of the urethra). The trigone is attached to the floor of the pelvis, so that as urine fills the bladder, it expands anteriorly and superiorly within the pelvis. Emptying the bladder, voiding, through the process of urination, may result in reflux of urine into the ureter if the trigonal ureterovesical flap is underdeveloped.

The female bladder lies between the symphysis pubis and the bordering vagina and uterus (Figure 18.7). The male bladder lies between the symphysis pubis and the rectum (Figure 18.8). The most inferior border of the bladder normally lies at the level of the symphysis pubis. Therefore, all urinary images should include the symphysis pubis.

URETHRA

The urethra has an internal and external sphincter (sfingk´ter). The external sphincter is controlled voluntarily. If the external sphincter is not relaxed voluntarily, the internal sphincter remains closed. Loss of voluntary control over the external sphincter results in **incontinence** (involuntary release of urine). The female urethra is 1 1/2 inches (4 cm) in length and has the sole function of transporting urine from the bladder to the external environment. The male urethra is 7 to 8 inches (17–20 cm) in length and is subdivided into the prostatic, membranous, and penile portions. The male urethra is also part of the male reproductive system as it is the conduit for passing sperm. The length of the male urethra acts as a natural barrier to external bacteria and the urine remains sterile, whereas the female urethra's shortness and close proximity to the anus leads to easier access to external bacteria. The entrance of bacteria into the urethra and up into the bladder causes **cystitis** (sĭs-tī´tĭs). If the bacteria are refluxed into the kidneys, a serious kidney infection can ensue. Urinary tract infections (UTIs) are a common malady in female patients. Reflux with a kidney infection is common in the female child who often has less well-developed trigonal ureterovesical flaps.

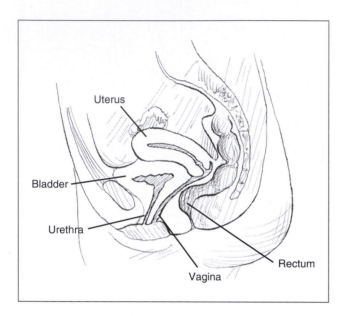

FIGURE 18.7   Bladder in female patient.

RADIOGRAPHIC CONSIDERATIONS

The radiographic examination of the urinary system images the two distinct phases of renal function: (1) the nephrogram phase, as the blood is being filtered, and (2) the collection/transport phase, as urine is being channeled and eliminated from the body. The most commonly requested radiographic study of the urinary system is the intravenous pyelogram (IVP). However, the prefix pyelo- refers only to the renal pelvis and is therefore a misnomer when used to order a study of the entire urinary system. The proper term is IVU (urogram) because it refers to the entire urinary system. Specific imaging procedures for the filtering phase of the nephron (nephrograms) and bladder and urethra studies (cystograms, voiding cystograms or voiding cystourethrograms [VCUGs]) are also part of a general radiology department's repertoire for studying the urinary system.

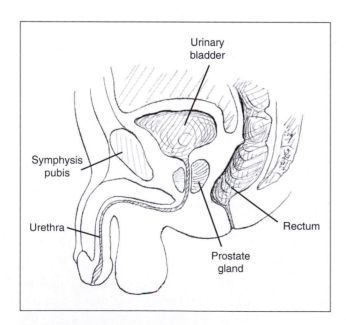

FIGURE 18.8   Bladder in male patient.

ANTEGRADE VERSUS RETROGRADE

During an IVU the contrast is traveling in the normal excretory direction of flow, in other words, antegrade. Therefore another descriptive term for the IVU is antegrade IVU or antegrade excretory urography. The differentiation of antegrade urography is important because certain clinical situations (discussed later in this chapter) dictate the use of retrograde urography. The retrograde (against normal flow or direction) method requires catheterization of the bladder and ureters with injection of contrast media through the catheters for a direct filling of the renal calyces, pelvis, ureters, and bladder.

CLINICAL INDICATIONS AND CONTRAINDICATIONS

The most common indications for ordering a radiographic study of the urinary system include trauma, severe flank pain, **hematuria** (hē´´mă-tū´rē-ă) and hypertension.

Contraindications include a known allergy to radiographic contrast media. Premedication with steroids over several days before the study may be useful in diminishing allergy risks when the examination is absolutely indicated. Additional contraindications include renal failure or dysfunction, **anuria** (ăn-ū´rē-ă), **multiple myeloma**, and pregnancy.

PATIENT PREPARATION

Patient preparation for the otherwise healthy adult patient includes a bowel cleansing routine. Although preferences for particular products vary, the ultimate goal is to create a bowel free of fecal matter and gas because either may obscure the urographic images. Each radiology facility provides instructions for preparation of the patient, including (1) identification of the allowed contents for the meal prior to the study, usually a light or liquid meal the night before the examination; (2) directions for the administration of a non–gas-forming laxative the evening before the study (over-the-counter cathartics may be identified); (3) a prestudy enema or cathartic suppository; and (4) NPO after midnight, which induces a mild dehydration so there is less dilution of the radiographic contrast media.

SPECIAL POPULATIONS

If a patient is diabetic, geriatric, or pediatric, these preparations can aggravate existing conditions or seriously dehydrate the patient. Therefore, many radiology facilities alter pre-exam preparation in the following manner.

Pediatric Patients

Laxatives are excluded and liquids are allowed up to 2 to 6 hours before the examination depending on the child's age. Often, the less invasive renal ultrasound (sonogram) is substituted for the IVU for pediatric patients.

Diabetic and Geriatric Patients

These patients are counseled individually on pre-exam preparation but are normally well hydrated to decrease dehydration and the chance of contrast-induced renal failure.

The amount of contrast used on these three patient populations will also vary because the risk of contrast-induced kidney failure is proportional to the volume of contrast media administered.

TECHNICAL ASPECTS

Contrast Media

The adipose capsule of the kidney and the surrounding muscle create enough subject contrast to allow imaging of a kidney silhouette on an abdomen radiograph. However, the nephron and collecting system cannot be visualized without the use of a radiopaque contrast material. Two types of contrast media are available for intravenous use—ionic and nonionic iodinated contrast media. The heavy element of iodine in the media is radiopaque and permits the enhanced imaging of the urinary system. Whether or not a patient is administered ionic or nonionic contrast will be determined by the institution's protocols and ultimately by the radiologist who considers patient history for allergies, past contrast studies, and renal function. The nonionic media produce fewer adverse reactions overall among the general population (Katayama, 1990). However, the nonionic media are up to ten times as expensive as the ionic media. In evaluating risk versus cost, it must be considered that the adverse reaction rate to the ionic media is still very low (4/10,000) and considered safe in the average patient population (Levin, 1990).

Contrast is administered intravenously either by a **bolus** injection or by a gravity-flow infusion. The contrast material is filtered by the nephron and is concentrated in the collecting system for imaging of the entire excretory system. The volume or dosage of contrast media administered to the patient depends on the weight and age of the patient. The status of the patient's renal function may limit the contrast dosage or cancel the examination because contrast media will aggravate renal insufficiency. Checking a patient's **blood urea nitrogen** (BUN) will indicate the status of renal function (normal range is 9–25 mg/mL).

Contrast used in cystourethrography and cystography is generally the same contrast media used in a department's IVUs, although in a diluted form.

Adverse Reactions to Radiographic Contrast Media

Adverse reactions to intravenously injected contrast media may range from mild nausea and a metallic taste to severe shock, which can cause a rapid death. The risk of any one patient having a severe reaction is very small; however, there are risk factors and precautions that all radiology facilities must consider.

In an attempt to address risk, most facilities have patients sign a consent form after an explanation of contrast reaction risks. Even the use of nonionic media does not eliminate the risk. The risk information and consent form includes a clinical history questionnaire. The information provided by the patient is used by the department to determine overall risk and to decide whether or not to use nonionic contrast. Generally, questionnaires include requests for allergy history for shellfish (iodine containing) and hay fever (general allergies). Information on past radiographic studies is requested because all injected radiographic contrast media are similar, and a previous nonreaction contrast study would indicate less risk for severe reactions. Even when a history dictates low risk, the patient must be monitored for systemic reactions and reassured when mild discomfort occurs. The technologist should be prepared for both mild reactions, with an emesis basin, blood pressure cuff, and stethoscope, and severe reactions, with a stocked drug cart in the room and an on-call emergency team. Table 18.1 summarizes potential reactions and the appropriate technologist response.

Preparation

Room preparation varies according to the department's procedures. The routine IVU requires radiographic films of the abdomen and a contrast injection. If the routine requires nephrotomograms, then a radiographic/tomographic room is required and prepared for both imaging procedures.

Before beginning an IVU, the technologist should ensure that a drug cart and emergency supplies are available (Figure 18.10).

TABLE 18.1 CONTRAST REACTION/RESPONSE

Patient Reaction	Technologist Response
Mild Reactions	
Nausea, heat flash, metallic taste	Reassure patient that these are normal occurrences and that they will pass. Slow deep breaths may help control nausea.
Vomiting	Prevent aspiration by rolling patient to the side (Figure18.9).
Urticaria (ŭr-tĭ-kā´rē-ă) or hives	Monitor for development of new hives.
Moderate Reactions	
Exorbitant number of hives or giant hives	Call for medical assistance—medication may be required (normally antihistamine-allergy medications). Comfort and monitor patient.
Tachycardia (tăk´´ē-kăr´dē-ă) (rapid heartbeat)	Call for medical assistance—medication may be required. Comfort and monitor patient.
Severe Reactions	
Dyspnea (dĭsp-nē´ă) Sudden hypotension Loss of consciousness Cardiac arrest	Call for emergency medical assistance; assist medical team and record events.

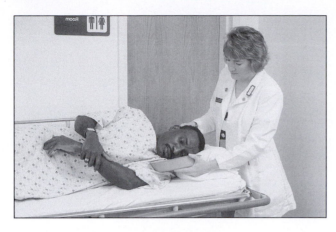

FIGURE 18.9   **Proper use of emesis basin.**

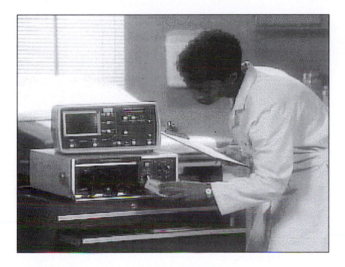

FIGURE 18.10   **Fully stocked emergency cart.**

The technologist prepares the room for a scout film(s):

1. Has the patient empty the bladder
2. Has the patient dress in a radiolucent patient gown
3. Has the patient remove all undergarments
4. Obtains a clinical history from the patient and explains the procedure and possible contrast-induced sensation
5. Prepares the appropriate contrast media and equipment for injection (see injection/instillation of contrast)
6. Takes scout radiograph(s) and checks for adequacy
7. Prepares room for first postinjection radiograph

Postinjection Serial Radiographs

Intravenous urography is a radiographic examination of the entire excretory process of the urinary system and requires filming at different times during the transport of contrast-containing urine to the calyces, the renal pelvis, the ureters, and bladder. The timing for the postinjection radiographs begins at the beginning of the injection.

The specific intervals for filming are determined by the patient's pathology and pre-existing conditions. However, typical adult transit time for contrast to well define the calyces is 5 minutes, with contrast delineating the ureters in 10 to 15 minutes, and delineation of the bladder in 15 to 30 minutes. Pediatric patient filming intervals are much shorter, with 1-minute, 5-minute, and 15-minute intervals common.

A hypertensive IVU requires radiographs at 1, 2, 3, 4, and 5 minutes postinjection. Because the timing for the postinjection radiographs starts at the beginning of the injection and a bolus injection can take 30 to 60 seconds, the technologist must be completely prepared to radiograph the patient immediately following the injection. The hypertensive IVU aids in the diagnosis of renal hypertension.

Tomograms of the kidneys taken within the first 6 minutes from the time of contrast injection visualize the nephron phase of excretion. Known as nephrotomograms, these films are commonly part of a routine adult IVU. Additionally, tomograms may be used to image the kidneys without superimposed bowel gas or feces in a nonprepared or ill-prepared patient.

Injection/Instillation of Contrast Media

Bolus Injection Setup   Equipment required for injection of radiographic contrast media (Figure 18.11):

1. Sterile syringe, usually 50 mL
2. Needle for loading contrast, usually 19 gauge
3. Ionic or nonionic contrast media

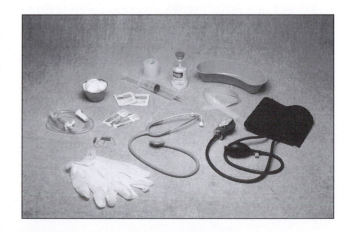

FIGURE 18.11   **Bolus injection equipment.**

4. Alcohol wipes
5. Variety of butterfly needles (18-21 gauge)
6. Paper tape
7. Protective latex gloves
8. Towel (rolled for extension of elbow for antecubital injection)
9. Tourniquet
10. Sterile cotton balls
11. Band-Aids
12. Emesis basin
13. Blood pressure cuff and stethoscope
14. 50-mL saline drip setup (optional)

Procedure The technologist, using sterile technique, fills the syringe with the appropriate contrast agent. All equipment used for the injection should be made accessible to the individual administering the contrast through a butterfly needle. The time at the beginning of the contrast bolus injection should be noted. After the needle has been secured and the contrast has been injected, the technologist connects the butterfly to the infusion saline drip if the protocol dictates. A slow drip rate is set to keep the intravenous line open.

Infusion Contrast Injection Setup

Equipment required for injection of radiographic contrast media (Figure 18.12):

1. Infusion radiographic contrast media
2. Connector tubing for contrast bottle

Items #4 through #13 from the bolus injection setup.

Procedure The technologist, using sterile technique, inserts the tubing into the contrast bottle and allows the fluid to replace all the air in the tubing. The cap on the end of tubing is replaced to maintain it in sterile condition. Make all equipment accessible for the individual administering the contrast. Following needle placement the infusion drip contrast is connected

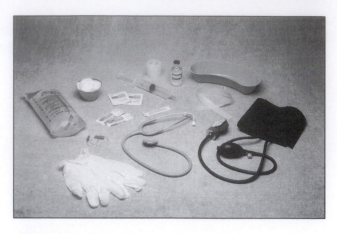

FIGURE 18.12   **Infusion injection equipment.**

to the butterfly. Department protocols will dictate the rate of infusion drip. The time at the beginning of contrast infusion should be noted.

Film Markers

Although film markers are essential for all radiographs, they are critical when doing serial radiography of the urinary tract. Accurate interpretation of the radiographic images depends on information provided by appropriate markers. In addition to correctly placed "R" or "L" markers, the following markers should be used when appropriate:

- "Upright"—for films taken with the patient erect
- Number identifying the fulcrum level—on tomographic images
- Time of film in relation to contrast administration—for serial films taken after administration of contrast
- "Postvoid"—for contrast films taken after the patient has voided

ROUTINE AND ALTERNATIVE POSITIONS/PROJECTIONS

Part	Routine	Page	Alternative	Page
Intravenous urogram (IVU)	AP abdomen (scout)	678		
	AP serial postinjection	680	Nephrotomograms	685
	Oblique	682		
	AP bladder	684		
			Upright postvoid AP	686
			Oblique bladder	688

SCOUT ABDOMEN OR KUB

Exam Rationale   The preliminary or scout film demonstrates specific anatomy of the patient for subsequent images and evaluation of technique. Both kidneys and the bladder (symphysis pubis) must be imaged on the scout film. Radiopaque stones may be seen on this film that are later obscured by radiographic contrast.

Technical Considerations

- Regular film/screen
- Bucky/grid
- kVp range: 70–80
- SID: 40 inch (100 cm)

Radiation Protection

 Male patients. Not possible for female patients

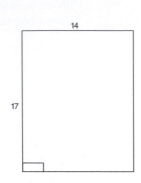

AEC (Phototiming)

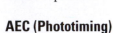 N DENSITY

Patient Position   Supine with sponge support under the knees; MSP centered to the long axis of the table; symphysis pubis placed at the bottom of the film or film centered to the iliac crest (Figure 18.13).

Central Ray   Perpendicular to the film and centered at the iliac crest and at the MSP.

Patient Instructions   "Take in a breath, let it out. Don't breathe or move."

Evaluation Criteria (Figures 18.14 and 18.15)

- Entire urinary system should be imaged (kidneys and symphysis pubis).
- The psoas muscles should be imaged.
- The spine is centered to the film.

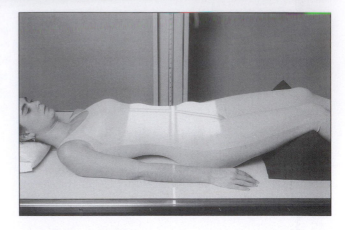

FIGURE 18.13   KUB scout.

- There is no rotation as evidenced by:
  —Symmetrical iliac alae
  —Visualization of ischial spines equally on both sides
  —Symmetrical rib cage
- No respiratory motion.

Tips

1. To find the iliac crest, first palpate the ASIS and center the film 4 inches (10 cm) above the ASIS at the iliac crest.
2. To find the symphysis, have the patient internally rotate the foot and palpate for the greater trochanter. Place the bottom of the film 1 inch (3 cm) below the trochanter.
3. If the symphysis pubis is always included on the scout and patient is too long for the film to image the entire system, a film of the kidneys, on an 11 × 14 inch (28 × 36 cm) crosswise film may need to be done on each subsequent film. *This extra kidney radiograph allows gonadal shielding on all patients,* whereas an extra bladder shot would increase gonadal dose.

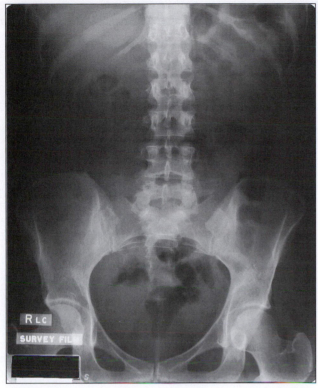

FIGURE 18.14   KUB.

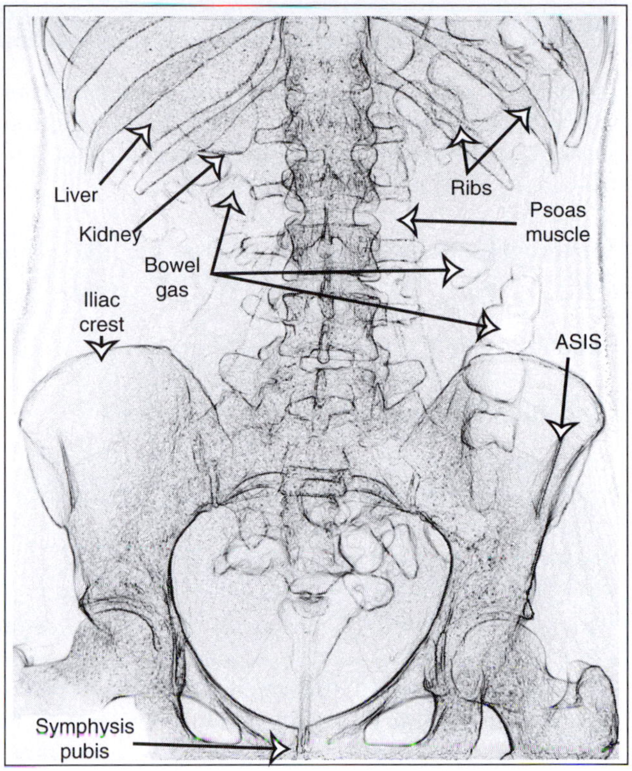

FIGURE 18.15   KUB.

AP SERIAL POSTINJECTION RADIOGRAPHS

Exam Rationale Radiographs taken at various intervals following injection of the contrast media demonstrate the calyces, the renal pelvis, the ureters, and the bladder in various stages of filling.

Technical Considerations Same as for the scout IVU

Patient Position Adjust for any errors on the scout

Evaluation Criteria (Figures 18.16 and 18.17)

- See scout criteria.
- Adequate contrast media in the calyces, renal pelvis, ureters, and bladder.
- Markers accurately identify serial film.

Tip Compression may be *carefully* used on the distal ureters to obstruct the flow of contrast media and increase the filling of the renal calyces and pelvis. Decompression must be done carefully and gradually (Figure 18.18).

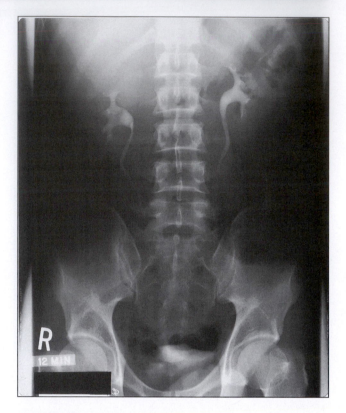

FIGURE 18.16   AP IVU.

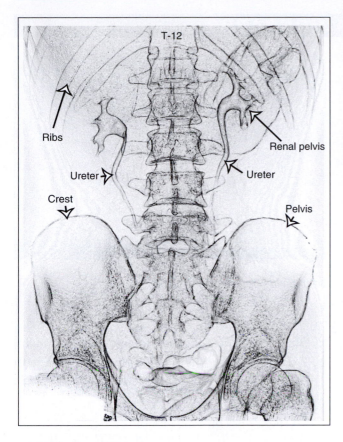

FIGURE 18.17 AP IVU.

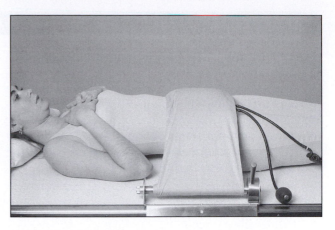

FIGURE 18.18 Positioning of IVU compression device.

OBLIQUE POSTINJECTION RADIOGRAPHS

Exam Rationale   The patient is rotated 30° to place a kidney parallel to the film and image it with less distortion. The kidney away from the film will be the one parallel to the film. The obliques provide another perspective of the urinary system and often eliminate overlap of anatomy. Both obliques are done for comparison and are normally taken in the middle of the examination (10–20 minutes).

Technical Considerations

* Regular film/screen
* Bucky/grid
* kVp range: 70–80 (increase +40% mAs or +4–6 kVp from AP)
* SID: 40 inch (100 cm)

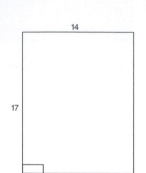

Radiation Protection

   Male patients. Not possible for female patients

Patient Position   Supine with knees flexed and ipsilateral arm across chest; spine is centered to the film and at the same transverse plane identified on the scout to include the entire urinary system (Figure 18.19).

Central Ray   Perpendicular to the film; center at the same transverse plane as on the AP and at the spine.

Patient Instructions   "Take in a breath, let it out. Don't breathe or move."

Evaluation Criteria (Figures 18.20 and 18.21)

* Entire urinary system should be imaged (kidneys to bladder).
* The kidney away from the table should be viewed without shape distortion and should not superimpose the spine.
* The ureter closest to the film should not superimpose the spine.

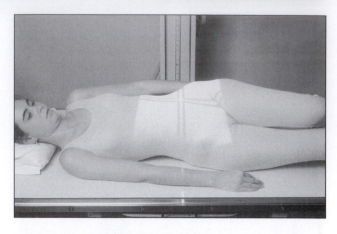

FIGURE 18.19   Posterior oblique IVU.

* Film density is adequate to visualize the radiographic contrast media in the calyces, renal pelvis, ureters, and bladder as you progress from the beginning of the injection.
* The spine is centered to the film.
* No respiratory or body motion.
* Markers identify side down (closest to the film).

Tips

1. The patient's entire body should be moved laterally from the KUB position 4 inches (10 cm) away from the side that will be down on the oblique. Then the patient can be rolled uniformly along the long axis for an unvarying 30° rotation. (Do not flex or extend the spine on rotation.)
2. A radiolucent sponge may be used to support the patient in the oblique position.

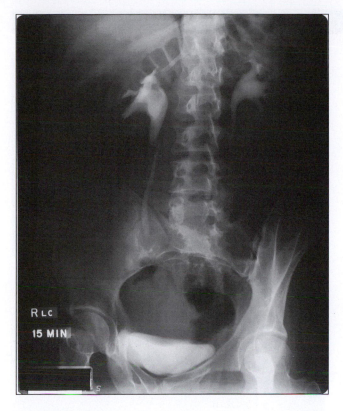

FIGURE 18.20   Posterior IVU oblique.

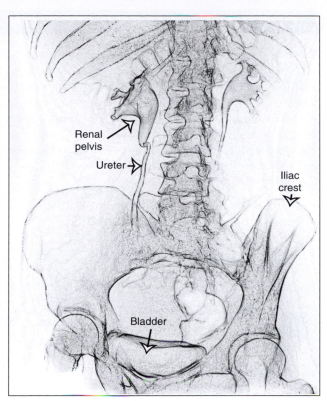

FIGURE 18.21   Posterior IVU oblique.

BLADDER—AP PROJECTION

Exam Rationale   This film is taken at the end of the radiographic examination to ensure maximum filling of the bladder. It provides another perspective of the bladder, often imaging the distal ureters and the ureterovesical junction. The bladder film may identify lesions of the bladder or it may provide etiologic factors involved in pathology of the ureters and kidneys.

Technical Considerations

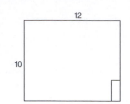

- Regular film/screen
- Bucky/grid
- kVp range: 70–75
- SID: 40 inch (100 cm)

Radiation Protection

   Male patients

AEC (Phototiming)

  N DENSITY

Patient Position   Supine with a sponge support under the knees; MSP centered to the longitudinal axis of the table; centered at the ASIS and the MSP (Figure 18.22).

Central Ray   Perpendicular to the film; centered at the ASIS and MSP.

Patient Instructions   "Take in a breath, let it out. Don't breathe or move."

Evaluation Criteria (Figures 18.23 and 18.24)

- Entire bladder is imaged.
- Spine is centered to the film.
- There is no rotation as evidenced by visualization of ischial spines equally on both sides.
- No body motion.

Tips

1. The entire symphysis pubis should be visualized on the male patient to ensure inclusion of the prostate gland.
2. Some protocols call for a 10° to 20° caudal angle of the central ray.

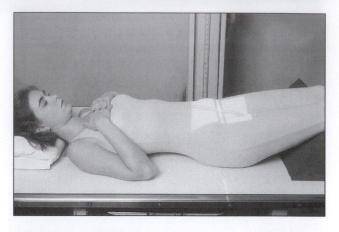

FIGURE 18.22   AP bladder.

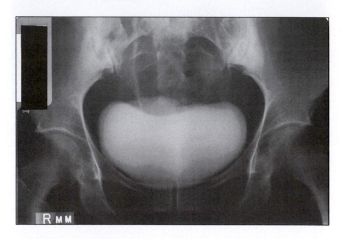

FIGURE 18.23   AP bladder.

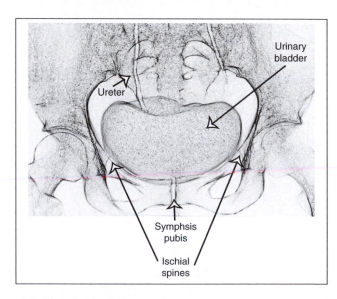

FIGURE 18.24   AP bladder.

NEPHROTOMOGRAMS

Exam Rationale Tomograms are taken to demonstrate the nephron phase of excretion. Nephrotomograms are taken within the first 6 minutes from the contrast injection. Tomograms taken at later phases of excretion are used to image the urinary system of an ill-prepared patient. In hypertensive studies, films are taken at 1, 2, 3, 4, and 5 minutes postinjection.

Technical Considerations

Tomographic Equipment Setup (linear or multidirectional):

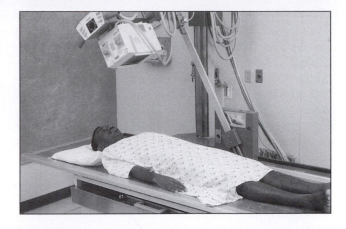

- 1-cm cuts are taken through the full thickness of the kidneys
- 11 × 14 crosswise
- Regular film/screen
- Bucky/grid
- kVp range: 70–75
- SID: 40 inch (100 cm) or appropriate for the tomographic equipment

Radiation Protection

FIGURE 18.25   Tomography setup.

Patient Position Supine with a sponge support under the knees (Figure 18.25).

Central Ray Perpendicular centered to the MSP midway between the xiphoid process and the iliac crest.

Patient Instructions "Take in a breath, let it out. Don't breathe or move."

Evaluation Criteria (Figures 18.26 and 18.27)

- Both kidneys fully visualized.
- Spine is centered to the film.
- There is no rotation as evidenced by symmetrical rib cage.
- No respiratory motion.
- Markers of tomographic level, time, and left/right are visible.

Tip

1. To ensure patient understanding and cooperation, thoroughly explain the length of the exposure and tube movement to the patient before the tomographic study.
2. Set time for Tomo Arc Time

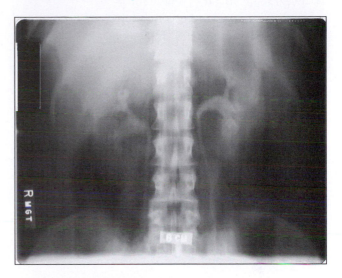

FIGURE 18.26   Nephrotomogram.

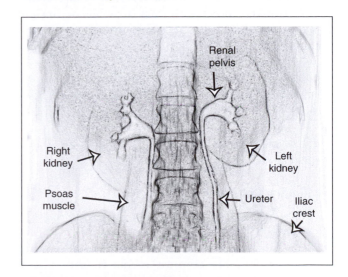

FIGURE 18.27   Nephrotomogram.

UPRIGHT POSTVOID AP PROJECTION

Exam Rationale   This projection provides information from both the upright position and the postvoid procedure. The upright position determines if the kidney's mobility is beyond normal limits and provides information about the bladder's position, possible **prolapse**, or an enlarged prostate. The postvoid film provides information about the ability of the bladder and the urethra to empty. By combining these factors, radiation is limited while providing both the upright and postvoid information.

Technical Considerations

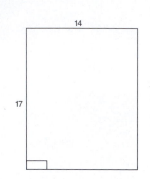

- Regular film/screen
- Bucky/grid
- kVp range: 70–80 (Technique may need to be increased; increase +40% mAs from AP technique, depending on how much abdomen falls into the field of view.)
- SID: 40 inch (100 cm)

Radiation Protection   Not possible on this projection.

AEC (Phototiming)

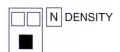

Patient Position   Patient should void before radiograph is taken; erect with back to table or upright Bucky; centered to the long axis of the film (Figure 18.28).

Central Ray   Perpendicular to the film and centered to the MSP at a level 1 inch (3 cm) below the iliac crest.

Patient Instructions   "Take in a breath, let it out. Don't breathe or move."

Evaluation Criteria (Figure 18.29)

- Entire urinary system should be imaged (kidneys to bladder).
- Film density and contrast are adequate to visualize the radiographic contrast media in the calyces, renal pelvis, ureters, and bladder.

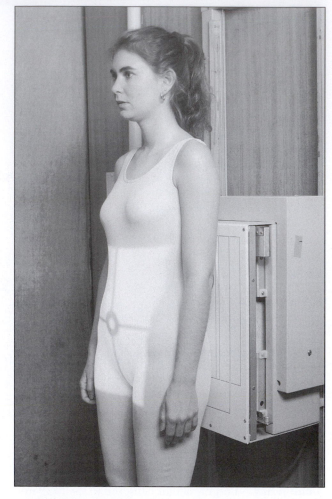

FIGURE 18.28   Upright position for IVU postvoid.

- Spine is centered to the film.
- No rotation as evidenced by:
  —Symmetrical iliac alae
  —Visualization of ischial spines equally on both sides
  —Symmetrical rib cage
- No respiratory or body motion.
- Markers upright, postvoid and right or left are visible.

Tips

1. The entire symphysis pubis must be included because the bladder may fall inferiorly and the male prostate gland should be fully visualized.
2. The kidneys will normally drop, so additional films for the hypersthenic patient are not necessary.

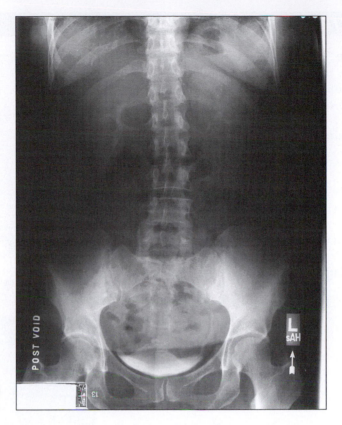

FIGURE 18.29
IVU upright postvoid.

OBLIQUE BLADDER POSITION

Exam Rationale   The oblique provides another perspective of the urinary bladder. It often eliminates overlap of anatomy and visualizes the ureterovesical junction. Either the LPO or RPO may be done.

Technical Considerations

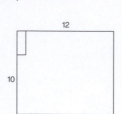

- Regular film/screen
- Bucky/grid
- kVp range: 70–75
- SID: 40 inch (100 cm)

Radiation Protection   None

AEC (Phototiming)

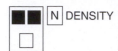

Patient Position   Rotated 45° to 60° up from supine; moved 4 inches (10 cm) from side of the desired posterior oblique (LPO or RPO) (Figure 18.30).

Central Ray   Perpendicular to the film and centered at the level of the ASIS and 2 inches (5 cm) medial to the side-up ASIS.

Patient Instructions   "Take in a breath, let it out. Don't breathe or move."

Evaluation Criteria (Figures 18.31 and 18.32)

- Entire bladder is included.
- Spine and sacrum are centered to the film.
- Entire symphysis pubis is included in the male patient.

Tips

1. The leg on the side down may be flexed for support or a radiolucent sponge may be used for support. Do not bend the leg on the side up as the upper thigh may superimpose the bladder.
2. Technique should be increased to compensate for more restrictive collimation.

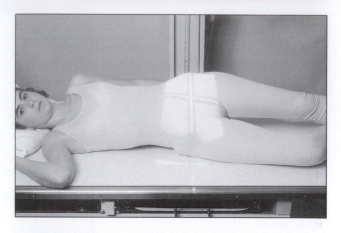

FIGURE 18.30   Position for oblique bladder.

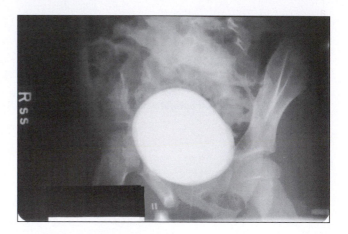

FIGURE 18.31   Oblique bladder.

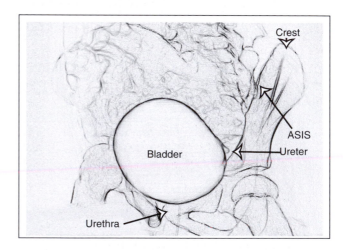

FIGURE 18.32   Oblique bladder.

Other Procedures

RETROGRADE UROGRAPHY

Retrograde urography, or retrograde pyelography, is done with less frequency because of the improved contrast media and techniques used in excretory urography. The retrograde method requires catheterization of the bladder and ureters in an aseptic environment and is usually done by a urologist. Because catheterization of the ureters is extremely uncomfortable, retrograde urography is usually a surgical procedure and is done under general anesthesia. The advantage of retrograde urography is the complete distended filling of the renal calyces, pelvis, and ureters with controlled amounts of contrast media. Often, the retrograde procedure is done subsequent to inadequate filling of the upper urinary tract on an antegrade urogram. The retrograde urogram is used when there is renal insufficiency and for evaluating tumors, lesions, and stones in the renal calyces and pelvis. The retrograde pyelogram is deemed safe for patients allergic to radiographic contrast because less contrast is used (10 mL) and there is very little absorption (1%) by the urinary tract.

The patient is placed on a radiographic/cystoscopic table. The cystoscopic table has leg rests that maintain the legs in a slightly flexed and abducted position or a modified lithotomy position (Figure 18.33). The technologist is responsible for producing a scout AP radiograph before the instillation of radiographic contrast media. The scout visualizes the placement of the catheters and necessary adjustments in patient positioning and technique selection for subsequent radiographs (Figure 18.34). Following the instillation of contrast (or during the instillation) the technologist produces AP radiographs of the distended renal pelvis and calyces. Subsequent to this imaging of the renal pelvis and calyces, the urologist withdraws the catheters into the distal ureter while injecting more contrast media. The technologist produces another AP as the ureters are distended (Figure18.35). Frequently during these final radiographs, the cystoscopic table will be placed into the **Trendelenburg** (trĕn-dĕl´ĕn-bŭrg) **position** to enhance the filling of the entire system. The urologist will determine if additional films or projections are needed while the patient is on the table and under anesthesia.

Following the procedure a catheter may be left in place in the ureters or bladder to ensure drainage.

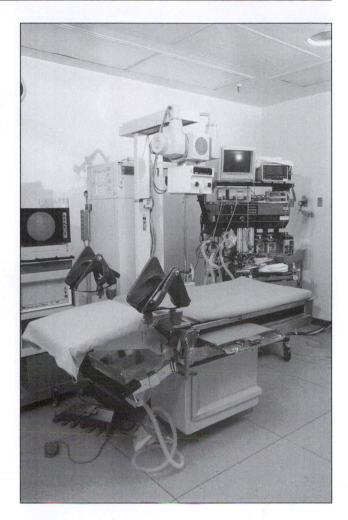

FIGURE 18.33   Cysto table prepared for patient in lithotomy position.

CYSTOGRAPHY

Cystography refers to retrograde filling of the bladder with subsequent radiographs. The diagnostic quality of retrograde cystography is superior to an excretory cystogram with inadequate filling. The retrograde procedure requires catheterization of the bladder and gravity-flow filling of the bladder. Pressure is never applied when filling the bladder due to the possibility of rupture. The cystogram aids in the diagnosis of tumors, stones, diverticula, **fistulas**, obstructive processes, and vesicoureteral reflux. The contrast media

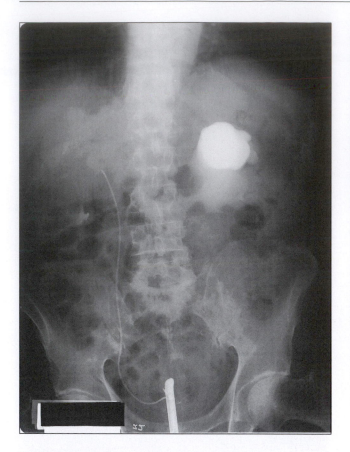

FIGURE 18.34   Scout retrograde kidney study film.

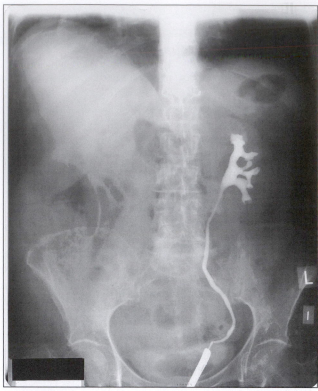

FIGURE 18.35   Retrograde kidney study (KUB).

is a diluted form of the same media used in the IVU. The diluted form is available in prepared sterile containers so there is no need to dilute contrast and risk contamination.

Unless the patient has a bladder infection, the bladder and urine are sterile. Therefore, the catheterization of the bladder must be conducted under strict aseptic conditions. The only patient preparation necessary is voiding or draining the catheter before the radiographic contrast media is instilled. Patients are normally catheterized before they come to the radiology department. If not, the person who catheterizes the patient in the radiology department will require sterile catheters and a catheterization tray.

The instillation of contrast is conducted under fluoroscopy so that the dynamics of reflux can be observed and documented with spot films. The bladder is filled until the patient cannot tolerate additional filling—usually 150 to 200 mL of contrast.

Following the end of gravity-flow instillation of contrast, overhead films are taken. An AP (Figure 18.36) and both RPO and LPO of the bladder are the com-

mon protocol (see page 688). Afterward, the patient is allowed to void, and a postvoid AP bladder radiograph is obtained to evaluate urine retention.

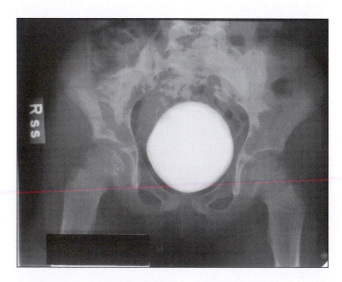

FIGURE 18.36   Filled AP bladder from a cystogram.

VOIDING CYSTOURETHROGRAPHY

The radiographic demonstration of micturition is obtained in a voiding urethrogram. The procedure requires the instillation of contrast and is always conducted following cystography, hence the study is called voiding cystourethrography (VCUG). This study aids in the investigation of incontinence, enlargement of the prostate, diverticula, and fistulas.

The patient is catheterized and cystography is performed (see page 689-690). Following cystography, the table is brought into a semi-upright position (45°–60°) so that the contrast eliminated during micturition will not pool on the table and obscure the radiographic images of the urethra. A radiolucent vessel or absorbent pads (towels) are placed to "catch" the eliminated contrast. The patient is monitored with fluoroscopy so that the dynamics of micturition can be documented on spot films. Several spot films are obtained in an oblique or AP position for the female patient. For the male patient, the table can be supine or elevated not more than 45°. The male patient is placed in a 30° RPO position with the urethra superimposed over the thigh. Again, the radiographic study is done with fluoroscopy and spot films (Figure 18.37).

Adult patients have difficulty urinating in a foreign environment, so the dignity of the patient must be foremost in the mind of the radiology personnel. The patient should be properly covered at all times and a minimum of personnel should be allowed in the room. Thorough explanation of the procedure, proper environmental controls, and a relaxed atmosphere will aid in the success of the study. Postvoid radiographs may be included in a department's protocol. All other films are usually taken under fluoroscopic control (Figures 18.38 and 18.39).

Patient Position

When doing voiding cystourethrography films, the film should be centered 3 inches (8 cm) below the ASIS at the MSP. This is lower than for a cystogram to ensure inclusion of the entire urethra.

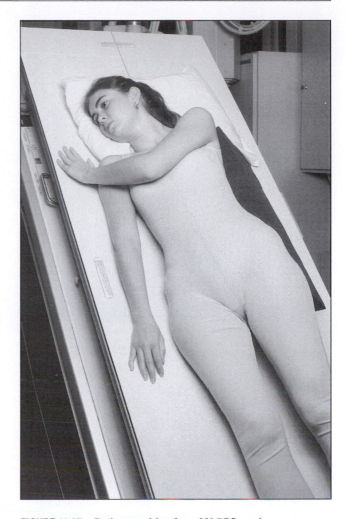

FIGURE 18.37   **Patient position for a 30° RPO urethrogram.**

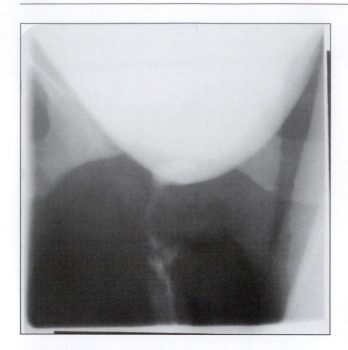

FIGURE 18.38   Female urethrogram.

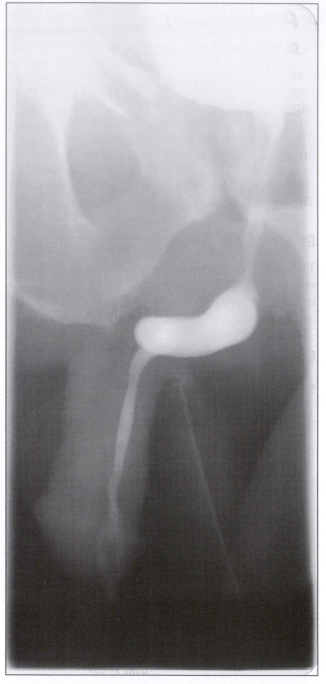

FIGURE 18.39   Male urethrogram.

Special Considerations

PEDIATRIC CONSIDERATIONS

Motion is always a concern when imaging the pediatric patient, and sedation and immobilization may be required. However, success without the use of sedation or immobilization can often occur if the child can communicate. The technologist can elicit the cooperation and support of the child and the attending caregiver through thorough, low-stress communication that eases fear and fosters understanding and trust.

Pediatric patients who have not had a bowel cleansing preparation may be given 2 to 10 oz of a carbonated drink (depending on age). The carbon dioxide distends the stomach and moves the bowel inferior to the kidneys, thereby acting as a "window" through which the kidneys can be viewed radiographically.

Never leave a pediatric patient unattended, even if the patient appears calm, comfortable, and communicative. The rational state of the pediatric patient is a result of the technologist's or parent's presence.

GERIATRIC CONSIDERATIONS

The serial radiographs of an IVU require the patient to remain on a cold, hard radiographic table for an extended period of time. The use of radiopaque sponges to ease the pain of pressure points and generally striving to make the patient comfortable and warm will ease the discomfort caused by this procedure and will attain more patient cooperation. Less rigorous patient preparation is often warranted (see contrast media).

COMMON ERRORS

Supine and Oblique Projections

1. Cutting off the symphysis pubis or the superior border of the kidney. If the symphysis pubis is always included on the scout film and the patient is too long for the film to image the entire system, a film of the kidneys may need to be done on each subsequent film. This extra kidney radiograph allows gonadal shielding on all patients, whereas the extra bladder shot increases gonadal dose. (Figure 18.40)
2. Inadequate radiographic density because the technique was not increased sufficiently for rotation or contrast.
3. Too much or too little rotation (Figures 18.41 and 18.42).

SELECTED PATHOLOGY

Urinary Tract Calculus (Kidney Stone)
A kidney stone or **calculus** is a concretion in the urinary tract (Figure 18.43). Usually composed of calcium minerals, stones are found in the pelvicalyceal system, ureters, and bladder. Theories about the cause of renal stones include the metabolic disease process that causes increased calcium excretion or increased dietary calcium and lack of dilution of renal filtrate. Men have kidney stones at twice the rate of women; 90% of calculi are radiopaque.

Ureterovesical Reflux
Retrograde flow of urine from the bladder back into the ureters occurs in 1% to 3% of all children under 11 years of age who have a UTI and is a common indication for VCUG. In cases of chronic reflux, the patient may have chronic **pyelonephritis** with subsequent scarring of the renal parenchyma. The VCUG images reflux on micturition (Figure 18.44) but the nuclear medicine VCUG is more sensitive to this finding (Figure 18.45). The renal ultrasound has become the preferred imaging modality for suspected pyelonephritis (Figure 18.46).

CORRELATIVE IMAGING

Anatomic detail of the collecting system is often better visualized on a CT infusion IVU with compression (Figure 18.47).

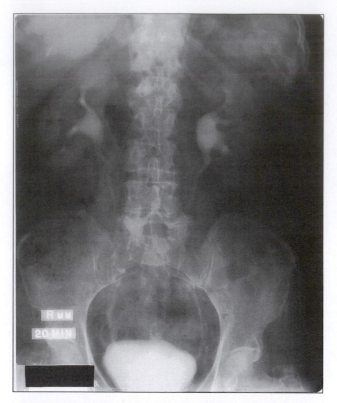

FIGURE 18.40   AP film with contrast without symphysis.

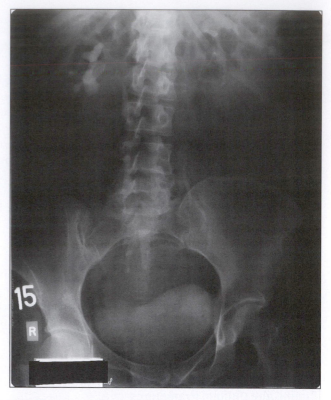

FIGURE 18.41   Oblique, underrotation.

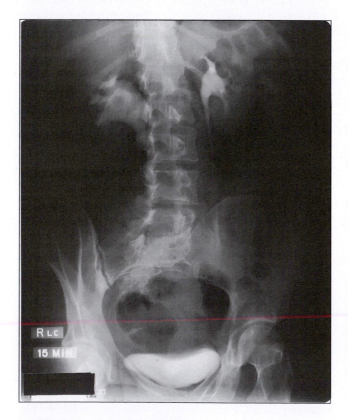

FIGURE 18.42   Oblique, overrotation.

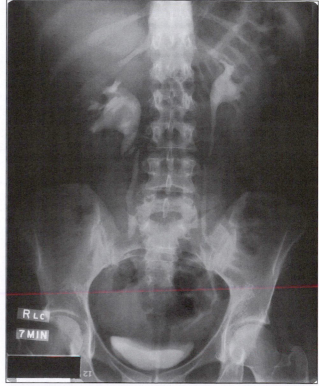

FIGURE 18.43   IVU with stone.

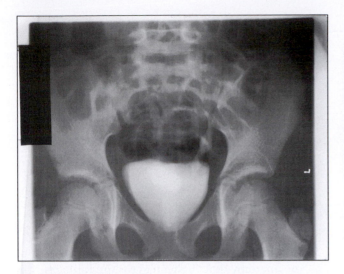

FIGURE 18.44   VCUG with reflux.

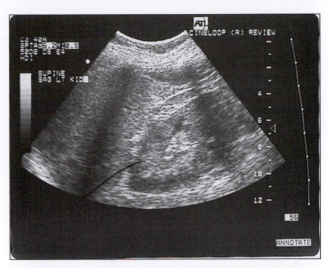

FIGURE 18.46   Sonogram of pylonephritis.

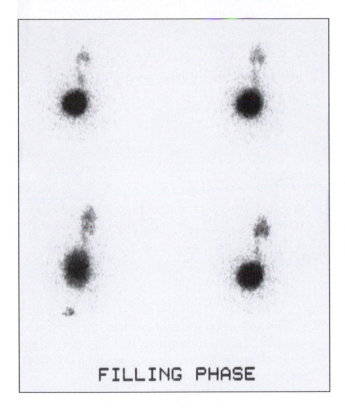

FIGURE 18.45   Nuclear medicine study of the bladder with reflux.

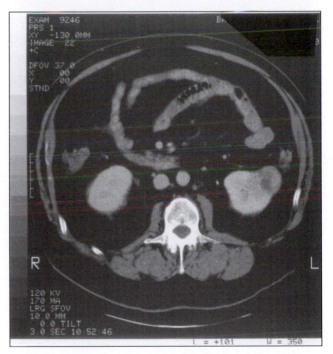

FIGURE 18.47   CT urogram of the kidneys.

Review Questions

1. Which of the following is a part of the kidney?

   1. calyces
   2. cortex
   3. nephron
   4. urethra

   a. 1 and 2
   b. 1, 2, and 3
   c. 1, 2, and 4
   d. 1, 2, 3, and 4

2. The kidney is involved in filtration and maintenance of the body's _____ balance.

   a. bilirubin
   b. electrolyte
   c. fat
   d. protein

3. Which of the following is a common indication for an IVU?

   1. flank pain
   2. hematuria
   3. hypertension

   a. 1 only
   b. 2 only
   c. 3 only
   d. 1 and 2
   e. 1, 2, and 3

4. The two main categories of radiographic contrast media used to study the urinary system are:

   1. oil based
   2. water based
   3. ionic
   4. nonionic

   a. 1 and 2
   b. 2 and 3
   c. 3 and 4
   d. 1 and 4

5. Which of the following factors might influence the amount of contrast administered for an IVU?

   a. patient's age
   b. patient's weight
   c. patient's BUN value
   d. a and b
   e. all of the above

6. Moderate reactions to contrast media include which of the following?

   1. giant hives
   2. tachycardia
   3. dyspnea
   4. hypotension

   a. 1 and 2
   b. 2 and 3
   c. 1 and 4
   d. 1, 2, and 3
   e. 1, 2, 3, and 4

7. At the one-minute postinjection IVU, the part of the anatomy that "lights up" on the radiograph is the:

   a. nephron unit
   b. renal capsule
   c. renal pelvis
   d. renal pyramid

8. In a normal adult undergoing an IVU, the bladder will fill with contrast _____ minutes following injection of contrast.

   a. 2–5
   b. 5–10
   c. 10–12
   d. 15–30

9. When positioning for an oblique IVU, the patient is rotated _____ from the supine position.

   a. 15°
   b. 30°
   c. 45°
   d. 60°

10. A pediatric patient is often not given a bowel cleansing preparation for an IVU. In this case, the patient may be given _____ to eliminate superimposition of the bowel on the kidneys.

    a. barium sulfate
    b. carbonated drink
    c. milk
    d. water

11. The most common clinical indication for a pediatric VCUG is:

    a. bladder cysts
    b. bladder reflux
    c. renal stones
    d. tumor

12. The left kidney is generally situated higher than the right.

    a. true
    b. false

13. The kidneys are firmly anchored within the abdomen and do not move during respiration.

    a. true
    b. false

14. Oblique postinjection radiographs should include the kidneys and the bladder.

    a. true
    b. false

15. The central ray for a scout KUB is perpendicular to the film to the MSP at the level of the ASIS.

    a. true
    b. false

16. With the patient semi-supine, the oblique IVU produces less distortion of the kidney away from the film because it is parallel to the film.

    a. true
    b. false

17. The ureters enter the bladder _____ and _____ .

18. For an oblique bladder, the patient is rotated _____ to _____ degrees from the _____ position.

19. Following instillation of contrast during a cystogram, the central ray should be directed perpendicular to the film at the MSP at the level of the _____ .

20. Write out the term represented by the following acronyms.

    a. IVP
    b. IVU
    c. VCUG

21. List two reasons for taking tomograms during an IVU.

22. List the routine positions/projections for an IVU at your clinical facility.

References and Recommended Reading

Amis, E. S., & Newhouse, J. (1991). *Essentials of uroradiology.* Boston: Little, Brown.

Ballinger, P. W. (1995). *Merrill's atlas of radiographic positions and radiologic procedures.* (8th ed., Vol. 2) St. Louis: Mosby-Year Book.

Bontrager, K. L. (1997). *Textbook of radiographic positioning and related anatomy* (4th ed.). St. Louis: Mosby-Year Book.

Elkin, M.(1980). *Radiology of the urinary system.* Boston: Little, Brown.

Katayama, H. (1990). Adverse reactions to ionic and nonionic contrast media: A report from the Japanese Committee on the Safety of Contrast Media. *Radiology, 175,* 621.

Laudicina, P., & Wean, D. (1994). *Applied angiography for radiographers.* Philadelphia: Saunders.

Levin, D. (1990, November). Nonionic agents: Okay they're safer—but how much safer and at what cost to society. *Administrative radiology,* 97–106.

Martini, F. (1992). *Fundamentals of anatomy and physiology* (2nd ed.), NJ: Prentice Hall.

Novelline, R., & Squire, L. F. (1987). *Living anatomy—A working atlas using computed tomography, magnetic resonance and angiography images.* St. Louis: Mosby.

Slovis, T. L,. (1989). *Imaging of the pediatric urinary tract.* Philadelphia: Saunders.

Solomon, E. P., & Davis, P. W., (1978). *Understanding human anatomy and physiology.* New York: McGraw-Hill.

Sutton, D. (1994). *Radiology and imaging for medical students* (6th ed.). New York: Churchhill Livingstone.

Witten, D. (1977). *Emmett's clinical urography: An atlas and textbook of roentgenologic diagnosis.* (Vol. I). Philadelphia: Saunders.

SECTION
VII

SPECIAL RADIOGRAPHY

CHAPTER 19

Mobile and Intraoperative Radiography

M. FERELL JUSTICE, BSRT(R)(ARRT)

OBJECTIVES

At the completion of this chapter, the student should be able to:

1. List and describe basic principles of mobile radiography.

2. Describe additional fundamentals of mobile radiography when performed intraoperatively.

3. List and explain the stages of perioperative radiography.

4. Explain the surgical suite setup and special considerations.

5. List and explain principles of aseptic technique.

6. List and describe principles of radiation protection with respect to mobile and intraoperative radiography.

7. List and describe surgical specialties and the radiographic procedures typically performed for each.

Principles of Mobile Radiography

The radiology department is equipped with mobile radiographic units as well as fixed units. Mobile units are used for radiography of patients at the bedside. Studies done with these units are typically referred to as "portable" examinations. This is an inaccurate term because portable refers to being carried (few units are transported by this mode). The intent when the term "portable" is used is the capability to be moved around. Therefore, mobile is a more proper term for these radiographic examinations. **Mobile radiography** is requested when a patient's condition makes transportation to the radiology department difficult or when radiographic procedures are performed in an area of the hospital other than radiology, such as an emergency trauma room or surgery (Figure 19.1).

Special considerations are required with mobile radiography. The technologist must have a keen awareness and good understanding of nonradiology equipment when performing mobile radiography, intraoperatively and on patient floors. It is important to know the function of equipment such as the ventilator, bed warmer/cooler, bed controls, suction units, intravenous and arterial line regulators, and so forth.

Specific alarm sounds are associated with certain medical equipment and should be recognized by the technologist to ensure proper action is taken. The technologist needs only to have an understanding of this equipment, not the responsibility of resetting alarms or troubleshooting errors. These actions are the responsibility of the individual with the proper training for that particular piece of equipment. It is the technologist's responsibility to leave equipment in the position in which it was found and return items to their original location before leaving the area.

Mobile radiography, especially intraoperative, presents the technologist with situations that make it difficult or impossible to obtain standardized positions. A knowledge of acceptable positioning variants and an experienced clinical background are necessary to overcome positioning obstacles. Although innovative positioning techniques are necessary and acceptable, the technologist should strive to perform the requested procedure as standard as possible. Examples include obtaining two projections of an extremity at 90° to each other, erect chest radiography and PA chest when possible, and so forth. It is also important to remove artifacts such as personal items, covering layers, medical lines, tubes, and leads, from the area of interest.

Automatic exposure controls (photo timing) are available for mobile units; however, manual technique is used most often. Establishing manual technical factors for each mobile unit is a common practice. Variables to consider when establishing such a chart for each unit include kV, mAs, distance, grid ratio, and film/screen combinations.

Mobile C-arm image intensifiers (fluoroscopic units) are frequently used within the intensive care units and the surgical suite for unique situations. All mobile radiography considerations and regulations are applicable to mobile fluoroscopy (Figure 19.2).

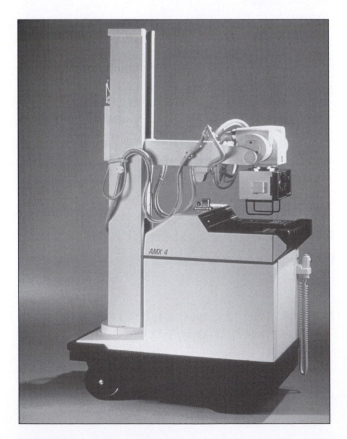

FIGURE 19.1   Mobile radiographic unit (Courtesy of GE Medical Systems, Milwaukee, WI).

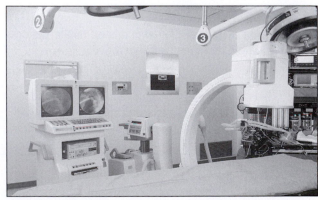

FIGURE 19.2   Mobile C-arm unit.

Common Mobile Radiographic Procedures

Virtually any anatomic area can be radiographed by mobile techniques. The most commonly performed procedures would include chest, abdominal, and orthopedic radiography.

CHEST

The most common projection of the chest performed using mobile radiography is the AP projection. Yet, PA projections are not uncommon along with lateral decubitus, cross-table lateral, and apical lordotic positions. Positioning for these views would be the same as for those described in Chapter 2, with the exception of the limitation factors that are common in mobile radiography. The limitations mobile radiography present for this anatomic area include decreased SID, kV, kVp and mAs factors, and the lack of the use of a reciprocating grid.

ABDOMEN

Abdominal radiographs and the abdominal acute series can be performed on critically ill patients who are unable to be transported to the radiology department. Many of the same technical considerations, positioning, and centering instructions discussed in Chapter 3 apply to mobile radiography. The critically ill patient may be receiving additional medical care (e.g., respirator, urinary catheter, feeding tube, sutures); therefore, accessory equipment must be carefully monitored to ensure nothing is damaged or accidentally dislodged. Objects, such as catheters and electrocardiographic wires, should be carefully moved out of the area of interest.

Supine Abdomen

For a general survey of the abdomen, the mobile examination is identical to one performed in the department. A strap-on grid or gridded cassette is highly recommended for mobile abdomen examina-

tions. The cassette may be placed in a plastic bag or pillowcase to avoid soilage. Care must be taken to avoid unnecessary manipulation of catheters, tubes, and other equipment.

Decubitus Abdomen

This examination is a routine projection in a mobile abdominal acute series. The patient must be *carefully* placed on the left side. Careful monitoring of patient, catheters, wires, and respirator tubing is essential. The cassette may be held in position by placing tape, connected to both sides of the bed, across the cassette. To avoid grid cutoff, the cassette and grid must not be tilted and the central ray must be directed perpendicular to the cassette.

AP Chest

For a mobile abdominal acute series, this projection replaces the PA chest. The patient is placed as upright as possible. Positioning and centering is the same as the AP chest examination discussed in Chapter 2.

ORTHOPEDIC

Orthopedic procedures are frequently requested to be performed as mobile studies and may include examinations of the upper and lower extremities, the cervical, thoracic, or lumbar spines, and the head. These procedures are performed as close as possible to the standard projections. However, variant positioning projections and techniques may be required to obtain an acceptable mobile radiograph.

Many times mobile orthopedic procedures present a unique challenge for the radiographer. Obstacles such as traction bars and weights, halos, spine supports, casts, and other immobilizing devices increase difficulty. These devices, along with decreased SID, alternate film-screen combinations, and the like, limit the radiographer in routine positioning projections.

Intraoperative Radiography

The role of the radiographer within the operating room setting requires a high degree of technical skill, including the ability to function under the direction of a surgeon versus a radiologist. Furthermore, intraoperative radiography has increasingly become a more specialized area considering the advances of today's technology being used in the operating suite. To fully comprehend the specific radiographic and

fluoroscopic studies performed by the intraoperative radiographer, the technologist must possess strong skills in aseptic technique, principles of mobile radiography, radiation protection, anatomic landmarks, pathologic findings, and the ability to perform efficiently and accurately with the highest level of service provided to the patient and the surgeon.

Intraoperative radiography is specifically defined as those radiographic procedures, either plain film or fluoroscopic, performed during surgery under aseptic technique. Intraoperative radiography is usually only one phase of a surgical patient's medical imaging experience. In a broader sense, three phases of radiography, called **perioperative radiography** practices, exist for a surgical patient. The stages of perioperative radiography are **preoperative**, **intraoperative**, and **postoperative radiography**.

The preoperative phase begins with the patient receiving radiographs before surgery. These examinations may include a chest radiographic examination or x-rays of the anatomic area of interest, which may not be limited to plain film radiography (i.e., CT, MRI, angiography, sonography, etc.). The intraoperative phase encompasses the radiographic procedures performed during surgery. The final phase, postoperative radiography, begins in the recovery room or when the sterile field has been terminated.

Surgical suites possess fixed radiographic generators; however, the majority of intraoperative radiography is performed with a mobile radiography unit or a mobile C-arm image intensifier. Special considerations are addressed when performing intraoperative mobile radiography. The most obvious and critical is performance in a sterile environment and practicing aseptic technique. Many times the sterile drapes prevent the technologist from viewing the area being radiographed (Figure 19.3). Therefore, a comprehen-

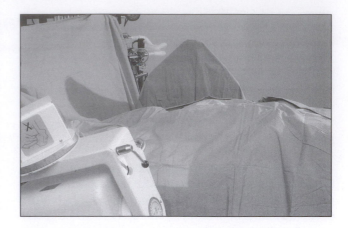

FIGURE 19.3   **Intraoperative mobile radiography; cross-table lateral position of the cervical spine.**

sive knowledge of anatomy, a thorough understanding of the operative procedure being performed and the radiographer's role during the operation are of great importance.

Effective communication between the radiographer, surgeon, anesthesia personnel, and other personnel in the surgical suite is necessary because timing is critical for many procedures. For example, anesthesia's role is important when performing many intraoperative radiographs due to their ability to regulate the patient's breathing.

Surgical Suite

The **surgical suite** is the actual room in which an operation is performed. The department, hence the suite, is a controlled area. Access is limited to those persons and items that have a reason to be present. It is important for the radiographer to be familiar with items, both sterile and nonsterile, in the surgical suite. Radiographers often find themselves in situations that require relocating items for the radiographic equipment to function effectively. Items the technologist may come in contact with include: automatic tourniquet, **bovie** and **electric coagulation** monitor, **Mayo stand**, operating room table, back table, anesthesia equipment, ring stand, kick bucket, suction bottles, and other special equipment for particular cases (Figure 19.4).

It is imperative for the technologist to communicate with the circulating nurse of the surgical suite when equipment needs to be relocated to accommodate the x-ray equipment. Items or equipment should

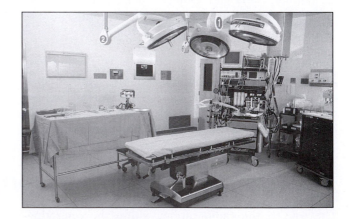

FIGURE 19.4   Surgical suite.

not be moved without consulting the surgical suite circulating nurse. The radiographer should also know the location of frequently needed items within the suite, such as electrical outlets, intercom systems, telephones, x-ray viewing illuminators, overhead light controls, and supply cabinets.

Because of the controlled environment, the wardrobe for personnel in this area is also controlled. Individuals who enter a surgical suite must wear surgical attire, often called **scrub clothes**, made available specifically for the operating room. If a radiographer must leave the operating room, for example, to receive a radiologist's reading for a case, the scrub clothes must be covered by a long-sleeved, full-length lab coat or gown. If this practice is not followed, then scrub clothes must be changed when the person re-enters the operating room. Items that complete a surgical attire suit include a cap to cover hair or a hood to prevent hair falling from long sideburns and facial hair. Masks are worn in designated areas and within the surgical suite. Shoe covers should be worn to reduce contamination to the surgical suite and provide additional protection to the wearer.

Aseptic Technique

One of the fundamental skills of intraoperative radiography is knowledge of aseptic technique. **Aseptic technique** is the method used to achieve and maintain a sterile field. **Sterile** is defined as free from all living organisms (Figure 19.5). To ensure proper aseptic technique, application of the following principles must be practiced by the intraoperative radiographer. First, the radiographer must don scrub attire with cap, mask, and shoe covers. Second, nonsterile persons must avoid contact with all sterile individuals and items. To ensure adherence to this principle, the radiographer must maintain effective communication and a **safe margin**—the distance required to avoid accidental contact, which will vary with the size of the area. Third, movement within the surgical suite should be held to a minimum and must not cause contamination. The area between the instrument table and the draped patient is known as the **sterile corridor** (Figure 19.6). This area is occupied by those individuals wearing sterile gowns and gloves and should never be entered by the intraoperative

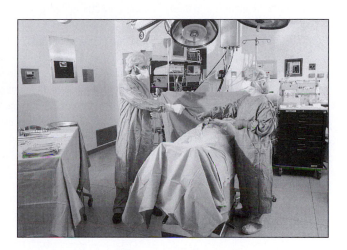

FIGURE 19.6 Sterile corridor—the area between the instrument table and the patient.

radiographer. Fourth, nonsterile persons should not reach over sterile surfaces and should handle only nonsterile items. Fifth, cassette transfer to a sterile cover is performed by the radiographer and the scrub nurse or surgical technician. To cover the cassette properly the sterile individual folds back the edges of the sterile cover and holds them open while the radiographer places the cassette inside. The sterile individual folds the edges back over the opening ensuring a closed sterile package. Caution must be used by both individuals to not contaminate the outside of the sterile cover and to review the sterile cover to make sure it has no holes (Figure 19.7). Sixth, precautions must be taken by the radiographer to ensure proper cleaning and draping techniques of the radiography equipment. This action aids in preventing dust and other microscopic particles from falling into the sterile field. Postoperative cleaning of the radiography equipment is of the utmost importance for

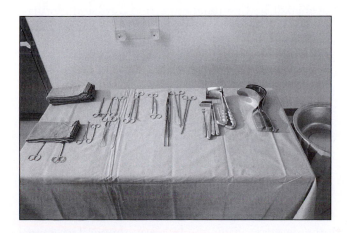

FIGURE 19.5 Instrument table.

maintaining aseptic technique. Other important actions and methods to consider to ensure aseptic technique are:

- If the sterility of an item is in question, the item is considered contaminated.
- The radiographer must be aware of what is and is not sterile.

- Breaks in the sterile field should be reported immediately.

Aseptic technique is a discipline of the intraoperative radiographer that is as equally important as one's radiography technical skills (Table 19.1).

TABLE 19.1 PRINCIPLES OF ASEPTIC TECHNIQUE

1. Proper surgical suite attire and accessories must be worn.
2. Sterile individuals and items contact only sterile items; nonsterile individuals or items contact only nonsterile items.
3. The sterile corridor is occupied only by sterile individuals and items.
4. Movement within the surgical suite must be held to a minimum and not cause contamination.
5. Nonsterile individuals should not reach over a sterile field or item.
6. Caution should be used when performing cassette transfer to a sterile cover or draping.
7. After each case, radiography units and accessory equipment should be cleaned to reduce dust and microscopic particles.
8. All items and areas of doubtful sterility must be considered contaminated.
9. The edges of a sterile package or container are considered contaminated when opened.
10. Gowns are considered sterile only from table level to shoulder and in front and the sleeves to 2 inches (5 cm) above the elbow.
11. Only the horizontal surface of the instrument table is considered sterile.
12. A break in the sterile field should be reported immediately.

(Portion courtesy of Phippen, M. I., & Wells, M. P. (1994). *Perioperative nursing practice*, copyright 1994 by W. B. Saunders Company).

Common Surgical Radiographic Procedures

The operating room provides services to many medical specialties, many of which require radiology services intraoperatively, either scheduled or unscheduled. It is important to be familiar with each specialty and the medical interest it represents. The medical specialties most likely to require intraoperative radiography are cardiac, general, gynecology, neurology, oncology, orthopedics, pain management, pediatrics, thoracic, urology, and vascular surgeries. These specialties may request either plain film mobile radiography, mobile fluoroscopy, or both.

Plain film mobile radiography in the surgical suite may be required during any stage of the perioperative procedure—preoperatively, intraoperatively, or postoperatively for final visualization and reading from the radiologist. All three phases may be performed within the surgical suite. The use of plain film radiography depends on the surgical specialty and the procedure being performed. Uses may include localization, pathologic recordings, or confirmation of the presence of a foreign body.

CARDIAC SURGERY

Cardiac surgery relates to those surgical procedures pertaining to the heart and the major blood vessels directly connected to the heart. The most common procedures using intraoperative radiography are pacemaker and automatic internal cardiac defibrillator (AICD) insertions. These procedures require fluoroscopy and usually an AP projection of the chest for fixation documentation postoperatively and to rule out a pneumothorax or other complications that can be detected radiographically. Coronary artery bypass grafts (CABG) are frequently performed and require a postoperative mobile AP chest radiograph. Refer to Chapter 2 for positioning guidelines for an AP projection of the chest.

GENERAL SURGERY

Procedures falling within this area that may require intraoperative radiography are appendectomies, cholecystectomies, exploratory laparoscopy, and gastric bypass. Intraoperative cholangiograms (Figure 19.8) are often performed during a cholecystectomy (see Chapter 17 for procedure details). These may be done by using plain film or fluoroscopy. Abdomen radiographs are obtained to rule out surgical sponges or instruments either intentionally or unintentionally left in the abdominal cavity. See Chapter 3 for positioning guidelines of the abdomen.

GYNECOLOGIC SURGERY

The surgical area of **gynecology** deals with the female genital tract. The physician may request intraoperative radiography of the pelvis during a tandem and ovoid procedure. This operation is performed for treatment of the ovaries and cervix using radioactive implants. An AP and lateral of the pelvis is obtained. A dosimetrist uses measurements acquired from these radiographs to determine the specific implant site (Figure 19.9). See Chapter 5 for positioning guidelines of the pelvis.

NEUROSURGERY

Neurosurgery includes the surgical treatment of diseases of the nervous system, head and spinal cord injuries, and brain and spinal cord tumors. Specific plain film intraoperative examinations performed for this specialty include, but are not limited to, cross-table lateral lumbar, thoracic, and cervical spines; AP and cross-table lateral skull projections; and PA lumbar, thoracic and cervical spines. Refer to Chapters 7 through 13 for specific positioning guidelines. When performing the lateral cervical spine view, the radiograph must demonstrate the base of the skull. This anatomic structure provides a landmark when counting the vertebral bodies (Figure 19.10). Mobile fluoroscopy may be requested for the same areas previously mentioned. Surgical procedures to be familiar with for this specialty would be cervical, thoracic, and lumbar **laminectomies** (lăm´´ĭ-něk´tō-mēz) and **discectomies** (dĭsk-ĕk´tō-mēz); spinal fusion; **discograms**; shunt placements; and **transphenoidal** (trăns-phĕ-noy´dăl) cases.

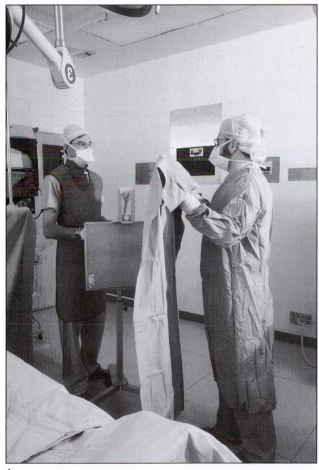

A

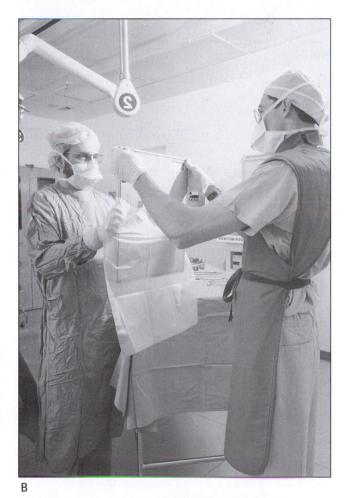

B

FIGURE 19.7 **Sterile cover for cassette. (A) scrub nurse draping cassette with a sterile cover; (B) technologist placing cassette in sterile drape held by scrub nurse.**

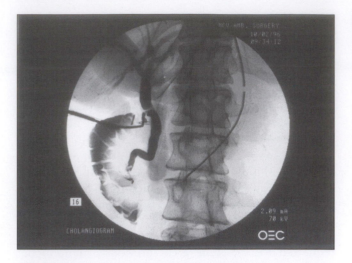

FIGURE 19.8 X-ray; intraoperative cholangiogram.

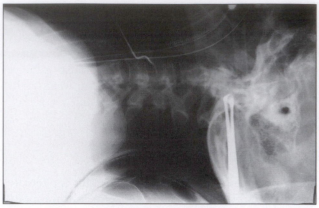

FIGURE 19.10 Intraoperative cross-table lateral cervical spine.

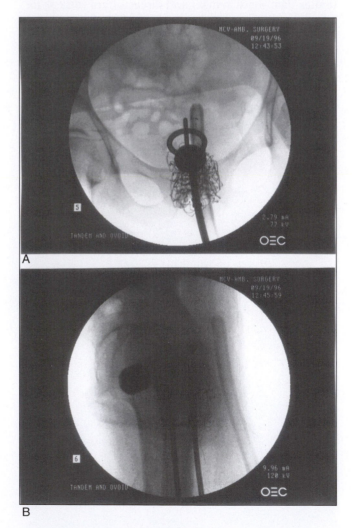

FIGURE 19.9 Tandem and ovoid placement; (A) AP and (B) cross-table lateral.

ONCOLOGY

Oncology is the area of medicine related to the study of tumors. Many times intraoperative radiography is used in the form of fluoroscopy for the placement of a catheter. These catheters come in many forms—Hickman, central line, Porta Cath, and Groshung. The radiographer's role is the same for each type of catheter placement. The surgeon will use fluoroscopy for guidance to place the catheter at the appropriate location. A postoperative AP chest film is usually obtained for final placement documentation and to rule out a pnuemothorax or any other complications that can be detected radiographically.

ORTHOPEDIC SURGERY

Orthopedic surgery deals with prevention and restoration of disorders of the musculoskeletal system. This specialty uses intraoperative radiography perhaps the most. **Open reduction internal fixations** (ORIF), the reduction of a fracture or dislocation after an incision, of various anatomic areas are by far the most common procedures. These procedures use fluoroscopy with plain film radiography at the end of the case for documentation. **Closed reductions**, the manipulation of a fracture or dislocation without an incision, are common as well. Both plain film and fluoroscopy are needed for closed reductions. Other orthopedic surgical procedures to become familiar with are arthroscopy (ăr-thrŏs′kō-pē) and joint replacements (Figure 19.11). Many times the orthopedic surgeon's idea of an optimal radiograph is different from that of the radiographer. Therefore, it is important to learn the surgeon's preferences.

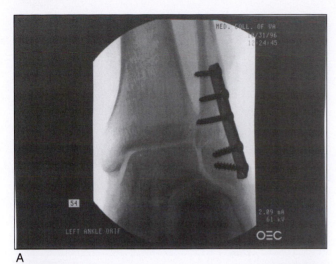

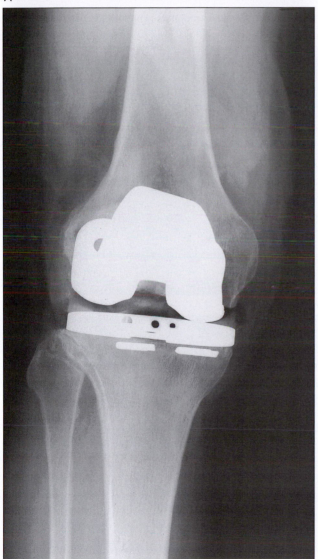

A

B

FIGURE 19.11   (A) open reduction; (B) joint replacement.

PAIN MANAGEMENT

Pain management relates to the measures used to provide relief from pain. An analgesic drug is administered by an anesthesiologist. Fluoroscopy is most often used for injections into the spinal facet, sacroiliac joint(s), caudal region, or at a specific nerve root. The lumbar spine is the most frequent target site, but injections to the cervical and thoracic spines are not uncommon. These procedures are sometimes done in the surgical suite; however, many times the procedure is performed under aseptic technique in a pain management suite or clinic.

PEDIATRIC SURGERY

Pediatrics is the branch of medicine dealing with the development of children and the diseases and treatments associated with the patient. Catheter placements are the most frequent procedures using intraoperative radiography. Other procedures to be familiar with, which will use either fluoroscopy or plain film, are foreign body removals and **esophageal** (ē-sŏf´´ă-jē´ăl) **dilatation** studies.

THORACIC SURGERY

Thoracic surgery pertains to surgical procedures involving the chest cavity. Anatomical structures include the lungs, heart, great vessels, trachea, esophagus, and rib cage. The most common thoracic surgery procedure using intraoperative radiography is bronchoscopy (brŏng-kŏs´kō-pē). This procedure requires fluoroscopy and an AP projection of the chest postoperatively.

UROLOGY

Urology pertains to the urinary system of females and the genitourinary system in males. Intraoperative urinary tract radiography is performed in a surgical suite commonly referred to as the "cysto room" (Figure 19.12). Surgical radiography of the urinary system may be divided into four groups: **cystography** (sĭs-tŏg´ră-fē), **percutaneous nephrolithotomy** (pĕr´´kū-tā´nē-ŭs nĕf´´rō-lĭth-ŏt´ō-mē) (PCNL), **retrograde pyelography** (rĕt´rō-grād pī´´ĕ-lŏg´ră-fē), and **urethrography** (ū-rē-thrŏg´ră-fē). All studies of this service use a form of catheter, stent, or guidewire that requires direct visualization with fluoroscopy. Plain film radiography is used for timed injections and documentation. The technologist must understand the procedure and anticipate the surgeon's need for a radiographic exposure.

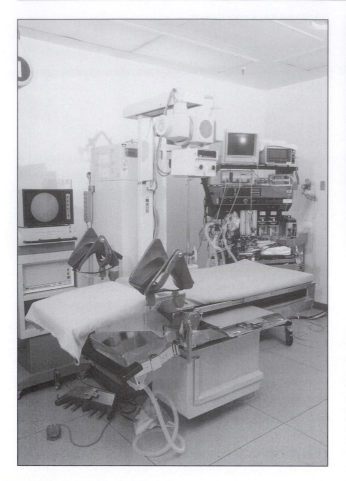

FIGURE 19.12   Cysto room.

Coordination between the surgeon, anesthesiologist, and the radiographer are of the utmost importance due to the use of direct contrast infusion (Figure 19.13).

VASCULAR SURGERY

Vascular surgery is the branch of medicine pertaining to the blood vessels. Both mobile plain film and C-arm fluoroscopy may be used when performing studies for this specialty. Femoral and lower leg arteriography is the most common surgical examination performed by the vascular surgeon using intraoperative radiography. Other procedures performed by this service that may require intraoperative radiographs are aortic aneurysm repair/resection, **arteriovenous** fistulas, declotting and revision of arteriovenous grafts, organ harvest and transplantation, and Greenfield filter placements. The technologist and surgeon must communicate effectively to obtain the radiograph at the most optimal time or at peak opacification, depending on the study being performed (Figure 19.14).

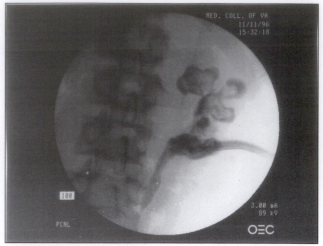

FIGURE 19.13   X-ray; percutaneous nephrolithotomy.

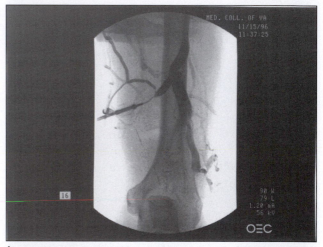

A

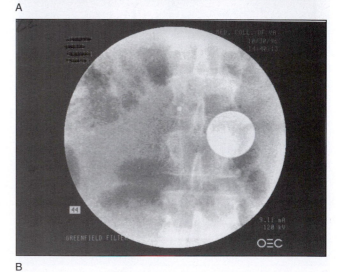

B

FIGURE 19.14   X-ray; (A) upper extremity arteriography; (B) Greenfield filter.

Radiation Protection Considerations

Mobile radiography and fluoroscopy have the highest occupational exposure potential for diagnostic x-ray personnel, other health care providers, and patients. This is due to the uncontrolled areas in which the equipment is used and the absence of stationary protective barriers. It is the technologist's responsibility to practice the highest level of technical skill and keep exposure to a minimum for everyone, including patients and health care workers.

To ensure radiation protection for all, these rules should be followed:

1. The mobile unit should not be used as a shield.
2. Protective lead aprons should be located with every mobile unit, both radiographic and fluoroscopic.
3. Protective lead aprons should be available for others in the surgical suite and for the patient.
4. When situations allow, the radiographer should extend the exposure control cord to the maximum distance when making exposures. If maximum distance is not achievable from the patient, then the exposure cord on a mobile unit must be at least 6 feet long.
5. Announcement of the intent to make an exposure should be made loudly and clearly and in sufficient time to allow individuals to leave the area.
6. A medical staff member's hand should not be placed in the primary beam without a protective (lead or tin) glove.
7. Gonadal shielding should be provided to all patients when possible.

8. Personnel monitoring badges should be worn properly at all times—outside the lead apron, proper side to the front and at the level of the collar.
9. Each cassette should be carefully labeled to avoid repeat examinations.
10. The cardinal rules of radiation protection are to maximize distance from the source, minimize exposure time, and use proper shielding materials.

Mobile image intensifying (fluoroscopic) units are popular in the surgical suite. The same considerations for mobile units should be followed for mobile fluoroscopic units. Other considerations that apply to mobile fluoroscopy are:

1. Maintain a minimum 12-inch source-to-skin distance.
2. Federal law requires a 5-minute, audible timer be installed.
3. Use collimators, shutters and minimize magnification when appropriate.
4. Be aware that the primary source of scatter radiation exposure to the surgeon, radiographer, and others around the surgical area is the patient (the lowest level of scatter occurs at a 90° angle to the incident beam).

It is the radiographer's duty to make each individual aware of the presence of diagnostic x-ray equipment and its potential for use. No exposure should be made unless everyone (regardless of their status) complies with proper radiation protection procedures—either by leaving the area or wearing a lead apron (Table 19.2).

TABLE 19.2 PRINCIPLES OF RADIATION PROTECTION

1. The mobile unit should not be used as a protective shield.
2. Lead aprons should be located with each mobile unit.
3. Lead aprons should be available for personnel in the surgical suite and for the patient.
4. The exposure cords on mobile units should be extended a minimum of 6 feet. The cord's maximum stretch length is most desired.
5. The intent to make an exposure should be announced loudly and clearly and in sufficient time to allow individuals to leave the area.
6. Never place the anatomic areas of staff members in the primary beam.
7. Patients should be shielded whenever possible.
8. A personnel monitoring badge should be worn by individuals working in the area where radiation is being administered.
9. Each cassette should be labeled carefully to avoid repeat examinations.
10. When using mobile fluoroscopy, in addition to the above:
    - A 12-inch source-to-skin distance must be maintained.
    - Appropriate collimation and shutter devices should be used.
    - Magnification should be reduced when possible.
    - Be aware the highest level of scatter occurs at a 90° angle to the incident beam.
    - Be aware the patient is the primary source of scatter radiation exposure.

Summary

Mobile radiography requires the radiologic technologist to move throughout the hospital. Patients being radiographed may be in critical condition or in a specific situation that warrants an alternate care plan. It is important for the radiographer to communicate clearly and effectively with personnel encountered and be aware of accessory equipment and critical care devices that may be present.

The successful intraoperative technologist will have a thorough understanding of the surgical suite and its contents, possess an extended knowledge of aseptic technique, and have excellent communication skills. The intraoperative radiographer needs to be efficient, and accurate, needs to work well in high-stress situations, and needs to perform well under the direction of the surgeon. The radiographer's relationship with the patient may begin before the patient enters the surgical suite, leading to performance during the actual surgical procedure and often ending postoperatively. Radiography within the surgical suite is performed with mobile plain film radiography, mobile fluoroscopy, or stationary radiographic units. A thorough understanding of the many different surgical departments, their specialty involvement, and the radiographer's role in the procedure being performed are important ingredients to success in the surgical suite. The goal is always optimal radiograph of the anatomic area of interest. However, it is important to keep in mind that the surgeon's needs may require the radiographer to deviate from the standard guidelines.

The mobile radiographer is in a prime environment to disseminate radiation protection principles to other health care providers and the public and to serve as a resource. Radiation safety for the patient, radiographer, nurses, anesthesia personnel, physicians, scrub technicians, and other members of the health care team becomes an integral role when performing radiography on the patient's floor or in the operating suite.

Review Questions

1. Cystography, nephrolithotomy, and retrograde pyelography are procedures generally required by which medical specialty?

   a. gynecology
   b. oncology
   c. urology
   d. vascular surgery

2. Which of the following positions/projections of the chest might be done as a mobile examination?

   1. AP
   2. PA
   3. lateral decubitus
   4. lordotic

   a. 1 and 2
   b. 1 and 3
   c. 1, 2, and 3
   d. 1, 2, 3, and 4

3. A tandem and ovoid procedure typically involves which of the following radiographic examinations?

   a. abdomen
   b. chest
   c. pelvis
   d. upper or lower extremity

4. The surgical treatment of diseases of the nervous system, of head and spinal cord injuries, and of brain and spinal cord tumors refers to which of the following medical specialties?

   a. neurosurgery
   b. orthopedic surgery
   c. pain management
   d. vascular surgery

5. The goal in mobile and operative radiography is to produce an image as close to the routine standard as possible.

   a. true
   b. false

6. Because of the severity of injury/illness of most patients undergoing mobile radiography examinations, it is not necessary to remove artifacts from the area to be imaged.

   a. true
   b. false

7. If there is any uncertainty about the sterility of an object, it should be considered contaminated.

   a. true
   b. false

8. If a radiographer accidentally contaminates a sterile field, he/she should wait until a suitable break in the procedure occurs to report it.

   a. true
   b. false

9. Most surgical suites have their own fixed x-ray generators.

   a. true
   b. false

10. An open reduction internal fixation (ORIF) refers to the reduction of a fracture or dislocation after _____ .

11. Define the following terms.

    a. sterile

    b. safe margin

    c. sterile corridor

12. List and briefly describe the three phases of perioperative radiography.

13. List at least five factors of aseptic technique in the surgical suite.

14. List at least three skills or specific areas of knowledge needed by a radiographer to be successful in the surgical suite.

References and Recommended Reading

Carlton, R. R., & Adler, A. M. (1996). *Principles of radiographic imaging: An art and a science*. Albany, NY: Delmar.

Ehrlich, R. A., & McCloskey, E. D. (1993). *Patient care in radiography*. St. Louis: Mosby-Year Book.

Fuller, J. R. (1981). *Surgical technology principles and practice*. Philadelphia: Saunders.

Marlow, J. E. (1983). *Surgical radiography*. Baltimore: University Park Press.

Phippen, M. L., & Wells, M. P. (1994). *Perioperative nursing practice*. Philadelphia: Saunders.

Glossary

aseptic technique   area of patient care meant to minimize the transmission of infectious diseases.

abdominopelvic cavity   one of the cavities of the body. Divided into abdominal and pelvic portions. Most of the digestive organs are found within this cavity.

abduct   to move a part away from the central axis of the body.

acanthiomeatal line   line drawn between the junction of upper lip/nose and the EAM, used to adjust the position of the cranium.

acanthion   point where the upper lip joins the base of the nose.

acetabulum   the rounded cavity on the external surface of the innominate bone that receives the head of the femur.

acromion (acromial)   the lateral triangular projection of the spine of the scapula that forms the point of of the shoulder and articulates with the clavicle; the acromion process lies on the superior aspect of the scapula, projecting posteriorly and superiorly.

adduct   to move a part toward the central axis of the body.

algorithim   a mathematical progression that is programmed for a computer.

alveolar ducts   a branch of a respiratory bronchiole that leads to the alveoli of the lungs.

alveolar sacs   sacules where gases are exchanged during respiration.

alveoli   air cells of the lungs.

alzheimer's disease   a chronic, organic, mental disorder; a form of presenile dementia due to atrophy of frontal and occipital lobes.

anatomic position   refers to the body being erect, facing forward, feet together, and arms extended with palms turned forward.

anterior (ventral)   the forward or front part of the body or body part.

antra   any nearly closed cavity or chamber, particularly in a bone.

anuria   absence of urine formation.

arteriovenous   pertaining to the arteries and veins.

aseptic technique   method used to achieve and maintain a sterile field.

asthenic   small body type, comprising about 10% of the population.

atlas (C1)   circular in shape, this is the most atypical vertebrae in the body.

auricle   cartilage protecting the ear canal.

axial   positions in which the central ray is angled along the longitudinal axis of the body.

axis (C2)   cervical vertebrae, easily distinguished by its long body that extends superiorly.

bile   digestive juice secreted by the liver which aids in fat digestion.

blood urea nitrogen (bun)   nitrogen in the blood in the form of urea.

body habitus   the general shape and form of the human body.

bolus   a concentrated mass of a diagnostic substance given rapid intravenously, such as an opaque contrast medium, or an intravenous medication.

bovie   instrument powered by electrical current that incises and coagulates.

brachycephalic   having a short, broad head, with a cranial index of 81.0 to 85.4.

bronchioles   a smaller subdivision of the bronchiole tubes.

bursa   sacs of fluid that surround joints.

calculus   pathological concretions occuring in the kidneys.

canthus   point where the upper and lower eyelids meet.

capitulum (capitellum)   a small, rounded, articular end of a bone.

cardiac orifice   juncture where the esophagus enters the stomach.

cardiac sphincter   muscular ring that surrounds the cardiac orifice.

cardiac surgery   surgical procedures pertaining to the heart and the major great vessels.

carina   bony spur of cartilage in the trachea.

carpal tunnel   an area of the wrist, formed when the wrist is hyperextended, formed by the anterior aspects of the distal rows of carpals, forming a shallow concavity.

carpals   bones of the wrist. The wrist contains eight carpals.

carpus   also known as the wrist.

cathartic   an active purgative, producing bowel movements.

cholecystokinin   hormone secreted into the blood by the muscosa of the upper small intestine which stimulates gallbladder contraction and secretion of pancreatic enzymes.

cholelith   a precipitation of gallstones (usually caused by a long-term high-fat diet).

chyme   food that is chemically and mechanically prepared for digestion by the stomach; mixture of partly digested food and digestive secretions found in the stomach and small intestine during digestion of a meal.

clavicle   the collarbone.

closed reduction   manipulating a fracture without an incision.

colitis   inflammation of the colon.

colles fracture   a transverse fracture of the distal radius.

contralateral   relates to the opposite side of the body or part.

coracoid   beaklike projection on the anterior border of the scapula.

coronal plane   plane that passes vertically through the body from left to right, dividing the body into anterior and posterior portions.

coronoid process   process that extends anteriorly from the superior part of the ulna.

cortex   one of two internal regions of the kidney, comprised of a peripheral ring of parenchymal tissue.

costophrenic angle   pertaining to the ribs and diaphragm.

costotransverse   pertaining to the ribs; also the transverse processes of articulating vertebrae.

costovertebral   pertaining to a vertebra and a rib.

cystitis   inflammation of the bladder usually occuring secondary to ascending urinary tract infections.

cystography   radiography of the bladder after injection of radiopaque solution.

decubitus   position in which the patient is recumbent while a radiograph is taken with a horizontal beam. The position is named by the side that is dependent.

diaphragm   the muscular structure that separates the thorax from the abdomen.

discectomy   excision of an intervertebral disk.

diskogram   study of the intevertebral disk spaces following the injection of radiopaque media.

distal   away from the origin of a part or away from its center or midline.

diverticulitis   inflammation of a diverticulum in the intestinal tract, esp. in the colon, causing pain and stagnation of feces in little distended sacs of the colon (diverticula) and pain.

diverticulosis   diverticula (a sac or pouch in the walls) in the colon without inflammation or symptoms.

dolichocephalic   having a skull with a long anteroposterior diameter.

dorsal recumbent   supine or lying on the back.

dorsum   refers to the anterior surface (or top) of the foot; in general, however, it refers to the posterior aspect of the body.

duodenal bulb   the area of the duodenum just beyond the pylorus of the stomach.

duodenum   10-inch tube that comprises the first part of the small intestine and connects the pylorus of the stomach to the jejunum.

dyspepsia   imperfect or painful digestion.

dyspnea   air hunger resulting in labored or difficult breathing, sometimes accompanied by pain.

electric coagulation   effect produced on tissues by the application of a bipolar current delivered by a needlepoint.

emphysema   a chronic disease involving the destruction and loss of elasticity of the walls of the alveoli, causing enlargement of the alveolar sacs and interference with an exchange of oxygen.

endocrine   a ductless gland which secretes hormones directly into the lymph or blood systems. Endocrine glands include the pituitary gland, thyroid, and the gonads. A portion of the pancreas is classified as an endocrine gland.

epicondyle   the eminence at the articular end of a bone above a condyle; the roughened areas of the bone just superior to the condyles.

epidural   hematoma above the dura mater.

epiglottis   specialized flap of skin that covers the trachea so food can pass into the esophagus and not enter the respiratory system.

epiploic appendages   numerous small fat-filled sacs in the large intestine.

erect   sitting or standing in an upright position.

esophageal dilatation   stretching the esophagus beyond the normal dimensions.

esophagus   muscular tube, approximately 10 inches long, that extends from the pharynx to the entrance of the stomach; food passageway.

evert   movement of the foot when the ankle is turned outward.

exocrine   a gland which secretes its chemical substances through a duct. The pancreas is also considered an exocrine gland by virtue of the presence of the pancreatic duct.

extend   to straighten a joint, increasing the angle between adjacent bones.

external auditory meatus   opening of the external ear canal.

fissures   a groove or natural division.

fistula   abnormal tubelike passage from a normal cavity or tube to a free surface or to another cavity; may be due to congenital incomplete closure of parts or may result from abscesses, injuries, or inflammatory processes.

flex   to bend a joint, decreasing the angle between adjacent bones.

foramen magnum   large opening in the inferior portion of the occipital bone through which the spinal cord enters the cranial cavity.

frenula   two lips on either side of the ileocecal valve which create membraneous ridges in the cecum.

frontal   projections referring to all AP and PA projections.

glabella   smooth, flat surface just above the midpoint of the eyebrows.

glabellomeatal line   line drawn between the glabella and the EAM, used to adjust the position of the cranium.

glenoid cavity   the socket that receives the head of the humerus below the acromion at the junction of the superior and axillary borders.

glomerulus   one of the small structures in the malpighian body of the kidney made up of capillary blood vessels in a cluster and enveloped in a thin wall.

glucose   a carbohydrate (sugar) of the body important for metabolism. A source of energy for the body.

glycogen   the storage form of glucose. Glycogen is stored within the liver and is converted to glucose as necessary.

gonion   junction of the mandibular body and ramus.

gynecology   area of medicine pertaining to the female genital tract.

haustration   folds in the wall of the large intestine.

hematoma   a swelling or mass of blood (usually clotted) confined to an organ, tissue, or space and caused by a break in a blood vessel.

hematuria   blood in the urine.

hemidiaphraghm   one half of the diaphragm. Often divided into left and right hemidiaphragm.

hemorrhage   abnormal, severe internal or external discharge of blood.

hemorrhoids   varicose veins in the rectum or anus.

hemothorax   presence of blood in the pleural cavity.

hernia   a protrusion of intestine through the abdominal wall.

hilum   area where the primary bronchi enter the lungs.

hilus   the long, narrow depression or "pocket" of the concave curve of the kidneys.

homeostasis   state of equilibrium of the internal environment of the body that is maintained by dynamic processes of feedback and regulation.

hyperextend   extreme extension of a joint.

hyperflex   extreme flexion of a joint.

hypersthenic   large body type, comprising about 5% of the population.

hyposthenic   a modification of the more extreme asthenic type, comprising about 35% of the population.

ileocecal valve   muscular sphincter that guards the opening of the ileum into the cecum and prevents digested materials from re-entering the small intestine.

ileum   third segment of the small intestine; approximately 11-foot long section that connects the jejunum to the cecum of the large intestine.

incontinence   involuntary release of urine, caused by loss of voluntary control over the external sphincter.

inferior (caudal)   part away from the head of the body, or , more generally, below some reference point.

infraorbitomeatal line   line drawn betwen the infraorbital margin and the EAM, used to adjust the position of the cranium.

infraspinous fossa   a depression lying below the spine of the scapula.

inion   external protuberance on the occipital bone.

intercondylar eminence   a prominence or projection, especially of a bone, located between the condyles.

intercondylar fossa   notch located between the condyles.

interphalangeal joints   classified as hinge type joints, they are found between middle and distal phalanges and between proximal and middle phalanges.

interpupillary line   line drawn between the pupils, used to adjust the position of the cranium.

intraoperative radiography   second stage of perioperative radiography; these are radiographic procedures, either plain film or fluoroscopic, performed during surgery under aseptic technique.

intussusception   the slipping of one part of the intestine into another part just below it.

invert   movement of the foot when the ankle is turned inward.

ipsilateral   relates to the same side of the body or part.

jaundice   the yellowing of all body tissues, caused by the backing up of bilirubin into the intestinal fluids when it is unable to be removed from the blood.

jejunum   second segment of the small intestine; approximately 8-foot long section that connects the duodenum to the ileum.

kyphoscoliosis   a combination of kyphosis and scoliosis occurring to the thoracic spine.

kyphosis   abnormal accentuation of the convex curvature of the spine or lumbar.

laminectomy   excision of the posterior arch of a vertebra.

laryngopharynx   posterior to the epiglottis, serves as a passage for both food and air.

larynx   located in the upper airway, it prevents food from entering the air passages and permits air through the lungs. It also has a role in voice production.

lateral   away from median plane of body or away from middle of a part to right or left; position named by the side of the patient that is placed closest to the image receptor.

lateral rotation (external rotation)   rotation of a limb away from the midline.

laxative   food or chemical substance that acts to facilitate passage of bowel contents at time of defecations, and, therefore, to prevent or treat constipation.

left lateral recumbent   lying on left side.

leteral malleolus (fibula)   the distal end of the fibula.

lobar bronchi (secondary)   division of the primary bronchi in the lungs; three on the right, two on the left.

longitudinal plane   plane that passes lengthwise through the body. Sagittal and coronal planes are also longitudinal planes.

lordosis   abnormal accentuation of the concave curvature of the lumbar spine.

manubrium   the easily palpable jugular notches on the sternum, at T2-T3 level.

mayo stand   accessory tray commonly used in a surgical or sterile environment.

mcburney's point   a useful surgical approximation for the location of the appendix, located by drawing a line between the umbilicus and the anterior superior iliac spine; the point is one third of the distance along the line starting from the anterior superior iliac spine.

medial   toward median plane of body or toward middle of a part from right or left.

medial malleolus (tibia)   the distal end of the tibia.

medial rotation (internal rotation)   rotation of a limb toward the midline.

mediastinum   the mass of organs and tissues separating the lungs, including the heart, esophagus, trachea, etc.

medulla   one of two internal regions of the kidney, comprised of an internal band of densely packed collecting ducts.

meningioma   a slow-growing tumor that originates in the arachnoidal tissue.

mental point   tip of the chin.

mentomeatal line   line drawn between the tip of chin and the EAM, used to adjust the position of the cranium.

mesocephalic   having a medium-sized head, with a cranial index of 76.0 to 80.9.

metacarpals   a bone of the hand that comprises the palm.

micturition   process by which the urethra, when the bladder is full, conducts the urine to the external environment; urination.

midcoronal plane   plane that passes vertically from right to left through the coronal suture of the skull, dividing the body into equal anterior and posterior portions.

midsagittal plane   plane that passes vertically through the midline of the body from front to back, dividing the body into equal left and right portions.

mobile c-arm image intensifier   x-ray tube and fluoroscopic image intensifier mounted on opposite ends of a C-shaped movable gantry.

mobile radiography   radiographic studies performed at the patient's bedside or in a department other than radiology in which fixed radiographic generators are not used.

mouth   opening at the beginning of the GI tract where mastication of food occurs.

multiple myeloma   a neoplastic disease characterized by the infiltration of bone and bone marrow by myeloma cells forming multiple tumor masses.

multiple sclerosis   an inflammatory disease of the central nervous system in which infiltrating lymphocytes, predominantly T cells and macrophages, degrade the myelin sheath of the nerves.

nasion   point where the right and left nasal bones meet.

nasopharynx   division of the pharynx; serves as a passageway for air and is posterior to the nasal cavity.

neoplastic disease   new, abnormal tissue formation.

nephron   parenchyma or working/filtering unit of the kidney.

neurologic deficit   the existence of a problem in the neurological system resulting in decreased neurologic functions.

neurosurgery   surgical treatment of diseases of the nervous system, head and spinal cord injuries, and brain and spinal cord tumors.

oblique   position in which the patient is rotated somewhere between a frontal and lateral position. Oblique positions are identified by the side closest to the image receptor.

occipital condyles   oval processes located lateral and anterior to the foramen magnum, which articulate with the first cervical vertebra to form the occipitoatlantal joint.

occiput   most posterior surface of cranium.

olecranon process   large and roughened portion of the ulna, posterior to the elbow; one of the most palpable of the ulnar processes.

oncology   area of medicine related to the study of tumors.

open reduction internal fixation (orif)   reduction of a fracture after creating an incision into the fracture site.

orbitomeatal line   line drawn between the outer orbital margin and the EAM, used to adjust the position of the cranium.

oropharynx   division of the pharynx, serves as a passage for both food and air, posterior to the oral cavity.

orthopedic surgery   branch of surgery that deals with prevention and restoration of disorders of the musculoskeletal system.

ossified   turned into bone.

osteoarthritis   a progressive, degenerative disease primarily caused by wear and tear at joints.

paget's disease   skeletal disease of the elderly with chronic inflammation of bones, resulting in thickening and softening of bones, and bowing of long bones.

pain management   field of medicine that relates to the measures used to provide relief from pain.

palmar   the palm of the hand.

papilla of vater   the duodenal end of the drainage systems of the pancreatic and common bile ducts.

paralytic/adynamic ileus   paralysis of the intestines accompanied by abdominal distention and pain.

pathogen   a disease producing microorganism.

pediatrics   branch of medicine dealing with the development of children and the diseases and treatments associated with children.

percutaneous nephrolithotomy (pcnl)   surgical procedure performed by entering through the skin and removing renal calculi by cutting through the body of the kidney.

perioperative radiography   patient's overall radiography experience as it relates to surgical procedures.

peristalsis   involuntary wave-like contractions that propel masticated food throughout the gastrointestinal tract.

peritoneum   serous tissue consisting of layers covering various organs and structures within the abdominal cavity.

peritonitis   inflammation of the peritoneum.

petrous pyramid   very dense bone, triangular in shape, that contains the structures of the middle and inner ear.

phagocytic cell   a cell that digests and destroys substances such as bacteria, cell debris, and protozoa.

phalanges   bones located in the finger, there are 14 in each hand.

pharynx   common area from the base of the skull to approximately the sixth cervical vertebra where air passes from the nasal cavity to the trachea and food passes from the mouth to the esophagus.

pharynx   passageway for air from nasal cavity to larynx and food from mouth to esophagus.

plantar   posterior surface (or sole) of foot.

pleura   continuous double-walled serous membrane that encases each lung separately and folds around the root of the lung.

pneumonia   inflammation of the lungs caused primarily by bacteria, viruses, and chemical irritants.

pneumoperitoneum   condition in which air or gas is collected within the peritoneal cavity.

pneumothorax   presence of free air in the thoracic cavity, caused by trauma; presence of air in the pleural cavity.

position   the term used to describe the patient's placement when both the entrance and exit points of the central ray are not defined.

posterior (dorsal)   the back part of the body or body part.

postoperative radiography   third and final stage of perioperative radiography; radiographic procedures performed after surgery is completed.

preoperative radiography   first stage of perioperative radiography; radiographic procedures performed before surgery.

projection   describes the path of the central ray in the process of recording a body part on an image receptor by indicating entrance and exit points. The term is restricted to description of the central ray. Projection is the opposite of view.

prolapse   falling or dropping down of an organ or internal part, such as the uterus or rectum.

pronate   to turn down the palm of the hand.

prone   lying face down.

proximal   closer to the origin of a part or closer to its center or midline.

psoas muscle   along with the diaphraghm, the psoas is one of the two primary abdominal muscles. These two large muscles can be found on both sides of the vertebral column.

pyelonehpritis   inflammation of kidney substance and pelvis.

radius   one of two long bones of the forearm, the other being the ulna.

rectal plexus   network of nerves or of blood or lymphatic vessels associated with the rectum.

recumbent   any reclining position.

reflux   backflow of urine into the kidney.

retrograde pyelography   radiography of the kidney and ureters after the structures have been filled backward with a contrast solution.

retrosternal   behind the sternum.

rheumatoid arthritis a relatively common inflammatory disease of the joints that can cause severe deformity as well as limit flexibility.

right lateral recumbent lying on right side.

rotation motion of the head around the longitudinal axis.

rotator cuff four tendons surrounding the shoulder joint.

rugae folds found in the mucosa of the stomach.

safe margin distance required to avoid accidental contact with sterile items within a surgical suite.

sagittal plane plane that passes vertically through the body from front to back, dividing the body into left and right portions.

scapula the shoulder blade.

sclerosis hardening within the nervous system, esp. of the brain and spinal cord, resulting from degeneration of nervous elements, such as the myelin sheath.

scoliosis abnormal lateral curvature of the thoracic spine or lumbar.

scrub clothes surgical suite attire.

sella turcica saddle-shaped, centrally located depression on the superior surface of the body that houses the pituitary gland (hypophysis).

serous pertaining to a membrane which produces a serous (lubricating) fluid. The fluid moistens the surface of serous membranes.

sesamoid bone occasionally found in the tendon of the hand.

sims' position a semi-prone position with patient on left side, knees flexed with right knee and thigh drawn well up in front of the left, left arm along patient's back, and chest inclined forward so patient rests upon it; used for insertion of enema tip.

sinusitis inflammation of a sinus, esp. a paranasal sinus.

sphincter of oddi a circular band of muscle at the terminal end of the common bile duct.

spina bifida failure of the laminae to fuse and form the spinous process.

standard precautions precautions developed in 1996 by the Centers for Disease Control (CDC) that augment Universal Precautions, providing a wider range of protection. They are designed to protect all health care providers, patients, and visitors.

stereoscopy three dimensional radiography; an impression of solidity or depth of objects created by combining images of two pictures.

sterile free from all living organisms.

sterile corridor area between the instrument table and the draped patient.

sthenic the "average" body type, comprising about 50% of the population. It serves as a reference point for others.

stomach organ of digestion; sac-like portion of the alimentary canal that is below the esophagus; food enters through the cardiac orifice and exits through the pylorus; masticated food digests into chyme here; varies in size according to body habitus.

styloid process rounded, disk-shaped head of the ulna and radius.

subdural hematoma located beneath the dura, usually the result of head injuries.

superciliary ridge/arch ridge of bone at the eyebrow.

superior (cephalic) part toward the head of the body or, more generally, above some point of reference.

supinate to turn up the palm of the hand.

supine lying on back, face up.

supraorbital groove depression in bone above the eyebrow.

supraspinous fossa a depression lying above the spine of the scapula.

surgical suite actual room in which an operation is performed.

suture the immovable joints between the bones of the skull.

symphysis pubis the bony eminence under the pubic hair; the junction of the pubic bones.

tachycardia abnormal rapidity of heart action, usually defined as a heart rate over 100 beats per minute in adults.

taeniae coli longitudinal muscle bands in the large intestine.

tangential positions in which the central ray skims a body part to demonstrate it in profile, free of superimposition.

terminal ileum most distal part of the ileum just before it enters the cecum.

thecal sac pertaining to a sheath; baglike part of an organ.

thoracic pertaining to the chest or thorax.

thoracic surgery surgical procedures involving the chest cavity, including anatomic areas of the lungs, heart, great vessels, trachea, esophagus, and rib cage.

tibial tuberosity roughened area of bone at the most superior edge of the anterior border extending upward from the shaft of the Tibia.

tilt when the longitudinal axis of the head is no longer aligned with the longitudinal axis of the body, the cranium is tilted.

trachea tubular structure extending from the larynx into the thoracic cavity.

tragus   cartilage flap at the opening of the EAM.

transphenoidal   pertaining to across or beyond the sphenoid bone (an irregular wedge-shaped bone at the base of the skull).

transverse plane   any plane that passes through the body at a right angle to the sagittal or coronal plane.

trendelenburg position   position in which the patient's head is low and the body and legs are on an elevated and inclined plane.

trigone   triangular-shaped muscle mass at the floor of the bladder.

trochanter   either of the two bony processes below the neck of the femur.

trochlear (trochlea)   crescent shaped structure on the medial, distal surface of the humerus.

tubercle   a small rounded elevation or eminence on a bone.

ulna   one of two long bones of the forearm, the other being the radius.

urethrography   radiography of the urethra after the injection of radiopaque solution.

urology   branch of medicine pertaining to the urinary system of females and the genitourinary system in males.

urticaria   a vascular reaction of the skin characterized by the eruption of pale evanescent wheals, which are associated with severe itching.

vascular surgery   area of operative medicine pertaining to the blood vessels.

ventral recumbent   prone or lying face down.

vertebral foramen   the hollow space enclosed by a vertebral arch.

vertex   most superior surface of cranium.

view   describes the representation of the image from the perspective of the image receptor. View is the opposite of projection.

villi   very small vascular network that lines the small intestines and absorbs the nutrients of digested food into the bloodstream.

viscera   internal organs enclosed within a cavity.

volar   the palm of the hand or the sole of the foot.

volvulus   twisting of a loop of bowel on itself.

whiplash   injury to the cervical vertebrae resulting from the head being forced into hyperflexion.

xiphoid   located at T10 on the thoracic spine.

zygapophyseal joints   the amphiarthrodial joints between the articular processes

Index